ADJUVANT THERAPY OF CANCER

ADJUVANT THERAPY OF CANCER

Proceedings of the International Conference on the Adjuvant Therapy of Cancer held in Tucson, Arizona, U.S.A., March 2-5, 1977.

Editors
Sydney E. Salmon, M.D.
and
Stephen E. Jones, M.D.

NORTH-HOLLAND PUBLISHING COMPANY
AMSTERDAM · NEW YORK · OXFORD

ISBN: 0 7204 0642 0

Publishers:
Elsevier/North-Holland Biomedical Press
335 Jan van Galenstr., P.O.B. 211
Amsterdam, The Netherlands

Sole distributors for the U.S.A. and Canada:
Elsevier North-Holland Inc.
52 Vanderbilt Avenue
New York, N.Y. 10017

First edition: 1977
Second printing: 1979

Library of Congress Cataloging in Publication Data

International Conference on the Adjuvant Therapy of Cancer, Tucson, Ariz., 1977.
Adjuvant therapy of cancer.

Includes index.
1. Cancer--Chemotherapy--Congresses. 2. Adjuvants, Immunological--Congresses. 3. Antineoplastic agents--Congresses. 4. Immunitherapy--Congresses. I. Salmon, Sydney E. II. Jones, Stephen E. III. Title.
RC271.I45I57 1977 616.9'94'061 77-8306
ISBN 0-7204-0642-0

PRINTED IN THE NETHERLANDS

Preface

One of the most important new directions in clinical cancer management is the development of effective adjuvant therapy for micrometastases which can be used in conjunction with surgery and or irradiation as initial combined modality therapy. Single agent and combination chemotherapy, as well as immunotherapy and hyperthermia all appear to show promise as adjuvants. This publication is composed of the submitted papers which were presented at the first International Conference on the Adjuvant Therapy of Cancer organized by the Section of Hematology and Oncology and the Cancer Center of the University of Arizona, and held in Tucson, March 2-5, 1977. The express purposes of this meeting were to summarize the scientific rationale for adjuvant therapy, to assess the current status of ongoing clinical research in the field, to consider the future potential of adjuvant therapy, and to foster interdisciplinary communications. In order to maximize the opportunity for presentation of a diversity of clinical research, a call for competitive papers was widely advertised to complement a series of invited papers from internationally recognized specialists. The response to our announcement of this conference was impressive: both in terms of the number of abstracts proferred and the number of registrants at the conference. There were over 600 registrants in attendance who came from 17 countries.

The editors decided to publish all submitted papers with only minimal editing. Except for Sections I and X which deal with rationale and general considerations respectively, each Section on specific types of cancer is organized with respect to the type of clinical trial. Accordingly, we have placed reports of concurrent randomized trials before historically controlled studies. Last in each section are pilot studies. Every effort was made to present as many papers as possible, but even then, only 75% of submitted abstracts could be accepted for presentation and publication.

Depending on the progress in the field, subsequent conferences are planned at two year intervals. The co-chairmen are grateful to those who were so willing to participate in the program and to those who came to listen and question the participants.

Success of the conference was insured by major financial support by Adria Laboratories, the Arizona Division of the American Cancer Society, and by a research conference grant from the National Cancer Institute (CA-21134). Additional support for this conference was also provided by Bristol Laboratories, Burroughs-Wellcome Co., Eli Lilly & Co., and Hoffman La Roche. The co-chairmen also give their special thanks to Ms. Margo Walter of the Cancer Center Staff who served as the conference coordinator. Finally, the readers should recognize that in order to publish the proceedings for rapid dissemination to the medical community, it was necessary for the authors to provide their completed manuscripts at the time of the conference in the camera-ready format. Accordingly, we wish to thank Drs. J. Geelen and his staff at Elsevier/North-Holland Biomedical Press for their endeavors to facilitate rapid publication of the proceedings.

Sydney E. Salmon, M.D.

Stephen E. Jones, M.D.

Section of Hematology & Oncology and the Cancer Center
University of Arizona, College of Medicine

Contents

SECTION III - LUNG CANCER

SECTION V - GENITOURINARY AND GYNECOLOGIC CANCER

SECTION VI - PEDIATRIC CANCER

SECTION VII - SARCOMA AND MELANOMA

Section I

THE RATIONALE FOR ADJUVANT THERAPY OF CANCER

Adjuvant Therapy of Cancer, S.E. Salmon and S.E. Jones eds.

EXPERIMENTAL BASIS FOR ADJUVANT CHEMOTHERAPY

F.M. Schabel, Jr.
Southern Research Institute
Birmingham, Alabama 35205

SUMMARY

Laboratory studies with transplantable metastatic lung, breast, and colon carcinomas and melanotic melanoma, and with a spontaneous breast carcinoma of mice, all of which are uniformly fatal if untreated, have shown that: (1) the incidence of metastatic disease is directly related to tumor mass, (2) surgical cure rates drop as tumor mass at surgery increases, (3) grossly evident primary tumors are generally not curable by drug treatment, and (4) surgical adjuvant chemotherapy increases the long-term cure rates with all of these tumors and significantly increases the life span of treatment failures.

Effective surgical adjuvant chemotherapy is both dose-responsive and related to the body burden of metastatic tumor at time of drug treatment. The effectiveness of surgical adjuvant chemotherapy decreases (1) as tumor staging is advanced prior to surgery, (2) as interval from surgery to start of effective chemotherapy is increased, and (3) as drug doses are reduced. Additionally, and of critical importance to treatment planning, some drugs that are marginally effective or ineffective against the presurgical total body burden of tumor cells are curative in some to all mice with metastatic disease if given shortly after surgical removal of the primary tumor.

INTRODUCTION

Cancer arises when one normal cell changes into a malignant neoplastic cell, either by spontaneous mutation or following chemical, viral, or radiation induction.[1] Once this oncogenic event takes place, successive doublings of the tumor cell and all its progeny to nearly one billion cells in a single focus is necessary for clinical recognition.[2] Considering the natural history of tumor growth from origin to host death, all tumors are advanced when first detected. Cancer is curable by either surgery or radiation treatment, in the main, only if it has not metastasized when it is first detected. Among the nearly 700,000 new cases of cancer in the United States each year, more than 50% will have metastatic disease at the time of diagnosis or will have a high risk of recurrence following the best presently available surgical, radiological, or drug treatment.[2]

These metastatic foci are the proper target for the medical oncologist using drugs and/or immunity mechanisms. Anticancer drugs spread throughout the body, with the exception, at least for some drugs, of certain pharmacologic sanctuaries such as the brain, and are able to kill drug-sensitive cancer cells wherever in the body they may be. Drug effectiveness is limited by many factors, chief among which is that drugs kill tumor cells by so-called first-order kinetics. Simply stated, this means that a constant percentage of tumor cells is killed by treatment with an effective drug, irrespective of the size of the tumor cell population, as long as that population is metabolically homogenous and all tumor cells receive drug exposure that is equal in both concentration and duration.[1,3] This principle seems illogical to many biologists, but not to bacteriologists who recognize first-order cell kill kinetics of bacteria by germicides, or to radiologists who recognize first-order cell kill kinetics of cells by radiation. It seems more reasonable to assume that a dose of drug that will kill more than 9,990,000 of a population of 10 million cancer cells should easily, under identican conditions, kill all of a population of 100,000 cancer cells, but such is not the case.[1,3] Therefore, the total body burden of drug-sensitive tumor cells at start of drug treatment is probably the most important single factor influencing cure.

Current failure to cure over 90% of clinically recognized metastatic (systemic) cancer with available drugs is due, in the main, to a total body burden of tumor cells at the start of drug treatment which is greater than the selective cell kill potential for tumor cells over vital normal cells of the most effective drugs we have presently available. Until we develop new drugs with orders of magnitude greater selective tumor cell kill potential than those we now have, improved long-term cure rates for systemic cancer in man will be primarily dependent upon reduction of the total body burden of tumor cells facing the chemotherapist by early surgical removal and/or radiation kill of grossly evident and accessible primary tumors. There are extensive data from studies with a number of metastatic and uniformly fatal animal tumors upon which the above statements are based.

DIRECT RELATIONSHIP BETWEEN PRIMARY TUMOR MASS AND METASTATIC BODY BURDEN OF TUMOR CELLS

There is a direct relationship between the size of the primary tumor in carcinoma of the breast in women and both the surgical cure rates and likely metastatic tumor cell body burden; the larger the primary tumor at time of surgery, the lower the long-term cure rates and the shorter the duration of life among the surgically curative failures.[4,5,6] Similar relationships have been observed with at least four metastasizing and uniformly fatal transplantable solid tumors of mice:[7] Lewis lung carcinoma, C3H mammary carcinoma, colon carcinoma, and B16 melanoma. Figures 1 and 2 show the cumulative mortality in groups of mice in which progressively larger subcutaneously (s.c.) implanted mammary carcinoma (Fig. 1) or colon carcinoma (Fig. 2) were removed by surgery. All deaths were from metastatic disease only. There was a low incidence of metastasis in mice bearing primary tumors up to 250 mg. The incidence of fatal metastatic disease exceeded 50% if the primary tumors were between 250 and 500 mg and was 80% or greater if the primary tumors were larger than 500 mg at the time of surgical removal. Further, the total body burden of metastatic disease in dying animals increased as the primary mass increased, since the interval from surgery to death from metastatic disease was inversely related to tumor mass at time of surgery.

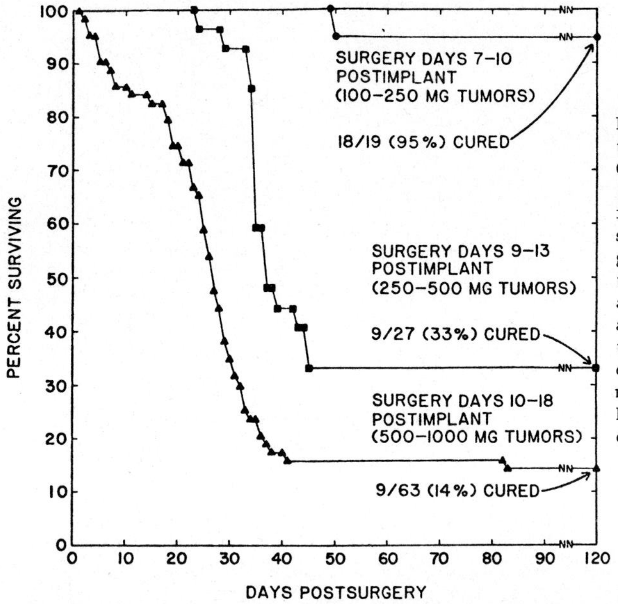

Fig. 1. Cumulative mortality from metastatic C3H mammary carcinoma (Line 44) following s.c. implant into C3H mice and surgical removal of progressively larger primary tumors. None of the animals showed grossly apparent tumor regrowth at the surgical site at time of death from demonstrated metastatic lesions. Reproduced with permission of Cancer.[7]

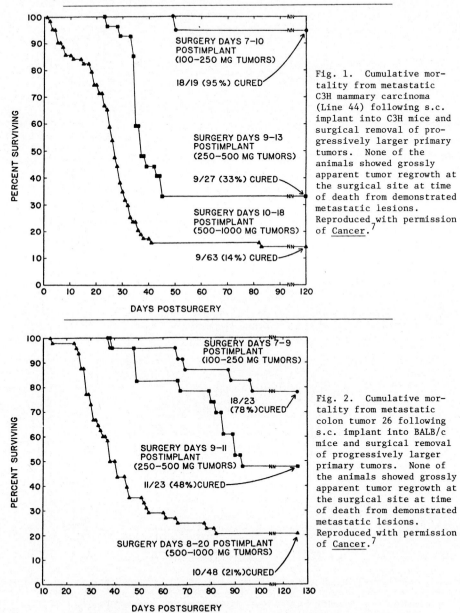

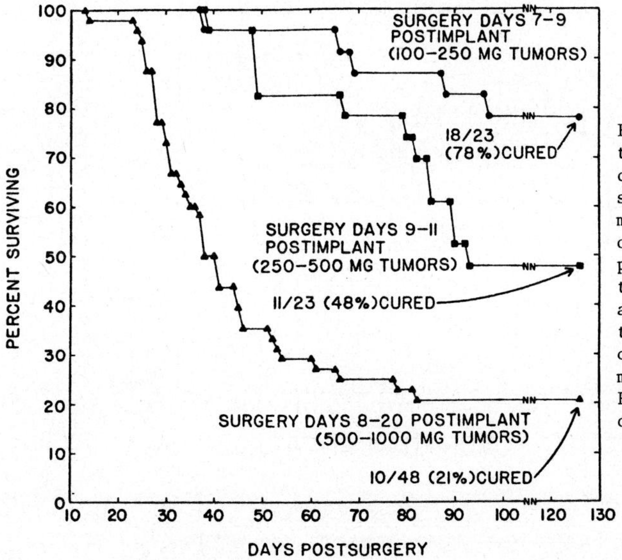

Fig. 2. Cumulative mortality from metastatic colon tumor 26 following s.c. implant into BALB/c mice and surgical removal of progressively larger primary tumors. None of the animals showed grossly apparent tumor regrowth at the surgical site at time of death from demonstrated metastatic lesions. Reproduced with permission of Cancer.[7]

These results mimic common experience with treatment of primary breast cancer in women, where surgical cure rates and median survival time of women with recurrent disease are directly but not invariably related to the size of the primary tumor at time of surgery.[4] With these murine tumors, death from metastatic disease followed surgical removal of small primary tumors (< 250 mg) in a few mice, and cure was accomplished by surgical removal of large primary tumors (up to one gram) in a few mice.

Similar results have been obtained following surgical removal of progressively larger primary tumors with B16 melanoma and Lewis lung carcinoma in mice.[7]

IMPROVED CURE RATES USING SURGICAL ADJUVANT CHEMOTHERAPY OF METASTATIC MURINE TUMORS

Improved cure rates of a number of metastatic (systemic) solid tumors of mice using surgical adjuvant chemotherapy have been reproducibly achieved by a number of different investigators. Examples of improved cure rates with surgical adjuvant chemotherapy obtained at Southern Research Institute are shown in Figures 3-7.

Lewis Lung Carcinoma: This tumor arose spontaneously as a carcinoma of the lung in a C57Bl mouse in 1951, and it has been maintained in continuous serial passage. It is a very anaplastic type of epidermoid carcinoma. It metastasizes, primarily to the lungs, within a few days after s.c. implant and kills by massive tumor growth in the lungs. Surgical removal of the primary after metastatic spread to the lungs does not increase life span.

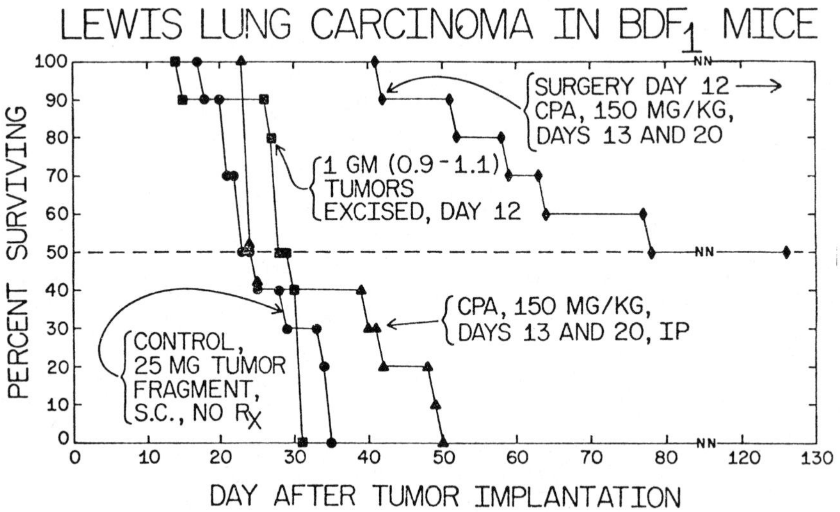

Fig. 3. Curative surgical adjuvant chemotherapy of Lewis lung carcinoma with surgical removal of the primary tumor (no cures); treatment with cyclophosphamide (CPA) on Days 1 and 8 after surgery (no cures); surgery followed by CPA (50% cured). Reproduced with permission of Am. J. Roentgenol.[1]

Curative surgical adjuvant chemotherapy with cyclophosphamide (CPA) and other drugs has been reported (published literature is reviewed in Reference 7). An example from our laboratory is shown in Figure 3. Surgical removal of the s.c. primary tumor 12 days after implant, or treatment with CPA on Days 13 and 20, failed to cure or to extend life span significantly; either surgery or CPA treatment when used alone was ineffective. However, surgical removal of the primary tumor on Day 12 followed by treatment with CPA on Days 13 and 20 cured 50% of the mice and significantly increased the life span of animals ultimately dying of metastatic disease.

C3H Mammary Adenocarcinoma (Line 44) (Fig. 4): This tumor was developed by Drs. T.H. Corbett and D.P. Griswold, Jr. of Southern Research Institute. It was established in transplant from a spontaneous mammary carcinoma in a C3H/HeN mouse. Its rate of metastasis was increased by selective s.c. transplant of naturally occurring metastatic foci from the lungs which produced a very anaplastic tumor. Surgical removal of the s.c. implanted tumor on Day 11 failed to cure more than 70% of the mice, and surgical removal on Day 13 or 14 postimplant failed to cure >90%. Treatment with N,N'-bis(2-chloroethyl)-N-nitrosourea (BCNU) plus CPA, or with *cis*-4-[[[(2-chloroethyl)nitrosoamino]carbonyl]amino]cyclohexanecarboxylic acid (CCCNU-*cis*) plus CPA on Days 15 to 18 postimplant failed to cure any mice, although therapeutic effectiveness based on increased life span was demonstrated.

BCNU + CPA treatment four days after surgical removal of the primary tumor on Day 11 increased the cure rate from about 30% with surgery alone to 100% with surgical adjuvant chemotherapy (Fig. 4A) and from less than 10% to about 50% with more advanced tumor (Fig. 4B). The data in Fig. 4C indicate that a reduction of about 33% in the doses of CCCNU-*cis* plus CPA reduced the cure rates with surgical adjuvant chemotherapy from >80% to <50%, with an accompanying decrease in life span of drug-treated mice dying of metastatic disease. Dose-response data such as these are commonly obtained in surgical adjuvant chemotherapy trials in animals, and they emphasize the importance of adequate drug treatment to obtain maximum cure rates with adjuvant chemotherapy, at least under laboratory conditions.

Colon Tumor (Line 26) (Figs. 5 and 6): This is a metastasizing, transplantable colon tumor of mice that is uniformly fatal if untreated.[8] Surgical removal of primary tumor on Day 15 postimplant failed to cure 65% of the mice (Fig. 5A), and removal on Day 18 failed to cure any (Fig. 5B). Treatment with N-(2-chloroethyl)-N'-(*trans*-4-methylcyclohexyl)-N-nitrosourea (MeCCNU) four days after surgery increased the cure rate from about 35% with surgery alone to 65% (Fig. 5A), and treatment with CCCNU-*cis* three days after surgery increased the cure rate from zero with surgery alone to 50% (Fig. 5B). Treatment with either drug alone increased the life span of tumor-bearing mice only to a limited degree.

Surgical adjuvant chemotherapy of this colon tumor with MeCCNU plus 5-fluorouracil (5-FU) is also very effective against the metastatic disease (Fig. 6).

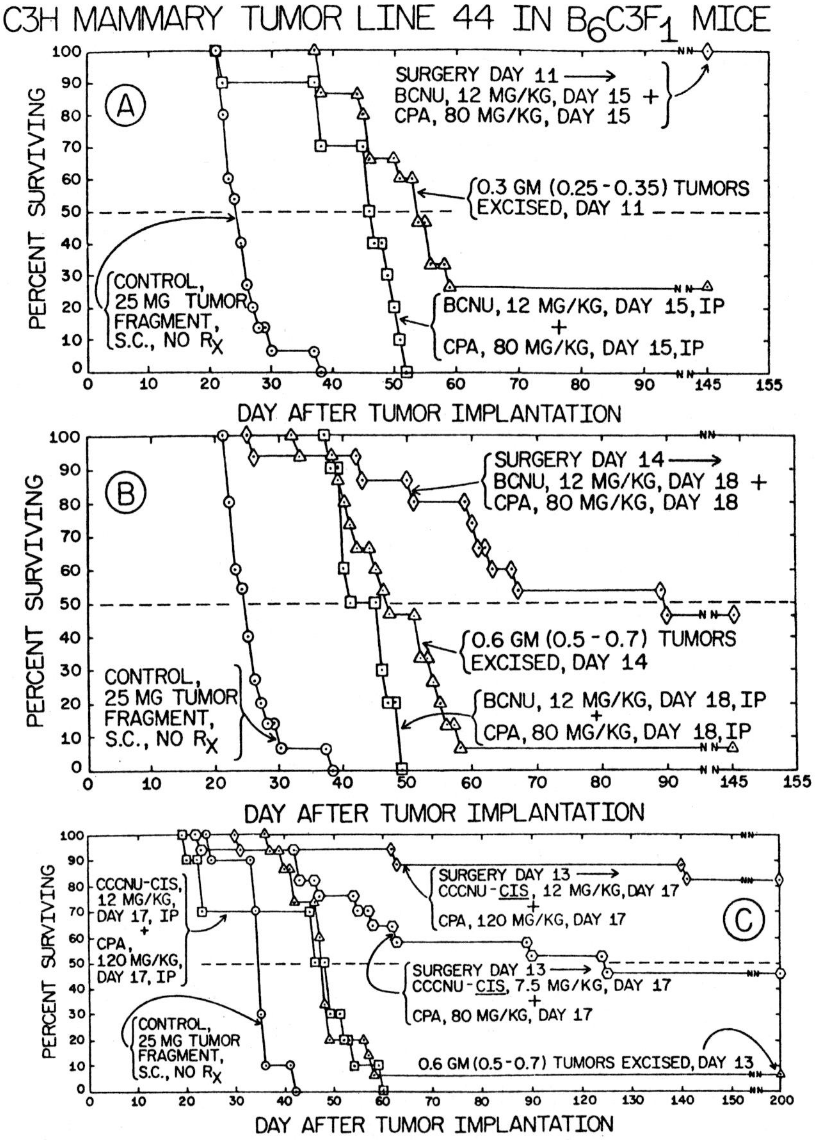

Fig. 4. Curative surgical adjuvant chemotherapy of C3H mammary adenocarcinoma. Influence of tumor staging and drug dosage on cure rates. (A) Surgery on Day 11 (about 30% cured) or BCNU + CPA on Day 15 (no cures); surgery followed by adjuvar drug treatment (100% cured). (B) Surgery delayed to Day 14 (less than 10% cured) or BCNU + CPA on Day 18 (no cures); surgery followed by adjuvant drug treatment (about 50% cured). (C) Surgery on Day 13 followed by drug treatment (CCCNU-cis + CPA) on Day 17 (about 80% cured with high drug doses and 50% cured with lower drı doses). Reproduced with permission of Am. J. Roentgenol.[1]

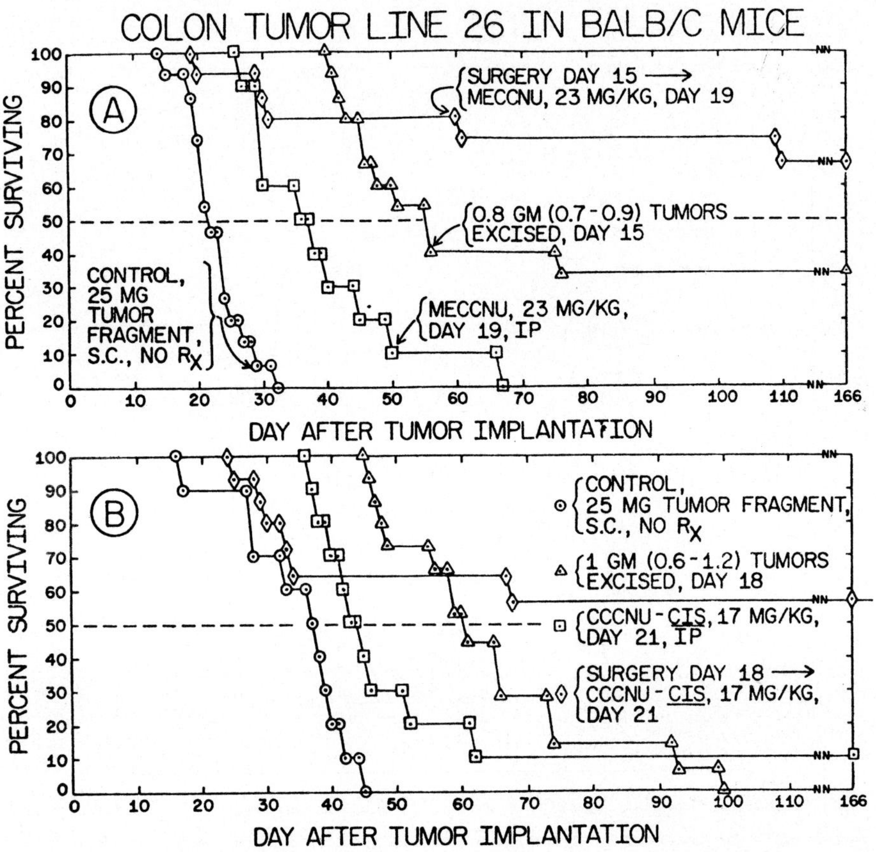

Fig. 5. Curative surgical adjuvant chemotherapy of colon tumor line 26. Influence of tumor staging on cure rates. (A) Surgery on Day 15 (35% cured) or MeCCNU on Day 19 (no cures); surgery on Day 15 followed by MeCCNU on Day 19 (65% cured). (B) Surgery on Day 18 (no cures) or CCCNU-cis on Day 21 (10% cured); surgery followed by CCCNU-cis (more than 50% cured). Reproduced with permission of Am. J. Roentgenol.[1]

Surgery alone on Day 15 cured less than 10% of the mice, and MeCCNU plus 5-FU on Day 15 without surgery failed to show therapeutic activity, while surgical adjuvant chemotherapy cured 40% of the mice and increased the median life span of animals dying of metastatic disease about 30 days beyond the median of those treated with surgery only. These results are of great interest, since MeCCNU plus 5-FU, with or without added vincristine, has been reported to be among the best drug treatment observed to date against advanced colorectal and gastric cancer in man.[9]

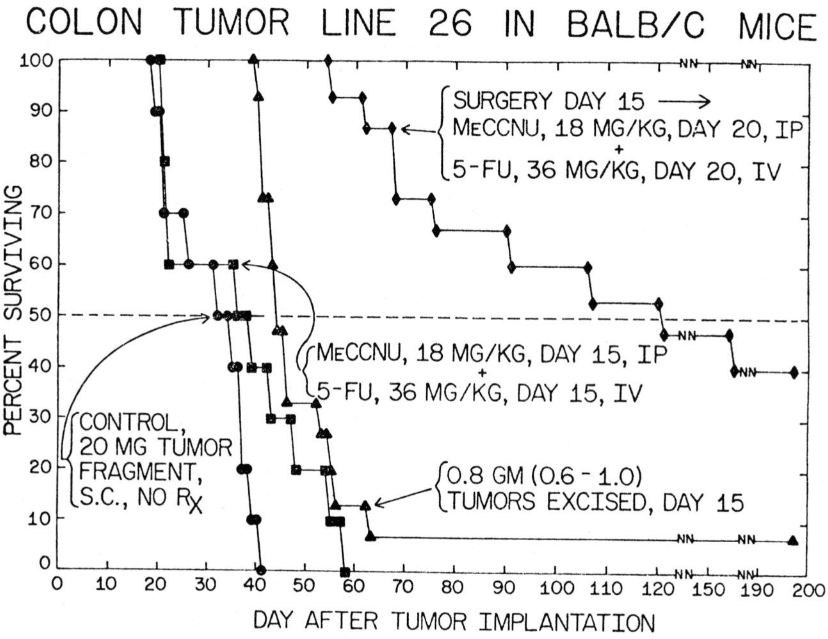

Fig. 6. Curative surgical adjuvant chemotherapy of colon tumor 26. Surgical removal of primary tumor on Day 15 (about 10% cured) or MeCCNU + 5-FU on Day 15 (no cures); surgery on Day 15 followed by adjuvant chemotherapy on Day 20 (40% cured and marked prolongation of life of those dying of tumor).

B16 Melanoma (Fig. 7): This is a transplantable melanotic melanoma that arose spontaneously in the skin at the base of the ear of a C57Bl/6 mouse in 1954 and has been maintained since by serial s.c. transplant. The rate of metastasis was increased by selective s.c. transplantation of naturally occurring metastatic foci from the lungs. This tumor has an 80% to 90% mortality rate from associated metastatic disease following surgical removal of the primary tumor on Days 12 to 15 postimplant. Treatment of the advanced primary tumor (1 gm) with MeCCNU alone was not curative, but it did increase life span to a limited degree. Surgical adjuvant chemotherapy increased the cure rate from 20% to 70% when given 24 hours after surgical removal of the primary tumor on Day 11 postimplant (Fig. 7A). When surgery was delayed to Day 15 postimplant, adjuvant chemotherapy only increased the 10% cure rate by surgery alone to 20%, but did significantly increase the life span of dying animals over that obtained with surgery alone (Fig. 7B). These data clearly indicate the importance of early postsurgical use of adjuvant chemotherapy (when the body burden of metastatic tumor cells is lowest) to obtain maximum cures.

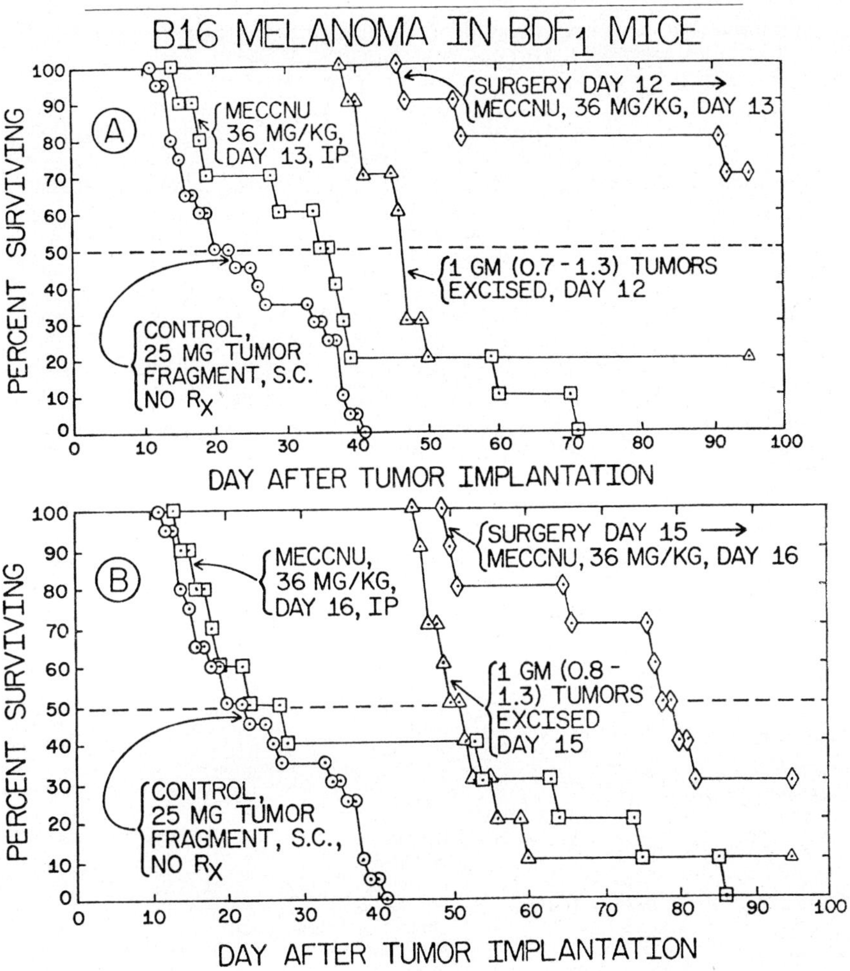

Fig. 7. Surgical adjuvant chemotherapy of B16 melanoma. Influence of tumor staging (body burden of tumor cells) on cure rates. (A) Surgery on Day 12 post-implant (20% cured) followed by single-dose treatment with MeCCNU 24 hr later. MeCCNU treatment without surgery was not curative. Surgery followed by MeCCNU raised cure rate to 70%. (B) Same as (A), except start of treatment was delayed to Day 15 postimplant. Surgical cure rate was reduced to 10%, and surgical adjuvant chemotherapy cure rate was reduced to 30%. Reproduced with permission of Am. J. Roentgenol.[1]

The results shown in Figures 3-7 are illustrative examples of increased cure rates obtained in the laboratory with surgical adjuvant chemotherapy of metastatic murine tumors. In Table 1, I have listed these and other improved cure rates with surgical adjuvant chemotherapy of naturally occurring or artificial metastases in mice that we and others have observed and reported. It is an impressive list,

TABLE 1
IMPROVED LONG-TERM CURE RATES WITH SURGICAL ADJUVANT CHEMOTHERAPY AGAINST METASTATIC MURINE SOLID TUMORS*

Tumor	Mouse	Clinical Staging of Primary Tumor Mass at Surgery	Treatment: Surgery Followed by	% "Cures" Surgery Only	% "Cures" Surgery→ Drug(s)
Lewis lung carcinoma	BDF_1	400 mg	CPA	0	10-90
			MeCCNU	0	40
		1000 mg	CPA	0	50
			MeCCNU	0	30
			CPA + MeCCNU	0	40
		2000 mg	CPA	0	5
			MeCCNU	0	10
			CPA + MeCCNU	0	20
C3H Breast Line 16 (Undifferentiated carcinoma)	C3H	1000 mg	ADR**	0-<20	15-50
			L-PAM**	<20	40
			ADR + CPA	<10	35
C3H Breast Line 44 (Undifferentiated carcinoma)	C3H	300 mg	BCNU + CPA	<30	100
		600 mg	BCNU + CPA	<10	45
			CCCNU-*cis* + CPA	<10	80
		1000 mg	BCNU	0	30
			BCNU + 5-FUdR**	ca 30	50
			CPA + 5-FUdR	0	10
Adenoca 755 (Carcinoma)	C57Bl	<100 mg	6-MP**	<5	46***
Adenoca RC (Carcinoma)	$CD8F_1$	<100 mg	6-MP	15	71***
Mammary Adenoca (Spontaneous) (Carcinoma)	$CD8F_1$	--	STEAM**	5	ca 30
Colon 26 (Undifferentiated carcinoma)	BALB/c	800 mg	MeCCNU	35	65
			CCCNU-*cis*	10	55
			CPA + CCCNU-*cis*	20	75
			BCNU + 5-FU	ca 20	75
			MeCCNU + PalmOara-C**	<10	70
			MeCCNU + 5-FU	<10	40
			CPA + PalmOara-C	<10	50
Colon 38 (Adenocarcinoma)	BDF_1	800 mg	CPA + CCCNU-*cis*	50	85
B16 Melanoma	BDF_1	500-1000 mg	MeCCNU	20	70
			CPA + MeCCNU	0	30
			PalmOara-C + MeCCNU	10	20
Sa180 (Sarcoma)	$CD8F_1$	<100 mg	6-MP	0	43***

*Published reports from which this table was prepared are listed in Reference 7

**ADR = adriamycin; L-PAM = L-phenylalanine mustard; 3[*p*-[bis(2-chloroethyl)-amino]phenyl]-L-alanine, HCl; 5-FUdR = 5-fluorodeoxyuridine; 6-MP = 6-mercaptopurine; STEAM = streptonigrin + 6-thioguanine + CPA + actinomycin D + mitomycin C; PalmOara-C = 1-β-D-arabinofuranosylcytosine, 5'palmitate—a depot form of ara-C

***Artificial metastases

including the major histologic types of human cancer with which surgical cure rates are often low and therapeutic response of advanced systemic disease is also poor. The drugs used as surgical adjuvants in Table 1 are predominantly alkylating agents, but a few antimetabolite drugs (5-FU, 5-FUdR, Ara-C) and those that bind to or intercalate with DNA (adriamycin) are represented.

DISCUSSION

Improved cure rates with a variety of histologic types of systemic and uniformly fatal solid tumors of mice, staged at start of treatment so that cures were infrequent or absent with either surgery or drugs used alone, have been reproducibly demonstrated, and this has been accomplished with a variety of clinically useful single drugs and combinations of drugs. The proper method of selection of candidate drugs for surgical adjuvant chemotherapy in man and the optimal treatment regimens (drug doses and schedules) have not been clearly shown. It seems obvious that drugs which are active but noncurative against the grossly evident advanced tumor would be most indicated for adjuvant chemotherapy. There are many theoretical indications, and a large and growing body of objective evidence from studies with animal tumors, indicating that failure of specific drug(s) to demonstrate effectiveness against advanced tumors probably should not deny their consideration for use as chemotherapeutic adjuvants to other treatment modalities, since marked therapeutic activity against small tumor cell populations has been repeatedly seen with drugs inactive against large tumor cell populations _in vivo_[1,3,10] (see Figs. 3, 6, and 7). Reduction of the total body burden of tumor cells by surgical removal or by radiological or chemical killing should increase the effectiveness of adjuvant drug treatment, since (a) this reduced body burden is more likely to be within the curative potential of drug treatment due to first-order cell kill kinetics of effective drugs; (b) reduced populations of residual viable tumor cells should be more drug-sensitive, especially to antimetabolite drugs, since smaller tumor cell populations have a higher proportion of cells in active anabolism (higher growth fraction) preparing for cell division and thus greater sensitivity to anticancer drugs with which lethal toxicity is due to the blocking of vital anabolic functions[3] (some anticancer drugs only kill tumor when they are actively anabolizing); (c) small numbers of cells from several different murine tumors will establish fatal disease _in vivo_ if implanted in the presence of radiation-killed tumor cells or normal cells,[3] and some radiation-killed tumor cells appear to support the growth of residual viable tumor cells in or close to the irradiated tumor target area; and (d) anatomical relationships allowing lethal exposure of tumor cells to effective anticancer drugs are more favorable in small tumor foci, such as micrometastases, than in large grossly apparent tumors, e.g. the greatest distance from the nearest capillary to the most distant viable tumor cell usually increases as the mass of each tumor focus increases. This is probably the major cause of progressive necrosis and a reduction of the growth fraction in a tumor focus as it increases in size, but it also undoubtedly influences drug response, because an otherwise effective drug will not kill a tumor cell it cannot reach in lethal concentration.

The logical, orderly, and objectively demonstrated concept, that at least some anticancer drugs which are essentially ineffective against advanced tumors should be and are effective (sometimes curative) against micrometastatic tumor foci, increases the drugs available for consideration for adjuvant chemotherapy. If surgical adjuvant chemotherapy data from metastatic murine tumor systems provide reliable indications for such considerations, then the number of candidate drugs that could be considered for use in the surgical or radiation adjuvant setting is sharply increased.

REFERENCES

1. Schabel, F.M., Jr. Concepts for treatment of micrometastases developed in murine systems. Am. J. Roentgenol. (1976) 126, 500-511.
2. DeVita, V.T., Young, R.C., and Canellos, G.P. Combination versus single agent chemotherapy: review of basis for selection of drug treatment of cancer. Cancer (1975) 35, 98-110.
3. Schabel, F.M., Jr. Concepts for systemic treatment of micrometastases. Cancer (1975) 35, 15-24.
4. Cutler, S.J., and Myers, M.H. Clinical classification of extent of disease in cancer of the breast. J. Natl. Cancer Inst. (1967) 39, 193-207.
5. Skipper, H.E. Kinetics of mammary tumor cell growth and implications for therapy. Cancer (1971) 28, 1479-1499.
6. Duncan, W., and Kerr, G.R. The curability of breast cancer. Br. Med. J. (1976) 2, 781-783.
7. Schabel, F.M., Jr. Surgical adjuvant chemotherapy of metastatic murine tumors. Cancer (1977) in press.
8. Corbett, T.H., Griswold, D.P., Jr., Roberts, B.J., Peckham, J.C., and Schabel, F.M., Jr. Tumor induction relationships in development of transplantable cancers of the colon in mice for chemotherapy assays, with a note on carcinogen structure. Cancer Res. (1975) 35, 2434-2439.
9. Moertel, C.G. Clinical management of advanced gastrointestinal cancer. Cancer (1975) 36, 675-682.
10. Schabel, F.M., Jr. The use of tumor growth kinetics in planning "curative" chemotherapy of advanced solid tumors. Cancer Res. (1969) 29, 2384-2389.

Adjuvant Therapy of Cancer, S.E. Salmon and S.E. Jones eds.

KINETIC RATIONALE FOR ADJUVANT CHEMOTHERAPY OF CANCER

Sydney E. Salmon, M. D.
Section of Hematology and Oncology
Department of Internal Medicine and the Cancer Center
University of Arizona College of Medicine
Tucson, Arizona 85724, U.S.A.

INTRODUCTION

The development of a rational approach to adjuvant chemotherapy of cancer is dependent upon (1) recognition that occult micrometastases frequently have already become established at distant sites prior to the time of primary field therapy with surgery or irradiation, (2) knowledge of drug sensitivity and kinetics of proliferation of the tumor stem cells (particularly after surgery or irradiation), (3) estimates of the residual tumor burden after surgery, and (4) availability of effective anticancer drugs, particularly those with a cycle-non-specific mode of action which will be lethal to G_o (resting) tumor stem cells as well as those in the proliferative cycle. At the present time, most investigators only consider adjuvant chemotherapy for patients with a greater than 50% risk of recurrence. However, the same approach would be reasonable (and perhaps even more effective) for patients at lower risk of recurrence if the treatment had only minor toxicity and was known to be effective in higher risk categories. In this analysis of the rationale for adjuvant chemotherapy, I will rely heavily on quantitative extrapolations relating to tumor kinetics and drug effects, and select kinetic parameters characteristic of cancers which might be difficult to eradicate. This approach permits projection of chemotherapeutic schedules and intensity of treatment which might prove necessary to achieve cellular cure (reduction in tumor burden to less than 10° (1 cell). The University of Arizona breast adjuvant program will be utilized to exemplify application of some of these principles.

TUMOR STEM CELLS

The most important cells in a cancer are undoubtedly the tumor stem cells. Tumor stem cells comprise the self-renewal system required for a cancer to grow. Additionally, tumor stem cells are the seeds of metastasis, have the capability of migration, and can therefore initiate new colonies at locations in the body which are distant from the primary neoplasm. Viewed from that perspective, rational design of adjuvant chemotherapy for cancer requires focus on the study of human tumor stem cells with respect to their kinetics of proliferation and unique susceptibilities to anticancer drugs. Studies of transplantable animal tumors or of long passage *in vitro* tumor cell lines may not accurately reflect the proliferative behavior of the small compartment of tumor stem cells of an individual patient's primary cancer or its micrometastases. I take this view because the established tumor cell systems are of limited diversity in comparison to the clinical situations which the clinician sees with cancers which differ in histopathology, proliferative behavior, and susceptibility to anticancer drugs. To overcome this problem, studies of human tumor growth from biopsy samples have recently been undertaken in immunodeficient mice[1] and *in vitro*. Very recently, Dr. Anne Hamburger and I developed an *in vitro* soft agar colony-forming system which supports the growth of a variety of human tumors from relatively small inocula (5×10^5 cells) obtained directly from patient biopsy samples[2]. Our experience to date has been obtained largely from advanced metastic neoplasms, but likely can be translated into the setting of primary tumors as well. Our initial colony-forming assay was developed for multiple myeloma[3]. For that cancer, we now regularly and routinely observe *in vitro* myeloma colony formation from bone marrow aspirates containing tumor cells, and have been able to directly measure the fraction of tumor stem cells in the S-phase of the cell cycle (with tritiated thymidine suicide studies) as well as initiate studies of the susceptibility of human myeloma stem cells to anticancer drugs such as melphalan and adriamycin. We have also successfully applied this system to colony formation by tumor stem cells from a number of patients with non-Hodgkin's lymphomas or ovarian carcinoma. Additionally, a few cases of other cancers studied (e.g., neuroblastoma) have also formed tumor colonies directly from biopsy samples. A typical ovarian cancer colony appears in Figure 1. There are distinct differences in morphology of colonies arising from different types of cancer and there are differences in the plating efficiency and growth rates for colonies from different human cancers *in vitro*. In most instances, tumor colonies of greater than 40 cells appear in the agar some 2-3 weeks after plating. From the kinetic standpoint, if a typical colony grows to 64 cells in size in 18 days, then the doubling time in this initial phase of growth of such an "*in vitro* micrometastasis" is 3 days.

Our work on drug sensitivity has thus far been limited to myeloma cases, but has already shown a 20-fold range in melphalan sensitivity by human myeloma stem cells from different patients. This result should be viewed in relation to results in transplantable mouse myeloma[4] wherein differences of that magnitude in drug sensitivity *in vitro* were observed between different myeloma cell lines and correlated with *in vivo* sensitivity to the same drugs. Thus, each individual myeloma patient's stem cells may be as different from the next patient's as one transplantable meyloma tumor system is from another. A reasonable extrapolation from current techniques to adjuvant therapy would include routine tests of drug sensitivity of tumor stem cells from high risk primary tumors resected at surgery. A feasible strategy would be to initiate a standardized adjuvant treatment for such patients, and then alter it, if needed, based on *in vitro* patterns of sensitivity or resistance. This approach is of course identical to the current strategy for management of difficult bacterial infections.

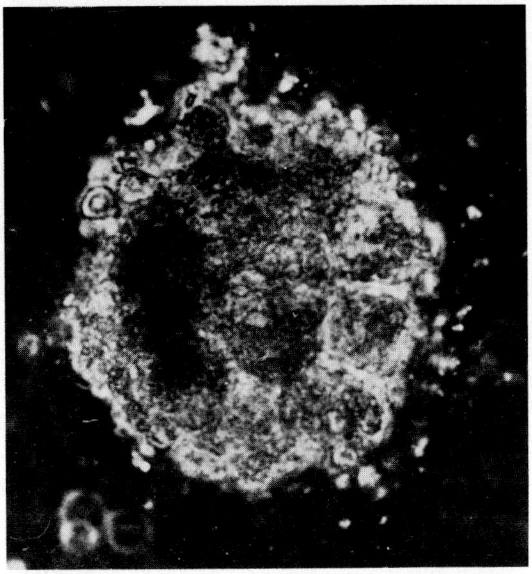

Figure 1. A 20-day-old human tumor colony in soft agar (200x). The tumor colonies were grown directly from cells in the ascitic fluid from a women with advanced ovarian carcinoma. Stained slides of such colonies show morphology characteristic of ovarian adenocarcinoma.

RESIDUAL TUMOR BURDEN AND TUMOR KINETICS

For the present discussion, I consider adjuvant chemotherapy to be limited to the setting wherein less than 10^4 tumor cells remain after surgery. While it is currently not possible to measure this small tumor burden directly, it is possible to back-extrapolate from data relating to the time to relapse for certain common tumors and estimate the residual burden of micrometastases after surgery. Such calculations require some knowledge of the cell cycle time and growth kinetics of the particular cancer.

This approach to kinetic analysis has been used effectively by Skipper and Schabel[5]. One important aspect of their analysis was the recognition that the characteristic relapse or relapse-free survival curve for patients with any given type of cancer provided valuable insights about the residual tumor burden after primary surgery or radiotherapy. They assumed that both the time to recurrence and death were related to the number of tumor cells surviving primary surgery and/or irradiation. A typical curve of cancer recurrences after primary local treatment manifests an initially constant rate of recurrence for 2-3 years after primary therapy, followed by a decreasing rate of recurrence, and then a relatively flat component thereafter, reflecting the prolonged survival of the cohort of patients who were likely cured by the primary treatment (Figure 2). Skipper and Schabel identified the change in slope just prior to the flat component as the "break" in the survival curve, and postulated that it reflected the time for a minimal tumor burden (less than 10^1 tumor cells) to repopulate and present as metastatic disease.

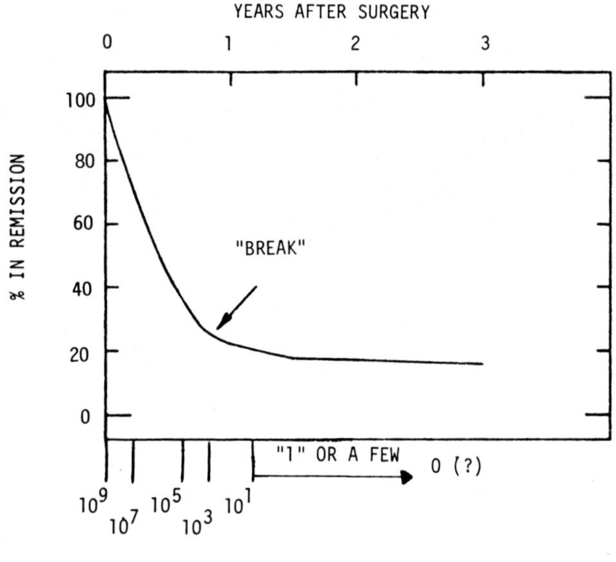

Figure 2. Example of a typical "break" in a remission curve and its postulated relationship to tumor burden. In this example, in which the median tumor doubling time is assumed to be 40 days, most patients who had only 10 tumor cells remaining after surgery still relapsed in about one year (reproduced with modification with permission of the authors (5))

Such curves were then related to tumor staging, and the relapse curve viewed as a titration of residual tumor burden after surgery (Figure 3). Additionally, it was proposed that if "just a few" tumor cells remain (e.g., 1-3 cells), the time to relapse may be exceptionally long because those few cells might not have typical growth characteristics, whereas if 10 or more cells remained, the chance of a cell remaining with growth characteristics typical for the original tumor would be rather high. They went on to assume that the doubling time was relatively constant from 10^1 to 10^6 cells, and calculated "median doubling times" (MDT's) for the repopulation phase so that they could then make predictions about the intensity of adjuvant chemotherapy which would be required.

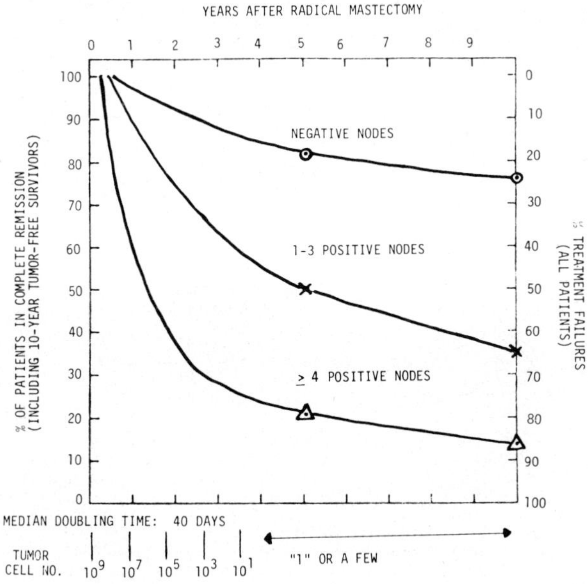

Figure 3. The presumed relationship between lymph node status, prognosis, and residual tumor burden after surgery for women with stage I or II primary breast-cancer who have undergone radical mastectomy. The numbers of residual tumor cells calculated to be present are based on an assumed median doubling time of 40 days (reproduced with modification from (5) with permission of the authors).

While such calculations of MDT's are reasonable, they are estimated to be 40-60 days, and are therefore considerably longer than the tumor cell generation time as measured with tritiated thymidine, or the *in vitro* doubling time for tumor cells in suspension cultures initiated at low dilutions. In these latter circumstances the tumor doubling times are closer to 2-5 days. The biochemical explanation for increasing doubling time with increasing cell mass is uncertain and may be related to feedback regulatory factors. Available evidence suggests that the level of regulation is on the fraction of tumor stem cells which are capable of entering the proliferative cycle. For purposes of illustration of rational design of adjuvant chemotherapy programs, I have used computer analysis and modeled a tumor with Gompertzian kinetics, selecting an initial doubling time (1 cell to 2) of 2.34 days (about 56 hours). The tumor growth curve is shown in Figure 4, while Table 1 shows the calculated doubling times at various cell burdens. This same "model tumor" will be used subsequently for designing a treatment schedule for adjuvant breast cancer treatment.

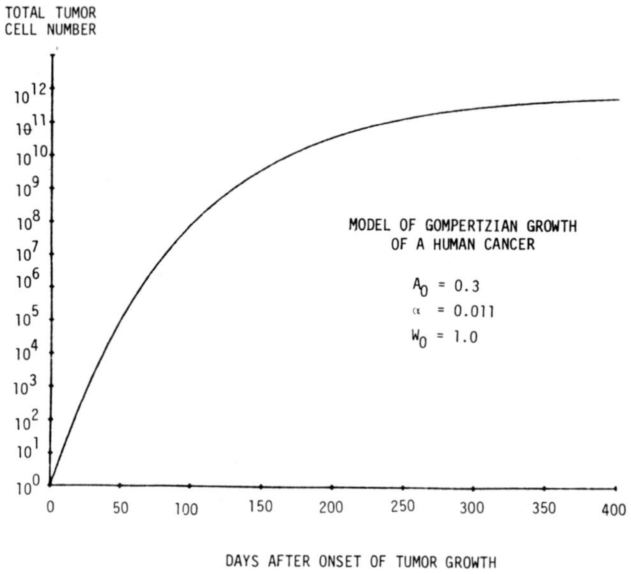

Figure 4. A Gompertzian growth curve for the "model" of micrometastasis of human breast cancer with a short initial doubling time (1 cell to 2 cells) of 2.34 days (about 56 hours). Doubling times and tumor mass at varying points along this curve are summarized in Table 1. The equation for the constants above is in ref. (6).

Table 1

Total Tumor Burden and Doubling Times for the Gompertzian Tumor Growth Curve Depicted in Figure 4

Cell Doubling	Log. No.	Mass*	Doubling Time
One to two	$1x10^0-2x10^0$	1 nanogram	2.34 days
One thousand to Two thousand	$1x10^3-2x10^3$	1 microgram	3.15 days
One million to Two million	$1x10^6-2x10^6$	1 milligram	4.31 days
One billion to Two billion	$1x10^9-2x10^9$	1 gram	10.2 days
One hundred billion to Two hundred billion	$1x10^{11}-2x10^{11}$	100 grams	40.1 days

* One cell is assumed to weigh one nanogram.

SELECTION OF ANTICANCER DRUGS AND ESTIMATION OF TUMOR CELL KILL

Over 40 anticancer drugs are now available for clinical use, all of which have efficacy in one or more types of cancer. Selection of the appropriate agents for adjuvant therapy is not easy, and takes a good deal of empiricism -- hopefully with some enlightenment. Certainly, it is logical to select agents capable of inducing remissions for advanced stages of the same type of cancer for which adjuvant therapy is contemplated. Other considerations also apply for adjuvant therapy. In general, we do not accept marked toxicity from adjuvant therapy programs because not all the patients treated assuredly have residual cancer. However, I believe that adjuvant programs should ideally be capable of reducing the size of the residual tumor stem cell population by 99% to 99.9% per course. In my opinion, major reliance should not be placed on cycle-specific drugs, because not all residual tumor stem cells are known to be in cycle or in the sensitive phase of the cycle at the time of drug administration. Cycle non-specific agents generally manifest a dose-dependent "fractional cell kill" of the tumor stem cells exposed.

The magnitude of this fractional kill of stem cells (e.g., 90%, or 99.9%) is grossly underestimated from tumor mass measurements in clinical trials in patients with advanced cancer. The conclusion that clinical tumor volume measurements grossly underestimate tumor stem cell kill is derived from several lines of evidence. Tumors are known to contain a number of components which contribute to volume but are not part of the tumor stem cell compartment. These include stromal elements such as blood vessels and connective tissue, differentiated tumor cells which have permanently lost capability of re-entry into the proliferative compartment, and grossly necrotic tissue. Indeed, after administration of chemotherapy there is a time delay of from days to months for physical dissolution of residual sterile tumor cells incapable of further division as well as for resorption of the dead and dying elements in the tumor nodule, and for involution of the stromal elements. Persistence of differentiated elements is perhaps best exemplified in testicular cancers which may be effectively cured with combination chemotherapy, but leave residual, non-malignant teratomas which may require subsequent surgical resection. Studies involving early transplantation of spontaneous animal tumors, as well as studies of primary human tumors transplanted into nude mice[1] and our recent studies of direct *in vitro* plating of human tumors[2] suggest that only a small fraction of tumor cells (generally less than 1%) are capable of giving rise to tumor colonies. Extrapolating this to effects of chemotherapy we might assume that a 10 gram tumor nodule (10^{10} cells) contains 1% tumor stem cells (10^8 stem cells). In this situation, 3 log kill (99.9%) in the tumor stem cell compartment (which only contains 0.1 grams) would be almost totally obscured initially by the remaining bulk of 9.9 grams of tumor which would be subject to clinical measurement (lymph nodes, pulmonary metastases, etc.). *In vivo* studies such as those which Dr. Schabel will discuss in his paper provide clear evidence that pharmacologically achievable concentrations of anticancer drugs cure animals with small tumor burdens and are sometimes capable of inducing multilog reductions in the number of tumor cells even in some tumors which may overtly appear to be resistant to treatment. However, drug sensitivity appears more important than tumor mass: choriocarcinoma in the female and ALL are often curable with chemotherapy even when they present at an advanced stage. Use of combinations of effective drugs for adjuvant chemotherapy seems most reasonable and if the agents are selected carefully, additive or synergistic lethality to tumor cells may occur.

An argument can be made for inclusion of cycle-active agents in adjuvant chemotherapy if a significant number of residual tumor stem cells are triggered into cycle after ablation of the primary tumor. Autoradiographic evidence for such kinetic behavior has been gathered by Simpson-Herren and associates for a transplantable animal tumor system[7]. Estimates of the fraction of tumor stem cells in cycle can also be achieved with *in vitro* tritiated thymidine suicide studies of tumor colony-forming units. The emergence of drug-resistant mutants is likely a smaller problem quantitatively in the adjuvant setting than with advanced cancer, but even in the adjuvant setting the existence of a single drug-resistant tumor stem cell could cause relapse. Use of non-cross resistant combinations of drugs with differing mechanisms of action should minimize the problem of repopulation by resistant mutants. Ideally, courses of treatment should be given sufficiently frequently to overcome apparent resistance which might be attributable to the kinetics of rapid tumor cell repopulation even by sensitive cells. Unfortunately, we do not have unequivocal data on tumor kinetics and the repopulation rates of specific human cancers over the range from one or a few viable tumor stem cells after surgery to a mass of 10^9-10^{10} cells which likely would be manifest as one or a few overt metastases ("macrocolonies"). Hopefully, this type of information will be available in the future with the development of better biological markers of tumor growth from very small numbers of cells. In the current analysis of the residual tumor stem cell problem, I assume that the initial doublings can be as rapid as they occur *in vitro*, and that characteristic Gompertzian growth applies to the repopulation which adjuvant chemotherapy must eradicate. In our previous biological marker studies of multiple myeloma[6] we have back-extrapolated from the clinical phase of tumor growth curves (from 10^{11} to 10^{12} cells) and predicted initial doubling times (10^0 to 2×10^0 cells) of 2-3 days. Our recent *in vitro* studies of myeloma colony doubling times now corroborate the earlier extrapolations from marker studies (e.g., Figure 4).

While many of these comments are general, they were useful in designing our adjuvant breast cancer chemotherapy program at the University of Arizona, which I will review as an example of the application of our scientific rationale to a clinical trial. We chose to combine the cycle-non-specific agents, adriamycin and cyclophosphamide, as in our own experience they were a very effective combination for use in advanced breast cancer and at several dosage levels induced a 60%-80% response rate, including about 15% complete responses[8,9]. In experimental tumor systems, this combination appeared to cause a 2-3 log reduction in the number of tumor stem cells for certain neoplasms, and was capable of curing some animals[10]. These data also suggested that this drug combination might be synergistic or potentiating,that is with the combination exerting a greater effect than maximum dosage of either adriamycin or cyclophosphamide alone. Using the kinetic parameters described earlier (Figure 4), we examined the effect of drug schedule, assuming that each course could induce a 99.7% cell kill. For these calculations we selected kinetics of an unfavorable tumor, with the view that the magnitude of the problem should not be underestimated.

As can be observed from the theoretical illustration in Figure 5, starting with 10^3 residual cells after surgery, cure could be obtained with 5 courses of treatment administered every 3 weeks. In striking contrast, the micrometastases could not be eradicated if the treatment interval was increased to 4 weeks. In fact, with a 4-week schedule, gradual increase in the number of tumor stem cells will occur. Even if the kinetics of repopulation of breast cancer are not as

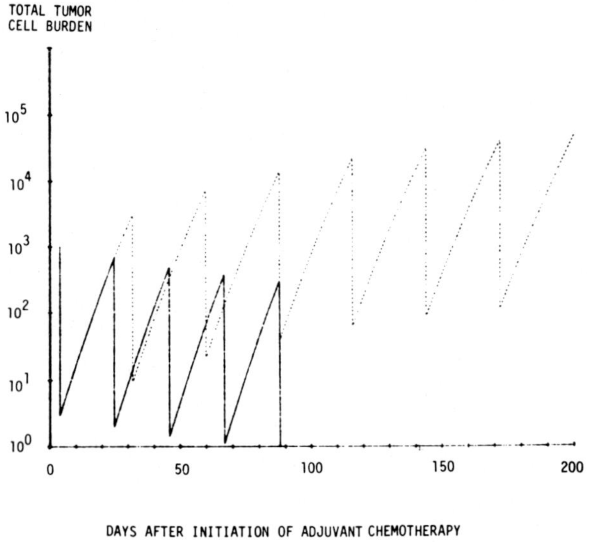

Figure 5. Model of the effect of treatment schedule (dose rate) on the outcome of adjuvant chemotherapy for micrometastases (10^3 cells) residual after primary surgery. The Gompertzian kinetic constants for tumor stem cell proliferation are identical to those shown in Figure 4. Each perpendicular line on the tumor growth curves is meant to reflect a tumor cell kill of 99.7% with each course of chemotherapy. This type of modeling was used in the development of the Arizona Adjuvant Breast Cancer Program. For this difficult tumor, treatment at the 3-week intervals resulted in cellular cure with 5 courses, while cure could not be achieved with a 4-week treatment interval regardless of the number of courses. (—— courses of chemotherapy every 3 weeks; --- courses of chemotherapy every 4 weeks).

vigorous as in the example we depicted, the effect of prolongation of the treatment intervals would nonetheless apply. Inasmuch as we did not have any direct measurements of the lethality of the adriamycin-cyclophosphamide chemotherapy regimen on human breast cancer stem cells, it appeared reasonable to us to rigidly standardize the treatment schedule to every 3 weeks, as this length of time was necessary for adequate repopulation of normal hematopoietic progenitors. We are hopeful that in the future *in vitro* bioassay of human tumor colony-forming cells will permit direct measurement of drug sensitivity on biopsy samples of the primary tumor. In light of Skipper and

Schabel's analysis of the relationship of lymph node involvement to the number of residual tumor cells after surgery (Figure 3), we chose to administer differing numbers of cycles of adjuvant chemotherapy based on lymph node (and primary tumor) status and risk of recurrence. Thus, patients with stage I breast cancer only receive 3 cycles of adjuvant chemotherapy (90 mg/m^2 of adriamycin), whereas patients with stage II disease receive 8 cycles of treatment (240 mg/m^2 of adriamycin), and complete adjuvant therapy approximately 6 months after mastectomy. As will be discussed later in this text by Dr. Neel Hammond [11], the early results of this program are quite encouraging, but we will need additional years of follow up to adequately assess the utility of this specific adjuvant program, particularly in the stage I cases. We utilize the same chemotherapy program in stage III cases, but also employ postoperative radiotherapy (4400 r) after the first two cycles of treatment in hope of further reducing the regional tumor burden. However, based on our own reasoning, it would appear likely that more potent systemic chemotherapy will also be required.

Similar rationale can likely be applied to development of adjuvant programs for a variety of other forms of cancer. In some instances, systemic or regional chemotherapy might be more appropriately started preoperatively. However, in that setting, early surgery should be contemplated because a large tumor burden exposed to chemotherapy may set the stage for the undesired selection of drug-resistant mutant colonies which could persist after surgery.

THE SANCTUARY PROBLEM

Even with effective anticancer drugs of adequate potency, certain neoplasms appear particularly prone to "the sanctuary problem" due to seeding of tumor stem cells to specific sites. This problem was first observed in childhood acute lymphocytic leukemia (ALL) wherein central nervous system (CNS) relapse was a major site of recurrent disease in patients in peripheral remission. This effect clearly appears to be due to the blood-brain barrier, and results from failure of adequate drug permeation to the meninges and brain substance. This problem has now been overcome in most ALL patients with intrathecal chemotherapy and whole brain radiotherapy administered prophylactically to eradicate a few occult stem cells. With the improvement in systemic therapy that is now observed in a variety of other neoplasms (e.g., oat cell carcinoma, diffuse histiocytic lymphoma, breast cancer) it has become apparent that the CNS sanctuary problem is important in these tumors as well, and will need to be addressed for a variety of cancers with known propensity for CNS metastasis. The extent to which CNS therapy becomes a part of adjuvant chemotherapy programs will undoubtedly be dependent on the patterns of recurrence that are observed in patients who relapse on some of the current adjuvant chemotherapy trials. While the testes also appear to represent a "sanctuary" for ALL cells (perhaps because of lower temperature), that site has not been a major site for relapse of other neoplasms. Sanctuaries such as the brain need not act only as a site of relapse. Conceivably, a site such as the CNS could serve as a reservoir for reseeding tumor stem cells to other systemic sites which offer more favorable growth conditions for tumor cells.

CONCLUSIONS

The idea of adjuvant chemotherapy of cancer is not new; and perhaps not too much rationale is necessary if it works. However, historically, initial progress in this field was slow, at least in part because perspectives were limited, and in part because some of the newer drugs were not available. However, as can be seen from my comments, the scientific foundation is now more concrete. New concepts, techniques for modeling tumor growth, and quantitative measurements, as well as a wealth of results from clinical trials in advanced cancer, have all emerged and have dramatically increased our interest and diversified our approach to adjuvant chemotherapy of cancer. Given this mixture and vigorous information exchange, the types of cancers which can be cured with combined modality therapy should increase in stepwise fashion.

ACKNOWLEDGEMENTS

I wish to thank Stephen B. Wampler, M. S., for the computer programming and operations necessary for the kinetic modeling, and Drs. Frank Schabel and Howard Skipper for allowing me to reprint Figures 2 and 3. The author's work was supported in part by USPHS grants CA 14102 and CA 17094.

REFERENCES

1. Shimosato, Y. et al. (1976) Transplantation of Human Tumors in Nude Mice J. Natl. Cancer Inst. 56 : 1251
2. Hamburger, A. and Salmon, S. (1977) Primary Bioassay of Human Tumor Stem Cells. Science (in press).
3. Hamburger, A. and Salmon, S. (1976) Primary Bioassay for Human Myeloma Stem Cells. Blood 48 : 995
4. Ogawa, M., Bergsagel, D. and McCulloch, E. (1973) Chemotherapy of Mouse Myeloma: Quantitative Cell Cultures Predictive of Response in Vivo. Blood 41:7
5. Skipper, H. and Schabel, Jr., F. (1977) Quantitative and Cytokinetic Studies in Experimental Tumor Systems. In Cancer Medicine (2nd ed.) (James F. Holland and Emil Frei, III, eds.), Lea and Febiger, Philadelphia (in press).
6. Sullivan, P.W. and Salmon, S.E. (1972) Kinetics of Growth and Regression of IgG Multiple Myeloma, J. Clin. Invest 51 : 1697
7. Simpson-Herren, L., Sanford A., Holmquist, J. (1976) Effects of Surgery on

the Cell Kinetics of Residual Tumor. Cancer Treat. Rep. 80 - Dec. (in press).

8. Jones, S., Durie, B. and Salmon, S. (1975) Combination Chemotherapy with Adriamycin and Cyclophosphamide for Advanced Breast Cancer. Cancer 36:90

9. Lloyd, R. et al. (1976) Randomized Trial of Low-dose Adriamycin and Cyclophosphamide ± Calusterone for Advanced Breast Cancer. Proc. Am. Assoc. Cancer Res. 17 : 126

10. Corbett, T. et al. (1975) Cyclophosphamide-Adriamycin Combination Chemotherapy of Transplantable Murine Tumors. Cancer Res. 35: 1568

11. Hammond, N., Jones, S.E., Salmon, S.E., et al. (1977) Adjuvant Treatment of Breast Cancer with Adriamycin-Cyclophosphamide with or without Radiation Therapy. In Adjuvant Therapy of Cancer (Sydney E. Salmon and Stephen E. Jones, eds.), Elsevier/North-Holland Biomedical Press (this volume).

Adjuvant Therapy of Cancer, S.E. Salmon and S.E. Jones eds.

EXPERIMENTAL AND RATIONAL BASES FOR IMMUNOTHERAPY AS CANCER ADJUVANT THERAPY

G. Mathé, O. Halle-Pannenko, I. Florentin, L. Olsson, F. Economides, P. Pouillart, M. Bruley-Rosset, M.C. Martyré, N. Kiger and C. Bourut

Institut de Cancérologie et d'Immunogénétique (INSERM), Hôpital Paul-Brousse, 94800-Villejuif, France.

1. We embarked on the cancer active immunotherapy (AI) adventure 15 years ago for the following reasons (1): a) with chemotherapy, in which the in vitro cell killing is correlated with dose, we can increase the number of cells killed until a certain dose is reached above which this number does not increase, and in vivo, it obeys first order kinetics (2,3,4), which need a logarithmic consideration of the cell killing, incomparably more pessimistic than the usual arithmetic one, the practical result being that chemotherapy does not kill the "last cell" (5); b) the mean inductive cell number of most of our experimental murine leukaemias is about 20 in normal mice, one in immunosuppressed animals, and between 10^3 and 10^5 in animals specifically pre-immunized or non-specifically "pre-stimulated" by what we called immunity systemic adjuvants ("immuno-prevention") (1).

Hence our first question was: are similar immuno-interventions efficient in prevention also efficient in therapy, which is to say after the tumour is established? We conducted experiments on several tumours [L1210 leukaemia (6,7), RC 19 (8), AkR (9)] and demonstrated that immunotherapy, that is the immuno-intervention applied after the tumour is established, is able to eradicate such tumours, at least in certain conditions which we will define.

2. Some of the conditions of action concern the modality of AI : the combination of irradiated tumour cells as the specific stimulus and of BCG as the adjuvant is often more active than BCG or leukaemic cells alone in the case of some tumours such as L1210 leukaemia(6,7).

Other conditions concern the cell population number of the tumour: AI is only able to cure mice that have received 10^5 leukaemic cells or less, and has no effect on those grafted with 10^6 or more (6), while some tumours, especially some leukaemias (EAkR) are only eradicated or delayed in their evolution by AI if the number of cells is $\leqslant 10^3$ (Fig. 1)$^+$ (10).

$^+$We only give in this paper the figures and tables which have not been previously published: the others can be found in Ref. 1.

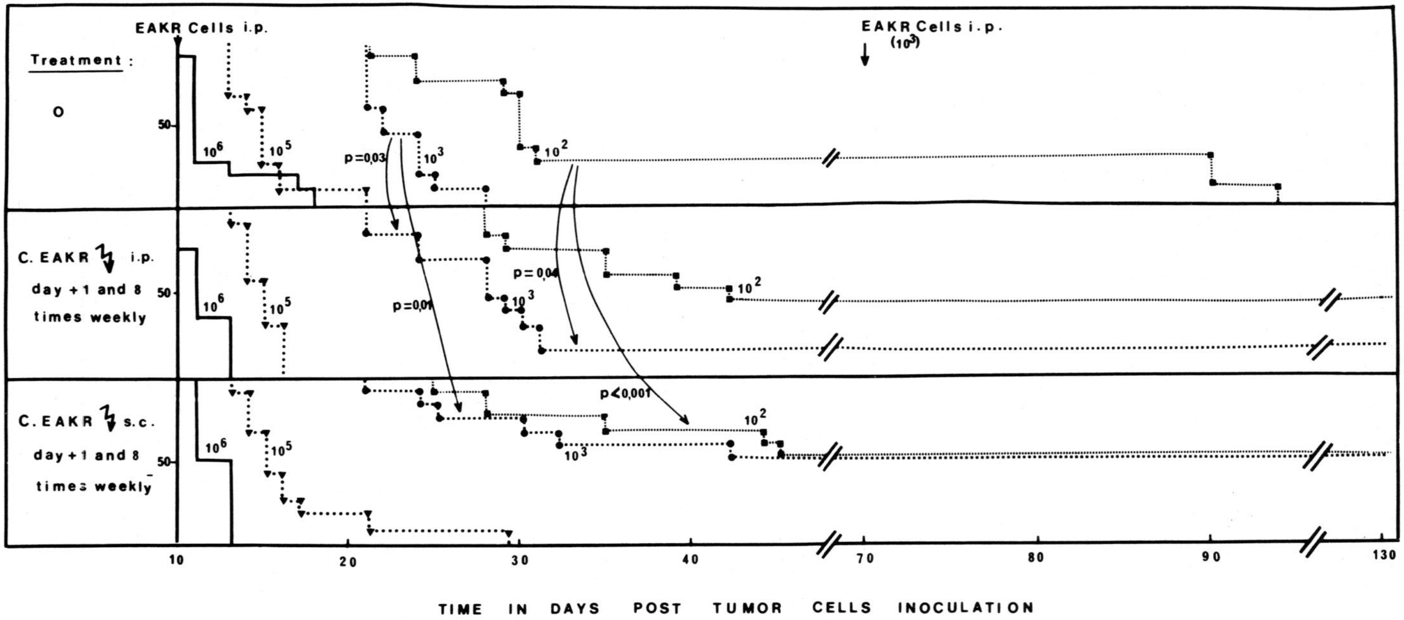

Fig. 1 Effect of a specific immunotherapy (using irradiated tumour cells) on the survival time of EAkR leukaemic mice according to the number of leukaemic cells grafted, and on their resistance to a challenge with viable tumour cells.

3. AI is a "double agent": it may induce growth enhancement(1). Even if applied in conditions respecting the above concept, it may enhance the growth of certain neoplasias, mainly solid tumours, especially Lewis tumour, which itself has been shown by Huchet (11) in our laboratory to induce an immunodepression in the host.

4. This quality of "double agent" of immuno-intervention makes it necessary to monitor the immune functions in order to follow the effects of immuno-intervention on the tumour-carrying subjects instead of only awaiting the effect on the tumour itself.

We compared (13) the effect of AI with BCG and cells in two groups of EAkR carrying mice, one in which it was effective, one in which it was not, and we could only correlate the antitumour efficiency with an increase of antibody-dependent cell-mediated cytotoxicity (Table I).

5. From the initial conclusion that AI is only efficient if the number of tumour cells is small, it was tempting to find out whether its effect was still present after the application of other cancer treatments, in other words, whether other treatments could be used before the immuno-intervention to reduce the number of tumour cells to the key number of 10^5-10^3. Not only does AI work after chemotherapy (Fig. 2) (13), radiotherapy (Fig. 3) (14), and surgery (Fig. 4) (15), but, in addition, a strong effect can be obtained by BCG given alone after these cell-reducing treatments.

Hence the application of AI is scientifically justified as a treatment complementary to the other cancer weapons in order to eradicate the few cells the other treatments usually leave and, in these cases, it may be limited to only the use of an efficient adjuvant such as BCG.

6. In most of the experiments mentioned above some mice were cured, but rarely 100%, even with the best conditions of AI application.

TUMOR CHARACTERISTICS IN RELATION TO THE TUMOR CELL (TC) CYTOTOXIC POTENTIAL OF ANTIBODIES AND LYMPHOID CELLS — Table I

PARAMETER	I		II		III	IV
	A	B	A	B		
TUMOR SIZE	↓	→	↓	→	→	CONTROLS
% TC IN PERITONEAL FLUID	↓	→	↓	→	→	CONTROLS
% LYMPHOCYTES AT DAY 13 AND 18	↑	→	↑	→	→	CONTROLS
% IMMUNOBLAST-LIKE CELLS AT DAY 13 AND 18	↑	→	↑	→	→	CONTROLS
COMPLEMENT-DEPENDENT ANTIBODY MEDIATED CYTOTOXICITY (CDAC)	+ +	+ +	+ +	+ +	+ (+)	0
INHIBITOR OF CDAC	+ +	+ +	+ +	+ +	+ +	-
SPLEEN	+ +	+ +	+ +	+ +	+ +	0
DIRECT LYMPHOCYTE CYTOTOXICITY (DLC)						
LYMPH NODES	0	0	0	0	0	0
SPLEEN	+ +	±	+ +	±	±	(+)
ANTIBODY-DEPENDENT CELL-MEDIATED CYTOTOXICITY (ADCM)						
LYMPH NODES	+ +	0	+ +	0	0	0

GROUP I : BCG ALONE
GROUP II : BCG plus IRRADIATED TUMOR CELLS
GROUP III : IRRADIATED TUMOR CELLS
GROUP IV : TUMOR-BEARING CONTROLS

Subgroup A : TUMOR SIZE BELOW CONTROLS
Subgroup B : TUMOR SIZE EQUAL TO CONTROLS
↓ lower than control values
↑ higher than control values
→ equal to control values

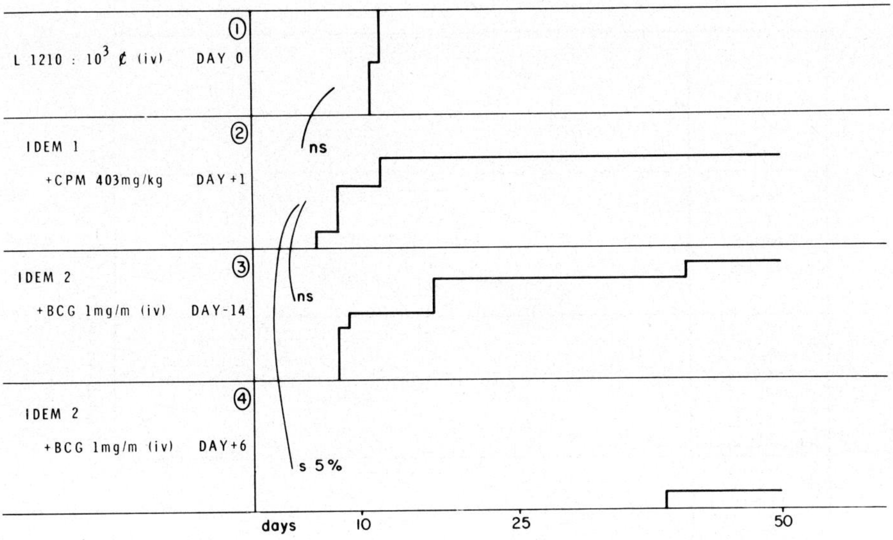

Fig. 2 Immunotherapeutic effect on L1210 leukaemia of BCG given 5 days after the injection of 403mg/kg of cyclophosphamide (CPM).

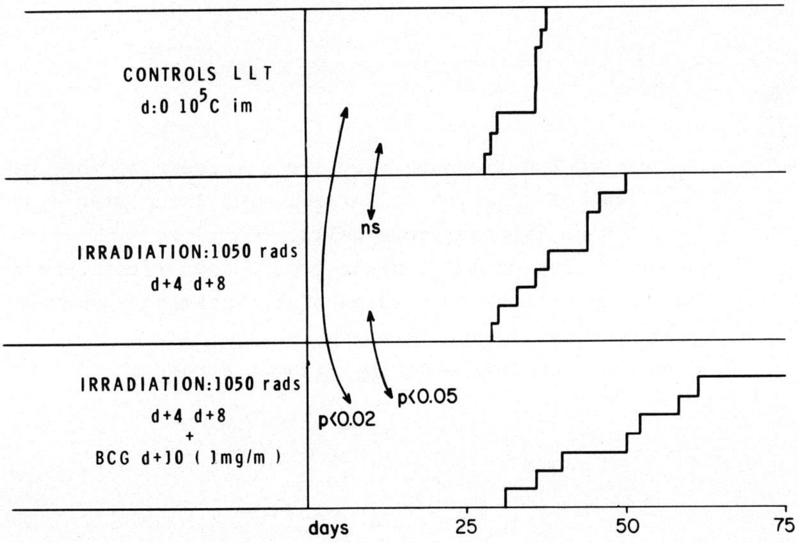

Fig. 3 Treatment of Lewis tumour in $C_{57}Bl/6$ mice by local radiotherapy followed by BCG.

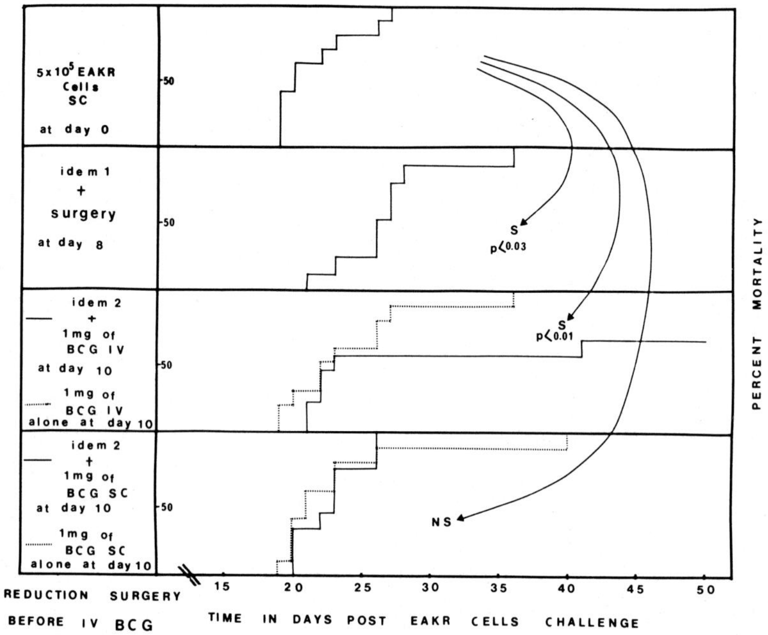

Fig. 4 Effect of BCG immunotherapy after surgery on the survival of (C_{57}Bl/6 x DBA/2)Fl mice inoculated with 5.10^5 EAkR lymphosarcoma cells.
(————) lmg of BCG i.v. or s.c. 2 days after surgery, which consisted of excision of the primary tumour and regional lymph nodes (Day 8).
(------) BCG immunotherapy without surgery.

Figure 5 (1) illustrates and explains this phenomenon. Following the tumour volume after AI in the case of s.c. grafted L1210 leukaemia, we observed three kinds of results: a decrease of the tumour volume and cure; an absence of effect on the tumour volume, which increases until death; a plateau in the tumour volume curve which eventually continues to ascend until death, suggesting an initial effect followed by immunoresistance. One should also note in Figure 5 the absence of effect of AI on the exponential phase (in which all the cells are in the cycle) and its effect only during the saturation phase.

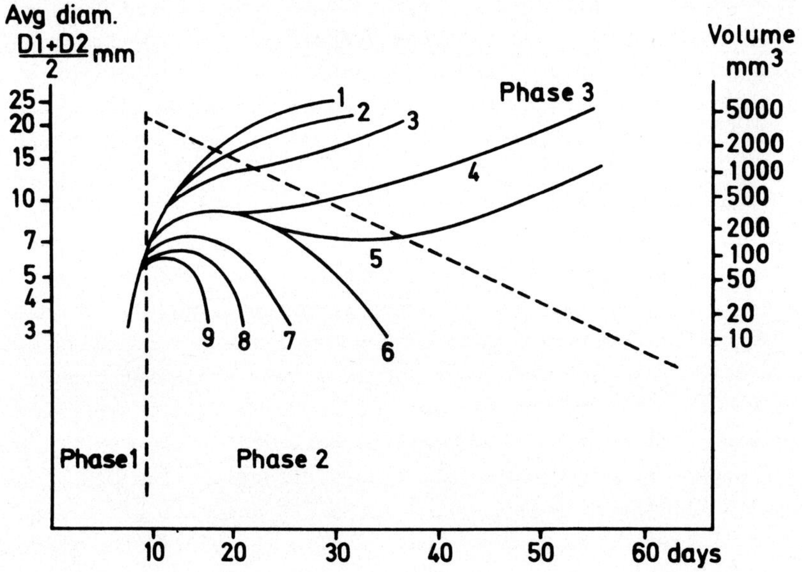

Fig. 5 Growth curve population of tumours obtained from mice treated with BCG and irradiated cells the day after injection with 10^4 cells L1210.

Figure 6 shows the results of AI on the cells at the different phases of the cycle that we studied and (16) explains this phenomenon more basically: AI only works on cells in Go and/or Gl.

These two experiments suggest the possible interest of interspersing AI and chemotherapy: a) to try to reduce (in the case of the experiment shown in Fig. 5) the number of cells when the tumour volume curve has attained the plateau to the number accessible to AI, i.e. 10^5 or 10^3; b) in order to increase the number of target cells, AI working only on cells in the Go-Gl phase (16) and chemotherapy mainly on cells in the other phases of the cycle (17,18).

7. Another reason in favour of interspersing AI and chemotherapy is the acceleration by immunity adjuvants, such as BCG, of blood cell restoration after chemotherapy (19). This suggests that such adjuvants act on stem cells, and we observed (20,21), using the techniques of colony-forming units in the spleen (CFUs) and colony-forming units in agar culture (CFUa) and the tritiated thymidine suicide method, that BCG increases the number of both types of stem cells in the S-phase.

8. Thus we were encouraged to intersperse cyclophosphamide (CPM) and BCG in the treatment of L1210 leukaemia on which we had previously seen that the sequence CPM→ BCG is much more efficient than CPM alone (13). But we were unpleasantly surprised (Fig. 7) to observe that two or three interspersion sequences of these two agents were no more efficient than CPM alone and much less efficient than the single sequence of one CPM and one BCG injection (22). The same result was observed for solid Lewis tumour.

As a single sequence CPM→ BCG is more effective than CPM alone, we wondered if the reverse sequence BCG→ CPM was less effective. As a matter of fact, Fig. 8 shows that this is the case: the sequence BCG→ CPM is significantly less efficient than CPM alone (23). As we had shown that the CPM effect is much poorer in immunodepressed animals (24), we wondered if BCG followed by CPM did not induce immunodepression as BCG pushes the lymphocytes in the cycle, rendering them more sensitive to the lymphostatic action of CPM, a cycle-dependent agent. An experiment on allogeneic skin grafting (23) demonstrated the value of this hypothesis: the sequence BCG→ CPM greatly prolongs allograft survival compared with CPM alone.

The problem was to investigate whether this phenomenon was true for all chemotherapy agents, or only for those that are known to be immunosuppressive (25). Hence, we performed a similar experiment

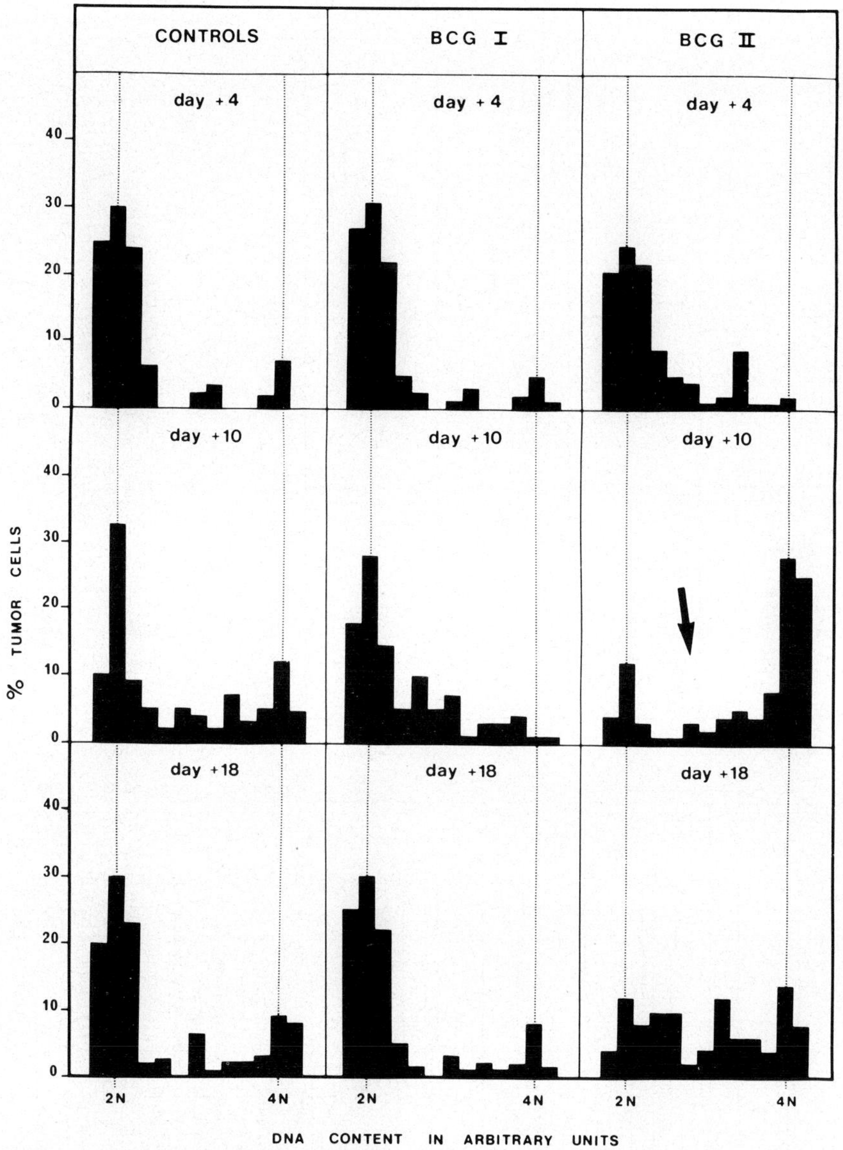

Fig. 6 Percentage distribution of ascitic tumour-cells as a function of single-cell DNA-content at various times after inoculation i.p. of 10^5 tumour-cells. 2N indicates the mean DNA-content of G_1 cells, and 4N the mean DNA-content of mitoses (and G_2-phase cells). Each value is the mean of 3-5 mice.
BCG I : BCG-treated mice with tumour load and tumour cell mitotic activity no different from controls.
BCG II : BCG-treated mice with a lower tumour cell number and a higher tumour cell mitotic activity than controls.

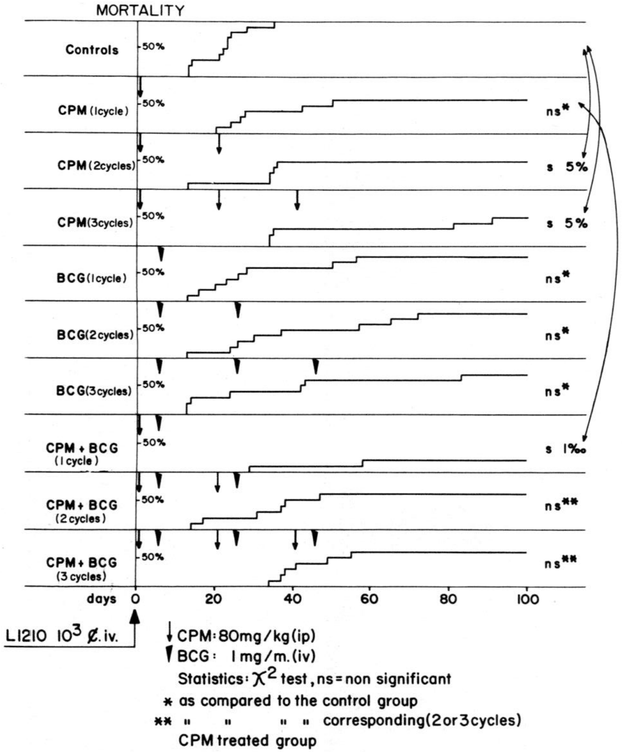

Fig. 7 Interspersion of cyclophosphamide (CPM) and BCG for treatment of L1210 leukaemia when their sequential combination is given 2-3 times: the effect is poorer than that obtained by one injection of CPM followed by one administration of BCG.

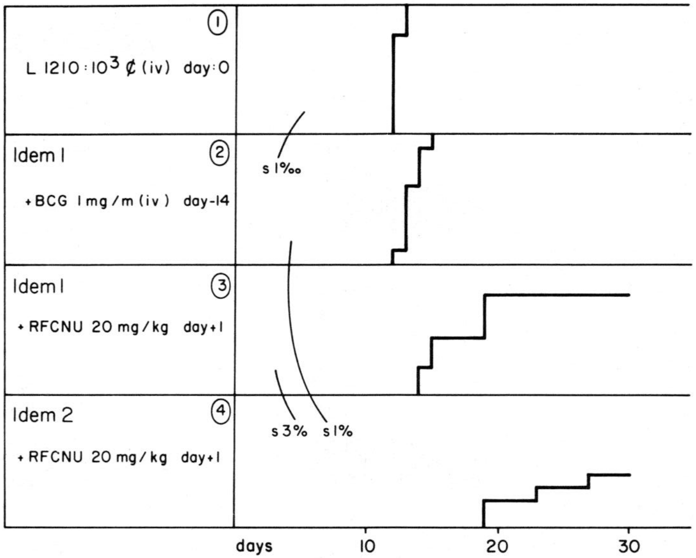

Fig. 8 The sequence BCG - RFCNU (a non immuno-suppressive drug) enhances the effect of both agents (contrary to the sequence of BCG-cyclophosphamide (an immunosuppressive agent) (see text).

using RFCNU [(chloro-2-ethyl)-1-ribofuranosyl-isopropylidene-2'-3' paranitrobenzoate-5')-3 nitrosourea], the only derivative of nitrosoureas which, among all those available in practice and a dozen sugar derivatives synthetized in Montpellier and shown to be strongly oncostatic by our experimental screening (26), is not immunosuppressive. Fig. 8 shows that the sequence BCG RFCNU is more efficient than BCG or RFCNU alone.

Thus we may conclude that the interspersion of immunotherapy and chemotherapy may be unfavourable or favourable depending on at least one factor: the effect on immunity of the chemotherapy used. Non-immunosuppressive cytostatics must be chosen according to the presently available experimental data. This effect on immunity does not eliminate the possible role of other factors, such as the time factor, the dose factor, the phase dependency of the cytostatics, or the adjuvant used for immunotherapy (1).

9. The above data on the possible enhancing effect of BCG applied before certain chemotherapy and the quoted dependency of chemotherapy action on the immune status of the host (24) led us to study the effect of immunotherapy applied before surgery. Figure 9 shows that BCG administered before tumour extirpation may significantly increase the effect of surgery. But the results of this experiment should be compared with those of others in which BCG was applied after surgery (Fig. 4): after surgery, BCG only works if injected i.v. and does not work if injected s.c. (as in all our experiments on systemic immunotherapy) (1) ; BCG applied before surgery does not work if injected i.v., and only works if injected s.c. in the region of the tumour (15). This regional presurgical immunotherapy, which is different from local immunotherapy (27,28,29, 30,31), consisting of intratumoral injection of the agents, may find many more clinical applications than local immunotherapy. An interesting finding concerning this regional immunotherapy is that it works better if the regional lymph nodes are not extirpated and does not work so well if they are (32).

10. These are some of the experimental data which we think indispensable to be known before setting up any clinical trial.

11. There are many more questions which the experimentalists have submitted to study; the answers to them may be useful for clinical trials.

a) Can we improve the efficacy of a specific immunotherapy using irradiated tumor cells by treating them with neuraminidase or other enzymes such as papain? We have not observed such a result on spontaneous

AkR leukaemia (9) and we have even noticed a growth enhancement on the EAkR leukaemia (33). Thus this manipulation of the cells, if it works, does not work in all conditions.

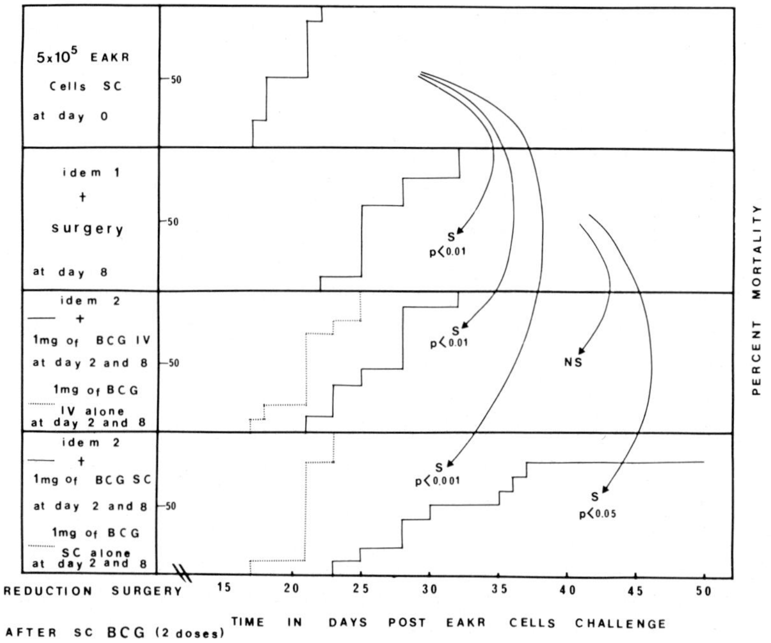

Fig. 9 Effect of repeated BCG injections, combined (or not) with surgery, on the survival of (C_{57}Bl/6 x DBA/2)F1 mice inoculated by 5.10^3 EAkR lymphosarcoma cells.
(————) 1mg of BCG, i.v. or s.c., 6 days before, and on the day of surgery, which consisted of excision of the primary tumour and regional lymph nodes (Day 8).
(-------) BCG immunotherapy on the same days as above, but without surgery.

The use of soluble tumour associated antigens, which may be very effective in some conditions, especially if administered very early (34), may be inefficient in others, for example, if injected later than in the preceding experimental condition.

These antigens may induce tumour rejection or tumour growth enhancement according to the modality of preparation (35).

b) Can we improve the efficiency of the non-specific manipulation made with adjuvants? Let us start by using the adjuvant that our experimental screening (36) has shown to be the most efficient, namely the fresh Pasteur preparation of BCG (37).

Let us also use, for this most efficient adjuvant, the routes of administration which have been shown experimentally to be efficient. A study on the mechanisms of action of fresh Pasteur BCG showed that most effects are only observed after systemic i.v. injection and not after local s.c. injection (38). This is clearly explained by the histological study conducted by Khalil and Rappaport (39) in our laboratory, which showed a strict correlation between the antitumour effect and the induction of a BCG septicemia of a given intensity: this septicemia is not obtained by the s.c. route.

As the i.v. route of administration of BCG is immunodepressive in man, we looked for other modalities of administration and found that application on scarifications or via the Heaf gun were efficient (Fig. 10) (40).

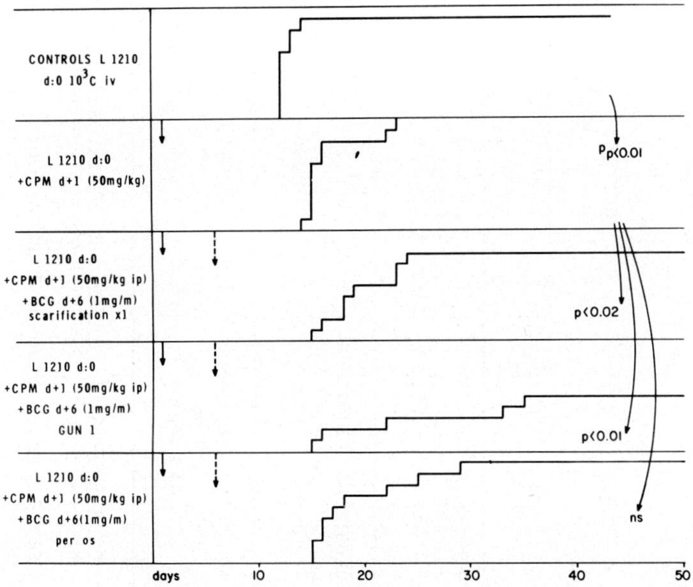

Fig. 10 Comparison of the activities of different routes of BCG administration in mice carrying L1210 leukaemia (application for active systemic immunotherapy after chemotherapy).

Table II

EFFECT OF TWO STRAINS OF BRUCELLA ABORTUS

(injection on day - 2.5 before antigen)

		JERNE		L1210		LLT	
		I_a	S_a	I_b	S_b	I_b	S_b
BRUCELLA ABORTUS S 500 /mice (strain B19S)	I.V.	0.95	N.S.	1.17	N.S.	1.11	N.S.
	S.C.	0.47	0.001 ↙	0.92	0.02 ↙	1.03	N.S.
BRUCELLA ABORTUS R 500 /mice (strain B19R)	I.V.	1.28	N.S.	0.92	N.S.	1.09	N.S.
	S.C.	1.98	0.05 ↗	0.92	N.S.	1.11	N.S.
BRUCELLA ABORTUS R 1500 /mice (strain B19R)	I.V.	2.82	0.02 ↗	1	N.S.		
	S.C.	2.4	0.05 ↗	1.19	0.05 ↗		

I_a = $\frac{\text{Mean number of plaque forming cells/spleen of treated mice}}{\text{Mean number of plaque forming cells/spleen of control mice}}$

S_a = Statistics : Student Fisher test   N.S. = Not significant

I_b = $\frac{\text{Median (days) of survival of treated mice}}{\text{Median (days) of survival of control mice}}$

S_b = Statistics = Wilcoxon's non-parametric test

IMMUNOPREVENTION EFFECT OF PYOCYANIC BACILLI (P.B.) ON L1210 LEUKAEMIA — Table III

INJECTION DAY BEFORE L1210		0.5 ml (P.B.)		0.2 ml (P.B.)		0.1 ml (P.B.)	
		I_a	S_a	I	S	I	S
- 10	I.V.	1	N.S.	1.14	0.01 ↗	1	N.S.
	S.C.	1	N.S.	1	N.S.	1	N.S.
- 7	I.V.	1.27	0.01 ↗	1	N.S.	1	N.S.
	S.C.	1	N.S.	1.27	0.01 ↗	1.25	0.01 ↗
- 4	I.V.	1.14	0.01 ↗	1.14	0.01 ↗	1	N.S.
	S.C.	0.91	N.S.	1.14	N.S.	1	N.S.
- 2.5	I.V	1.27	0.01 ↗	1	N.S.	1.27	0.01 ↗
	S.C.	1.27	0.001 ↗	1.27	0.01 ↗	1	N.S.

$I_a = \frac{\text{Median (days) of survival of treated mice}}{\text{Median (days) of survival of control mice}}$

S_a = Statistics: Wilcoxon's non-parametric test

N.S. = Not significant

Table IV

ACTION OF LIPOPOLYSACCHARIDE (L.P.S.)

IN E.O.R.T.C.-I.C.I.G. SCREENING FOR IMMUNITY SYSTEMIC ADJUVANT

(injection on day - 2.5. before antigen)

		JERNE		MACROPHAGE STIMULATION	L_{1210}		LLT	
		I_a	S_a		I_b	S_b	I_b	S_b
250 /mice	I.V.	5.23	0.001 ↗	71% (inhibition)	0.92	N.S.	0.84	0.03 ↘
	S.C.	6.55	0.001 ↗		0.92	N.S.	0.88	0.05 ↘

$I_a = \frac{\text{Mean number of plaque forming cells/spleen of treated mice}}{\text{Mean number of plaque forming cells/spleen of control mice}}$

S_a = Statistics: Student Fisher test

N.S. = not significant

$I_b = \frac{\text{Median (days) of survival of treated mice}}{\text{Median (days) of survival of control mice}}$

S_b = Statistics: Wilcoxon's non-parametric test

Another important parameter for BCG efficiency is the dose applied: if small doses ($\leqslant$ 0.5 mg/mouse) (41) are not efficient, neither are high doses, and the absence of action of high doses has been shown by Geffard and Orbach (42) working in our laboratory to be due to the increase of suppressor cells.

c) Can we replace living BCG by extracts? We have observed that if most extracts, including hydrosoluble ones, are efficient in an antibody production test, only methanol extraction residue fraction of tubercle bacilli (MER) is active on tumour growth inhibition (43). But its local tolerance is much poorer than that of living BCG.

d) What about other dead organisms? I shall not comment on Corynebacteria which have been studied extensively by many other workers (44,45): they have given us moderate and irregular anti-tumour effects (1). This may be explained by their known deteriorating effect on T-cell immunity in certain conditions (see 1), which makes their use imprudent until we have an operational monitoring of their effect.

Conversely, we are enthousiastic about the action of Brucella (46) which, in our screening summarized in Table II (47), again illustrates the importance of a phenomenon we noted for BCG, namely that the adjuvant action depends on the strain of micro-organism used: only the strain B19R is efficient, and only at certain doses, while the strain B19S is immunosuppressive and enhances tumour growth (48).

Finally, we have recently obtained very promising results with pyocyanic bacilli (Table III) (not published).

The possibility of tumour growth enhancement by certain modalities of immuno-intervention underlines the fact that immunotherapy is not homeopathy and must be based on experimental data: Table IV shows that a B-dependent adjuvant, i.e. Lipopolysaccharide (LPS) increases antibody production but enhances tumour growth.

In conclusion, there is a strong experimental background of knowledge for clinical immunotherapy which should be considered carefully before establishing any protocol for clinical trials.

SUMMARY

Systemic active immunotherapy (SAI) is able to cure mice inoculated with an experimental tumour usually only when the number of grafted cells is small ($\leqslant 10^5$), which suggested that its best situation in the strategy of cancer treatment be the residual minimum imperceptible diseases left by a first treatment.

SAI when applied alone is usually more efficient when consisting of BCG + cells than when consisting of BCG or cells only.

When applied after chemotherapy, BCG alone or C. parvum alone is usually strongly efficient. BCG may also be efficient when given after local radiotherapy or after surgery or surgery followed chemotherapy. As a growth of a tumour treated by SAI may became a plateau which finally gives way to relapse, as SAI kills only the cells in G1, one is tempted to interperse SAI and chemotherapy. This interspersion may be unfavorable when immunosuppressive cytostatics (CTS) are used, but favorable when non immunosuppressive CTS are used.

Regional AI may be efficient under the form of s.c. injection of BCG near to a tumour before its surgical removal.

These notions as well as the dose effect, and that of the differences of effects according to the immunomodulating materials and their combinations will be illustrated by results of personal experiments.

REFERENCES

1. Mathé G Active immunotherapy of cancer: its immunoprophylaxis and immunorestoration. An introduction. Heidelberg-New York, 1976, Springer Verlag.
2. Skipper H.E., Schabel F.M., Wilcox W.S. Cancer Chemoth. Reports 1964, 35, 1.
3. Skipper H.E., Schabel F.M., Wilcox W.S. Cancer Chemoth. Reports 1965, 45, 5.
4. Skipper H.E., Schabel F.M., Wilcox W.S. Cancer Chemoth. Reports 1967, 51, 125.
5. Mathé G. Presse Med., 1967, 75, 2591.
6. Mathé G. Rev. Fr. Et. Clin. Biol., 1968, 13, 881.
7. Mathé G., Pouillart P., Lapeyraque F. Brit. J. Cancer 1969, 23, 814.
8. Mathé G., Pouillart P., Lapeyraque F. Experientia 1971, 27, 446.
9. Mathé G., Halle-Pannenko O., Bourut C. Exp. Hematol., 1973, 1, 110.
10. Economides F., Bruley-Rosset M., Florentin I., Mathé G. Cancer Immunol. Immunoth., 1977 (in press).
11. Huchet R., Lheritier J. p. 65 in "Lymphocytes, macrophages and cancer " (G. Mathé, I. Florentin, M.C. Simmler, eds). Heidelberg-New York, 1976, Springer Verlag.
12. Olsson L., Florentin I., Kiger N., Mathé G. J. Nat. Cancer Inst. 1977 (submitted to).

13. Mathé G., Halle-Pannenko O., Bourut C. Europ. J. Cancer 1974, 10, 661.
14. Martin M., Bourut C., Halle-Pannenko O, Mathé G. Biomedicine 1975, 23, 337.
15. Economides F., Bruley-Rosset M., Mathé G. Biomedicine 1976, 25, 337.
16. Olsson L., Mathé G. Cancer Res., 1977 (in press).
17. Bruce W.R., Meeker B.E., Valeriote F.A. J. Nat. Cancer Inst., 1966, 37, 233.
18. Van Putten L.M., Lelieveld P., Kram-Idsenga L.K.J. Cancer Chemoth. Reports 1972, 56 (Part I), 691.
19. Mathé G. p. 124 in "Complications of cancer chemotherapy". (G. Mathé, R.K. Oldham, eds). Heidelberg-New York, 1974, Springer Verlag.
20. Pouillart P., Palangié T., Schwarzenberg L., Brugerie H., Lheritier J., Mathé G. Biomedicine 1975, 23, 469.
21. Pouillart P., Palangié T., Schwarzenberg L., Brugerie H., Lheritier J., Mathé G. Cancer Immunol. Immunoth., 1976, 1, 163.
22. Mathé G., Halle-Pannenko O., Bourut C. Europ. J. Cancer, 1977 (in press).
23. Mathé G., Halle-Pannenko O., Bourut C. Transplant. Proc., 1974, 6, 431.
24. Mathé G.,Halle-Pannenko O., Bourut C., Cancer Immunol. Immunoth 1977, 2, (in press).
25. Clarysse A., Kenis Y., Mathé G. Cancer Chemotherapy. Its role in the treatment strategy of hematologic malignancies and solid tumors. Heidelberg-New York, 1976, Springer Verlag.
26. Imbach J.L., Montero J.L., Moruzzi A., Serrou B., Chenu E., Hayat M., Mathé G. Biomedicine 1975, 23, 410.
27. Rapp H.J. Israel J. Med. Sci., 1973, 9, 326.
28. Zbar B. Nat. Cancer Inst. Monogr., 1972, 35, 341.
29. Zbar B., Bernstein I.D., Bartlett G.L., Hanna M.G.jr, Rapp H.J. J. Nat. Cancer Inst., 1972, 49, 119.
30. Zbar B., Ribi E., Rapp H.J. Nat. Cancer Inst. Monogr., 1973, 39, 3.
31. Zbar B., Tanaka T. Science 1971, 172, 271.
32. Economides F., Bruley-Rosset M., Mathé G. Biomedicine 1977 (in press).
33. Doré J.F., Hadjiyannakis M.J., Coudert A., Guibout C., Marholev L., Imai K. Lancet 1973, 1, 600.

34. Martyré M.C. Biomedicine 1976, 25, 360.
35. Martyré M.C., Weiner R., Halle-Pannenko O. p. 405 in "Investigation and stimulation of immunity in cancer patients" (G. Mathé, R. Weiner, eds). Heidelberg-New York, 1974, Springer Verlag.
36. Mathé G., Kamel M., Dezfulian M., Halle-Pannenko O, Bourut C. Cancer Res., 1973, 33, 1987.
37. Mathé G., Halle-Pannenko O., Bourut C. Nat. Cancer Inst. Monogr., 1973, 39, 107.
38. Florentin I., Huchet R., Bruley-Rosset M., Halle-Pannenko O. Mathé G. Cancer Immunol. Immunoth., 1976, 1, 31.
39. Rappaport H., Khalil A. Cancer Immunol. Immunoth., 1976, 1, 45.
40. Martin M., Bourut C., Halle-Pannenko O., Mathé G. Biomedicine 1975, 23, 339.
41. Mathé G. p. 67 in "The prediction of chronic toxicity from short term studies". Amsterdam, 1976, Excerpta Medica.
42. Geffard M., Orbach-Arbouys S. Cancer Immunol. Immunoth., 1976, 1, 41.
43. Mathé G., Hiu I.J., Halle-Pannenko O., Bourut C. Israel J. Med. Sci., 1976, 12, 468.
44. Halpern B., Fray A., Crepin Y., Platica O., Lorinet A.M., Rabourdin A., Sparros L., Isac R. p. 217 in "Immunopotentiation" (Ciba Foundation Symp. n°18) 1 vol., Amsterdam, 1973, Elsevier Excerpta Medica.
45. Woodruff M.F.A. p. 272 in "Investigation and stimulation of immunity in cancer patients" (G. Mathé, R. Weiner, eds). Heidelberg-New York, 1974, Springer Verlag.
46. Toujas L., Sabolovic D., Dazord L., Legarrec Y., Toujas J.P., Guelfi J., Pilet C. Europ. J. Clin. Biol. Res., 1972, 17, 267.
47. Mathé G., Halle-Pannenko O., Bourut C. (in preparation).
48. Mathé G., Halle-Pannenko O., Bourut C. (in preparation).

Adjuvant Therapy of Cancer, S.E. Salmon and S.E. Jones eds.
© *1977 Elsevier/North-Holland Biomedical Press, Amsterdam*

ADJUVANT CHEMOTHERAPY OF OSTEOGENIC SARCOMA:

PROGRESS AND PERSPECTIVES

Emil Frei III, M.D., Norman Jaffe, MB, BCh, Dip. Paed.
Howard E. Skipper, M.D.[x] and Michael G. Gero
Sidney Farber Cancer Institute
44 Binney Street
Boston, MA 02115

[x] Southern Research Institute
2000 Ninth Avenue South
Birmingham, AL 35205

In July of 1972, adjuvant chemotherapy studies were initiated at the Sidney
Farber Cancer Institute-Children's Hospital Medical Center. The following is an
analysis of our experience to date with the consideration of some of the problems,
interpretations, and perspectives.

The application of chemotherapy as adjuvant for a given category of neoplastic
disease depends upon the development of effective chemotherapy programs for overt
macrometastatic disease (Figure 1). Prior to 1970, the only agents of probable
but limited activity in overt osteogenic sarcoma (OGS) were the alkylating agents,
where response rates up to 20% were reported. In the early 1970's, adriamycin
was found to be effective in 30-40% of such patients.[1] At about the same time,
Jaffe and Djerassi, using a high-dose methotrexate-citrovorum rescue program,
demonstrated a similar response rate.[2,3] Methotrexate, because it is myelosuppressive, has been used intermittently at 3-week intervals to allow for recovery
from myelosuppression. However, with proper monitoring of the pharmacology of
methotrexate and of renal function and with the use of fluids and alkali, myelosuppression with high-dose methotrexate-citrovorum factor rescue (Mtx-CF) occurs
infrequently and it has been possible to deliver this program on a weekly basis
(Figure 1).[4] Consistent with the experimental evidence for a steep dose response
curve for Mtx, this program has produced an objective response in 80% of patients
with overt OGS.[5]

The first adjuvant program for OGS involved high-dose Mtx-CF every 3 weeks (Figure 2). Vincristine was given as a priming dose because of experimental evi dence that vincristine, at concentrations which are probably achieved _in vivo_, increases _in vitro_ uptake of tritiated Mtx. The efficacy of vincristine in thi setting has not been demonstrated in the clinical trial context. With increasi

Figure 1

Agent(s)	Objective Response[a] (%)
Alkylating Agents	20%
Adriamycin	35%
MTX-CF q. 3 Weeks	35%
MTX-CF q. 1 Week	80%

(a) >50% decrease in product of 2 diameters

Figure 2

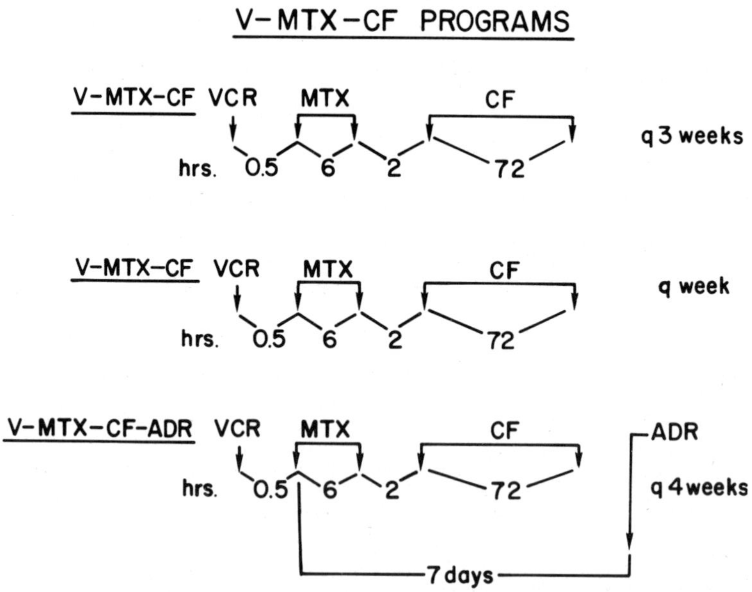

experience and compelling evidence that the high-dose Mtx-CF program could be delivered without myelosuppression and with the evidence that adriamycin was effective in advanced osteogenic sarcoma, our second protocol was developed which involved the use of both programs with minimal compromise in dose rate (second program in Figure 2). In the hematologic malignancies, major progress has been achieved with combinations of chemotherapeutic agents wherein full doses could be delivered because of lack of additive dose limiting toxicity.[6]

Figure 3 represents a summary of the categories of progression of OGS. It applies in general to most categories of neoplastic disease. The disease progresses from the primary to micrometastases and finally to overt metastatic disease. As above, the medical and pediatric oncologists are usually initially involved in the development of effective programs for overt metastatic disease. Once this is achieved and if micrometastatic disease represents a significant problem, such treatment is applied as adjuvant chemotherapy shortly after control of the primary. Since both control of the primary and control of micrometastatic disease are equally important, the term adjuvant is unfortunate and multi-modality treatment is perhaps better. However, the latter is insufficiently precise and adjuvant chemotherapy remains the popular term.

The results of our first two protocols of adjuvant chemotherapy of OGS are presented in Figure 4.[7] In the historical control curve, 80% of patients have relapsed by 12 months and the cure rate (leveling off of the curve) is between 15 and 20%. In our experience and in the experience of six institutions or groups who have recently carefully analyzed their data, there has been no change in the historical control curve as determined from two-year survival data over the years and up to the present time or to the time when adjuvant chemotherapy studies were initiated. There is one important exception to this experience wherein the control curve indicates a 45% survival at two years.

For the initial study, that is Mtx-CF, the curve has plateaued at 50% and the minimum follow-up for that group of patients is three years (Figure 4). For the second study (Mtx-CF plus adriamycin), the curve at three years is at 67% with a minimum of follow-up at 12 months and a maximum follow-up of 36 months.

Figure 3

EVOLUTION OF TREATMENT OF OSTEOGENIC SARCOMA

PRIMARY

PAST: AMPUTATION, RADIOTHERAPY
CURRENT APPROACHES:
INITIAL INTENSIVE CHEMOTHERAPY DESIGNED TO SHRINK PRIMARY
SUBAMPUTATIVE SURGERY

MICROMETASTASES

PAST: NO TREATMENT
CURRENT: SYSTEMIC (ADJUVANT) CHEMOTHERAPY, IMMUNOTHERAPY

OVERT METASTATIC DISEASE

PAST: PALLIATION
CURRENT:

1) SYSTEMIC CHEMOTHERAPY ± SURGERY ± XRT DESIGNED TO CREATE NED*
2) "ADJUVANT" CHEMOTHERAPY FOR MICROSCOPIC DISEASE

*NED - NO EVIDENT DISEASE (SEE TEXT).

Figure 4

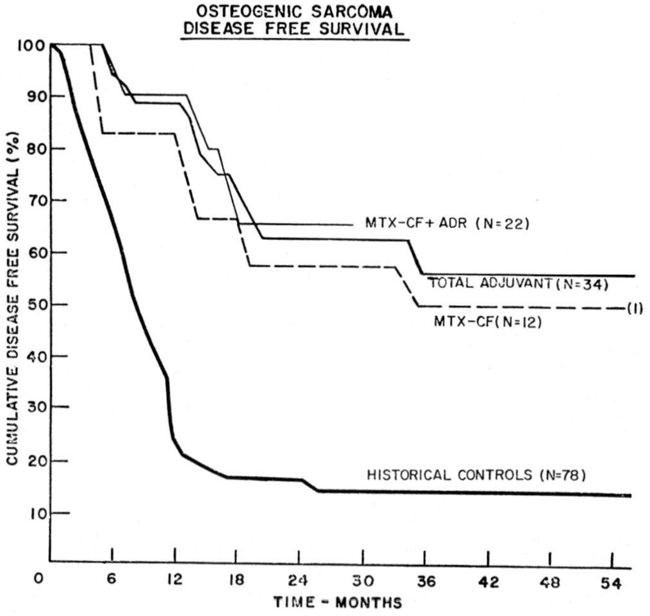

Similar results have been achieved in five other studies of adjuvant chemotherapy in OGS. Thus, the leveling off of the curve has been between 50% and 75% and late relapses have been infrequent. These results are consistent with the interpretation that the cure rate for OGS has been increased by adjuvant chemotherapy from 20% to 50-60%.

In order to achieve a better understanding of the dynamics of micrometastatic disease, we have extrapolated and applied cytokinetic data from experimental adjuvant chemotherapy studies. These extrapolations derive largely from the experimental work of Drs. Lloyd, Skipper, and Schabel at the Southern Research Institute.

Both intuitively and as a result of experimental adjuvant studies, it seems logical that the break in the untreated control curve in Figure 4 represents the time required for 1 or a very few clones of neoplastic cells to expand to a clinically recognizable number. This duration of OGS is 12 months. If one assumes that approximately 10^9 cells in the lungs would be roentgenographically evident then the calculations made for microscopic disease in Figure 5 are applicable. The number of doublings required to go from 1 to 10^9 cells is 30. If it takes 365 days to achieve this increase then the tumor cell doubling time would be 12 days. Approximately 1×10^{12} cells represent the number present in a patient with clinically evident acute leukemia. In OGS, metastatic disease is largely confined to the lungs and the lethal number is approximately 5×10^{11} (approximately 500 grams of neoplastic cells). The time from the development of roentgenographically evident pulmonary metastases to death is six months.[7] By direct analysis of the doubling time of pulmonary metastases on serial radiograms, Band has found the doubling time to be 25 days. From our calculations, a figure of 20 days is derived. These calculations, as presented in Figure 5, are consistent with the known Gompertzian dynamics of solid tumors, that is, that the doubling time of tumors decreases with increasing tumor size.

A kinetic interpretation of the adjuvant osteogenic sarcoma studies is presented in Figure 6. This approach involves the extrapolation of an approach which has proved effective in _in vivo_ adjuvant experimental models. In such systems, the number of persisting neoplastic cells following control of the primary can be

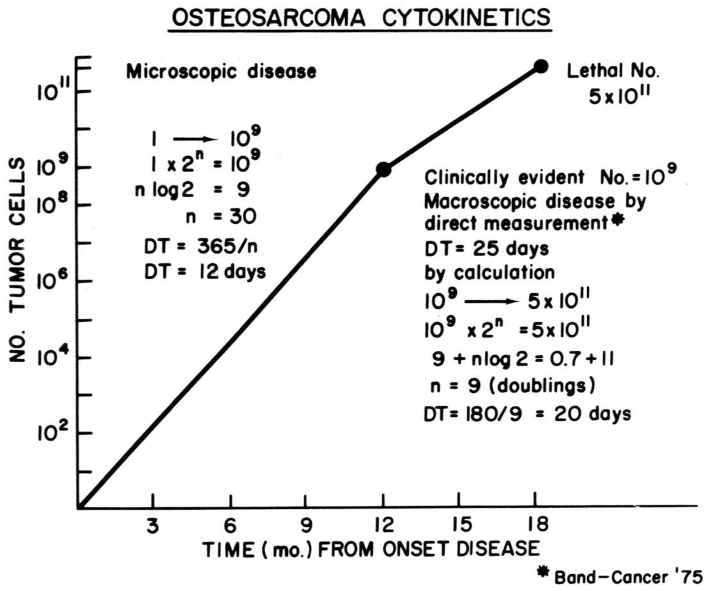

Figure 5

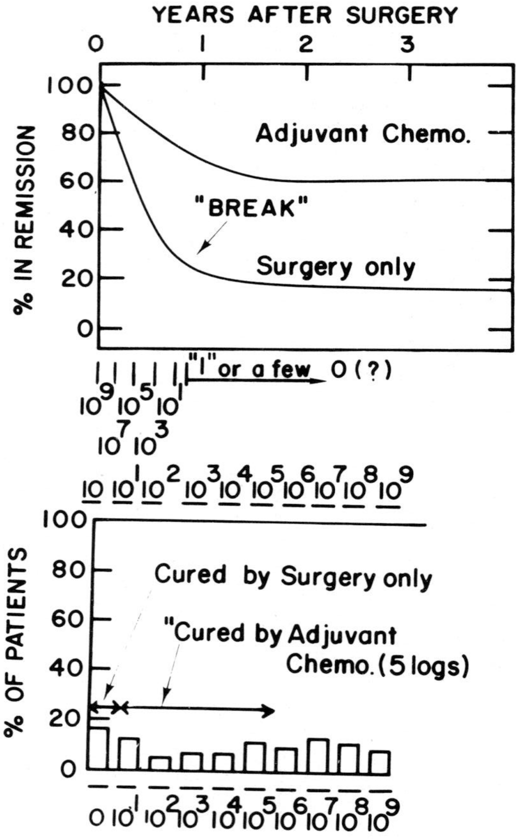

Figure 6

calculated with reasonable accuracy and confirmed by bio- assay from the nature of the survival curve. Thus, as indicated above, the break point in the curve is the time beyond which surviving patients are presumed to be cured. Such patients therefore, had no tumor cells capable of indefinite expansion and the production of relapse following control of the primary. For surgery-only curves, the curve plateaus at 16%. Patients with greater than 10^9 cells would have had clinically evident or roetgenographically evident disease by chest film. Therefore, the distribution of patients in terms of number of neoplastic cells persisting after amputation varies between 0 and 10^9. That distribution is determined from the nature of the descending portion of the disease-free survival curve. With adjuvant chemotherapy, the plateau of the disease-free survival curve is at 60% as compared to 16%. In order to encompass tumor cytoeradication in 60% of the patients, those patients having up to 10^6 cells would have to be cured. Assuming these calculations are correct, such chemotherapy would be capable of irradicating up through 5 logs of neoplastic cells.

An additional expression of the cytokinetic aspects of adjuvant chemotherapy of osteogenic sarcom is presented in Figure 7. In the top portion of the Figure, a schematic diagram of cytoreduction with intermittent chemotherapy is presented. There are two major components to the curve: 1) cytoreduction achieved by the course of chemotherapy and 2) proliferative recovery in the interval between courses of treatment. The overall effect of an intermittent treatment program is a function of these two variables. Lloyd's formula is presented in Figure 7. The total tumor cell kill in logs equals the total cell kill in logs minus the total cell recovery. The total log cell kill is the product of the log kill per course and the number of courses while the recovery between courses is inversely related to the doubling time and directly related to the number of courses and the interval between courses. From our previous analysis, a maximum of 5 logs of tumor are killed by adjuvant chemotherapy and the doubling time of micrometastatic OGS is 12 days. With these substitutions, the log kill per course is .9 and the percent cell kill per course is 79. While this is greater than can be achieved in patients with overt disease, it is not inconsistent with what might be expected in the kinetically

ADJUVANT CHEMOTHERAPY: KINETICS

Figure 7

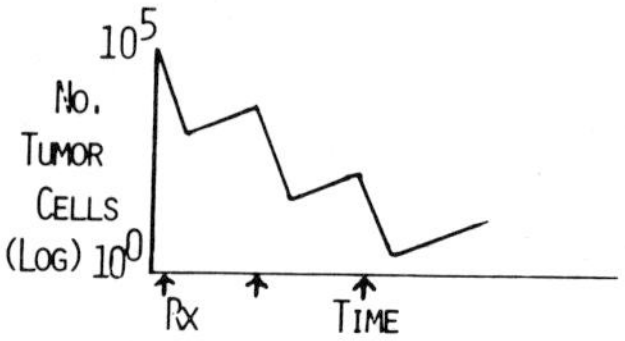

$$\text{Total Log Tumor Cell Kill} = \underbrace{\left[\text{Log Kill Per Course} \times N\right]}_{\text{Total Cell Kill}} - \underbrace{\left[\frac{\text{Log } 2}{DT}(N-1)I\right]}_{\text{Total Recovery}}$$

N = # Courses; DT = Doubling Time
I = Interval between courses

Osteosarcoma:
Adjuvant
Chemotherapy
60% "Cure"
1-5 Logs
(Max. 5)

$$5 = \left[X \times 12\right] - \left[\frac{\text{Log } 2}{12}(11)\ (21)\right]$$

X = 0.90 Log Kill/Course
= 79% Cell Kill/Course
(Max.)

ADJUVANT CHEMOTHERAPY: TREATMENT VARIABLES

$$\text{Total Log Tumor Cell "Kill"} = \underbrace{\left[\text{Log Kill Per Course} \times N\right]}_{\text{Total Cell Kill}} - \underbrace{\left[\frac{\text{Log } 2}{DT}(N-1)\ I\right]}_{\text{Total Cell Recovery}}$$

Figure 8

N=# Courses; DT=Doubling Time
I=Interval between courses

Total Cell Kill Varies
1) Directly with cell kill per course
   a) dose
   b) better drug(s)(*a)
   c) combinations(*b)
2) Directly with number of courses
3) Directly with doubling time
4) Inversely with interval(*c)

---

*a) AD-32 (Adriamycin analog)
*b) Mtx-CF q.3wk + Adriamycin
*c) Mtx-CF q.1wk

more active and thus, presumably more sensitive micrometastatic disease.

Further analyses are presented in Figure 8. Since total log cell kill sufficient to produce cure is the goal, the variables which influence this are separately analyzed. Total log cell kill varies directly with log cell kill per course. For experimental homogeneous populations of tumor cells, there is a linear-log relationship between dose and tumor cell kill. Thus, a two-fold increase in dose might double the log kill. Clearly, better drugs such as improved adriamycin might lead to an increased log cell kill per course. Finally, combinations of agents, particularly those wherein the dose rate of agents individually is minimally compromised would be expected to increase the log cell kill per course.

The total cell kill would vary directly with the number of courses. As indicated below, however, it seems unlikely that one can exploit this with respect to long term chemotherapy. AS one might anticipate the log cell kill varies directly with the doubling time. Thus, the shorter the doubling time, the greater the proliferative recovery in the interval between treatment. Finally, total cell kill varies inversely with the interval between treatments. This may be exploited in OGS by the use of weekly high-dose Mtx-CF programs wherein the interval between treatments is reduced by three-fold.

The above approaches have, in fact, been employed in the generation of our second and third adjuvant chemotherapy protocol for OGS.

The above approach involves a number of assumptions, the importance of which will become increasingly apparent with the application and adaption of a model to clinical trials and experimental data. One important variable involves drug resistance. It has been observed for a number of different tumor cells in culture that approximately 1 in 10^6 (10^{-6}) cells of a given population is resistant to a given drug. There is compelling _in vivo_ experimental evidence which supports this (Figure 9). In this study of L1210 mouse leukemia treated with ara-C, it is apparent that inoculum sizes of 10^5 cells can be cured by the drug. However, inoculum sizes of 10^7 cells are not cured by the same treatment and the cells recovered after the end of treatment are resistant to subsequent exposure to ara-C. Inoculum sizes of 10^6 are intermediate. These data are consistent with substantial

Figure 9

Overt metastatic osteogenic sarcoma

Treatment Strategy, Categories and Results

TREATMENT SEQUENCE	No.	NED Achieved	Continued
Surgery (Chemotherapy 2 + XRT) Chemotherapy 3	5	5	5
Chemotherapy 1 Surgery Chemotherapy 3	3	3	2
Chemotherapy 1 Surgery (Chemotherapy 2 + XRT) Chemotherapy 3	5	4	4
Chemotherapy 1 Chemotherapy 3	8	3	3
TOTAL	21	15	14

1 patient received adriamycin only

Chemotherapy 1: V-Mtx-CF q wk4 8

Chemotherapy 2: V-Mtx-CF q wk4

XRT - Radiation therapy

Chemotherapy 3) V-Mtx-CF q 2-3 w for 18 mos.
2 received concurrent adriamycin

Figure 10

OSTEOSARCOMA CELLS : DRUG RESISTANCE

ASSUME FRACTIONAL RESISTANCE = 10^{-6}

THEN:

CURE IMPOSSIBLE IF INITIAL CELL BURDEN $> 10^{6}$

ASSUME FRACTIONAL RESISTANCE OF DAUGHTER CELLS PRODUCED DURING TREATMENT = 10^{-4}

THEN:

CURE IMPOSSIBLE IF NO. OF DAUGHTER CELLS PRODUCED, AS CALCULATED FROM

$$\left[\frac{\text{Log } 2}{\text{DT}} (I)(N-1)\right], \text{ IS} > 10^{4}$$

in vitro data that 10^{-6} cells are drug resistant and this population is selected out by the treatment of native populations of 10^6 are larger.

When these data with respect to experimental studies of drug resistance are considered with respect to the data presented in Figure 6, it is titillating to speculate that 60% ceiling rate on disease-free survival is a function of the fact that 40% of patients have 10^6 or more cells which means that drug resistance in one or more cells would obtain and cure would not be achievable.

The above calculations obtain for drug resistant cells in the initial unexposed population. Most antitumor agents are variably mutagenic so that during the course of treatment, mutant daughter cells are produced which have a higher potential for being genetically drug resistant. Several *in vitro* studies indicate that such chemical mutants will increase the proportion of drug resistant cells by a factor of 100. Thus, for daughter cells produced during treatment, 1 in 10,000 (10^{-4}) will be resistant

These data are summarized in Figure 10. Thus, treatment failure due to drug resistance may occur if the initial population of micrometastatic cells is greater than 10^6 or if the number of daughter cells produced during treatment is greater than 10^4. This latter calculation has major implications for the duration of drug treatment. Thus, the longer the interval between courses of treatment and the longer the total duration of treatment required to produce tumor cytoeradication the greater the risk of the production of resistant duaghter cells. Conversely, intensive treatment involving a larger tumor cell kill per course, shorter intervals between treatment, and therefore, a reduced number of courses required to produce total cell kill would markedly reduce the risk of emerging resistant cells.

Our third chemotherapy adjuvant protocol for OGS started one year ago and is based upon some of the above considerations and is presented in Figure 11. As already indicated, weekly high-dose Mtx-CF is more effective in advanced disease than tri-weekly and presumably would affect a more rapid cytoreduction of micrometastatic disease and a decreased chance of the emergence of drug resistant cells. Accordingly, there is an initial period of intensification with weekly Mtx-CF.

Figure 11

OSTEOSARCOMA-ADJUVANT CHEMOTHERAPY

SFCI - CHMC STUDY III

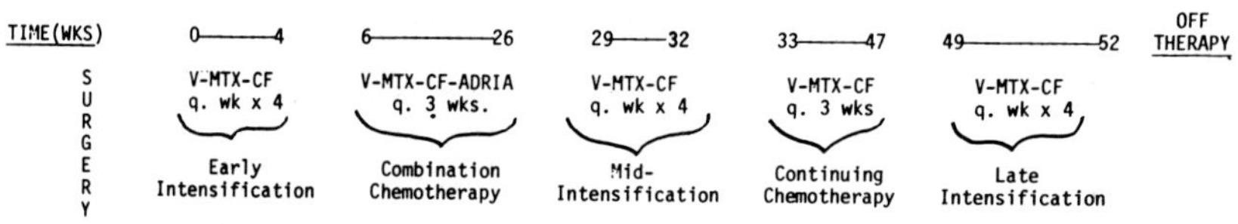

Figure 12

Typical results observed on treating L1210 leukemia with arabinosylcytosine (ara-C).

Number of leukemic cells at initiation of Rx	No. of courses of ara-C; q3hr (x 8); q4d	Resistance of leuk. cells to ara-C after end of Rx*	Animals "cured"
10^5	1	No	50%
10^5	2	–	90-100%
10^5	4	–	90-100%
10^7	1	Yes	0
10^7	2	Yes	0
10^7	4	Yes	0
10^7	6-12†	Yes	0

* Demonstrated by passage of cells after treatment and retesting response to ara-C. Such cells are not cross-resistant to other classes of drugs.

† Good increases in host survival time but all animals die during maximum tolerated treatment. After 2-4 courses, the die is cast; cure has been achieved or failure is inevitable.

For practical reasons, such treatment cannot be carried beyond 4 weeks. Following this, combination chemotherapy without compromising the dose rate of either program is delivered in the form of adriamycin and high-dose Mtx-CF tri-weekly. Further cases and follow-up will be required to evaluate the effectiveness of this program as compared to protocols 1 and 2.

If micrometastases are eradicated by adjuvant chemotherapy in a substantial proportion of patients, it seems reasonable to assume that the number of such metastases is reduced in patients who eventually have recurrent disease. Our preliminary studies indicate that this is, in fact, so. Also, the time to the development of overt metastatic disease in patients receiving adjuvant chemotherapy as compared to the non-adjuvant control patients is delayed. This fact plus the increasing effectiveness of systemic treatment has led to a multi-disciplinary, curative intent, treatment program for relapsing patients (Figure 12). The principle involves an initial combined chemotherapy and surgical attack on the pulmonary metastases designed to produce a state of NED (No clinical or roentgenographic Evidence of Disease). The chemotherapy cannot be specified since it will depend in part on the chemotherapy employed in the previous adjuvant treatment. Multi-modality treatment is initiated with chemotherapy or surgery depending upon the clinical circumstances. If chemotherapy is initiated, surgery is employed in order to achieve NED unless the chemotherapy itself has produced a complete remission. Once NED is achieved, it is assumed that micrometastatic disease persists and chemotherapy is continued for a period of 12 months. In 21 patients so treated NED was achieved in 15 (Figure 12). The survival of such patients is presented in Figure 13. Again, the control is historical. The time for the appearance of pulmonary metastases to death in such patients was plotted and the median was six months. For the multi-modality treated patients, the curve is at 65% at 18 months and 12 of the 21 patients continue NED. These results are preliminary but promising.[8]

The final arbiter of the effect of a treatment program for cancer is survival. We have previously discussed objective response rate, complete response rates, and tumor free survival. In Figure 14, the overall survival of patients with OGS

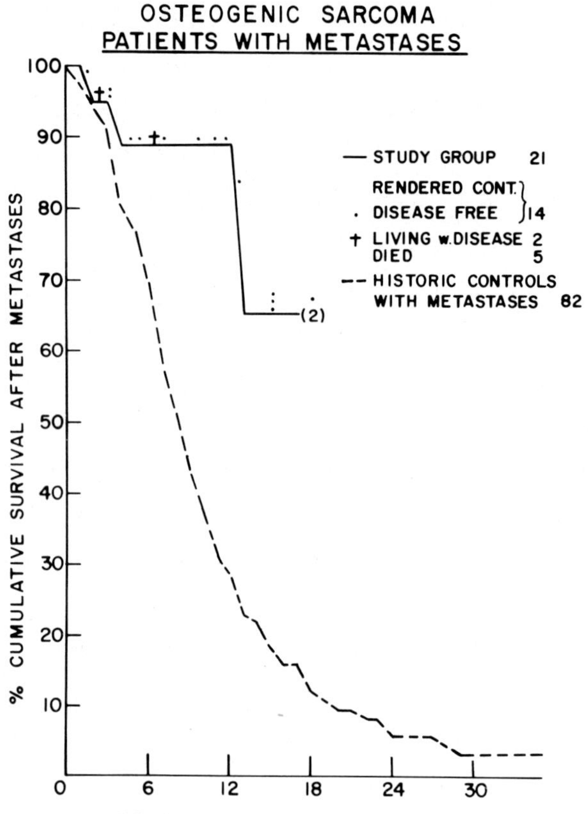

Figure 13

SURVIVAL OSTEOGENIC SARCOMA
ADJUVANT THERAPY

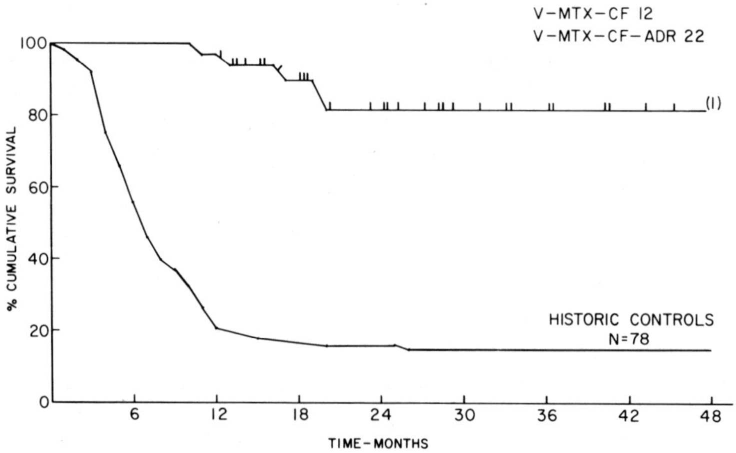

Figure 14

treated prior to July of 1972 and after that date at the Sidney Farber Cancer Institute-Children's Hospital Medical Center are presented. The lower curve is again the historical control patients where the plateau is at 16%. For the 34 patients treated on our first 2 adjuvant protocols (the third protocol was introduced only 1 year ago, too short to impact on survival) the curve levels off at 24 months and remains at 80% at 48 months. OGS is a relatively rare disease and even at a large center, case accrual is such that it is difficult to ask a quantitative therapeutic question. For example, while Mtx-CF is clearly highly effective in advanced OGS, there were only 12 patients included in the adjuvant study. In the second study, adriamycin was added to Mtx-CF. Again, the survival appeared to be superior to that of the historical control patients but the question as to whether the combination was superior to Mtx-CF only remains open because of insufficient follow-up. Finally, the multi-modality treatment of relapsing patients has produced positive but preliminary results. In short, while the results of three of these programs present problems primarily because of small case numbers and/or insufficient follow-up the overall impact has been very substantial as evidenced in Figure 14.

REFERENCES

1. Wang, J., Cortes, E., et al. (1971) Therapeutic Effect and Toxicity of Adriamycin in Patients with Neoplastic Disease. Cancer 28:837-843.

2. Djerassi, I. (1975) High-Dose Methotrexate (NSC-740) and Citrovorum Factor (NSC-3590) Rescue: Background and Rationale. Cancer Chemother. Rep. (Part 3) 6:3-6.

3. Jaffe, N. (1972) Recent Advances in the Chemotherapy of Metastatic Osteogenic Sarcoma. Cancer 30:1627-1631.

4. Pitman, S., Parker, L., et al. (1975) Clinical Trial of High-Dose Methotrexate (NSC-740) with Citrovorum Factor (NSC-3590)-Toxicologic and Therapeutic Observations. Cancer Chemother. Rep. 6:43-49.

5. Jaffe, N., Frei E, III, et al. (1977) Weekly High-Dose Methotrexate-Citrovorum Factor in Osteogenic Sarcoma: Pre-surgical Treatment of Primary Tumor and of Overt Pulmonary Metastases. Cancer 39:45-50.

6. Frei, E. III. (1972) Combination Cancer Therapy: Presidential Address. Cancer Res. 32:2593-2607.

7. Jaffe, N., Frei E. III, et al. (1974) Adjuvant Methotrexate and Citrovorum Factor Treatment of Osteogenic Sarcoma. New Engl. J. Med. 291:994-997.

8. Jaffe, N., Traggis, D., et al. (1976) Multidisciplinary Treatment for Macrometastatic Osteogenic Sarcoma. Brit. Med. J. 2:1039-1041.

Section II

BREAST CANCER

Adjuvant Therapy of Cancer, S.E. Salmon and S.E. Jones eds.

STUDIES OF THE NATIONAL SURGICAL ADJUVANT BREAST PROJECT (NSABP)

Bernard Fisher, M.D., Carol Redmond, Sc.D. and participating
NSABP investigators (Table 1)
National Surgical Adjuvant Breast Project Headquarters
University of Pittsburgh
Pittsburgh, Pa. 15261

INTRODUCTION

Despite expansive operative procedures with and without postoperative radiation for local and regional control of disease, noteworthy gains relative to survival and freedom from disease have not occurred during the past 3 or 4 decades. There is increasing awareness that, most if not all, patients have disseminated disease at diagnosis and that improvement in survival is only apt to result from employment of effective systemic therapy in conjunction with modalities used for local/regional disease control. The use of chemo-, immuno-, or hormonal therapy in conjunction with operation has been inappropriately designated as "adjuvant" therapy. Recent advances in knowledge support the contention that operation and/or radiation by reducing tumor burden could actually serve as the "adjuvant" to systemic therapy. Consequently, the term "combined modality" therapy seems more appropriate to describe the various conglomerate treatment regimens. None the less, because of its common usage and the general familiarity with its connotation, the term "adjuvant therapy" will be employed in this review.

As a consequence of this significant change in attitude toward the therapy of breast cancer, numerous clinical trials evaluating a multitude of systemic adjuvant therapies are in progress throughout the United States and in other countries of the world. Since 1958, the National Surgical Adjuvant Breast Project (NSABP) has been at the forefront of those investigations. In a trial initiated at that time, the efficacy of administering triethylenethiophosphoramide (Thio-TEPA; TSPA) in conjunction with "curative" cancer surgery was determined.[1] Patients were

TABLE 1 PARTICIPANTS IN CLINICAL TRIAL OF L-PHENYLALANINE MUSTARD FOLLOWING CONVENTIONAL OR MODIFIED RADICAL MASTECTOMY IN PRIMARY OPERABLE BREAST CANCER

Institution	Responsible Surgeon or Medical Oncologist	Responsible Pathologist
	NSABP	
Akron City Hospital	Marvin J. Sakol	L. B. Reyes
Denver General Hospital	George E. Moore	Joseph Preston
Downstate Medical Center, SUNY	Bernard Gardner	A. Nicastri
Georgia Baptist Hospital	A. Hamblin Letton	Lester Forbes
Greater Bakersfield Memorial Hospital	James E. Donovan	Robert Wybel
Group Health Medical Center	Robert Bourdeau	Charles E. Marshall
Hershey Medical Center	William E. DeMuth	Malcolm McGavran
Hotel-Dieu (Quebec City, Quebec)	Louis Dionne	Lagace Real
Huron Road Hospital	M. D. Ram	Edward Siegler
Kaiser Permanente (Portland, Oregon)	Andrew Glass	Richard Gourley
Letterman General Hospital	Harvey Conklin	William F. Doyle
	Michael Corder	
Lynn Hospital (Lynn, Massachusetts)	Bernard Willett	Emei Shen
Memorial Cancer Research	David Plotkin	Jacob Turner
Foundation of Southern California	Elliot Hinkes	
Mercy Hospital (Des Moines, Iowa)	Joseph Song	Joseph Song
Montreal General Hospital	John MacFarland	W. D. Duguid
Newark Beth Israel	Frederick B. Cohen	Alkiviadis Campbell
Roger Williams General Hospital (Providence, R.I.)	Jack Savran	Israel Diamond
Royal Victoria Hospital (Montreal, Quebec)	Henry Shibata	Thomas Seemayer
St. Luke's Hospital (Kansas City, Missouri)	Paul Koontz	John Rippey
Southern California Permanente (San Diego, CA)	Thomas Campbell	Marvin Nicola
University of Florida (Jacksonville, FL)	Neil Abramson	Ronald Rhatigan
University of Louisville	Condict Moore	William Christopherson
	Carl Knutson	
University of Mississippi	George V. Smith	Carl Evers
University of Pittsburgh	Bernard Fisher	Susan Rogers
USC-LA County Medical Center	Lewis Guiss	Peter Schwinn
Washington University	George J. Hill	Walter Bauer
West Suburban Hospital (Chicago, Illinois)	Everett Nicholas	Frederick Volini
White Memorial Medical Center	Samuel Fritz	George Kypridakis
	ECOG	
Cleveland Metropolitan Hospital	Edward Mansour	John Reid
Highland Hospital (Rochester, N.Y.)	Edwin Savlov	David Platt
Pennsylvania Hospital	Harvey Lerner	Santo Longo
Rush Presbyterian-St. Luke's Medical Center	Steven Economou	George Hass
	Charles Perlia	
Tufts-Pondville Hospital (Walpole, MA)	Leo Stolbach	Lalita Gandbhir
University of Alberta	Pierre Band	Gordon Bain
	COG	
Duke University Center	William Shingleton	Peter J. Dawson
Ohio State University	John P. Minton	William Holaday
Wilmington Medical Center	Robert W. Frelick	Patrick Ashley

randomized following conventional radical mastectomy so that they received either placebo or TSPA at the time of operation and on each of the first two postoperative days. It was anticipated that such a therapeutic regimen would destroy tumor cells dislodged into the blood and lymph during surgical manipulation. At the end of 5 years, there was a difference in the TSPA and placebo groups of premenopausal patients who had 4 or more positive nodes. The effect of TSPA in that category was best demonstrated by the observation that 50 percent of patients in the placebo series had recurrences by the thirteenth month after surgery, whereas recurrences did not occur in half of the TSPA patients until the forty-fifth month of follow-up. While the difference between the treated and control groups relative to treatment failure was no longer statistically significant after five years, it was 20 percent. A 33 percent difference in the survival rate that was significant, $P < 0.05$, was observed at that time between the TSPA treated and control groups: 56.5 percent for the former versus 24.3 percent for the latter. Recently results obtained from a ten year follow-up revealed a persistence of the difference.[2] After ten years, 21 percent fewer patients in the TSPA groups had treatment failures and 21 percent more of them survived. Thus, the initial suppression of treatment failures had a lasting effect that was reflected in patient survival. The data also suggested that the limited chemotherapy employed was more effective in patients in other subsets having smaller tumors. In retrospect, the findings with TSPA must be considered remarkable in view of the small amount of drug employed for only a brief interval.

Despite increasing support from the experimental laboratory and the clinic for the use of adjuvant chemotherapy, for a variety of reasons, mostly non-scientific, a hiatus of almost 10 years existed prior to the onset of another trial utilizing adjuvant chemotherapy. In late 1971, after extensive planning, a trial of <u>prolonged</u> adjuvant chemotherapy involving 37 member institutions of the NSABP and the Eastern Cooperative Oncology Group (ECOG) headed by Dr. Paul Carbone was implemented.

STRATEGY OF THE NSABP

The choice of a regimen to be employed for this first trial related to numerous considerations. First it was considered essential that the agent(s) employed should have had a beneficial effect in advanced breast cancer. Rightfully or wrongly, it was deemed at that time that surgeons and their patients were unlikely to accept a drug or drugs which produced the kind of toxicity observed and accepted in patients with advanced disease. Consequently, patient toxicity was of prime concern. In considering pharmacologic characteristics of the agent to be employed, it was felt that the ideal adjuvant would be one which could be taken orally. There was general agreement that if a single agent were to be employed, one which was cell cycle, non-stage specific offered the best choice for success. At that time there was a great deal of consideration given to the use of combination chemotherapy instead of a single agent since there was convincing evidence, both experimental and clinical, to indicate that the use of multiple agents produced a significantly greater remission rate in patients with advanced disease than did single agents. On the face of it, there was every reason to anticipate that combination chemotherapy would be extremely effective in the presence of a minimal tumor burden (micrometastases), and should be employed as adjuvant therapy. Because experimental evidence indicated that there existed the possibility that drugs moderately or only marginally effective when employed as single agents in advanced disease might be as effective as combinations in the adjuvant setting, a "game plan" was devised which started with the use of a single agent. This seemed to be a logical starting point. After determining its effectiveness, it would then seem proper to proceed with the evaluation of multiple agents in a logical step-wise fashion so that each new effort was based on sound biological hypothesis. The plan was to first compare a single agent with no treatment, then two agents versus a single one and eventually three versus two. Hopefully, it could thus be ascertained what is required to attain a maximal therapeutic effect with acceptable toxicity. Moreover, such an orderly approach should permit definition of subsets of patients who might be as responsive to a single agent as to combinations. In that regard, it cannot be too strongly emphasized that "breast cancer" is an eponym employed to designate a biologically heterogeneous group of cancers of the breast residing in a biologically heterogeneous group of women. Consequently, it is highly unlikely that uniformly quantitative and qualitative chemotherapeutic regimens will be required for every patient.

Aside from the important pragmatic aspects of a clinical trial, i.e., determining the worth of using a particular therapeutic regimen, each should ideally provide answers to important biological questions. Hopefully the NSABP series will comply in that regard. A question of utmost importance which remains to be answered is, "Do patients who have 1-3 positive axillary nodes and subsequently develop treatment failures (65% of such patients) have a residual tumor burden equivalent to that of those with $\geqslant$ 4 positive nodes who ultimately develop treatment failures (90% of patients), or is there a quantitative difference in the tumor burden of the 1-3 positive node patients? Expressed differently, do the proportion of patients with 1-3 positive nodes who develop treatment failures differ in their tumor burden following operation from those with $\geqslant$4 positive nodes who ultimately fail; or do they have the same tumor burden? Is there simply a smaller proportion of patients who fail in the 1-3 node group? Information in that regard is of fundamental importance in planning chemotherapy strategies. For, if the former is true, (there is less tumor burden in 1-3 positive node patients who fail), less intensive chemotherapy may be required to eliminate treatment failures in that group. On the other hand, if the second hypothesis is true, i.e., that there is simply a smaller proportion of patients who fail, no less chemotherapy will be necessary for the 1-3 positive node group than for those with $\geqslant$4 positive nodes.

A prime consideration leading to the formulation of the "game plan" was related to an unwillingness to ignore the lesson of history associated with breast cancer surgery. It may have been a blessing to women had

Halsted progressed in an orderly fashion from lesser operations to progressively more radical ones, as results dictated. He would thus have not closed doors which have taken at least 50 years to reopen. It is unfortunately more difficult to go backward! Should three or five drug therapy be effective, who would be willing to take the chance to find out if one or two drugs were equally as good?

EARLY RESULTS OF THE L-PAM VS. PLACEBO TRIAL (NSABP PROTOCOL #5)

The first NSABP trial (Protocol #5) of prolonged adjuvant therapy began patient accrual the end of September, 1972. Women with pathological Stage II breast cancer were randomized so that they received either L-PAM or Placebo. The specific aim of that study was to ascertain whether the administration of L-PAM (0.15 mg/kg/day for five consecutive days every six weeks) could prolong the disease free interval of patients with breast cancer. When after an average follow-up time of about 9 months, there was evidence that this had been achieved, a progress report of findings was presented.[3] At that time treatment failures had occurred in 22 percent of 108 patients receiving placebo and 9.7 percent of 103 women given L-PAM (P=0.01). A statistically significant difference (P=0.02) existed in favor of L-PAM relative to disease free interval.

In premenopausal women, the difference with respect to disease free interval of treated and control groups was highly significant (P=0.008). A treatment failure occurred in 30 percent of premenopausal patients receiving placebo and 3 percent of those treated with L-PAM (P= 0.008). Whereas a similar trend was observed in postmenopausal patients, the difference was not statistically significant.

Of interest was the finding that results were achieved with minimal alteration of the well-being of patients, despite the fact that 60 percent of women demonstrated myelosuppression (Grades 1 and 2 toxicity). Nausea and vomiting was reported in 30 percent of the L-PAM treated patients. Ten percent of all courses of therapy were associated with that discomfort.

ADDITIONAL NSABP TRIALS OF ADJUVANT CHEMOTHERAPY

With completion of patient entry into NSABP Protocol #5 (placebo vs. L-PAM), as part of our original plan, NSABP Protocol #7 was implemented. Utilizing the same criteria of patient acceptability and keeping all other aspects of the protocol comparable with Protocol #5, patient entry began in February, 1975. By March, 1976, 700 patients had been randomized between L-PAM and L-PAM plus 5-FU (PAM-FU) and patient entry was terminated. The L-PAM was administered as the only agent at a dose of 6 mg/M^2 by mouth. When combined with 5-FU, 4 mg/M^2 was given orally. The 5-FU dosage was 300 mg/M^2, iv. Drugs were given on 5 consecutive days every 6 weeks for 2 years. The toxicity of the 2 drug combination was only a little greater than L-PAM alone and was entirely acceptable.

With completion of patient accrual into Protocol #7, a third protocol (Protocol #8) of the series was begun comparing PAM-FU with PAM-FU plus Methotrexate (MTX). The dosage, times of administration of PAM-FU etc., are similar to those employed in Protocol #7. The Methotrexate (MTX), 25 mg/M^2, iv., is given on days 1 and 5 of each cycle. Since 600 patients have been randomized into that protocol (NSABP Protocol #8) in slightly less than a year, it will be terminated shortly. The time is too short for meaningful follow-up information. On May 1, 1977, two new NSABP protocols, #9 comparing PAM-FU with PAM-FU plus Tamoxifen (an anti-estrogen) and #10 comparing PAM-FU with PAM-FU plus C. parvum (an immunostimulating agent) will be begun. The Tamoxifen will be administered 10 mg, p.o., bid and the C. parvum, 2.5 mg/M^2, iv., on days 5 and 21 of each treatment cycle.

CONFIRMATION OF THE ORIGINALLY REPORTED L-PAM FINDINGS

Since the originally reported findings indicating the effectiveness of L-PAM were from a relatively small sample size, particularly in subgroups of patients, there may have been those who were skeptical of the significance of the results. The recent findings from Protocol #7 reaffirm the early observations. At a similar point in time of average follow-up (about 9 months), the findings from Protocol #7 with L-PAM and with the combination of PAM-FU revealed a reduction in treatment failure which, for the most part, is as good or better than that observed with L-PAM in the first protocol, lending credibility to the earlier findings (Table 2). Since larger numbers of patients are present in the subsets, the results are even more convincing. Of particular importance is the observation that these agents are indeed effective in significantly delaying the disease free interval of postmenopausal patients as well as those who are premenopausal.

AN UPDATE OF THE ORIGINAL L-PAM FINDINGS

A recent update of findings was reported. Life table summaries of patients at risk at specific times post mastectomy and % probability disease free were made available. There continued to exist overall a highly significant difference (P=0.009) between the treated and placebo groups. At 18 and 24 months, a 37 and 25 percent reduction in treatment failures was observed. Consideration of patients relative to age indicates that a more pronounced effect was obtained in those under 50 (P=0.007). In the older age group at 12 months, a difference of 10% in favor of those treated was noted. This represented an almost 50% reduction in treatment failure compared with a 68% reduction in those under 50. In the older patients, this difference subsequently diminished so that at 18 months the reduction in treatment failures was 23% and at 2 years, based on small numbers, 5%. Overall there existed no statistical significance between the groups. Similar patterns, as observed with age, were noted when patients were stratified by menopausal status. Relative to nodal status, the beneficial effects of L-PAM were seen in both patients with 1-3 positive nodes or $\geqslant$ 4 positive nodes (with the possible exception of data at 24 months), although the overall difference was statistically significant (P=.028) only in patients with 1-3 positive nodes. At 2 years, there was a 55% reduction in treatment failures as a result of the chemotherapy. Examination of results for patients classified simultaneously by age and nodal status revealed a most highly significant (P=.008) effect in young patients with 1-3 positive nodes, where after 2 years there was an 89% reduction of treatment

TABLE 2 REPETITION OF EARLY FINDINGS NSABP 2/28/77

		# PTS.	AV. MO. ON STUDY	% TF	P VALUE (VS. PLACEBO)
ALL PATIENTS					
PLACEBO	P-5	108	8.4	22.2	----
L-PAM	P-5	103	9.1	9.7	.01
L-PAM	P-7	309	8.9	7.4	<.001
PAM-FU	P-7	300	9.0	5.0	<.001
PREMENOPAUSAL					
PLACEBO	P-5	37	8.6	30.0	----
L-PAM	P-5	30	9.3	3.0	.008
L-PAM	P-7	64	10.1	10.9	.019
PAM-FU	P-7	67	10.7	4.5	<.001
POSTMENOPAUSAL					
PLACEBO	P-5	63	8.3	21.0	----
L-PAM	P-5	66	8.8	11.0	.15
L-PAM	P-7	94	10.8	6.4	.007
PAM-FU	P-7	91	10.8	8.8	.03
1-3 POSITIVE NODES					
PLACEBO	P-5	47	7.3	9.0	----
L-PAM	P-5	52	8.5	1.9	.15
L-PAM	P-7	168	8.9	2.4	.07
PAM-FU	P-7	156	9.1	1.9	.05
≥4 POSITIVE NODES					
PLACEBO	P-5	61	9.3	34.4	----
L-PAM	P-5	51	9.7	17.6	.04
L-PAM	P-7	141	8.9	13.5	.0008
PAM-FU	P-7	144	8.8	8.3	.00001
PRE- 1-3 POS. NODES					
PLACEBO	P-5	18	6.8	17.0	----
L-PAM	P-5	17	8.8	0.0	.250
L-PAM	P-7	35	10.6	2.9	.108
PAM-FU	P-7	33	10.9	0.0	.039
PRE- ≥4 POS. NODES					
PLACEBO	P-5	19	10.2	42.0	----
L-PAM	P-5	13	10.0	8.0	.08
L-PAM	P-7	23	9.8	21.7	.139
PAM-FU	P-7	24	11.3	4.2	.003
POST- 1-3 POS. NODES					
PLACEBO	P-5	27	7.6	0.0	----
L-PAM	P-5	32	8.0	3.0	.54
L-PAM	P-7	40	11.6	5.0	.35
PAM-FU	P-7	38	11.5	2.6	.58
POST- ≥4 POS. NODES					
PLACEBO	P-5	36	8.8	36.0	----
L-PAM	P-5	34	9.6	18.0	.14
L-PAM	P-7	42	11.0	9.5	.005
PAM-FU	P-7	42	10.8	16.7	.044

TABLE 3

NSABP 2/28/77

NSABP PROTOCOL NO. 5

	# PTS.	AV. MONTHS FOLLOW-UP	% TF	AV. MONTHLY TF RATE
ALL PATIENTS				
PLACEBO	169	24.0	31.4	1.71
L-PAM	179	24.0	23.5	1.12
P VALUE			.06	.009
PATIENTS ≤49				
PLACEBO	60	24.8	36.7	1.95
L-PAM	59	26.2	22.0	0.94
P VALUE			.06	.008
PATIENTS ≥50				
PLACEBO	109	23.6	28.4	1.57
L-PAM	120	22.9	24.2	1.23
P VALUE			.28	.22
1-3 POSITIVE NODES				
PLACEBO	87	21.6	19.5	1.04
L-PAM	97	23.9	11.3	0.50
P VALUE			.09	.02
≥4 POSITIVE NODES				
PLACEBO	82	26.6	43.9	2.46
L-PAM	82	24.1	37.8	2.02
P VALUE			.26	.16
≤49 - 1-3 POS. NODES				
PLACEBO	31	22.5	25.8	1.42
L-PAM	32	26.8	6.3	0.24
P VALUE			.04	.009
≤49 - ≥4 POS. NODES				
PLACEBO	29	27.3	48.3	2.48
L-PAM	27	25.6	40.7	2.01
P VALUE			.38	.26
≥50 - 1-3 POS. NODES				
PLACEBO	56	21.1	16.1	0.84
L-PAM	65	22.5	13.8	0.66
P VALUE			.46	.51
>50 - >4 POS. NODES				
PLACEBO	53	26.2	41.5	2.45
L-PAM	55	23.3	36.4	2.02
P VALUE			.36	.37

failures. A similar but less striking finding was observed in those under 50 with >4 positive nodes (P=.27). In older patients, in both nodal categories the early observed effect for L-PAM had decreased with time. Table 3 summarizes the proportion of treatment failures and the average monthly treatment failure rates for all patients and appropriate subsets.

Information regarding patient survival indicated that insufficient time has elapsed for there to be meaningful mortality in the control groups. At two years, survival in all L-PAM patients was 5.7% greater than those receiving placebo representing a mortality reduction of 36.0%. Survival was somewhat better in every subgroup for those receiving L-PAM although not statistically significant.

COMMENTS

(a) It has previously been pointed out that the most important aspect of the findings achieved with L-PAM and with CMF is not the statistical magnitude of the differences achieved, nor that they were obtained with acceptable toxicity, but that it has been demonstrated that the rationale for prolonged chemotherapy as an adjunct to operation is a sound one. Different agents alone or in various combinations, refinements of administration, sequencing of drugs with hormonal or immunostimulating agents, etc., will undoubtedly produce increasingly better results.[4]

(b) The next decade may represent a most critical and significant period in the history of breast (as well as other) cancer therapy. The present spectrum of combined modality trials throughout the world are setting the stage for a crisis situation. Should many or most of those trials fail to be continued to a point where meaningful data are obtained, or because of improper design or implementation, produce information of questionable credibility, valuable time will have been lost, patient resources will have been squandered and above all, therapeutic confusion and disenchantment will prevail. On the other hand, should a sufficient number of protocols be impeccably carried to completion and meaningful data obtained, the next 10 years could be even more crucial. For, there will result verification or repudiation of not only the concepts and principles upon which the use of adjuvant therapy is based, but the very worth of those modalities which, at present, represent our total therapeutic resources and hopes for cure of the disease.

(c) Since the findings indicate that therapeutic regimens may affect subsets of patients differently, they stress the need for obtaining results on those subsets rather than on the group as a whole. The need for adequate sample size in each subset requires that large numbers of patients be entered into a clinical trial. Moreover, since there is variation in the rate of occurrence of treatment failure or mortality among subgroups, the time for determination of therapeutic effectiveness may differ for the various subsets. Consequently, determination of effectiveness at the same time for the entire population or for each subgroup may be misleading. Such a consideration may be more important when evaluating the effectiveness of new regimens against those which may be partially effective in either all or some groups.

(d) While review of data may generate pessimism concerning the effect of the agents employed in postmenopausal patients, it is emphasized that during the early follow-up period the relative reduction in treatment failure in older women was similar to that observed in the younger age group. Further information from postmenopausal women in our on-going protocols should provide the data necessary to more firmly establish the effectiveness of the drug in older women. The seemingly different response in different subsets in this reviewer's opinion represent a major contribution and are extremely important. For, they indicate that breast cancer is indeed a heterogeneous disease and they give direction to an investigative course for the immediate future, i.e., to identify biological differences which have led to these findings. The simplistic approach may be to give subsets of patients who respond less well, greater, more complex and more prolonged regimens of chemotherapy. The possibility must be considered however, that such findings may be the result of a clonogenic cell populations, which will not be responsive to such an approach. In that regard, it is interesting to note that the medical oncologists are succumbing to the same temptations in thought for which they so fervently and rightfully criticized their colleagues in other disciplines. When the surgeon decided that radical surgery was not adequate, it seemed reasonable to him to proceed to extended radical or super radical operations which proved fruitless rather than to search for a biological explanation for his failure. When the radiation oncologist found that orthovoltage radiation was not as effective in the treatment of breast cancer as was claimed, he proceeded to enlarge "fields" as well as his equipment. The interest has been notorious for "shotgunning". Now there is a similar inclination on the part of the adjuvant "therapologist". They may just be right! Certainly the hypothetical justifications for their use need evaluation.

(e) At the time of first publication of the L-PAM findings, it was pointed out that many questions were raised by the findings which only time and additional protocols could resolve. We are, in terms of time, at least a step closer to answering many of them.

(f) A few comments are in order concerning the repeatedly asked question, "Should all patients with primary breast cancer and positive axillary nodes receive systemic chemotherapy?" Those of us who are responsible for the obtaining of this information have consistently strongly emphasized that our presentations are not to be construed as forums for the advocacy or rejection of a particular thesis. They have always been presented as results obtained as of a certain time from studies aimed at applying the scientific method to clinical problems solving. It is unfortunate that the significance of the data from ours and the Milan trials have been obtunded by non-scientific, superficial polemics gracing the editorial and "letters to the editor" pages of prestigious journals as well as throw away tabloids. It has been this reviewer's opinion that since systemic adjuvant chemotherapy represents such an important and promising aspect of clinical research, every patient, ideally, should be a participant in a <u>major</u> clinical trial employing such agents. Should that not be possible - and more often than not reasons for impossibility are less than convincing - such patients deserve the opportunity for such therapy but only by physicians who are entirely familiar not only with the use of such regimens, but who are aware of the "pros and cons" of such therapy, who are sufficiently current with the information being reported and who are prepared to "shift gears" without becoming despondent by temporary failures or uncertainties.

(g) The triad of factors which hold promise of making a major impact on the breast cancer problem in the immediate future are so closely interrelated that the benefit of each member, -early diagnosis, local/regional management and systemic adjuvant therapy-, cannot be appraised independent of the other two. The modest findings and undoubtedly the improved ones to come with adjuvant chemotherapy directly implicate the other two members of the triad. Since the rationale of modern chemotherapy is related to the hypothesis that such therapy is apt to be more effective and less drug may be required when fewer numbers of cells remain to be destroyed by systemic therapy, the impact of earlier diagnosis on the effectiveness of systemic therapy is obvious and early detection becomes more important. Moreover, it is not unreasonable to anticipate that the use of effective systemic therapy will make more remote the chance that a lesser surgical procedure, i.e., segmental mastectomy, will be putting a patient at a disadvantage. As a consequence, increased disease control may be accomplished together with better cosmesis.

Adjuvant chemotherapy has been demonstrated to prolong the disease free interval of all patients with positive nodes having primary breast cancer - some for a longer time than others. Effect on survival, on undesirable long-term sequellae and on "cost-benefit ratio" must await the passage of time. There is no justification for despondency. A major effort must be directed toward making systemic therapy work better.

BIBLIOGRAPHY

1. Fisher, B., et al. (1968) Surgical Adjuvant Chemotherapy in Cancer of the Breast: Results of a Decade of Cooperative Investigations, Annals of Surgery 168: 337-356.

2. Fisher, B., et al. (1975) Ten-Year Follow-up of Breast Cancer Patients in a Cooperative Clinical Trial Evaluating Surgical Adjuvant Chemotherapy, Surgery, Gynecology & Obstetrics 140: 528-534.

3. Fisher, B., et al. (1975) L-Phenylalanine Mustard (L-PAM) in the Management of Primary Breast Cancer: A Report of Early Findings, New England Journal of Medicine 292: 117-122.

4. Fisher, B. and Wolmark, N. (1975) New Concepts in the Management of Primary Breast Cancer, Cancer 36: 627-637 (Supplement 2).

Adjuvant Therapy of Cancer, S.E. Salmon and S.E. Jones eds.

ADJUVANT CHEMOTHERAPY WITH CMF IN BREAST CANCER WITH POSITIVE AXILLARY NODES

Gianni Bonadonna, Anna Rossi, Pinuccia Valagussa,
Alberto Banfi, and Umberto Veronesi
Istituto Nazionale Tumori, Milano
Italy

INTRODUCTION

The contemporary clinical research for resectable breast cancer is actively engaged in studying the effectiveness of various combined treatment modalities on the disease-free interval and the overall survival. The strategic approach involving a prolonged sistemic treatment for high-risk patients has both a scientific and a clinical rationale[1,2,3]. The early attempts have yielded inconclusive results[4,5]. More recently, modern concepts about natural history of operable breast cancer[6,7], growth kinetics of micrometastases[8], and efficacy of cyclic combination chemotherapy[9] have provided a more solid baseline for the design of new clinical trials.

TABLE 1

RATIONALE FOR ADJUVANT TREATMENT IN HIGH-RISK PATIENTS WITH OPERABLE BREAST CANCER

1.	The traditional surgical approach has been challenged.
2.	The role of routine postoperative radiotherapy has been seriously questioned.
3.	High incidence of micrometastases when the primary tumor involves the axillary nodes or infiltrates the intramammary lymphatics.
4.	Improved efficacy of cyclic chemotherapy. Its activity in the clinically apparent tumors may not predict optimal scheduling of the same drugs against micrometastases.
5.	Efficacy of combined local-systemic treatment in animal model systems as well as in some human neoplasias (e.g. pediatric tumors, lymphomas).

THE CMF ADJUVANT PROGRAM

The adjuvant study with prolonged combination chemotherapy in operable breast cancer (T_1 -T_2 -T_{3a}) having histologically positive axillary nodes (N+) was started in Milan on June 1, 1973. The details of the controlled trial (experimental design, selection of patients, treatment modalities, follow up studies and statistical methods) have appeared in previous publications[10,11,12].

The cyclic combination known as CMF (cyclophosphamide, methotrexate, fluorouracil) was selected because of its known efficacy in clinically advanced disease and its lack of severe toxicity[13,14,15]
The initial dose schedule was as follows:

cyclophosphamide (CTX)	po	100 mg/m2	from day 1 to 14
methotrexate (MTX)	iv	40 mg/m2	on day 1 and 8
fluorouracil (FU)	iv	600 mg/m2	on day 1 and 8

Treatment was recycled on day 29. A low dose schedule (MTX 30 mg/m2, FU 400 mg/m2) was employed in postmenopausal patients older than 65 years. A dose reduction schedule was utilized in the presence of myelosuppression (leukocyte count < 4,000 per cu. mm. and/or platelet count < 130,000 per cu. mm.) on day 1 and 8 of each cycle. In the absence of treatment failure (new disease manifestations in local, regional or distant sites) CMF was continued for 12 consecutive monthly cycles. In the control group, no further treatment was given after radical mastectomy. By September 11, 1975, a total of 386 patients (radical mastectomy, or control group: 179; radical mastectomy + CMF: 207) were considered evaluable for statistical analysis. Both groups were comparable in terms of extent of axillary lymph nodes (1 to 3 and ≥ 4) and menopausal status. In the large majority of patients the primary tumor was classified as T_2 (TNM staging system). Twenty nine patients (14%) received CMF with some protocol deviation[12]. In particular, 23 patients (11%) refused to complete their adjuvant treatment program. As of February 1, 1977, the mean time on study was 29.5 months (range 16.5-44 months).

Both treatment failure and survival rates were calculated by use of the standard life-table method, thus utilizing all information accumulated up to the time of present analysis. The data are presented at 36 months, at which time a consistent fraction of the whole series is exposed at risk.

TABLE 2

MAIN CHARACTERISTICS OF STUDY PATIENTS

	CONTROL	CMF
Total randomized	181	210
Total non evaluable	2	3
Total evaluable	179	207
Ductal infiltrating ca.	88.2%	86.9%
T_2 extent	75.9%	73.9%
Nodes: 1-3	70.4%	67.7%
≥4	29.6%	32.3%
Mastectomy: radical	73.2%	71.5%
extended	26.8%	28.5%
Premenopause	48.0%	49.7%
Postmenopause	52.0%	50.3%
Off protocol	1.7%	1.0%
Protocol deviation	0	14%
Mean time on study* (months)	29.5 (16.5-44)	

*from June 1, 1973 to February 1, 1977

COMPARATIVE TREATMENT FAILURE

The total failure time distribution curves for both treatment groups are shown in Figure 1. At 36 months from mastectomy the difference remains highly significant. In the large majority of patients (control 57 of 73 or 78%; CMF 35 of 46 or 76%) new manifestations of disease were documented in distant sites and particularly in the skeleton.

Figure 2 presents the 3-year recurrence rate for premenopausal patients. The advantage of CMF therapy is evident in both nodal groups. It is noteworthy the early recurrence rate of control patients with ≥ 4 axillary nodes. In postmenopausal women (Figure 3) the difference in the failure time distribution was appreciable (but not statistically significant) during the first 24 months in the subgroup with

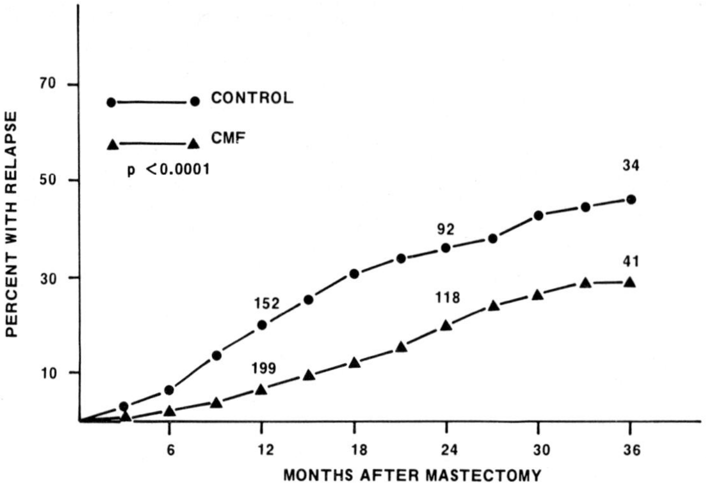

Fig. 1: Treatment failure time distribution in all patients.

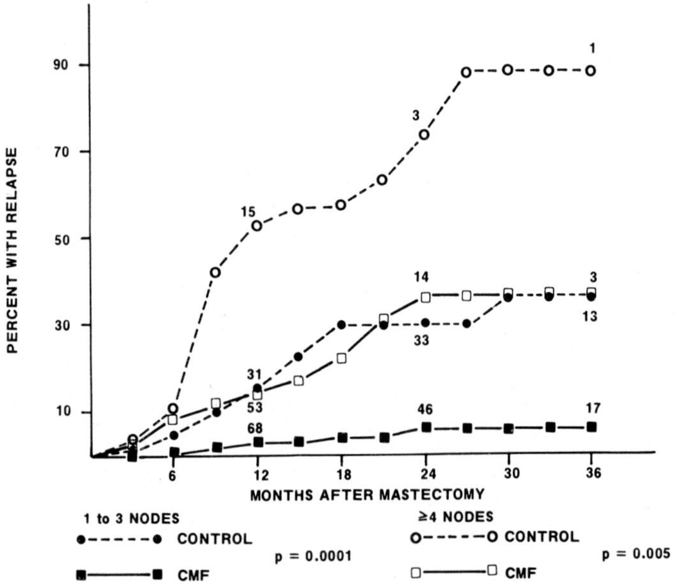

Fig. 2: Treatment failure time distribution in premenopausal patients related to degree of axillary involvement.

≥ 4 nodes. From this time on, the curves showed a progressive tendency to come closer to each other. However, it should be noted that the number of patients at risk for 36 months is very low, thus preventing a valuable comparison. In the subgroup with 1 to 3 nodes there was no difference during the first 3 years between the failure rate of control and that of CMF patients.

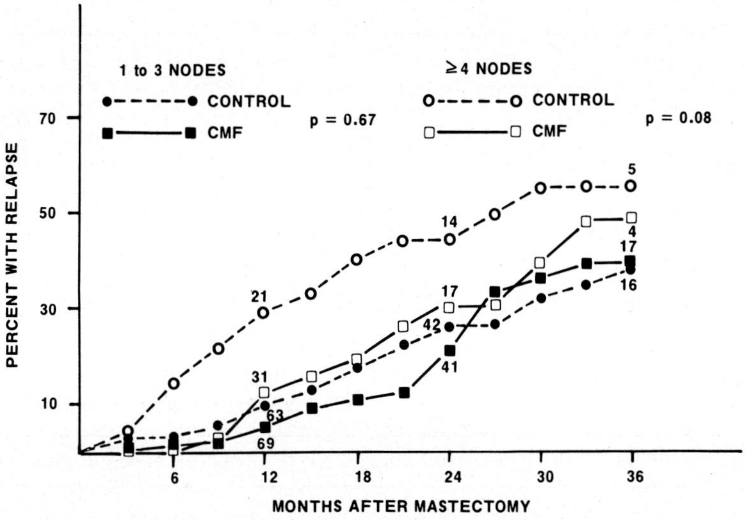

Fig. 3: Treatment failure time distribution in postmenopausal patients related to degree of axillary involvement.

Table 3 shows that in menstruating patients the incidence of relapse was not statistically influenced by CMF-induced amenorrhea.

TABLE 3

TREATMENT FAILURE AT 36 MONTHS RELATED TO DRUG-INDUCED AMENORRHEA

	%	±SE	
At risk without amenorrhea	27.2	9.9	P = 0.09
At risk with amenorrhea	10.6	3.8	

No statistical difference in treatment failure was also observed in pre and postmenopausal women receiving a high (≥75%) or a low (<75%) percent of optimal dose of CMF (Table 4).

TABLE 4

TREATMENT FAILURE AT 36 MONTHS RELATED TO PERCENT OF CMF ADMINISTERED

	%	±SE	P*
Total failure	29.2	3.9	
CMF ≥ 75%	24.6	4.9	0.09
CMF < 75%	34.5	6.4	
Premenopause			
Total failure	16.0	3.8	
CMF ≥ 75%	15.7	4.9	0.50
CMF < 75%	16.6	6.2	
Postmenopause			
Total failure	41.4	6.2	
CMF ≥ 75%	34.8	8.3	0.17
CMF < 75%	47.7	9.3	

*Calculated on time distribution SE: Standard Error

Upon relapse, secondary treatment for postmenopausal patients consisted of CMF for controls and adriamycin plus vincristine (AV) for those relapsing after CMF. In premenopausal patients castration was usually the treatment of choice followed by either CMF (controls) or AV (CMF failures). Due to particular clinical situations (e.g. brain metastases, age, performance status) or refusal to receive chemotherapy, local radiotherapy and/or additive hormonal therapy were also employed[12]. In evaluable patients, secondary systemic treatment produced complete plus partial response in 36.5% (control group) and in 22.2% (CMF group). In particular, endocrine therapy yielded the same response (21.4%) in both groups. In the control group, secondary treatment with CMF yielded complete plus partial response in 40.6% (13 of 32 patients).

The overall survival curves are presented in Figure 1. At this point of the analysis, the difference is statistically significant.

At 36 months, 20.4% of the control group have died of progressive cancer compared to 8.7% of CMF patients. The median survival of patients with relapse was similar in both groups (control 22 months, CMF 23 months).

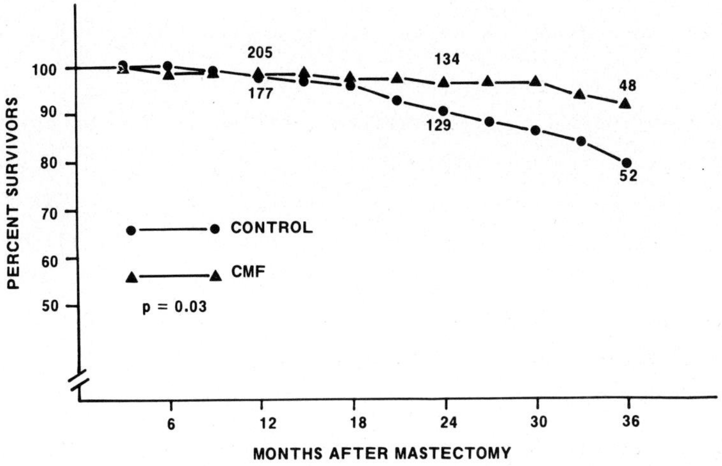

Fig. 4: Actuarial analysis of overall survival.

Table 5 presents a summary of the most important findings related to treatment failure and survival observed during the first 3 years from radical mastectomy. A second neoplasia was documented in two patients of the control group (cervical carcinoma in situ 3 months after mastectomy and melanoma after 20 months, respectively). A total of 3 patients (control 1, CMF 2) have died of cerebrovascular accident in absence of primary treatment failure.

SIDE EFFECTS

Most patients experienced gastrointestinal symptoms of nausea, vomiting and anorexia. Reversible hematosuppression represented the dose limiting factor in the large majority of patients. However, it is important to point out that marked leukopenia (leukocyte count below 2,500 per cu. mm.) occurred only in 7% of patients. Platelets fall below 75,000 per cu. mm. was observed in 19%. Stomatitis (19%) was always very mild. Transient chemical cystitis secondary to CTX occurred in 30% and hair loss in 69%. However, pronounced to almost complete alopecia was observed in only 5% of patients. CMF produced amenorrhea in 78% of menstruating women (≤ 40 years: 58%, > 40 years: 89%). In 20% suppression of menses was temporary (≤ 40 years: 63%, > 40 years 4%).

Despite a variety of side effects, prolonged CMF therapy was, in general, fairly well tolerated. The average percent of optimal dose administered to patients who have completed 12 cycles (CTX 74%, MTX 90%, FU 80%) supports the above mentioned statement. All patients received their treatment in the out patient clinic, most continued to work while on therapy, and none had to be readmitted to the hospital because of severe toxicity[12].

TABLE 5

PRIMARY TREATMENT FAILURE AND OVERALL SURVIVAL AT 36 MONTHS

(Actuarial analysis)

	CONTROL		CMF		P*
	%	±SE	%	±SE	
Total failure	46.2	4.2	29.2	3.9	< 0.0001
Nodes 1-3	37.8	5.0	23.2	4.4	< 0.01
≥ 4	67.0	7.6	42.8	8.4	< 0.001
Survival	79.6	3.9	91.3	3.0	0.03
Premenopause					
Total failure	48.0	5.9	16.0	3.8	< 0.00001
Nodes 1-3	36.0	6.6	6.3	3.1	0.0001
≥ 4	87.1	5.8	35.9	9.0	0.005
Survival	76.7	6.6	97.3	1.6	0.06
Postmenopause					
Total failure	44.0	6.1	41.4	6.2	0.17
Nodes 1-3	38.8	7.2	39.2	7.3	0.67
≥ 4	55.8	10.4	48.6	12.9	0.08
Survival	82.0	4.9	85.7	5.3	0.19

*Calculated on time distribution SE: Standard Error

COMMENT

Traditionally the role of chemotherapy in breast cancer was that of palliative treatment for patients with either recurrent disease after surgery and/or radiotherapy or with primary advanced neoplasia which have failed endocrine treatment. Based on the principles learned from experimental animal tumor models a more biological approach seems justified[3]. During the past few years most research clinicians have become convinced that the best chance to improve the cure rate is first to identy those patients with high probability of having distant micrometastases at the time of curative surgery and then to apply a prolonged systemic treatment. In fact, when the metastatic foci are small (10^8 or less) the chances of cure by adequate chemotherapy become high[8]. Adjuvant treatment should be carefully planned and, for the time being, the effects of any new therapy are best test ed under a controlled basis.

Present updated results confirm once more the therapeutic advantage of combined surgery and prolonged combination chemotherapy. Not only was the 3-year relapse rate markedly decreased, but the more recent findings have indicated that also the overall survival was significantly improved in patients given CMF compared to controls treated with the conventional surgical approach. The favourable effect of adjuvant treatment was not evident in all subsets. In premenopausal patients the free interval was significantly prolonged irrespective of the number of axillary lymph nodes. In contrast, postmenopausal patients appeared, in general, less responsive to systemic treatment. The subset showing aggressive disease (≥ 4 positive nodes) showed some advantage by treatment with 12 cycles of CMF, while the relapse rate in women with slow growing tumor (1 to 3 positive nodes) was not apparently influenced by the treatment schedule utilized in this study.

At the present moment, the actual reasons for the different response to CMF remain essentially unknown. As already mentioned, there is a possibility that the rapid growth rate of micrometastases during the first 3 years from mastectomy in the four node groups has played an important role in the response to chemotherapy. CMF could have been more efficacious in the subset showing a rapid progressive cancer compared to that with slow growing tumor. If this hypothesis is true then, contrary to what has been observed in the presence of gross metastatic disease, postmenopausal women would require a more aggressive and probably a more prolonged adjuvant chemotherapy. It is also conceivable that in premenopausal patients some, yet undefined, endocrine factors have favourably contributed to the therapeutic effect of CMF. However, present findings have not indicated a positive statistical correlation between incidence of amenorrhea and percent of recurrence. Clearly, only time and different types of controlled trials will provide a more definite answer to these questions.

The aim of our trial as well as that of NSABP[16] was to demonstrate that the biological concept of adjuvant therapy in high-risk patients with operable breast cancer had clinical validity. In our opinion, this concept was successfully tested. The information provided by our short-term follow up will certainly stimulate new controlled studies aimed to modulate therapy also in relation to menopausal status and number of axillary nodes. Many questions remain open, and they are not only related to the search of optimal treatment for any given subset of patients. In fact, the optimal treatment duration and the incidence of long-term effects are some practical questions to be answered.

As result of early findings observed in new adjuvant studies[10,12,16], modern oncologists can look at the treatment of primary breast cancer with a more strategic attitude. In fact, the conquest of minimal residual disease in high-risk patients appears to be a dominant factor in the contemporary strategic approach for most neoplastic diseases, including breast cancer. In pediatric neoplasias (Wilms's tumor, osteosarcoma, Ewing's sarcoma, rhabdomyosarcoma), in Hodgkin's disease, and probably also in malignant melanoma, there is a substantial evidence that the initial combined clinical efforts are significantly improving both the recurrence rate and the overall survival.

In breast cancer controlled clinical trials were started later and, therefore, long-term results from combined local-systemic approaches are not yet available. However, numerous studies are in progress all over the world, and it is logical to expect that, hopefully, within the next decade or so, a definite progress in the cure rate will be made.

For the time being, only patients with positive axillary lymph nodes are candidate for systemic adjuvant therapy. This treatment should be carried out by medical oncologists or, at least, closely supervised by qualified centers. At the present time, two factors obviate the use of adjuvant chemotherapy in patients with negative nodes. The first concerns the limited follow up period of patients currently being given adjuvant chemotherapy. Actually, the usefulness of systemic therapy should be evaluated at a minimum follow up period of 5 years. The second concerns the lack of clinicopathologic guidelines to select those patients with considerable risk for developing distant metastases. Prolonged systemic chemotherapy is not devoid of potential long-term dangerous effects; further, overtreatment must be avoided in women likely to have been cured by local methods. Recently, F.A. Nime et al.[17] have reported the results of a histopathologic study having potentially important therapeutic implications. The authors findings clearly indicate that in women treated by radical mastectomy with negative axillary nodes, 43% of those with tumor cells in intramammary lymphatic vessels developed visceral metastases compared to 4% of control women who had no intramammary tumor emboli. If this important observation is confirmed in a larger series, clinicians could base the selection of high-risk patients suitable for adjuvant chemotherapy on an objective prognostic parameter which can be applied within the context of routine histopathologic examination.

ACKNOWLEDGMENTS

The work reported herein was partially supported by Contract NO1-CM-33714 with DCT, NCI, NIH.

REFERENCES

1. Martin, D.S. et al. (1974) Cancer Chemother. Rep. 4, 13-24.
2. Carter, S.K. (1976) Cancer Treat. Rev. 3, 141-174.
3. Carbone, P.P. (1976) Int. J. Radiation Oncology Biol. Phys. 1, 759-767.
4. Bonadonna, G. et al. (1976) Breast Cancer: Trends in Research and Treatment (J.C. Heuson, W.H. Mattheiem, M. Rosencweig Eds) Raven Press, New York.
5. Tormey, D.C. (1975) Cancer 36, 881-892.
6. Fisher, B. et al. (1975) Surg. Gynecol. Obstet. 140, 528-534.
7. Valagussa, P. et al. (1977) Tumori (in press).
8. Schabel, F.M. Jr. (1975) Cancer 35, 15-24.
9. De Vita, V.T. et al. (1975) Cancer 35, 98-110.
10. Bonadonna, G. et al. (1976) N. Engl. J. Med. 294, 405-410.
11. Rossi, A. et al. (1977) Recent Res. Cancer Res. (in press).
12. Bonadonna, G. et al. (1977) Cancer (in press).
13. Canellos, G.P. et al. (1974) Br. Med. J. 1, 218-220.
14. Canellos, G.P. et al. (1976) Cancer 38, 1882-1886.
15. Brambilla, C. et al. (1976) Br. Med. J. 1, 801-804.
16. Fisher, B. et al. (1975) N. Engl. J. Med. 292, 117-122.
17. Nime, F.A. et al. (1977) Am. J. Surg. Pat. 1 (in press).

Adjuvant Therapy of Cancer, S.E. Salmon and S.E. Jones eds.

OVARIAN IRRADIATION AND PREDNISONE FOLLOWING SURGERY FOR CARCINOMA OF THE BREAST

J.W. Meakin, W.E.C. Allt, F.A. Beale, T.C. Brown,
R.S. Bush, R.M. Clark, P.J. Fitzpatrick, N.V. Hawkins,
R.D.T. Jenkin, J.F. Pringle, and W.D. Rider
Princess Margaret Hospital, Toronto, Canada
J.L. Hayward and R.D. Bulbrook
Imperial Cancer Research Fund, London, U.K.

SUMMARY

Following surgery and regional radiotherapy for operable carcinoma of the breast in premenopausal women, ovarian irradiation (2000 rads in 5 daily fractions) plus prednisone (7.5 mg per day) results in delayed recurrence and prolonged survival.

INTRODUCTION

Because some recurrent breast cancers regress following therapeutic castration, several clinical trials have been carried out to test the value of prophylactic ovarian ablation as part of primary treatment.

In the Manchester Trial[1] ovarian irradiation (450r in 1 fraction), in premenopausal patients with histologically negative and positive axillary nodes, delayed the appearance of distant metastases (P = 0.04) but did not significantly prolong survival (P = 0.07) at 10 years.

In the Oslo Trial[2] ovarian irradiation (1000r in 6 daily fractions) in premenopausal (histologically positive axillary nodes) and postmenopausal (histologically negative and positive axillary nodes) patients delayed recurrence and also prolonged survival at 7 years but the differences were small.

In the Trial of the National Surgical Adjuvant Breast Group[3] oophorectomy did not result in a significant delay in recurrence nor prolongation in survival during 3 to 5 years of follow up in premenopausal patients who had either histologically negative or positive axillary nodes.

Because of the ambiguity resulting from these trials the following study was begun in 1965 to test the hypothesis that prophylactic ovarian irradiation, with or without prednisone, could not only delay recurrence but also prolong survival.

MATERIALS AND METHODS

From 1965 to 1972, following mastectomy, premenopausal and postmenopausal patients, aged 35-70 years, with or without histologically positive axillary nodes, received irradiation to the chest wall and regional nodal areas. They were then randomized to receive no further treatment (NT), or ovarian irradiation to a dose of 2000 rads in 5 days (R), or (if 45 years or more) ovarian irradiation in the same dosage plus prednisone, 7.5 mg daily (R + P) for up to 5 years. Patients, entered on study, have been followed for up to 10 years. Patients were considered premenopausal if their last menses had occurred within 6 months of the date of surgery. Patients who had had a hysterectomy, but not an oophorectomy, were considered premenopausal up to the age of 50 years.

The generalized Wilcoxon Test[4] has been used to determine the significance of differences in the results.

RESULTS

Of 779 randomized patients 23 were ineligible by protocol and are omitted from all analyses. An additional 44 patients were eligible by protocol but did not receive the randomly-assigned treatment; analyses of the data with or without these patients included has not affected the results. Therefore the following data relate to 712 randomized patients who were eligible by protocol and did receive the assigned treatment.

For reporting the patients are divided into 3 groups: (a) premenopausal less than 45 years of age, (b) premenopausal 45 years or more in age, and (c) postmenopausal.

Premenopausal patients less than 45 years of age: In this group (35-44 years) only clinical stages (TNM) II and III were entered, and were randomized only between NT and R. The two groups were comparable for age and stage. Histologically positive axillary lymph nodes were identified in 87% of the NT group and in 98% of the R group.

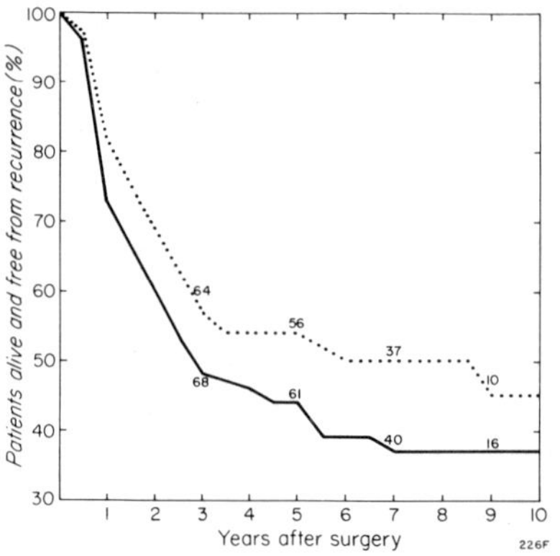

Fig. 1. Premenopausal patients less than 45 yrs. NT (70 patients)———
R (67 patients)......
(NT vs R, P = 0.21)

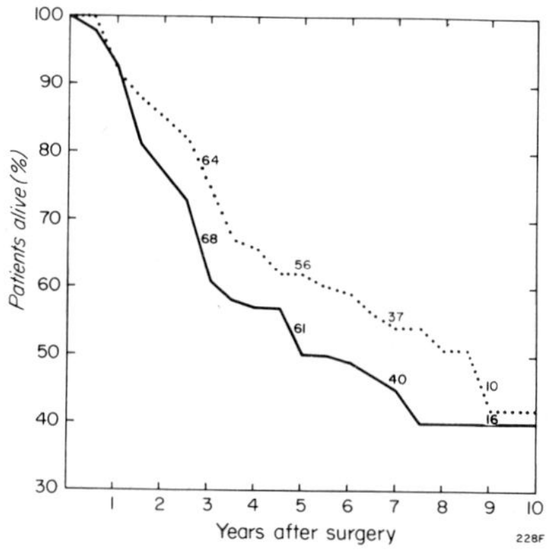

Fig. 2. Premenopausal patients less than 45 yrs. NT (70 patients)———
R (67 patients)......
(NT vs R, P = 0.21)

In Figures 1 and 2 are presented the recurrence-free and survival curves (actuarial). Numbers of patients followed to specific times are recorded on the graphs. While there is a persistent delay in recurrence and prolongation of survival the differences are not statistically significant (P = 0.21 for both Figures).

Separate analyses of the histologically node-positive patients only from Figures 1 and 2 reveals a similar degree of delay in recurrence and improvement in survival between the NT and R groups as follows: (a) Figure 1, P = 0.13; (b) Figure 2, P = 0.2

Premenopausal patients 45 years or more: In this group clinical stages (TNM) I, II, and III were randomized between NT, R, or R + P. The three groups were comparable for age and stage. Histologically positive axillary nodes were identified in 75% of the patients in all three groups.

The actuarial recurrence-free and survival curves are shown in Figures 3 and 4. Numbers of patients, followed to specific times, are recorded on the graphs.

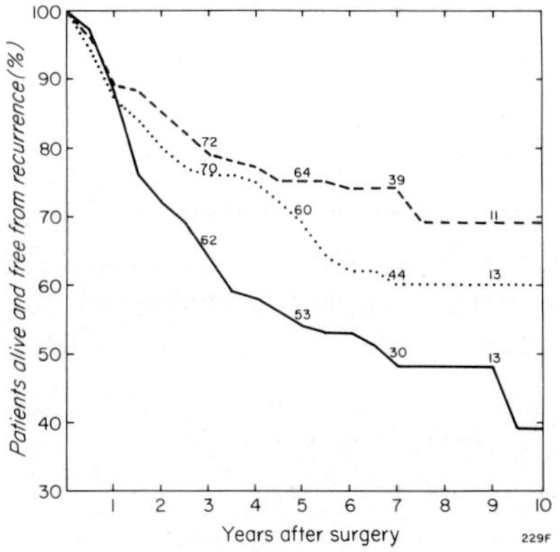

Fig. 3. Premenopausal patients 45 yrs. or more. NT (64 patients)———
R (71 patients)··········
R + P (73 patients)----------
(NT vs R, P = 0.15; NT vs R + P, P = 0.01; R vs R + P, P = 0.24)

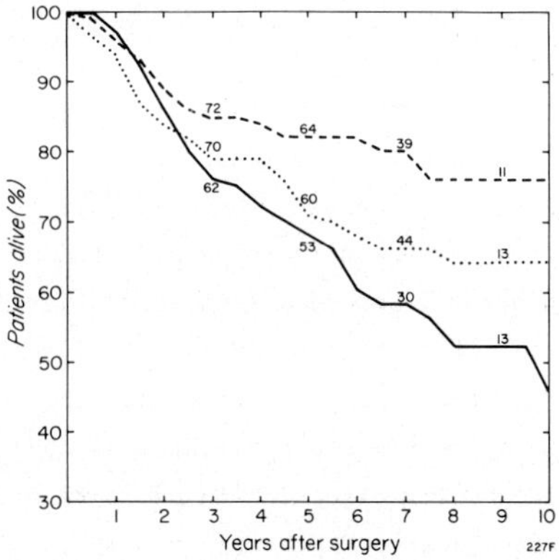

Fig. 4. Premenopausal patients 45 yrs. or more. NT (64 patients)———
R (71 patients)··········
R + P (73 patients)----------
(NT vs R, P = 0.46; NT vs R + P, P = 0.02; R vs R + P, P = 0.13)

In Figure 3 while R and R + P are delaying recurrence, only R + P is doing so to a statistically significant degree (NT vs R + P, P = 0.01).

In Figure 4 R and R + P are prolonging survival, but only R + P is doing so significantly over the NT group (P = 0.02).

If only the patients with histologically positive axillary nodes (75% in each group) from Figures 3 and 4 are analyzed the significance of the differences between the NT and R + P groups decreases to: (a) Figure 3, P = 0.03; (b) Figure 4, P = 0.06

Postmenopausal patients: No differences in time to recurrence nor in survival could be demonstrated between the NT, R and R + P groups.

DISCUSSION

These data are in agreement with the Manchester[1] and Oslo[2] Trials in demonstrating an apparent delay in recurrence and prolongation of survival after adjuvant ovarian irradiation which were not statistically significant in this study.

The lack of agreement with the results of the NSABP[3] Trial of prophylactic oophorectomy is possibly the effect of chance, or that an irradiated ovary may result in a different physiologic state from that after a surgical oophorectomy. Alternatively, further follow-up data from the NSABP[3] Trial may demonstrate some value for surgical oophorectomy, for it may be noted that the effect of ovarian ablation in our study did not become firm until after 3 to 5 years of follow up.

However the data of this study indicate that the addition of small doses of prednisone to ovarian irradiation produces significant delay in recurrence and prolongation in survival in premenopausal patients. Whether the prednisone produced its effect by suppressing estrogen of adrenal origin, or by some other mechanism is not known. Other possible mechanisms include a reduction in prolactin secretion (perhaps mediated by reduced estrogen production), immunological factors, or direct anti-tumour effects. Again it is emphasized that the effect of ovarian irradiation plus prednisone did not become definite until after 3 to 5 years of follow up.

One of the important features of these data is that ovarian ablation and prednisone were effective in patients with histologically positive axillary nodes to a degree comparable to the published data for adjuvant melphalan[5] in premenopausal patients. Thus it would seem rational in future studies to examine the role of adjuvant hormonal therapy, both as a complement to, and as an alternative to adjuvant chemotherapy.

ACKNOWLEDGEMENTS

The authors are grateful to the Ontario Cancer Treatment and Research Foundation and the Imperial Cancer Research Fund for their financial support of this study. We thank Dr. G. DeBoer, Mrs. J. Reid and colleagues for their statistical and clerical assistance.

REFERENCES

1. Cole, M.P. (1968) In Forrest, A.P.M. and Kunkler, P.B. (Eds.) Prognostic Factors in Breast Cancer, pp. 146-156 (from Proceedings of First Tenovus Symposium, Cardiff). Edinburgh: E & S Livingston.
2. Nissen-Meyer (1968) in Forrest; A.P.M. and Kunkler, P.B. (Eds.) Prognostic Factors in Breast Cancer, pp. 139-163 (from Proceedings of First Tenovus Symposium, Cardiff). Edinburgh: E & S Livingston.
3. Ravdin, R.G. et al. (1970) Surgery Gynec. Obstet. 131: 1055.
4. Gehan, E.A. (1965) Biometrika 52: 203.
5. Fisher, B. et al. (1975) New Eng. J. Med. 292: 117.

Adjuvant Therapy of Cancer, S.E. Salmon and S.E. Jones eds.

THE EFFECT OF ADJUVANT CHEMOTHERAPY ON ENDOCRINE FUNCTION IN PATIENTS WITH OPERABLE BREAST CANCER

R.D.Rubens, R.D.Bulbrook, D.Y.Wang,
R.K.Knight, J.L.Hayward, H.Bush,
D.George, D.Crowther, R.A.Sellwood.

Imperial Cancer Research Fund Breast Cancer Unit,
Guy's Hospital, London;
Department of Clinical Endocrinology,
Imperial Cancer Research Fund Laboratories, London;
Departments of Medical Oncology and Surgery,
University of Manchester:
England

INTRODUCTION

Optimism has been engendered that the prognosis of operable breast cancer may be improved by adjuvant chemotherapy. Promising results have been shown with L-phenylalanine mustard (L-pam)[1] and cyclophosphamide, methotrexate and 5-fluorouracil in combination (CMF)[2]. The authors of these reports have been careful to stress that their results, at the present concerned only with the short-term recurrence-free interval, are preliminary.

Considerable difficulties exist in finding the optimum adjuvant chemotherapy for breast cancer because clinical trials are based on empirical and theoretical considerations and many years must elapse for effects on survival to be shown or for long-term toxic effects of the therapy to be identified. Furthermore, it is now known that some forms of prophylactic endocrine treatment lead to a significant improvement in both the recurrence-free interval and survival in patients with operable breast cancer[3].

It is important that, during the course of clinical trials of adjuvant therapy, attempts should be made to identify underlying mechanisms of action. One approach is to study the effect cytotoxic drugs may have on endocrine function and to determine whether any beneficial results from chemotherapy might be partially explained by such effects. L-pam has been shown to result in a significant lengthening of recurrence-free interval in pre-menopausal patients only[1], suggesting that the drug's effect may be mediated by suppression of ovarian function. A similar trend has now been reported with CMF[4]

Because L-pam is administered orally, is relatively free from subjective side-effects, and the results reported have been unexpectedly good[1] (in view of the relatively poor activity of L-pam in advanced disease[5]), this study requires confirmation. A trial to undertake this was started at Guy's Hospital in May 1975 which, in March 1976 was combined with a similar study in Manchester; concurrent endocrine investigations are being done.

PATIENTS AND METHODS

Patients with T_{1a}-$T_{3a}N_{1b}M_0$ breast cancer[6] are randomised, after mastectomy with axillary clearance, to receive either no further treatment or courses of L-pam 6mg/m^2 daily for 5 days every 6 weeks, starting on the 12th post-operative day and continued for 2 years or 16 courses (whichever is sooner). In Manchester this forms part of a trial comparing no treatment, L-pam and CMF.

Pre-operatively, 10 days post-operatively, and on the first day of the 3rd, 6th and 12th courses of L-pam, blood is taken for the estimation of serum oestrone, oestradiol, progesterone, free dehydroepiandrosterone and its sulphate, testosterone, Δ_5-androstene-3β-17β-diol, Δ_4-androstene-dione, cortisol, follicle-stimulating hormone, luteinising hormone and prolactin. All assays are carried out by standard radioimmunoassay.

In this paper, preliminary results for serum oestradiol, progesterone and prolactin are reported. The oestradiol and progesterone results are given in pg/ml and ng/ml respectively. The prolactin results are expressed in mU/L using the Medical Research Council (UK) working standard 71/222 which may be converted to ng/ml by dividing by a factor of 20.

RESULTS

At the 31st December, 1976, 149 patients had entered the trial with a mean follow-up time of 7.8 months (range $<$1-19). It is, therefore, premature to report results on recurrence-free interval or length of survival.

1. Prolactin. The serum prolactin levels in pre-menopausal women in the control and L-pam groups are compared in Fig.1. There are no apparent effects of L-pam on peripheral prolactin concentrations and a similar lack of effect was found in post-menopausal women (Fig.2). It is striking that, in both the control and treated patients, there is an unexpected increase in the number of high prolactin values following mastectomy.

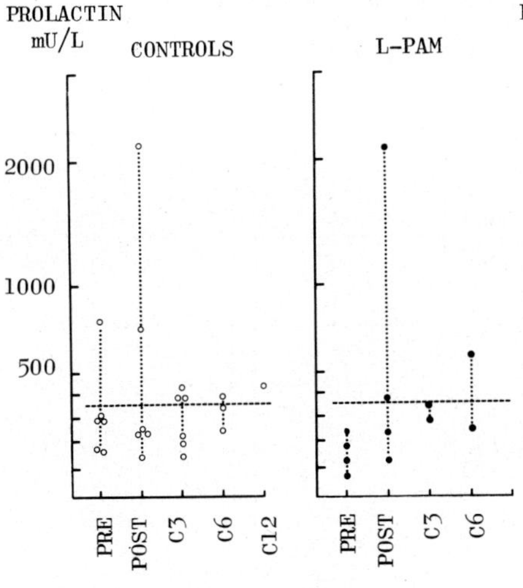

Fig.1. Serum prolactin levels in pre-menopausal women*

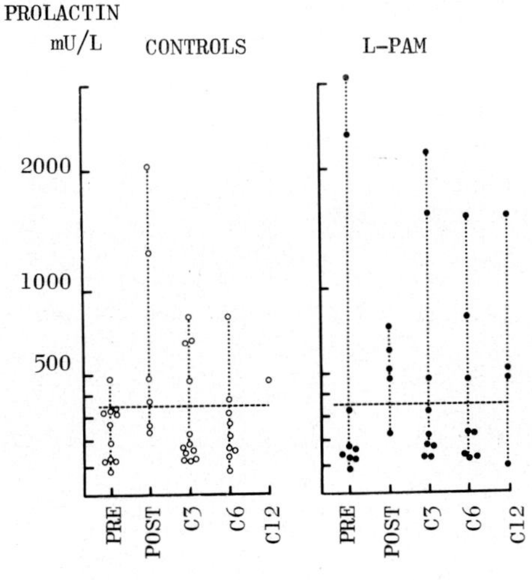

Fig.2. Serum prolactin levels in post-menopausal women*

*'Pre' and 'Post' refer to 1 day before and 10 days after mastectomy: 'C3', 'C6' and 'C12' indicate day 1 of the 3rd, 6th and 12th courses of L-pam and the same follow-up times in control patients. The horizontal line shows the upper limit of the normal range.

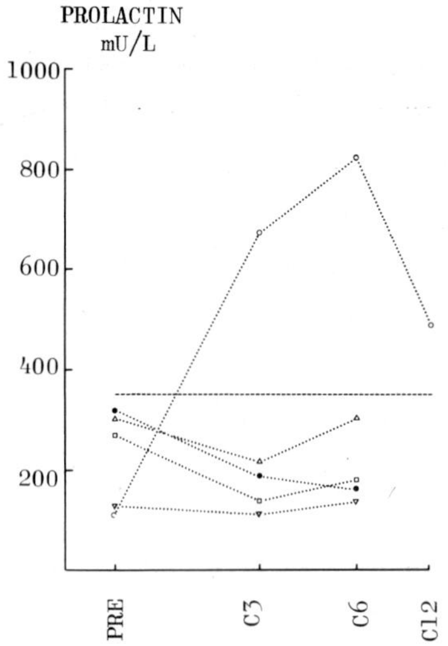

Fig.3. Serial prolactin levels in control patients*

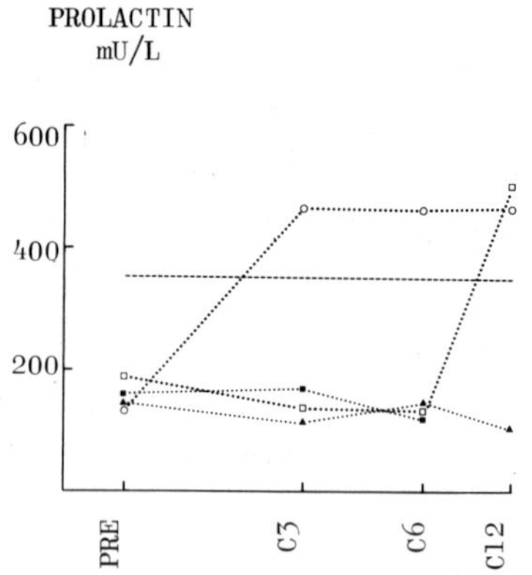

Fig.4. Serial prolactin levels in patients treated with L-pam*

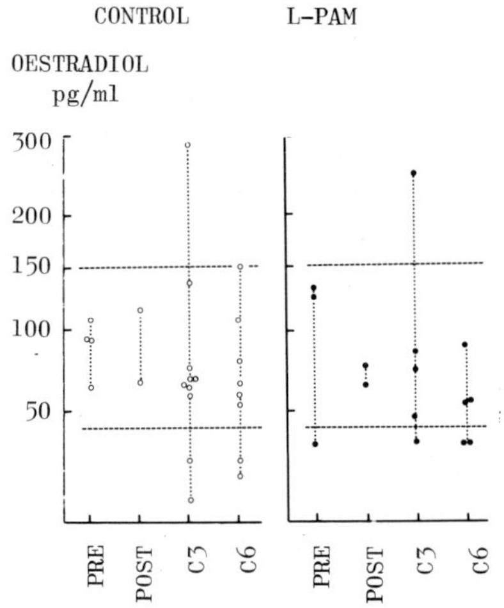

Fig.5. Serum oestradiol levels in pre-menopausal women*

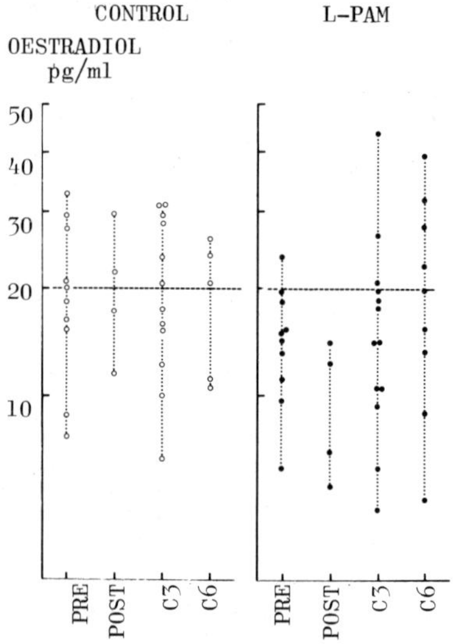

Fig.6. Serum oestradiol levels in post-menopausal women*

---

*See footnote on previous page.

In 9 patients, sequential serum analyses have been completed. These are shown in Figs 3 and 4 which show that, in both the control group and patients treated with L-pam, serum prolactin levels remained unchanged in most, but that one patient in each group showed a marked and sustained increase in these levels.

2. Oestradiol. L-pam had no discernable effect on the levels of plasma oestradiol in pre-menopausal women (Fig.5). Since the blood specimens were obtained at any time in the menstrual cycle, it is difficult to determine what the normal range should be, but levels between 40 and 150 pg/ml would be compatible with normal ovarian function. The majority of the results fall between these limits in both the treated and control groups. There is thus no evidence, so far, that L-pam depresses ovarian function as far as oestradiol is concerned.

The results of serum oestradiol determinations for post-menopausal women are shown in Fig.6. Again, there is no evidence of any effect of L-pam on peripheral levels of this oestrogen. The range for plasma oestradiol in normal post-menopausal women is 0-20 pg/ml[6]. In the control and L-pam treated groups, the majority of the values fall within this range, but in both groups a substantial number of values lie above this range.

3. Progesterone. Because of the small numbers and the uncontrolled time at which blood specimens were taken during the menstrual cycle, it is not possible to state with certainty what effect L-pam has on progesterone levels in pre-menopausal women. However, 3 out of 12 control women had levels indicative of corpus luteum activity ($>$3ng/ml) during the treatment period compared to none in 6 patients treated with L-pam.

In post-menopausal women 68 progesterone estimations were done and there was no indication that treatment with L-pam had any effect on progesterone production.

4. Incidence of amenorrhoea. Information concerning menstrual function for 24 patients, pre-menopausal at operation (13 controls and 11 receiving L-pam), is available. The control patients have all continued to menstruate in contrast to those receiving L-pam, 7 of whom ceased to menstruate within 5 months of operation.

DISCUSSION

Endocrine function of 33 patients in a controlled study of adjuvant chemotherapy in breast cancer has been studied. It is too early to draw definitive conclusions but the preliminary findings do not show that L-pam has any marked effect on the serum levels of prolactin or oestradiol in either pre- or post-menopausal women. If the prolactin levels, before mastectomy, of the pre- and post-menopausal women are considered together (Figs 1 and 2), only 2 of 17 patients in the control group and 2 of 13 in the L-pam group had prolactin levels above the upper limits for a normal population. After operation, 18 if the 44 control values were raised as were 16 of the 34 values for women treated with L-pam. Similarly in post-menopausal patients, 13 of 40 post-mastectomy serum oestradiol values were above the normal range (Fig.4). These unexpected findings need further investigation.

In contrast to the lack of effect of L-pam on the above hormone levels, the incidence of amenorrhoea in patients receiving L-pam is higher than in controls suggesting that this drug may indeed affect ovarian function. The preliminary results of progesterone assays are compatible with this suggestion. The possibility of the induction of ovarian failure by cytotoxic drugs has previously been discussed[8] and it is notable that the preliminary results of adjuvant CMF have suggested that the beneficial results in pre-menopausal women, were greater when amenorrhoea occurred[4]. Furthermore, it is now apparent that prophylactic oophorectomy results in an improvement both in recurrence-free interval and survival after mastectomy[3]. It is therefore, reasonable to speculate that the preliminary beneficial results of adjuvant chemotherapy so far obtained[1,2], could be attributable in part to a suppressive effect of cytotoxic drugs on ovarian function. The lack of effect for post-menopausal women is similarly explained.

Current knowledge about the effects of cytotoxic chemotherapy on endocrine function in patients with breast cancer is fragmentory, and the endocrine studies currently in progress with the Guy's/ Manchester trial of adjuvant chemotherapy might clarify the situation.

SUMMARY

The preliminary results of endocrine studies in 33 patients on a controlled trial of L-pam as an adjuvant in the treatment of operable breast cancer are described. This drug has not been demonstrated to have any effect on serum oestradiol or prolactin levels, but there appears to be a higher incidence of amenorrhoea in patients receiving L-pam compared with controls.

REFERENCES

1. Fisher, B. et al (1975) New Engl. J. Med., 292, 117
2. Bonadonna, G. et al (1976) New Engl. J. Med. 294, 405
3. Meakin, J.W. (1977) in this volume
4. Bonadonna,G. et al (1977) Cancer, in press
5. Canellos, G.P. et al (1976) Cancer, 38, 1882
6. TNM Classification of Malignant Tumours, UICC,Geneva, 1974
7. Bulbrook,R.D. et al (1976) Europ. J. Cancer, 12, 725
8. Schein, P.S. and Winokur, S.H. (1975) Ann. intern. Med. 82,84

Adjuvant Therapy of Cancer, S.E. Salmon and S.E. Jones eds.
© 1977 Elsevier/North-Holland Biomedical Press, Amsterdam

ADJUVANT CHEMOTHERAPY AND CHEMOIMMUNOTHERAPY FOR BREAST CANCER

Frank C. Sparks, Beth E. Meyerowitz, Kenneth P. Ramming, Richard W. Wolk, Myron H. Goldsmith, Stephen R. Lemkin, Irene K. Spears and Donald L. Morton

Division of Oncology, Department of Surgery
University of California, Los Angeles, CA 90024, U.S.A.

INTRODUCTION

Adjuvant chemotherapy can delay early recurrence after operation in stage 2 carcinoma of the breast.[1,2] Our own adjuvant program is designed to determine if adjuvant chemoimmunotherapy is more effective than chemotherapy alone in reducing recurrence and improving survival.

Why have we combined immunotherapy with chemotherapy? Numerous studies suggest that a woman's immune response to her breast cancer may be an important factor in determining survival. The natural history of breast cancer suggests a host-immune response. Some patients have a 10- to 20-year tumor-free interval followed by the sudden appearance of rapid tumor growth. Tumor-associated antigens have been found in human breast cancer. Antibodies against these antigens have been shown by several techniques and have been found to correlate with the clinical course.[3] Lymphoid infiltration of the primary tumor and sinus histiocytosis or the regional nodes also correlate with survival.

Immunotherapy with BCG given after operation has been shown to increase the survival rate in both animals and humans. The anti-tumor activity of BCG is probably mediated by nonspecific stimulation of the immune system. In our experience, the intratumor injection of BCG appears to be an effective method for controlling local recurrence of breast cancer in selected patients.

Chemoimmunotherapy with anticancer drugs and BCG is a logical combination of 2 forms of therapy that have different mechanisms of action and no overlapping toxicity. Immunotherapy also has the potential of reducing the immunosuppressive effects of chemotherapy. In patients with stage 3 breast cancer, chemoimmunotherapy with 5-fluorouracil, adriamycin, and cytoxan (FAC) plus BCG is thought to be more effective than FAC alone.[4]

MATERIALS AND METHODS

All women who underwent a conventional or modified radical mastectomy for potentially curable breast carcinoma and who had histologic proof of metastases in

1 or more axillary nodes were considered eligible for adjuvant treatment. Since publication of our preliminary results,[3] a third arm has been added to our protocol such that patients are now randomized to receive cytoxan, methotrexate, and 5-fluorouracil (CMF), CMF plus BCG, or CMF plus BCG plus an irradiated allogeneic tumor cell vaccine.

Specific details of the program have been given elsewhere.[3] Twelve cycles of CMF are given over 64 weeks. The first 4 cycles are repeated at 4-week intervals and the last 8 cycles at 6-week intervals. Dosage modification is made for age and myelosuppression. Chemotherapy is started within 10 weeks of operation. In compliance with federal and local guidelines for informed consent, nonstudy alternatives are discussed with each patient.

Tice strain BCG is given by the multiple-puncture tine technique as described every week for 11 weeks and then every other week for 2 years. The tumor cell vaccine consists of 3.5×10^7 cells from each of 3 breast carcinoma cell lines: MDA-MB-231, MDA-MB-157, and NBL-374B. These cell lines were all derived from malignant pleural effusions in women with breast cancer. Cells are grown in tissue culture, mixed, divided in ampules of 1.05×10^8 cells, program frozen in liquid nitrogen at 1^oC/min to -150^oC, irradiated with 10,000 r, and stored in liquid nitrogen at -196^oC. The tumor cell vaccine is then thawed in a 37° water bath and given intradermally every week for 11 weeks and then every other week for 2 years.

Followup studies included physical examination and liver function tests every 8 weeks. Chest roentgenograms and bone scans were obtained every 4 months. The end point of the study was the first evidence of treatment failure, represented by the development of a second primary carcinoma in the contralateral breast, distant metastases, or local recurrence from the chest wall or in the axilla.

The first 100 patients to enter our study are fairly evenly divided between those who are premenopausal (47) versus those who are postmenopausal (53) and those with 1 to 3 positive nodes (48) versus 4 or more positive nodes (52). The great majority of the patients have received a modified radical mastectomy (80) and no postoperative radiation therapy (91)

RESULTS

Table 1 lists the results of the first 100 patients. The average followup after operation is 14 months with a range of 2 to 32 months. The followup is shorter in the patients who have received CMF alone since that arm of the protocol was added in the past year. Seven patients have developed recurrence and 6 of these have 4 or more nodes involved with metastases. Four patients under the age of 50 have developed recurrence compared to 3 patients who were 50 or more years of age. Four patients have died from metastases.

TABLE 1

RECURRENCE : FIRST 100 PATIENTS

Treatment	Number of Patients	Followup (months)	Nodes		Age		Total
			1-3	≥4	<50	≥50	
CMF	13	7 (2-10)	0	0	0	0	0
CMF+BCG	49	15 (2-30)	0	2	1	1	2
CMF+BCG+TCV	38	16 (3-32)	1	4	3	2	5
Total	100	14 (2-32)	1	6	4	3	7

Table 2 compares the recurrence rate in our patients with that reported by Bonadonna et al.[1] The average followup after operation was 14 months in each study. The recurrence rate in our study is comparable to that reported by Bonadonna in his patients treated with CMF. In both studies, the recurrence rate in patients treated with CMF with or without immunotherapy is lower than in the control group. This is especially noticeable in the patients with 4 or more nodes where the recurrence rate in the control group was 41% compared to 9% and 12% in Bonadonna's and our patients respectively.

More recently Bonadonna, now with an average followup after operation of 22 months, reported that in postmenopausal patients there was no longer a significant difference between the control patients and those treated with CMF alone. This observation brings Bonadonna's date more in line with that reported by Fisher[2] wherein the increase in probability of remaining disease-free in postmenopausal women approached but did not reach statistical significance. Our own data do not yet show a difference between pre- and postmenopausal women.

TABLE 2

PERCENT RECURRENCE AFTER ADJUVANT THERAPY

Study Group	Nodes		Age		Total
	1-3	≥4	<50	≥50	
Control[1]	17	41	23	25	24
CMF[1]	4	9	6	4	5
UCLA	2	12	8	6	7

Why is adjuvant chemotherapy with thiotepa, L-PAM, and CMF more effective in premenopausal than in postmenopausal women? These drugs may decrease ovarian but not adrenal estrogen output. Both Bonadonna and Fisher have discussed and discounted this possibility. Indeed, the NSABP prospective randomized study showed that prophylactic oophorectomy did not convey significant advantage. Other evidence suggests that there may be a role for adjuvant hormonal therapy, at least in postmenopausal women. Dao[5] reported that adjuvant adrenalectomy delayed recurrence in postmenopausal women. Estradiol receptor protein is found more frequently and in greater quantity in breast cancer of postmenopausal women.

Another alternative explanation for the increased effectiveness of adjuvant therapy in premenopausal women has been suggested by Salmon at this symposium. Estrogen may increase the growth fraction of breast cancer, thereby making chemotherapy with cell-cycle-specific agents more effective. In support of this is the positive correlation between high growth fraction as expressed by thymidine index and the complete response rate in adult acute leukemia.

Tumor cell growth kinetics indicate that the growth fraction is inversely related to population size. The growth of solid tumors is characterized by a progressively longer tumor-doubling time as the tumor increases in size. The theoretical implication of this observation is that cure by chemotherapeutic drugs is more likely in an adjuvant setting with microscopic disease than when the tumor has clinically recurred.

Bonadonna's data on postmenopausal women suggests that at least in these patients there may be no substance to this theory. Fifty-three percent of women with metastatic breast carcinoma responded to combination chemotherapy with CMF with a median duration of remission of 25 weeks. If the response rate and duration of remission with CMF in the adjuvant setting is the same as in the treatment of metastatic disease, one would expect data similar to that which Bonadonna reported.

What then will immunotherapy do to an adjuvant chemotherapy regimen? If immunotherapy increases the duration of remission then we would expect to see a greater delay in recurrence than that observed by Bonadonna with chemotherapy alone. Our own study should answer this question after an additional followup of approximately 24 to 36 months.

Has the delay in recurrence compensated for the toxicity, inconvenience, and expense of chemotherapy and chemoimmunotherapy? The side effects from the chemotherapy and chemoimmunotherapy have been discussed in detail previously. These include fatigue, anorexia, nausea, vomiting, weight gain, alopecia, and myelosuppression. The expense of a CMF program in our area runs between $2,500 and $3,500 per patient for the first year. The widespread use of adjuvant chemotherapy following Holland's recommendation has had a significant impact upon our nation's health bill. One can postulate that 20 to 40% of the 70,000 women each year who develop breast cancer are receiving adjuvant chemotherapy. The cost of chemoimmunotherapy is even greater. The long-term effects of adjuvant chemotherapy has yet to be determined. This information and the preliminary data already reported suggest that adjuvant chemotherapy in breast cancer should remain in an investigational setting.

We have studied the social and psychological impact of adjuvant chemotherapy and found that 87% of women described the fatigue associated with chemotherapy emotionally distressing and behaviorally inhibiting. Unexplained nervousness, irritability, or tearfulness was reported by 70% of the patients. Physical symptoms resulting from chemotherapy and immunotherapy were disruptive factors in the daily lives of 54% of the patients. Side effects that were most commonly reported as disruptive were alopecia (46%), changes in weight and appetite (38%), flu-like symptoms (30%), vomiting following chemotherapy (28%), and local irritation at the site of immunotherapy (22%).

Thirty-one percent reported having to give up activities they were engaged in regularly prior to adjuvant chemotherapy. Seventy-five percent claimed that adjuvant therapy had some negative influence on work-related activities (job and/or housework). One-third of the patients were employed outside the home. Sixty-one percent of these women reported having to miss work an average of 11.5 days a year as a direct result of the physical side effects of treatment. Seven women complained that their job status had been negatively influenced since beginning the program, e.g., having to leave work entirely, take less responsible positions, or pass up promotions. Fifty-six percent of the sample reported that participation in adjuvant therapy had created a financial burden due both to loss of income and to increased medical expenses.

Responses in the area of marital/family relationships were somewhat different. Twenty-one percent reported that their family lives had changed for the worse since operation, but an equal number reported positive improvements in their home lives. These stressful experiences, operation plus adjuvant chemotherapy, thus can lead to or at least correlate with increased closeness and support. No woman felt that her sexual life had improved while 30% of the women involved in sexual relationships at the time of the interview reported that they experienced greater difficulty. How much of this was due to operation and how much to adjuvant chemotherapy is impossible to judge.

In spite of the widespread distress and disruption related to adjuvant chemotherapy, 69% of the women said they were glad to have the opportunity to participate. They felt their anxiety and fears concerning their health would have led to still greater distress had no adjuvant treatment been prescribed. Furthermore, 78% of the patients claimed that they would tell a friend in a similar situation to "definitely" participate in the program if given a chance. No woman reported that she would discourage a friend, in spite of the stress of participation.

ACKNOWLEDGEMENT

Investigation Supported in Part by Contract CB-43917
Awarded by the National Cancer Institute, DHEW

REFERENCES

1. Bonadonna, G., Brusamolina, E., Valagussa, P., et al. (1976) N. Engl. J. Med. 294 : 405-410.
2. Fisher, B., Carbone, P., Economou, S.G., et al. (1975) N. Engl. J. Med. 292 : 117-122.
3. Sparks, F.C., Wile, A.G., Ramming, K.P., et al. (1976) Arch. Surg. 111 : 1057-1062.
4. Gutterman, J. U., Blumenschein, G.R., Hortobagyi, G., et al. (1976) Breast 2: 29-34.
5. Dao, T.L., Nemoto, T., Chamberlain, A., et al. (1975) Cancer 35: 478-482.

Adjuvant Therapy of Cancer, S.E. Salmon and S.E. Jones eds.

ADJUVANT CHEMOTHERAPY OF NODE-POSITIVE BREAST CANCER IN THE COMMUNITY

John T. Carpenter, Jr., William A. Maddox, Henry L. Laws,
David Wirtschafter, John R. Durant, Seng-jaw Soong
University of Alabama in Birmingham
P.O. Box 193, University Station
Birmingham, Alabama 35294

The use of adjuvant chemotherapy following mastectomy has reduced the recurrence rate substantially in two major trials.[1,2] Both of these studies were done principally in academic centers or groups of such centers. Little or no information is available about the use of such regimens by practicing community physicians. In Alabama, surgeons and physicians have entered their patients into a prospective trial of adjuvant chemotherapy in a statewide network known as the Alabama Breast Cancer Project (ABCP). We submit here an interim analysis of the early results from that trial.

PATIENTS AND METHODS

Practicing surgeons and physicians in the State of Alabama and those at the University of Alabama in Birmingham admitted patients to this trial. Ninety percent of patients were entered by private practitioners. All patients had a radical or modified radical mastectomy done by a surgeon who was a member of the Alabama American College of Surgeons and/or board-certified in surgery. Criteria for patient eligibility into the adjuvant chemotherapy trial are listed below in Table 1.

TABLE 1

CRITERIA FOR ELIGIBILITY

Signed Informed Consent

Tla, Tlb, T2a, T2b, T3a, T3b with No, Nla, Nlb and Mo

Age 70 or less

One or More Pathologically Positive Axillary Nodes
with No Distant Metastasis

WBC $>$ 4,000 and Platelets $>$ 150,000

Serum Creatinine $\leq$ 1.5 mg/dl

Non-pregnant

No Previous or Concurrent Second Primary Cancer

Therapy Must Begin Within 2 Months of Mastectomy

Pathology slides on all patients were reviewed by Dr. Tariq Murad at the University of Alabama. In cases where there was a difference of opinion, they were reviewed again by Dr. Paul Peter Rosen of the Memorial Sloan-Kettering Cancer

Center, New York, New York. Patients with one or more positive axillary nodes then received eight cycles of melphalan (MPL) or 24 cycles of cyclophosphamide, Methotrexate, and 5-fluououracil (CMF), depending on their month of birth (odd months CMF, even months MPL). The duration of each these regimens was approximately one year. Patients were then followed at three-month intervals without further therapy. No postoperative radiation was administered. Patients whose primary lesion was fixed to deeper tissue, i.e., T1b, T2b or T3b were entered into the trial but were stratified separately. After entry in the trial patients were considered to be disease-free until the first evidence of treatment failure, either local or distant recurrence. Biopsy was done of recurrent lesions for confirmation when possible.

Patients received one of the following two regimens:

melphalan 7 mg/M^2 by mouth daily for five days; the treatment was repeated every six weeks for a total of eight cycles;

OR

cyclophosphamide	300 mg/M^2 IV	The treatment was repeated every two weeks for a total of 24 cycles.
Methotrexate	30 mg/M^2 IV	
5-fluorouracil	300 mg/M^2 IV	

Chemotherapy was started within two months of the date of mastectomy. Dosage was delayed if the white blood cell count was below 4,000 or the platelet count was below 150,000 on the day of the scheduled treatment. If these counts had risen to the above levels, two weeks after treatment was delayed, treatment was then resumed in full dosage. If the white cell and platelet counts had not risen to normal levels four weeks after the administration of CMF or eight weeks after the administration of MPL, the treatment was given in half dosages and subsequently escalated to the maximum tolerated level. Doses were reduced 25-50% if necessary for stomatitis (Methotrexate) or nausea (all drugs). A chest x-ray and blood chemical studies (SMA-12 or equivalent) were done every three months while the patient received therapy to monitor for toxicity or recurrent disease.

Visit-by-visit instructions were sent to the participating community physicians utilizing the Consultant-Extender System[3] developed by the Clinical Information Systems Group, U.A.B. These instructions were incorporated into a multi-copy progress note form, which prompted monitoring of the patient's status, displayed appropriately calculated dosage(s), and indicated the protocol's dosage adjustment rule for the specific clinical situation of that visit. These forms were exchanged by mail before each visit to provide concurrent monitoring and modification of the chemotherapy. Correct dosages were given more than 97% of the time.

After the completion of chemotherapy, patients were seen by their own physicians at three-monthly intervals at which time there were examined for recurrent disease.

RESULTS

Table 2 presents the characteristics of patients entered into the trial. No significant difference is present in either group when examined for menopausal status, nodal involvement, or type of operation. Although it is not distributed evenly among the two treatment groups, age does not seem to influence the recurrence of disease in this study (See Table 3). For two patients the exact

TABLE 2

PATIENT CHARACTERISTICS

	CMF	MPL	TOTAL	p VALUE
Number of Patients	40	53	93	
Age				
<50	24(60%)	19(36%)	43	0.02
≥ 50	16(40%)	34(64%)	50	
Menopausal Status				
Premenopausal	20(50%)	20(38%)	40	0.25
1-5 Years Postmenopausal	8(20%)	9(17%)	17	
>5 Years Postmenopausal	11(27%)	24(45%)	35	
Other	1(3%)	0(0%)	1	
Nodes Involved				
1-3	15(37%)	25(47%)	40	0.88
4 or More	12(30%)	16(30%)	28	
Unknown	1(3%)	1(2%)	2	
Not Yet Reviewed	12(30%)	11(21%)	23	
Surgery				
Modified Radical Mastectomy	21(52%)	30(57%)	51	0.79
Radical Mastectomy	18(45%)	23(43%)	41	
Other	1(3%)	0(0%)	1	
Fixation-No Fixation				
Fixation	2(5%)	2(4%)	4	0.11
No Fixation	33(82%)	50(94%)	83	
T1a	15	13	28	
T2a	15	28	43	
T3a	3	9	12	
Other	5(13%)	1(2%)	6	
Median Duration of Follow-up	8 Months (1-20 Months)	8 Months (1-20 Months)		

number of nodes involved is unknown, although at least one node was known to be involved. In twenty-three patients the number of involved nodes has not been determined as of this writing pending review of the project pathologist.

Figure 1 portrays the disease-free interval for all patients entered into the trial. The probability of remaining disease-free at fourteen months was 0.85. Figure 2 compares the disease-free intervals for the groups receiving CMF and MPL. The groups are further broken down in Figure 3 according to the type of surgical procedure. Figure 4 contains the disease-free interval curves for premenopausal and postmenopausal women. It is interesting that the small number of patients who are 1-5 years postmenopausal remains free of recurrence to date. If patients whose tumor was fixed to deeper tissue (T1b, T2b, T3b) are excluded from the analysis, the disease-free intervals for the CMF and Melphalan groups are as shown in Figure 5; in these groups the probability of remaining disease free at fourteen months is 0.88. None of these figures shows any significant difference between the groups compared. The disease-free curves were calculated based on the method of Kaplan and Meier, and a generalized Wilcoxon test was used for testing the significance of any differences.[4] Exclusion of patients with fixed tumors makes this set of patients comparable to other major trials.

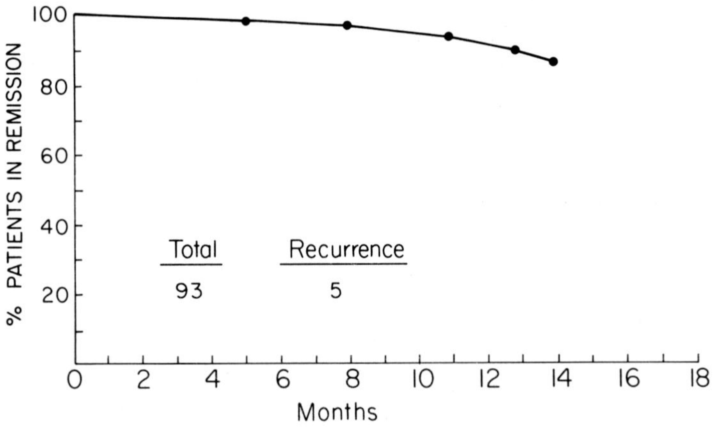

Figure 1.
Disease-Free Interval
All Patients

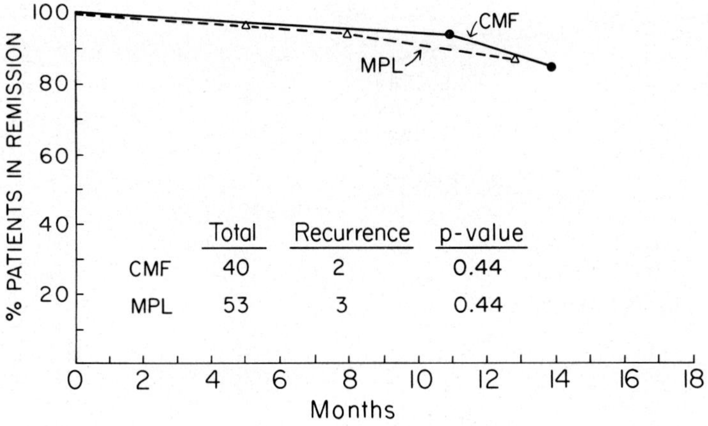

Figure 2.
Disease-Free Intervals:
MPL vs. CMF

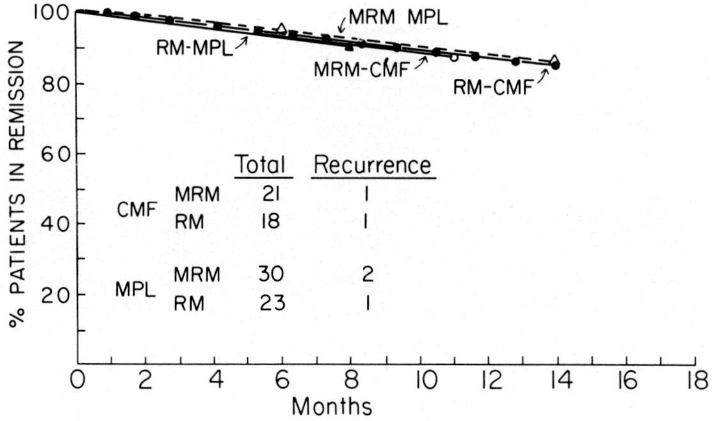

Figure 3.
Disease-Free Intervals:
Surgical Procedure and
Adjuvant Therapy

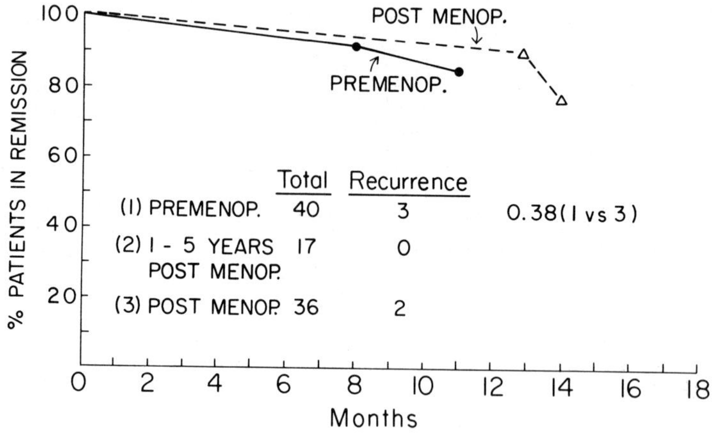

Figure 4.
Disease-Free Intervals
by Menopausal Status

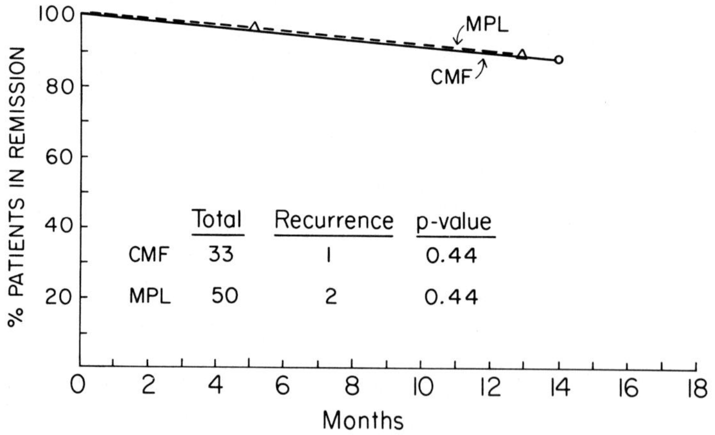

Figure 5.
Disease-Free Intervals,
Excluding Patients With Tumor
Fixed to Deeper Tissue

Toxic manifestations were principally gastrointestinal and hematologic. Table 3 shows the incidence and severity of toxicity.

TABLE 3

TOXICITY DATA

	CMF	MPL
Nausea and Vomiting	54%	23%
Severe	46%	17%
Platelet		
100,000-150,000	23%	27%
$<$100,000	3%	11%
WBC		
3,000-4,000	21%	28%
$<$3,000	5%	21%

One patient who received MPL withdrew from the study because of nausea and vomiting, while five patients in the CMF group did so. No patient in either group was hospitalized for hemorrhage or infection due to hematologic depression from therapy during the 20 months of this trial.

The characteristics of patients with recurrent disease are listed in Table 4 below. Both local and distant recurrences have occurred; they are distributed evenly between the two groups of patients.

TABLE 4

CHARACTERISTICS OF PATIENTS WITH RECURRENT DISEASE

	CMF	MPL	TOTAL
Age $<$ 50 Years	1	2	3
Age $\geq$ 50 Years	1	1	2
Local Recurrence Only		2	
Distant Recurrence Only	2		
Local and Distant Recurrence		1	

DISCUSSION

The interim results presented above indicate that 1) adjuvant chemotherapy can be delivered by private practicing physicians if appropriate guidelines and supervision are provided and 2) no difference in relapse rates has beem demonstrated so far between the MPL and CMF regimens. The effect of these regimens on survival cannot be determined at present. These early results are comparable to those in other trials[1,2]; subsequent results will provide more definitive comparisions between these two regimens and between our overall results and those trials done in major centers.

REFERENCES

1. Fisher, B., et al., 1-Penylalanine Mustard (L-PAM) in the Management of Primary Breast Cancer, N Engl J Med 292:117-122, 1975.
2. Bonadonna, G., et al., Combination Chemotherapy as an Adjuvant Treatment in Operable Breast Cancer, N Engl J Med 294:405-410, 1976.
3. Wirtschafter, D.D., et al., The Consultant-Extender System: Experience with Adjuvant Chemotherapy for Primary Operable Breast Cancer. Proceedings of the Sixth Annual Conference of the Society for Computer Medicine, Boston, Mass., November 11, 1976.
4. Gross, A., et al., Survival Distributions: Reliability Applications in the Biomedical Sciences, John Wiley and Sons, New York, 1975.

ACKNOWLEDGEMENTS

This work was supported by National Cancer Institute Contract No. NO1-CN-45129 and grant No. 1R-18-CA-16409. Dr. Carpenter is an American Cancer Society Junior Faculty Clinical Fellow. We thank Mrs. Diane Richards, Mrs. Mary Bolling, Ms. Joanie Pigford, Mrs. Sandy Wolanski, and Ms. Lucia Threeton for their invaluable assistance.

Adjuvant Therapy of Cancer, S.E. Salmon and S.E. Jones eds.
© 1977 Elsevier/North-Holland Biomedical Press, Amsterdam

L-PHENYLALANINE MUSTARD (L-PAM) VS. COMBINATION CHEMOTHERAPY AS ADJUVANT THERAPY IN OPERABLE BREAST CANCER

Allan Lipton, Charles Antle, William Demuth, Richard Dixon, Robert Gottlieb, Robert Heckard, Robert Kane, Michael Kukrika, Ross Moquin, David Nahrwold, Lewis Patterson, Joseph Ricci, William Shaver, John Stryker, Samuel Ward, Deborah White, Harold Harvey and Elliott Badder
The Central Pennsylvania Oncology Group
Hershey, Pennsylvania 17033

SUMMARY

Prolonged L-Phenylalanine Mustard (L-PAM) administration was compared with a cyclic oral 4-drug program as an adjuvant to mastectomy in primary breast cancer with positive axillary lymph nodes.

After 28 months of study, 91 patients have been entered on this protocol. The median duration of follow-up is 10 months. Sixteen patients have relapsed. The initial new clinical manifestations occurred in distant sites in 14 relapsed patients.

The comparative effectiveness of L-PAM and the 4-drug program was examined in several subgroups of patients. The two treatments have thus far had approximately the same effect on the chance of a relapse in premenopausal patients, in postmenopausal patients, in patients with a small primary tumor, in patients with a large primary tumor, and in patients with more than 4 nodes involved with disease. Only two relapses have occurred in patients with 1-3 nodes involved with disease; both of those relapses were in the L-PAM group.

The most significant result thus far is that patients for whom a reduction in either therapy was required due to toxicity had less chance of relapse. Additionally, in those patients for whom a dose reduction was required, L-PAM appears more effective. However, the 4-drug program was more effective for those patients for whom no dose reduction was required.

INTRODUCTION

In two recent studies the recurrence rate after mastectomy has been decreased in high risk patients treated with anticancer drugs. Prolonged treatment with L-Phenylalanine Mustard (L-PAM) resulted in a statistically significant decrease in recurrent malignancy when compared with placebo[1]. Prolonged cyclic combination chemotherapy with cyclophosphamide, methotrexate and 5-FU also resulted in a statistically significant reduction in recurrence rate during the first 27 months after radical mastectomy when compared with placebo treatment[2].

PATIENTS AND METHODS

Patient Selection: The study was carried out on patients admitted to hospitals within the Central Pennsylvania Region.

All patients had a modified radical mastectomy for potentially curable breast cancer and were found to have one or more axillary nodes positive on histologic study. All pathologic specimens were reviewed by a pathologist (S.W.). In all cases the tumor was confined to the breast and axilla. All patients had negative chest x-ray, liver scan, bone survey or scan, peripheral white-cell count >4,000 and platelet count >150,000. Patients were informed that they would receive either single agent or combination agent chemotherapy. Signed consent was obtained.

Patient Entry: Following surgery patients were selected to receive or not receive radiation therapy by their own physician. They were then stratified according to menopausal status. Patients were then randomized to receive Alkeran therapy or 4-drug combination chemotherapy.

Patients were ineligible if they were over age 75; pregnant or lactating. Other criteria for exclusion from this study were previous treatment for malignancy; T_{3b}-T_4 lesions (i.e. fixation to underlying pectoral fascia or muscle, or with fixation to chest wall or skin) or N_2-N_3 extent (i.e. homolateral axillary nodes fixed to one another or to other structures, or homolateral supraclavicular or infraclavicular nodes or edema of the arm); inflammatory carcinoma; presence of lymph nodes elsewhere suspected of containing tumor; and poor-surgical-risk patients having non-malignant systemic disease and therefore unsuitable for prolonged follow-up observation.

The first patient was entered into the study on October 1, 1974, and to date 91 patients have been entered and randomized. The present analysis of our experience was performed in January 1977. The median period of follow-up for all patients is 10 months.

The end point of the study used for statistical analysis was the first evidence of treatment failure, represented by local, regional or distant recurrence. Whenever possible, the presence of tumor was confirmed by biopsy.

Drug Administration: Patients randomized to L-PAM received 0.15 mgm per kilogram per day for five consecutive days every six weeks. Patients randomized to 4 drug combination chemotherapy received: Leukeran 8 mgm p.o. daily x5 days; Methotrexate 5 mgm p.o. daily x5 days; Prednisone 60 mgm p.o. daily x5 days and 5-Fluorouracil 15 mgm per kilogram p.o. each week. This cycle was to be repeated each month. This 4-drug program was designed to be easy to administer and non - toxic. In each case, treatment was begun no later than eight weeks following surgery and was to be continued until there was documented evidence of treatment failure, or for two years, whichever occurred first.

Drug dose was modified according to the presence and degree of toxicity. Hematopoietic toxicity was assessed on the first day of each drug course. L-PAM dose modifications were those used by the NSABP[1]. Multiple agent chemotherapy modifications were as follows: If WBC is less than 4,000 or platelet count is less than 150,000 give one-half above 5-FU, Leukeran and Methotrexate dose. If WBC is less than 3,000 or platelet count is less than 100,000 stop 5-FU, Leukeran and Methotrexate until counts recovered, then restart therapy at full dosages. (If BUN above 30 give one-half suggested Methotrexate dose; if BUN above 60mgm% omit Methotrexate).

End Point: Treatment failure, which is the major end point of this study, is defined as the presence of tumor in local, regional, or distant sites, confirmed by biopsy when possible or by acceptable clinical, pathological, radiologic or radioisotopic evidence.

Pathology: All material relative to tumor and lymph nodes was subject to independent pathological review at Hershey Medical Center by one of the authors (S.W.) after examination by the responsible pathologist at each hospital. In no case did the review change the diagnosis or the nodal pathologic diagnosis.

Statistical Analysis: A detailed discussion of the data analysis is contained in a technical report[3] by Charles Antle and Robert Heckard of the Department of Statistics, The Pennsylvania State University. The analysis included the use of Gehan's modification of the Wilcoxon test and a Bayesian approach. (The technical report is available from the Department of Statistics upon request). These two methods of analysis gave similar results.

PATIENT CHARACTERISTICS

Menopausal Status: When the 91 patients used for analyses were grouped according to their menopausal status 35% were premenopausal and 65% were postmenopausal.

Nodal Status: Forty-three per cent of patients had 1-3 nodes involved with tumor while 57% had involvement of 4 or more nodes. Thus, our treated patient population is more like the NSABP control population (55% with 4 or more positive nodes) than the Milan[2] control population (30% with 4 or more positive nodes).

Patients were not stratified according to nodal status. 28/45 (62%) of patients treated with Alkeran had 4 or more involved nodes; 24/46 (52%) of patients treated with 4 drugs had involvement of 4 or more nodes (Table 1).

Radiation Therapy: Patients were not stratified according to radiation therapy. This was left to the discretion of the referring physician due to the strong feelings regarding this mode of therapy.

Thirty-two patients received post-operative radiation therapy (23/32 had 4 or more positive nodes in the mastectomy specimen). Seventeen patients treated with Alkeran and 15 with 4 drug therapy also received radiation therapy (Table 1).

Follow-up Status: Forty-four of 45 patients randomized to receive Alkeran are evaluable. One patient elected to discontinue therapy. Thirty-nine of 46 patients randomized to receive the 4-drug protocol are evaluable. One patient died of CVA. Four elected to discontinue therapy due to undue toxicity (nausea, vomiting, dizziness) and two decided they did not want to receive any further treatment.

TABLE 1

CHARACTERISTICS OF 91 STUDY PATIENTS

	Alkeran (45 patients)	4 Drugs (46 patients)
Menopause:		
Pre	16	16
Post	29	30
Nodes:		
1-3	17	22
$\geq$ 4	28	24
Size of Primary Tumor:		
$\leq$ 3.5 cm.	21	27
> 3.5 cm.	24	19
Radiation Therapy:		
No RT	28	31
RT	17	15
Median duration on study in months	10	10

RESULTS

Alkeran vs. 4-Drug Therapy: Thus far 16 patients have relapsed. Ten of the 45 patients on Alkeran have relapsed while 6 of the 46 patients on the 4-drug program have relapsed. Figure 1 illustrates the survival curves for the two treatment groups. No statistically significant differences between these two survival curves was found using both Gehan's modification of the Wilcoxon test (P = .43) and a Bayesian approach.

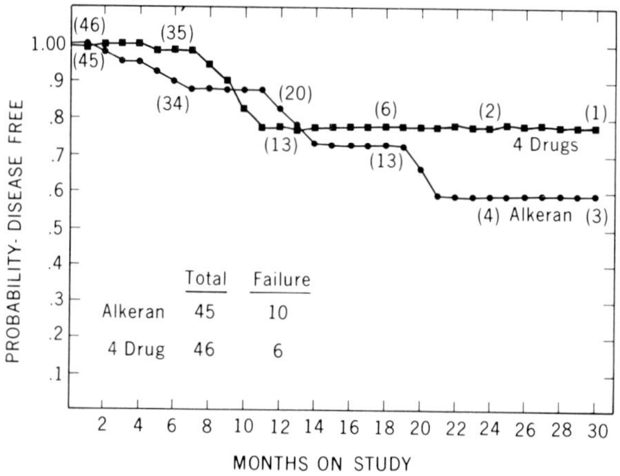

Fig. 1 - Treatment - Failure Time Distribution in All Evaluable Patients

The two therapies were compared in several subgroups of the patients. In premenopausal patients, Alkeran and the 4-drug program had approximately the same effect on failure rate. The two treatments also performed about equally in postmenopausal patients.

When patients were classified by nodal status, no significant difference between the treatments was found in patients with 4 or more involved lymph nodes. In patients with 1-3 nodes involved with tumor, the probability of disease-free survival appears greater in those patients treated with 4 drugs (P= .11) [Figure 2]. A striking feature of Figure 2 is that only 2 of the 39 patients with 1 - 3 nodes involved have had a relapse. Both of these patients were in the Alkeran group.

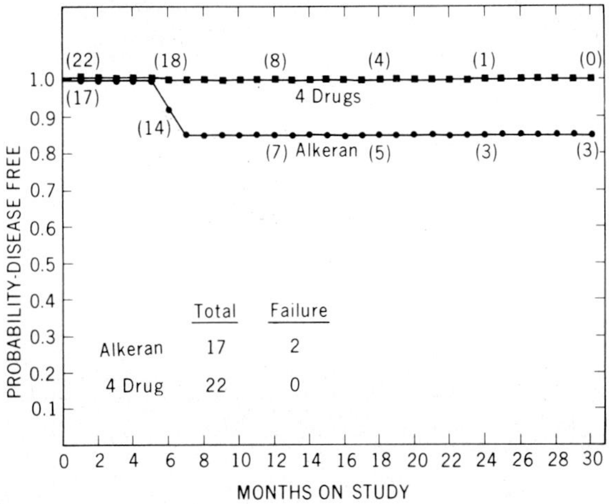

Fig. 2 - Treatment - Failure Time Distribution of Patients with One to Three Positive Axillary Lymph Nodes.

In patients with a large primary tumor (>3.5 cm in greatest diameter), no difference between the two treatments was uncovered. Similarly, no difference between the two drug therapies was found in patients with a small primary tumor (<3.5 cm in greatest diameter).

Toxicity: Leukopenia (+ thrombocytopenia) represented the most frequently encountered sign of toxicity. In all cases, this was reversible within 2 weeks. There was no life-threatening infection or bleeding. Nausea and vomiting was more frequent in those patients treated with the 4-drug program. Side effects of therapy were seen more often in these patients (Table 2). Four of these patients stopped the medication because of side effects.

TABLE 2

TOXICITY DUE TO THERAPY

	Alkeran (45 patients)	4 Drugs (46 patients)
Leukopenia	15	17
Thrombocytopenia	4	2
Diarrhea	1	2
Nausea $\pm$ vomiting	3	9
Chills	1	0
Thrush	1	0
Mouth ulcer	1	3
Diabetes	0	1
Taste Change	0	1
Dizzy	0	1
Asthmatic Symptoms	0	1
Psychiatric Symptoms	0	1
Patients with no toxicity	28	21
Patients with dose reduction	13	20

Figure 3 shows survival curves for patients who had reductions in their therapy due to to toxicity (usually leukopenia) and for those who did not. Patients for whom a dose reduction was necessary had a significantly smaller chance of relapse than patients for whom no dose reduction was required (P = .05). In patients for whom no dose reduction was required, the 4-drug program was more effective (P = .18). However, in those patients for whom a dose reduction was required, Alkeran appears more effective than the 4-drug program (P = .16).

Site of Recurrence: Fourteen of the 16 relapses have been in distant sites. Ten of the 10 relapses in the Alkeran group have been in distant sites while 4 of the 6 relapses on 4-drug chemotherapy have been in distant sites.

Radiation Therapy: The survival rate of the group of patients treated with radiation therapy was approximately the same as the survival rate of the group of patients who were not treated with radiation therapy. Radiation therapy had little effect on disease-free survival in patients with 4 or more involved lymph nodes. In patients with fewer nodes, there is a suggestion that radiation may improve the disease-free rate. This group is, however, quite small and these results are not statistically significant at this early date.

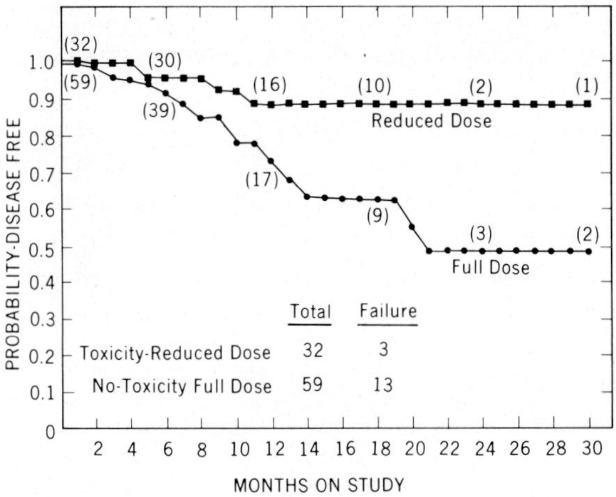

Fig. 3 - Treatment - Failure Time Distribution of Patients with Dose Reduction Due to Drug Toxicity

DISCUSSION

Since the intial reports of success of adjuvant chemotherapy in treating patients with breast cancer, this concept has been widely accepted. In many areas CMF has become standard therapy for all patients following mastectomy, despite disappointing follow-up reports in both early major series.[1,2]

Our purpose in presenting this preliminary analysis of our data is to see if any trends are emerging which would be useful at this time - either in treating patients or in planning future protocols.

At this time in our study there does not appear to be any advantage in treating most patients with multiple agent chemotherapy. Most patients treated with Alkeran alone appear to be doing as well as those treated with this 4-drug program. The use of multiple agents adds toxicity as well as long-term theoretical risk of second malignancy. The one possible exception at this time is the group of patients with 1-3 positive nodes. Here, there is an early suggestion that multiple agent therapy may be beneficial. More aggressive therapy may be useful in patients with lesser amounts of disease. Further study is needed.

In this protocol radiation therapy does not enhance disease-free survival. Most recurrences were in distant sites and were multiple. This would again support the concept that patients with positive axillary nodes have disseminated microscopic foci of disease at the time of surgery and are not benefited by a local form of therapy. No deleterious effect of radiation therapy was seen.

An unexpected finding was an improved disease-free survival in those patients who had a dose reduction in their medication - either Alkeran or the 4-drug program. This would imply that many patients are being underdosed and perhaps an improved survival could be obtained by more aggressive treatment with only Alkeran.

Our 4-drug program does not coincide with the schedule used to administer CMF.[2] In addition, for convenience sake, our 5-FU was administered orally. None the less, at this time we wish to warn against the widespread adoption of a multiple drug approach as an adjuvant in breast cancer. There is no direct evidence as yet available showing that multiple agents will help all patients. It is our belief that individualization of therapy will come to pass when the results of the many ongoing studies are available.

REFERENCES

1. Fisher, B., Carbone, P., Economon, S.G., Frelick, R., Glass, A., Lerner, H., Redmond, C., Zelen, M., Band, P., Katrych, D.L., Wolmark, M., and Fisher, E.R. (and other cooperating investigators). New Engl. J. Med. 292:117-122, 1975. L-Phenylalanine Mustard (L-PAM) in the Management of Primary Breast Cancer. A Report of Early Findings.
2. Bonadonna, G., Brusamolino, E., Valagussa, P., Rossi, A., Brugnatelli, L., Brambilla, C., DeLena, M., Transini, G., Bajetta, E., Musumeci, R. and Verowesi, U. New Engl. J. Med. 294:405-410, 1976. Combination Chemotherapy as an Adjuvant Treatment in Operable Breast Cancer.
3. Antle, C., Heckard, R., and The Central Pennsylvania Oncology Group. Technical Report 33, Department of Statistics, The Pennsylvania State University. Statistical Analysis of CPOG Adjuvant Breast Cancer Study.

Adjuvant Therapy of Cancer, S.E. Salmon and S.E. Jones eds.

ADJUVANT RADIOTHERAPY AND CHEMOTHERAPY IN STAGE II CARCINOMA OF THE BREAST

Dr. H. Abu-Zahra, Dr. B. McDonald, Dr. J. Maus,
Dr. G. Mok and Dr. S. Yoshida
The Ontario Cancer Foundation
Windsor Clinic
2220 Kildare Road
Windsor, Ontario
Canada

INTRODUCTION

The rationale and use of adjuvant chemotherapy in patients with primary carcinoma of the breast and nodal involvement (Stage II) have been discussed earlier in this conference by other participants. To date, the use of postoperative radiotherapy in this disease has reduced the rate of local recurrence with little apparent effect on patient survival or the development of distant metastases[1-3].

In an attempt to control local residual tumor and distant micro-metastases in these patients, a pilot study was designed to test the sequential use of radiotherapy and combination chemotherapy adjuvant to modified radical mastectomy. In this report, we present the preliminary data of our findings.

PATIENTS AND METHODS

This study was carried out on patients referred to the Ontario Cancer Foundation Windsor Clinic between June 1975 and December 1976. All patients, who had had modified radical mastectomy with complete removal of the primary tumor and involved lymph node(s) and who consented to enter this study, were included. Other major criteria of the protocol were as follows: the diagnosis of carcinoma of the breast and lymph node(s) involvement was proven histologically; the primary tumor and lymph nodes were mobile and not fixed to skin or underlying structures; there was no evidence of distant metastases or involvement of the other breast as shown radiologically or by appropriate scanning; patients with inflammatory carcinoma, skin ulceration greater than 2 cms. or with peau d'orange involving more than one-third of the skin of the breast were excluded.

Except for two patients who were already under treatment by radiotherapy, all other patients were selected randomly for one of two intensive regimens given within approximately twenty weeks following mastectomy. The remaining patients were allocated to either group A: four cycles of chemotherapy were given before and after radiotherapy or group B: radiotherapy was given primarily followed by eight cycles of chemotherapy. Treatment was started two weeks after mastectomy unless local or systemic post-operative complications were present. Delay of adjuvant therapy was not allowed beyond four to six weeks after surgery. At the end of intensive treatment and after a two week rest period, identical intermittent chemotherapy was given to each group for an overall elapsed period of twelve months or until relapse.

The chemotherapeutic agents and their dosages are outlined in (Table I). 5-Fluorouracil 400 mg./m^2 and Methotrexate 20 mg./m^2 were given intravenously weekly for eight cycles and then every two weeks. Cyclophosphamide 100 mg./m^2 was given orally for forty-two days and then during days one to fourteen starting at the beginning of each cycle. A two week rest period intervened before and after radiotherapy in group A and after radiotherapy in group B and then between the cycles of chemotherapy during the intermittent phase.

TABLE I

The chemotherapeutic agents and their dosages

DRUGS	DOSE mg/m^2	ROUTE	FREQUENCY Intensive	FREQUENCY Intermittent
5-Fluorouracil	400	i.v.	Weekly x 8	Every 2 weeks
Methotrexate	20	i.v.	Weekly x 8	Every 2 weeks
Cyclophosphamide	100	p.o.	42 days	1-14 days

Radiotherapy was given using both Cobalt 60 and deep x-ray at 280 Kilo Volts Peak and 3.5 mm. of copper Half Value Layer. Medial and lateral tangential fields were used to treat the chest wall by the x-ray unit. The parasternal area was also treated with x-rays using a single, anterior field covering both internal mammary lymph node chains. The supraclavicular fossa and the axilla were treated with Cobalt through a single anterior field. The tumor dose to the chest wall, supraclavicular fossa and axillary regions averaged 4,000 rads. in four weeks. A skin dose of 4,000 rads is given to the parasternal field, also in four weeks.

During treatment, a reduced dose of chemotherapy was given in the presence of myelosuppression. Hemopoietic toxicity was classified according to the drop in the neutrophil or platelet counts determined on the day of or the day before treatment. At the beginning of each treatment, the neutrophil count must have exceeded 1,000 per cu.mm. and platelet count 50,000 per cu.mm. The grades of toxicity per neutrophil and platelet count and dose modifications are outlined in (Table II).

TABLE II

Grades of hematological toxicity and dose modifications

GRADE	PMN	PLATELET	DOSE (%)
0	>2000	100,000	100
1	1999-1500	99000-75000	75
2	1499-1000	74000-50000	50
3	<1000	50,000	0

Methotrexate was omitted entirely when oral ulceration and/or mucositis developed. In the presence of hemorrhagic cystitis, Leukeran would replace Cyclophosphamide.

Pre-study and follow up investigations were carried out as outlined in the protocol.

RESULTS

The characteristics of the patients in each group are outlined in Table III.

TABLE III

Patient characteristics in each group

CHARACTERISTIC	GROUP A	GROUP B
Number of patients	10	12
Age; median	51 (39-66)	53 (37-79)
Menopause		
Pre	3	2
Post	7	10
Lymph nodes		
1-3	3	9
≥4	7	3
Mastectomy		
mod. Rad.	10	11
Pathology		
Lobular	2	0
Ductal	6	10
Anaplastic	2	0
Carinoma - not specified	0	2

Twenty-two patients were entered into the study. The median age was 51 and 53 for group A and B respectively. More patients with extensive node involvement (over 4) were in group A than B. All patients had had modified radical mastectomy.

Three patients were not evaluable and were excluded from the present analysis. The reasons for exclusion were as follows: one patient from group A received initial chemotherapy but refused to continue with radiotherapy; similarly one patient from group B had post-operative radiotherapy but refused to continue with chemotherapy. One patient from group B was excluded because of a delay of chemotherapy for five weeks. She had had three cycles of chemotherapy and developed severe toxicity with a sharp drop in the neutrophil count associated with fever. A detailed analysis of nineteen evaluable patients is shown in Table IV.

TABLE IV

Results of adjuvant radiotherapy/chemotherapy in carcinoma of the breast (Stage II)

	GROUP A	GROUP B
Number of patients	10	12
Not Evaluable	1	2
Evaluable	9	10
Recurrence	0	2 (9½ mon. & 18 mon.)
Local	0	0
Liver	0	x
Bone	0	xx
Pleura	0	0
Death	1 (8 mon.)	0
Follow-up		
Completed Ex	4	3
36-52 (wks)	2	3
24-35 (wks)	2	3
12-23 (wks)	0	1
Less 12 wks	0	0

Seven patients, four from group A and three from group B have completed the designed course of adjuvant radiotherapy/chemotherapy as of December 1976. The follow-up period after completed treatment ranged from one to six months. For the entire group the median follow up period was twelve months. Two patients from group B showed evidence of relapse after nine and a half months and eighteen months respectively. Evidence of metastases was shown in bone and liver in one patient and in bone alone in the other. None showed evidence of local or regional recurrence. Another patient (group A) presented with right pleural effusion after eight months of treatment. Sanguineous fluid was drained but malignant cells were not seen histologically. At the time of the examination, the patient had an extensive pericardial rub which persisted until death. She was believed to have relapsed and treatment was discontinued. Autopsy, however showed no evidence of metastases anywhere. Acute and chronic hemorrhagic fibrinous pericarditis and epicarditis were demonstrated with bilateral pleural effusions. The immediate cause of death was upper gastrointestinal hemorrhage due to esophageal varices and severe thrombocytopenia. Initially chemotherapy had been delayed for six weeks because of poor healing of the surgical wound requiring skin grafting. Subsequently, her tolerance to treatment was poor and she was admitted to hospital on several occasions for treatment of infection and bleeding.

Hematological Toxicity: Grade III neutropenia (neutrophil count less than 1,000 per cu.mm.) occurred in seven patients during intensive treatment. In three patients this was associated with infection and two required treatment in hospital. In most patients, the neutrophil count reached its nadir in five to six weeks following radiotherapy. A representative neutrophil count observed in two patients, one from each group as well as the relationship to treatment was plotted in a semilog scale. Figure I clearly demonstrated this trend.

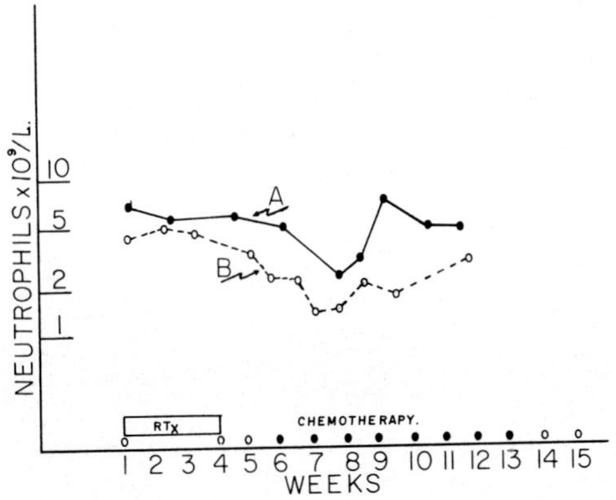

Fig. 1. The relationship of the neutrophil count to adjuvant therapy during the intensive phase in group A and B patients.

Thrombocytopenia was rarely seen in this series. Grade III thrombocytopenia (less than 50,000 per cu.mm.) occurred in two patients during intermittent chemotherapy and in one patient during radiotherapy. Only one patient required a platelet transfusion for treatment of bleeding.

Subjective Toxicity: All patients experienced partial or complete hair loss. Nausea and vomiting were invariably present but were easily controlled with antiemetic drugs. Four of five menstruating women developed amenorrhea sometime after treatment. Mucositis was observed in three patients. None of the patients developed hemorrhagic cystitis nor was there evidence of liver or renal insufficiency as determined biochemically.

Radiation pneumonitis was suspected in three patients but only in one patient acute symptoms of dyspnea, cough, fever and response to steroid treatment were documented. One patient developed herpes zoster infection of the first branch of the left trigeminal nerve eleven months after mastectomy and in the absence of myelosuppression.

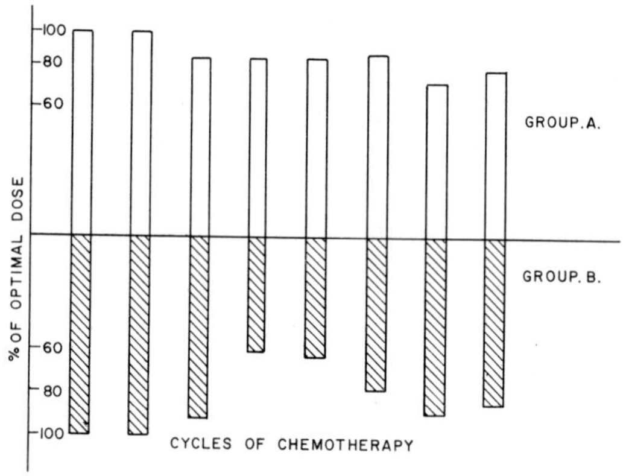

Fig. 2. The optimal dose of chemotherapy given during intensive treatment.

As shown in Fig. 2, a sudden decrease in the average dose administered to 75% was noted in course seven of group A patients. This reflected the fall in neutrophil count four weeks after ending radiotherapy. In group B, a dose reduction to 69% was noted in course four and to a lesser degree in five and six. This also reflects the fall in the neutrophil count five to six weeks after radiation. In both groups, the average total dose given was almost identical, 87.3% and 86% for group A and B respectively. But, the time for treatment administration during the intensive phase was shorter in A with a median of 16 weeks (range of 14-18 weeks), than in B with a median of 18 weeks (range of 14-20 weeks), exceeding in each group the planned time of 14 and 13 weeks respectively.

COMMENT

This preliminary report deals with the immediate toxicity and the pattern of treatment-failure in patients with carcinoma of the breast and axillary nodal involvement who received radiotherapy and triple-drug chemotherapy adjuvant to modified radical mastectomy. In a small number of patients and a relatively short follow-up period, no definite conclusion can be made. However, a certain trend of toxicity and treatment failure was observed. Two of nineteen patients showed evidence of distant metastases involving liver and/or bone but without evidence of local or regional recurrence. The severity of neutropenia observed in this series, five to six weeks after radiation, is of a prime concern and required special attention by the attending physician. This was associated with systemic infection in two patients requiring aggressive treatment by appropriate antibiotics intravenously.

In both treatment regimens, close to 85% of the optimal dose was given during the intensive phase. Yet the planned time of treatment administration was exceeded in both instances, less so in group A than B. With radiotherapy being sandwiched between cycles of chemotherapy with a two-week rest period intervening before and after radiotherapy, this may have allowed more time for bone marrow recovery in group A patients. Thrombocytopenia was not a frequent complication in our series. Only one patient during intermittent chemotherapy required platelet transfusions to control local bleeding. Gastrointestinal symptoms were a constant complaint by most patients but were easily controlled by anti-emetic drugs. Hair loss, partial or complete was transiently experienced by most patients. In most instances, hair regrowth was observed despite continued chemotherapy.

Radiation pneumonitis was suspected in three patients. Only one patient presented with acute symptoms including fever, dyspnea, cough and radiological changes in the lung, all of which were reversed following the administration of steroids and antibiotics. The development of herpes zoster in one patient after eleven months of treatment may have been due to immunosuppression for no evidence of myelosuppression was noted at the time of onset. Whether or not this underlines a delayed effect of the treatment is an open question.

Finally, the long term consequences of this approach remain unanswered and its value has to be tested within the context of a controlled cooperative trial.

We would like to express our gratitude to Mrs. J. Benedet and Mrs. P. Jahn for their secretarial help.

REFERENCES

1. Murrary, J.G., et al: Management of Early Cancer of the Breast; report on an international multicentre trial supported by the Cancer Research Campaign. British Medical Journal 1:1035-1038, 1976.
2. Weichselbaum, R.R., et al: The Role of Post-operative Irradiation in Carcinoma of the Breast. Cancer 37:2682-2690, 1976.
3. Fisher, B., et al: Postoperative Radiotherapy in the Treatment of Breast Cancer; Results of the NSABP Clinical Trial. Ann. Surg. 172:711-732, 1970.

Adjuvant Therapy of Cancer, S.E. Salmon and S.E. Jones eds.
© 1977 Elsevier/North-Holland Biomedical Press, Amsterdam

ADJUVANT CHEMOIMMUNOTHERAPY FOLLOWING REGIONAL THERAPY IN BREAST CANCER

A. U. Buzdar, G. R. Blumenschein, J. U. Gutterman,
C. K. Tashima, G. N. Hortobagyi, W. Wheeler*, E. Gehan, E. J. Freireich, E. Hersh
University of Texas M. D. Anderson
Hospital and Tumor Institute, Houston, Texas

SUMMARY

Combination of 5-Fluorouracil, Adriamycin, Cyclophosphamide and BCG was evaluated as an adjuvant treatment in Stage II and Stage III breast cancer patients with positive axillary nodes at the time of surgery. After 32 months of study, treatment failure occurred in 5.3% of 75 treated patients as compared to 40% of 152 comparable matched control patients (p=.016). The advantage appeared statistically significant in all subgroups of patients. Chemotherapy was well tolerated with acceptable toxicity. Results look very encouraging but long term side effects and survival remain unknown.

INTRODUCTION

Surgery and radiotherapy have been two main forms of treatment for operable breast cancer. These two modalities of treatment have not altered the overall survival and cure rates in the last few decades. The poor prognosis of patients with positive axillary nodes is apparent and is due to clinical occult dissemination in early stages of the desease, prior to definitive treatment for local disease. Chemotherapy regimens have been applied as postoperative adjuvant for many years. The clinical benefit of these adjuvant programs has been modest in most instances, because single drugs were used in ineffective doses and schedules. The low growth fraction and long cell cycle time of breast cancer and limited success of earlier short term chemotherapy suggested that more prolonged chemotherapy will be necessary to eradicate the microscopic disease (1).

Two major postoperative adjuvant studies, Fisher'ssingle drug chemotherapy with L-PAM (2) and combination chemotherapy by Bonadonna with Cyclophosphamide, Methotrexate and 5-Fluorouracil (CMF) (3),have been published recently and have been shown to have limited success, only in premenopausal woman.

Recently, we reported that a 3 drug combination including 5-Fluorouracil, Adriamycin and Cyclophosphamide (FAC) resulted in a remission rate of 75% for

*Present address Riverside Hospital, Columbus, Ohio 43214.
The authors are indebted to Kathy Calahan for secretarial help in preparing this manuscript.
Supported by NCI Contract 33888 from National Cancer Institute, NIH, Bethesda, Maryland.
Dr. Gutterman is recipient of Public Health Research Career Development Award CA 71007-03.

patients with advanced breast cancer (4). The addition of immunotherapy with BCG in that regimen resulted in a significant prolongation of remission duration and survival (5). In January 1974 we initiated a trial of adjuvant chemoimmunotherapy for operable breast cancer. For this, we selected our best chemoimmunotherapy regimen, based on the demonstration that most effective regimens for minimal disease in experimental systems are those which are most effective for advanced tumors (6).

SELECTION OF PATIENTS

All patients who had mastectomy for potentially curable breast carcinoma and who had one or more axillary nodes positive on histological studies were considered eligible for this study, provided they satisfied the following protocol: The tumor was confined to the breast and axilla, radiological studies were negative (chest x-ray, mammogram of opposite breast, skeletal survey, liver scan and bone scan), adequate bone marrow function as demonstrated by peripheral white count greater than 3,000 and platelet count greater than 150,000, blood urea nitrogen under 25mg%. Patients were informed of the investigational nature of the study in compliance with federal and local institutional guidelines. Other treatment options were considered with each patient and a written informed consent was obtained. Patients with bulky local disease considered as Stage III, if technically operable, were included in this study. Pregnancy, lactation, age over 75 or any prior chemotherapy for previous or concomitant neoplasm except successfully treated squamous or basal cell carcinoma of the skin precluded entry in the study. Any patient with a co-existent serious medical disorder that would make the patient a poor risk for aggressive chemotherapy was not included in this study.

EXPERIMENTAL DESIGN AND TREATMENT

Seventy-five patients were entered on the study from January 1974 until December 1975, 74 females and one male. Their median age was 52 years with a range of 26-73 years. Fifty-seven patients received postoperative irradiation. Eighteen patients were entered into the study without radiation therapy. The chemoimmunotherapy program was started within 10 weeks after surgery and consisted of 5-Fluorouracil 400mg/M^2 IV on day 1 and 8, Cyclophosphamide 400mg/M^2 IV on day 1 and Adriamycin 40mg/M^2 IV on day 1. Connaught BCG was given by scarification (6×10^8 viable units) on days 9, 16 and 23 of the 28 day cycle. After a total dose of 300mg/M^2 of Adriamycin, the patients were changed to the maintenance chemoimmunotherapy. The maintenance regimen, included 5-FU 500mg/M^2 PO on day 1 and 8, Methotrexate 30mg/M^2 IM on day 1 and 8 and Cyclophosphamide 500mg/M^2 on day 2. BCG was continued by scarification on day 9, 16 and 23 of every 28 day cycle. The total chemoimmunotherapy program lasted for 24 months.

If severe leukopenia (granulocyte less than 1,000 and/or platelet under 75,000) developed as a result of chemotherapy, the dosage of all 3 drugs was decreased by 20%. The appearance of unexplained EKG changes or a decrease of QRS voltage in the standard 6 leads by more than 40% was considered as an indication to discontinue Adriamycin. BCG dose reduction was carried out by half log if patient had severe local or systemic reaction lasting greater than 48 hours.

FOLLOW-UP STUDIES

Patients were followed with weekly CBC,platelet,differential. SMA-12, EKG and urinalysis were repeated before each cycle of chemotherapy. Chest x-ray, bone scan, liver scan and skeletal surveys were done every 4 months or earlier if indicated by the clinical course. Mammograms on the remaining breast were done yearly.

TABLE I

COMPARABILITY OF CONTROL AND FAC-BCG GROUPS

Characteristics	Control	FAC-BCG	P Value Control vs. FAC-BCG
Total patients	152	75	
Age < 50	49 (32%)	28 (37%)	0.54
≥ 50	103 (68%)	47 (63%)	
Size of Primary *T_1	47 (31%)	11 (15%)	0.02
T_2	66 (43%)	44 (59%)	
T_3	39 (26%)	20 (27%)	
No involved nodes			
1-3	60 (39%)	20 (27%)	
4-10	54 (36%)	25 (33%)	0.05
≥ 10	38 (25%)	30 (40%)	
Stage *II	91 (60%)	49 (65%)	0.51
III	61 (40%)	26 (35%)	

* According to UICC classification of breast cancer.

SURGICAL CONTROL GROUP

In order to compare the results of adjuvant FAC-BCG to conventional methods of treatment, a group of control patients was defined in the following manner. All patients with diagnosis of breast cancer who were treated with curative intent at M. D. Anderson Hospital between January 1972 and December 1973 (the years immediately preceeding the initiation of FAC-BCG study) were used as historical controls provided these patients had Stage II or Stage III disease and had at least one lymph node involved at time of surgery; 152 patients comprise this control group.

STATISTICAL ANALYSIS

Statistical analysis was carried out both on total proportions of treatment failures and time distribution. Tests for differences in distribution of various patient characteristics between treated and control groups were carried out by

Chi-square test. A generalized Wilcoxon test was used to compare the distribution of time to disease recurrence and survival between various groups.

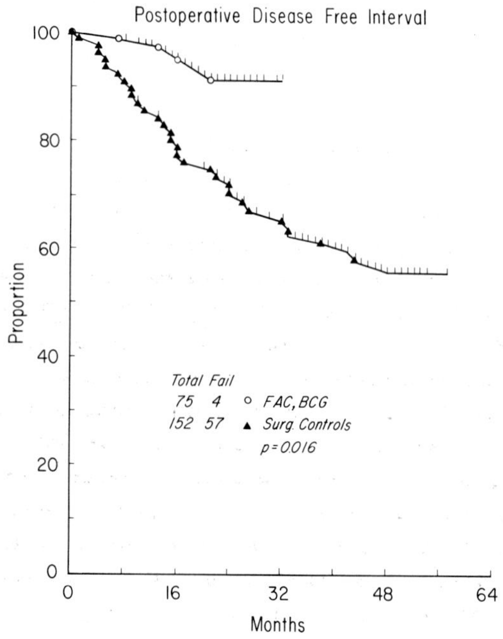

Fig. 1. Postoperative disease-free interval.

RESULTS

Table I shows the comparability of control and FAC-BCG groups by various prognostic indicators. Both groups were comparable except for the higher percentage of patients with ten or more nodes and with larger primary tumors in the FAC-BCG group as compared to the control group. Thus the control population by the various prognostic criteria was slightly more favorable as compared to the FAC-BCG group. As shown in Figure 1, 5.3% of the FAC-BCG patients have relapsed at 32 months (median 18 mos.) as compared to 40% of control patients (p 0.016). Table II gives the percentage of patients disease-free at one and two years after surgery by treatment group and characteristics related to prognosis. Patients receiving FAC-BCG have significantly fewer recurrences per unit of time, regardless of their menopausal status, age, stage of disease and the size of the primary tumor. The difference in time to recurrence was not statistically significant between the control and the FAC-BCG group for those patients who had a primary tumor less than 3cm or 1-3 positive nodes. The patients with less favorable prognostic factors

TABLE II

TIME TO RECURRENCE FOR CONTROL AND FAC-BCG PATIENTS BY ENTERING CHARACTERISTICS

Charact.	Trt.	No. Pts.	Total No. Recurr.	% Pts. Disease-free by year of study 1 YR.	2 YR.	P Value Wilcoxon Test 2-tailed
Menopausal Status *						
Pre	Control	39	19	65	56	<.01
	FAC-BCG	34	3	97	85	
Peri-Post	Control	113	38	92	74	.04
	FAC-BCG	40	1	98	98	
Age						
< 50 yrs.	Control	49	24	72	59	.01
	FAC-BCG	28	3	97	81	
≥ 50 yrs.	Control	103	33	91	75	.02
	FAC-BCG	47	1	98	98	
Size of Primary						
< 3cm	Control	47	18	91	70	.21
	FAC-BCG	11	0	100	100	
3-5cm	Control	66	20	86	76	.02
	FAC-BCG	44	2	98	94	
> 5cm	Control	39	19	76	58	.03
	FAC-BCG	20	2	92	85	
Number Involved Nodes						
1-3	Control	60	17	93	78	.31
	FAC-BCG	'20	1	94	--	
4-10	Control	54	19	83	70	.03
	FAC-BCG	25	1	93	88	
> 10	Control	38	21	75	55	<.01
	FAC-BCG	30	2	94	93	
Stage						
II	Control	91	28	91	76	.04
	FAC-BCG	49	2	98	94	
III	Control	61	29	76	61	.01
	FAC-BCG	26	2	94	88	

* One male patient

who received FAC-BCG did have significantly longer disease-free intervals as compared to control. It is also apparent that patients with 4-10 and 10 or more nodes have significantly prolonged disease-free intervals with FAC-BCG as compared to the surgery alone group. Figure 2 gives the survival curves for the patients in FAC-BCG and control groups. The estimated percentage of patients surviving two years in the control group was 87%. All patients followed for 2 years were still surviving in FAC-BCG group. The one death in the FAC-BCG group occurred at 28 months. The overall difference in survival curves between the groups was highly statistically significant (p 0.02).

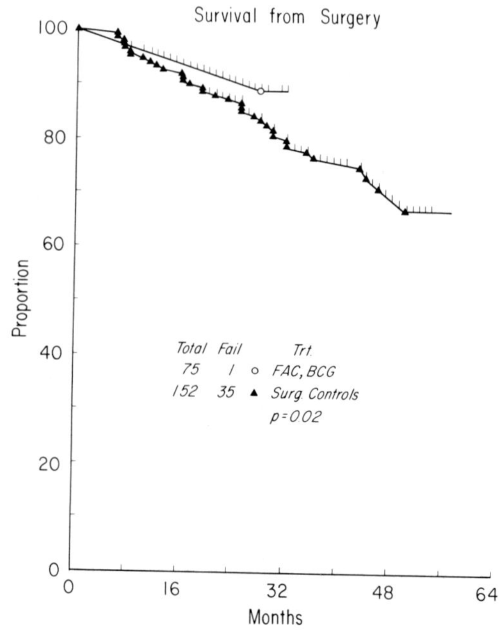

Fig. 2. Survival from surgery.

TOXICITY

Nausea and vomiting occurred in the large majority of patients within a few hours of intravenous chemotherapy, as shown in Table III. Usually nausea and vomiting lasted 24 to 48 hours after administration of combination of Adriamycin, Cytoxan and 5-FU. The second most common complication was total alopecia which was reversible once Adriamycin was discontinued. In one patient at the dose of $240 mg/M^2$, EKG changes in the form of voltage reduction and slight increase in cardiac size (on chest x-ray) were noted. Adriamycin was discontinued and the patient has been observed for over a year, with no resulting evidence of congestive heart failure. Hematological toxicity is shown in Table IV. The median lowest absolute granulocyte count was 2,400 with range of 1,000 to 4,700. Median lowest platelet count was 260,000 with a range of 63,000 to 400,000 and there is no apparent cumulative toxicity of the chemotherapy on the bone marrow. Infectious complications were very rare in spite of leukopenia. There were three episodes of pneumonia, two episodes occurred in one patient. Amenorrhea was observed in 71% of the premenopausal patients. Six patients refused further chemotherapy after receiving one or more cycles of chemotherapy.

TABLE III

FAC-BCG ADJUVANT

NON-HEMATOLOGICAL TOXICITY

Manifestations	No. of Patients	Percent
Nausea, Vomiting	70	93.3%
Total Alopecia	73	97.3%
Oral Mucositis	1	1%
Amenorrhea	20 of 28	71.5%
Adriamycin Skin Infiltration	1	1%
Non-specific EKG changes	1	1%
Pneumonia	2	2.6%
Severe BCG Reactions	4	5.3%

TABLE IV

FAC-BCG ADJUVANT

HEMATOLOGICAL TOXICITY

Course		1	2	3	4
Nadir Absolute Granulocyte	Median	2.7	2.6	2.4	2.1
	Range	1.0-4.7	1.2-3.5	1.4-4.5	1.6-4.3
Nadir Platelet	Median	240	268	159	270
	Range	98-400	92-283	63-212	144-311
% Drugs Administered		100	95	90	90

DISCUSSION

The data indicates that intensive postoperative chemoimmunotherapy results in a statistically significant reduction in recurrence during the first 32 months after mastectomy for Stage II or III breast cancer. At the present time this advantage from chemoimmunotherapy appears statistically evident in all subgroups of patients except those with 1-3 positive nodes and T_1 or small primary. Since the patients in these favorable prognostic groups have shorter follow-up it is possible that with longer follow-up a statistically significant advantage could arise in these two subgroups. This is the first reported study to demonstrate that survival after surgery has been significantly prolonged by use of post-operative adjuvant treatment compared to regional therapy for breast cancer. At the present time the advantage of FAC-BCG appears statistically significant in most subgroups including pre and post menopausal as well as patients with 4 or more positive nodes. Long term treatment has been associated with acceptable rate of toxic manifestations. While we have not seen clinical cardiac toxicity, long term effects of Adriamycin on the heart remain to be determined. We would hope that by discontinuing this drug well below the acceptable cumulative levels, permanent damage will not result.

REFERENCES

1. Young, R. C., et al: Cell Cycle Characteristics of Human and Solid Tumor in Vivo. Cell Tissue Kinet. 3: 285-290, 1970.
2. Fisher, B., et al: l-Phenylamine Mustard (L-PAM) in Management of Primary Breast Cancer. A report of early findings. N. Eng. J. Med. 292: 117-122, 1975.
3. Bonadonna, G., et al: The CMF Program for Operable Breast Cancer With Positive Axillary Nodes. Presented at the Symposium on Breast Cancer. A Report of the Profession. November 22-23, 1976.
4. Blumenschein, G. R., et al: FAC Chemotherapy for Breast Cancer. Proceedings of American Society of Clinical Oncology, March 27, 1974, Abstract #829.
5. Gutterman, J. U., et al: Chemoimmunotherapy of Advanced Breast Cancer Prolongation of Remission and Survival with BCG. Brit. Med. J. 2: 1222-1225, 1976.
6. Schabel, F. M., Jr.: Concept for Systemic Treatment of Micro-Metastasis. Cancer 35: 15-24, 1975.

Adjuvant Therapy of Cancer, S.E. Salmon and S.E. Jones eds.

ADJUVANT CHEMOIMMUNOTHERAPY OF STAGE IV (NED) BREAST CANCER

G. R. Blumenschein, A. U. Buzdar, C. K. Tashima,
G. N. Hortobagyi and J. U. Gutterman
The University of Texas System Cancer Center, M. D. Anderson Hospital
and Tumor Institute, 6723 Bertner Avenue, Houston, Texas 77030

INTRODUCTION

The occurrence of an isolated metastatic focus of breast cancer distant in location and time from the site of the regional therapy for primary disease implies that the patient has disseminated metastatic disease.[1,2] These isolated first recurrences or metastases have been treated with local resection and/or irradiation with varying degrees of success in terms of the duration of disease free survival to subsequent recurrences of metastases.[3,4] The duration of the disease free interval between the first clinically apparent metastasis and the second appears to be related to the stage of the primary disease and probably is a reflection of the growth rate of the breast cancer.[5] Because only 21% of patients survive 5 years from the discovery of an initial single metastasis despite aggressive regional treatment and because essentially no patients are cured by such regional therapy, we considered these patients an ideal population for the investigation of intensive adjuvant chemoimmunotherapy. These patients have been termed Stage IV, no evidence of disease (NED).

MATERIALS AND METHODS

Between January 1974 and October 1976, fifty-six patients who met the criteria of having an initial site of recurrence which was either surgically resectable or curable by irradiation were entered into the study. When it was considered advisable the combination of surgery and irradiation were used. All patients were staged with complete history and physical examination, blood counts, serum chemisteries, bone marrow aspiration and biopsy, skeletal x-ray survey, chest x-ray, bone scan, liver scan, and mammogram of the opposite breast. Following regional therapy of the initial site of metastases, all patients were clinically free of metastatic breast cancer and were begun on a program of 5-Fluorouracil (400mg/M^2 IV on days 1 and 8 of each course), Adriamycin (40mg/M^2 IV on day 1) and Cyclophosphamide (400mg/M^2 IV on day 1) (FAC). Courses of chemotherapy were repeated every 28 days. BCG (Lyophilized Tice or Pasteur strain) nonspecific immunotherapy in a dose of 6×10^8 infective units was administered by scarification on days 9, 16 and 23 of each course. This chemotherapy program was continued until patients had received a total of 450mg/M^2 of Adriamycin, at which time IM Methotrexate was substituted for the antracycline antibiotic. Patients then received Cyclophosphamide (500mg/M^2 PO on day 2), Methotrexate (30mg/M^2 IM on days 1 and 8) and 5-Fluorouracil (500mg/M^2 PO on days 1 and 8) (CMF) until a total of two years of treatment had elapsed. BCG immunotherapy was continued on days 9, 16 and 23 of each 28 day CMF course. Dose escalation or de-escalation was performed in order to maintain the granulocyte nadir between 1,000 and 2,000 counts per cubic millimeter and the platelet count nadir above 50,000. Documented infection and/or hemorrhage required a dose reduction of 25% regardless of blood counts. Clinical evidence of congestive heart failure prompted the discontinuation of Adriamycin. Excessive local inflammation, disseminated skin-satellite lesions or protracted severe systemic reactions from BCG caused an initial 50% reduction in BCG dose and if persistent, a 90% reduction. Patients were restaged at 4-month intervals for clinical evidence of metastatic disease.

Disease free survival between initial metastasis and second occurrence of metastasis was measured from the day of regional therapy to the day of clinical appearance of a second metastasis. The duration of survival was measured from the time of the regional treatment of initial recurrence to time of death.

A control group was selected by reviewing all charts of breast cancer patients seen at M. D. Anderson Hospital between January 1969 and December 1975 with identifiable isolated recurrence in a site which was treated either by surgery and/or radiation and who had no other clinical evidence of systemic metastatic disease. Sixty-seven patients met the criteria for this control group. Their disease free survival between the treatment of first recurrence and the appearance of a second metastasis and their overall survival were calculated and compared to the FAC-BCG treated Stage IV (NED) patients. The Stage IV (NED) FAC-BCG treated patients were comparable to the historical control patients as to sites of first recurrence (Table 1) and as to the type of regional therapy employed to treat the initial re-

TABLE 1

COMPARABILITY OF CONTROL AND IMMUNOCHEMISTRY PATIENTS AS TO SITE OF OCCURRENCE - STAGE IV (NED) BREAST CANCER

PARAMETER	CONTROL	FAC-BCG	P VALUE
Site of 1st Recurrence			
Chest Wall	41	31	0.51
Supraclavicular Nodes	14	9	0.49
Bone	6	6	0.74
Axillary Nodes	2	5	0.16
Scalp	1	0	--
Hilar Nodes	1	0	--
Lung	1	2	--
Brain	1	1	--
Endobronchial	0	1	--
Ovaries	0	1	--
TOTAL	67	56	

currence (Table 2). The study groups were similar as to initial stage of breast cancer (Table 3) and disease free interval between primary regional therapy and initial recurrence (Table 4).

TABLE 2

COMPARABILITY OF CONTROL AND IMMUNOCHEMOTHERAPY PATIENTS AS TO REGIONAL THERAPY OF FIRST RECURRENCE-STAGE IV (NED) BREAST CANCER

PARAMETER	CONTROL	FAC-BCG	P VALUE
Surgery	25	26	0.31
Radiotherapy	17	16	0.69
Both	25	14	0.14

TABLE 3

COMPARABILITY OF CONTROL AND IMMUNOCHEMOTHERAPY PATIENTS AS TO DISEASE FREE INTERVAL - STAGE IV (NED) (MEDIAN TIME IN MONTHS BETWEEN TREATMENT OF PRIMARY BREAST CANCER AND 1ST SOLITARY METASTASES)

FAC-BCG		CONTROL	
Median	24	Median	28
Range	2-106	Range	2-181

TABLE 4

COMPARABILITY OF CONTROL AND IMMUNOCHEMOTHERAPY PATIENTS AS TO STAGE AT PRIMARY DIAGNOSIS - STAGE IV (NED)

STAGE	FAC-BCG	CONTROL
I	11 (20%)	8 (12%)
II	39 (69%)	52 (78%)
III	6 (11%)	7 (10%)

The statistical methods used included a CHI-Square test for differences in disease free survival, a generalized Wilcoxon test with a one tailed analysis for testing differences in survival curves.[6] and the method of Kaplan and Meier for calculating and plotting survival curves.[7]

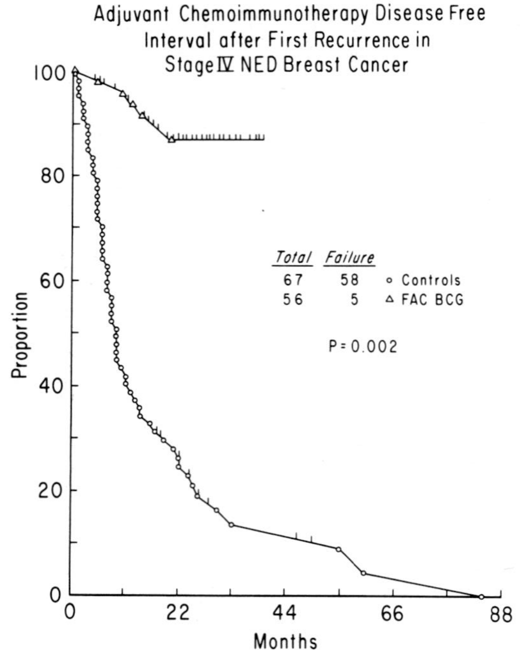

Fig. 1. Adjuvant Chemoimmunotherapy Disease-Free Interval After First Recurrence in Stage IV NED Breast Cancer

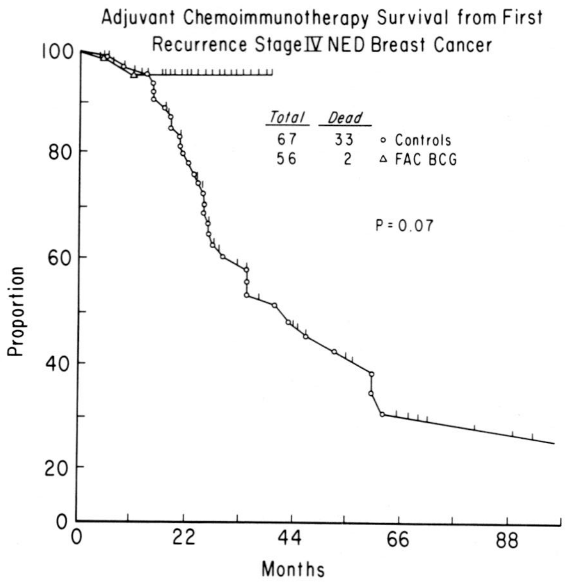

Fig. 2. Adjuvant Chemoimmunotherapy Survival from First Recurrence Stage IV NED Breast Cancer

RESULTS

At 32 months of study, with a median follow-up of 17 months, 5 of 56 FAC-BCG patients have developed clinical evidence of metastatic disease. In contrast the median disease free interval for control patients between the first and second recurrence was 9 months (P=0.002), and at a similar follow-up period of 17 months, 47 of the 67 control patients had evidenced recurrent metastatic disease (Fig. 1). During the same period of time two study patients have died of metastatic disease and one of unrelated causes. Six of the control patients had died from metastatic disease within a similar time period. Overall survival of the FAC-BCG treated patients approaches significance as compared to controls (P=0.07) (Fig. 2).

Toxicity to the chemoimmunotherapy was similar to that reported in detail for FAC-BCG.

DICUSSION

The failure of regional therapy alone for solitary first metastasis in breast cancer is well documented.[3,4] The 9-month median duration of disease free survival and the poor overall survival of the 67 historical control patients in this study is comparable to published reports of similarly treated patients.

While the disease free interval (DFI) and survival of patients from initial surgery is related to stage of primary disease,[9] the survival of patients following regional treatment of initial metastatic recurrence appears less related to initial stage and not related to DFI.[5,10]

We selected Stage IV (NED) breast cancer patients for intensive adjuvant chemoimmunotherapy because this patient population represented a clinical setting in which there was a nearly 100% probability for the presence of microscopic metastatic disease.

The populations of treated patients and control patients were small, and differed slightly as to intensity of staging for clinically evident metastatic disease and as to systemic therapy for treatment of disseminated metastases. The interval of study is too short to draw significant conclusions regarding the major question of improved overall survival and possible cure for adjuvant chemoimmunotherapy treated patients. The data does indicate that the use of intensive combination chemoimmunotherapy with FAC-BCG in patients with isolated recurrent metastatic disease, completely removed by either surgery or irradiation, can significantly prolong the disease free interval in these patients and improve survival for the short term. Whether this therapeutic approach can achieve sufficient tumor cell kill to eliminate all breast cancer in a significant proportion of this population of patients awaits continued observation.

REFERENCES

1. Spratt, J. (1967) Locally Recurrent Cancer After Radical Mastectomy. Cancer, 20:1051-1053.
2. Dao, T. and Nemoto, T. (1963) The Clinical Significance of Skin Recurrence After Radical Mastectomy in Women With Cancer of the Breast. Surgery, Gynecology & Obstetrics 117:447-453.
3. Chu, F. et al. (1976) Locally Recurrent Carcinoma of the Breast. Results of Radiation Therapy. Cancer 37:2677-2681.
4. Auchincloss, H. (1958) The Nature of Local Recurrence Following Radical Mastectomy. Cancer 11:611-619.
5. Devitt, J. (1971) The Enigmatic Behavior of Breast Cancer. Cancer 27:12-17.
6. Gehan, E. (1965) A Generalized Wilcoxon Test for Comparing Arbitrarily Single Censored Samples. Biometrika 52:203-223.
7. Kaplan, E. and Meier, P. (1958) Non-parametric Estimation from Incomplete Observations. Journal of the American Statistical Association 53:457-481.
8. Gutterman, J. et al. (1976) Chemoimmunotherapy of Advanced Breast Cancer Prolongation of Remission and Survival with BCG. British Medical Journal 2: 1222-1225.
9. Bond, W. (1975) Natural History of Breast Cancer. In Stoll, B., Ed., Host Defense in Breast Cancer. Chicago, William Heinemann Medical Books Ltd., 95-110
10. Papaioannou, A. et al. (1967) Fate of Patients With Recurrent Carcinoma of the Breast. Recurrence Five or More Years After Initial Treatment. Cancer 20:371-376

Adjuvant Therapy of Cancer, S.E. Salmon and S.E. Jones eds.

ADJUVANT TREATMENT OF BREAST CANCER WITH ADRIAMYCIN-CYCLOPHOSPHAMIDE WITH OR WITHOUT RADIATION THERAPY

Neel Hammond, M.D.
Stephen E. Jones, M.D.
Sydney E. Salmon, M.D.
Gerald Giordano, M.D.
Ralph Jackson, M.D.
Robert Miller, M.D.
Robert Heusinkveld, M.D., Ph.D.
Cancer Center Division
University of Arizona College of Medicine
Tucson, Arizona 85724

INTRODUCTION

Initial studies with the combination of adriamycin and cyclophosphamide (A-C) in human breast cancer began in 1973 at the University of Arizona. These trials were based on our exploratory observations in patients plus simultaneous observations in animal tumor systems which indicated that the combination of these two agents might be synergistic[1,2]. Indeed, in our first study we observed an overall objective response rate of 78% in 51 patients with advanced breast cancer who had not received prior chemotherapy. The high response rate, acceptable toxicity, and ease of administration of the drugs in patients with advanced disease encouraged us to employ this combination in an adjuvant breast cancer program. (The additional kinetic considerations of this trial have been summarized by Salmon elsewhere in this text[3].) Thus, in mid-1974 we initiated the Arizona Breast Cancer Adjuvant Program[4,5]. This report will summarize our preliminary results to date in this ongoing clinical trial.

PATIENTS AND METHODS

Since July 1974, patients undergoing recent surgery for breast cancer who are potentially eligible for adjuvant treatment have been referred for possible inclusion in the program. After referral, patients are evaluated for evidence of metastatic disease by means of a careful physical examination, routine laboratory work, chest radiograph, and bone scan. If the bone scan is abnormal, appropriate x-rays are obtained. Unless the x-rays confirm overt metastatic disease, patients are eligible for adjuvant treatment. Additional laboratory, radiographic, or nuclear diagnostic studies are performed when clinically indicated. Patients also have baseline cardiac examination with a battery of non-invasive tests of ventricular function (eg, systolic time intervals, echocardiography)[6].

The eligibility criteria for this study include initiation of chemotherapy within 2 months after surgery for infiltrating ductal adenocarcinoma of pathologic stage I, II, or III extent, no evidence of overt metastases, no prior breast cancer or heart disease, and informed written consent in accord with University of Arizona guidelines for protection of human subjects. The assignment of treatment depends on assessment of the potential risk of relapse, which, in turn, is predicated on knowledge of the stage of disease and nodal status (Table 1).

TABLE 1

ARIZONA BREAST CANCER ADJUVANT PROGRAM

TREATMENT PLAN BASED ON INITIAL STAGE OF DISEASE

Stage of Disease	Risk Category/ Treatment Plan*
Stage I (lateral lesion) (tumor < 4 cm; negative nodes)	"Low Risk" 3 courses of A-C
Stage I (medial lesion) or Stage II (tumor > 4 cm or 1-3 positive nodes or < 50% of removed nodes positive)	"Intermediate Risk" 2 courses of A-C ± radiation therapy + 6 courses of A-C
Stage II (≥ 4 positive nodes or > 50% of removed nodes positive) or Stage III (skin involvement, fixed tumor or nodes, infra- or supraclavicular nodes)	"High Risk" 2 courses of A-C + Radiation Therapy + 6 courses of A-C

*A-C = adriamycin and cyclophosphamide administered at 3-week intervals.

All patients entered to date have received chemotherapy in the schedule shown in Table 2. The doses employed in the adjuvant schedule represent 75% of the "full" doses originally employed in patients with advanced disease[1]. These lower doses were chosen to minimize toxicity in the adjuvant setting.

TABLE 2

DRUG DOSES AND SCHEDULE OF CHEMOTHERAPY

	Days 1	2	3	4	5	6
Adriamycin	30 mg/M^2 IV	—	—	—	—	—
Cyclophosphamide	—	—	150 mg/M^2 PO Q D x 4 days			

*Administered every 3 weeks.

Patients with stage I disease (negative axillary nodes and primary lesions of less than 4 cm in diameter) have been divided into "low" and "intermediate" risk groups according to the tumor location (Table 1). Lateral lesions are considered as "low" risk, and these patients receive 3 courses of A-C at 3-week intervals without irradiation. Medial lesions are treated as "intermediate risk" because of the unknown status of the internal mammary nodes. Medial stage I lesions and stage II lesions (1-3 involved axillary lymph nodes, or primary tumor more than 4 cm in diameter) are considered "intermediate" for risk of relapse. All patients in this category receive 8 courses of A-C at 3-week intervals. Half of these patients also receive radiation therapy commencing after the first 2 courses of A-C. Radiation therapy is administered at least 1 week after the second dose of adriamycin to a dose of 4400 rads to the chest wall, supraclavicular, axillary, and internal mammary lymph node chains[7]. Within 1-2 weeks after completion of the radiation therapy, another 6 courses of A-C are administered at 3-week intervals. Patients with matted or clinically fixed axillary lymph nodes, enlarged supraclavicular lymph nodes, or involvement of the muscles at the time of surgery are considered to have stage III disease and receive 8 courses of A-C with irradiation after the first 2 courses.

Following completion of the initial treatment, patients undergo a careful reexamination including bone scanning[8]. Subsequent followup is carried out at 3-month intervals. Repeat bone scans are performed at 6-month intervals if initially abnormal or if they have changed serially and otherwise at 12-month intervals. Relapse is confirmed histologically (if possible) or radiographically in all cases. Survival and relapse-free survival have been calculated by the method of Kaplan and Meier[9] and differences evaluated by the method of Gehan[10].

RESULTS

Between June 1974 and June 1976, 61 eligible patients with surgically resected breast cancer who were free of overt metastases were entered into this adjuvant program. Surgery consisted of either a modified radical mastectomy (40 patients), a standard Halsted radical mastectomy (18 patients), or a simple mastectomy (3 patients with stage III disease). All patients began chemotherapy within 2 months after surgery. The preliminary results are summarized in Table 3.

TABLE 3

PRELIMINARY RESULTS (JULY 1974 TO JANUARY 1977)

Stage of Disease	Number of Patients	Mean Time of Followup (months)	Number of Relapses
I	10	9	0
II	36	14	1
III	15	17	5
Total	61		6

With a mean followup time of 9 months from mastectomy, there have been no recurrences in the patients with stage I disease. Among the 36 patients with stage II disease (mean followup time of 14 months from mastectomy), a single recurrence has been observed. The major prognostic factors in this group of patients with stage II disease (which are comparable to the patients receiving adjuvant chemotherapy in other ongoing trials[11,12]) are summarized in Table 4. Approximately one half of these patients received radiation therapy in addition to chemotherapy.

TABLE 4
CLINICAL, PATHOLOGIC, AND TREATMENT FEATURES
OF 36 PATIENTS WITH STAGE II BREAST CANCER
RECEIVING ADJUVANT THERAPY WITH A-C (± RADIATION THERAPY)

Feature	Number of Patients
Menopausal Status:	
Premenopausal	12
Postmenopausal	24
Size of Primary Tumor	
$<$ 2 cm	7
2-5 cm	26
$>$ 5 cm	3
Number of Involved Axillary Lymph Nodes	
1-3	20
$\geq$ 4	16
Regional Radiation Therapy	19

The relapse-free survival curves for all patients entered on this study before June 1976 are given in Figure 1.

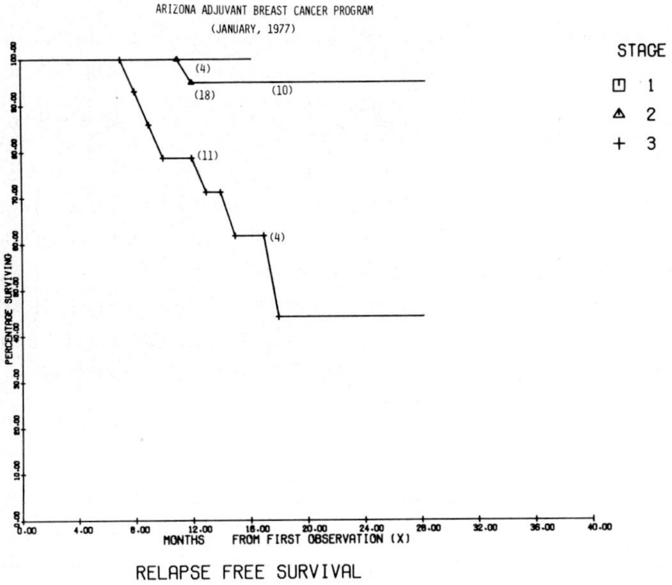

Figure 1. Disease-free survival according to initial stage of disease for 61 patients with breast cancer who received adjuvant chemotherapy with adriamycin-cyclophosphamide with or without regional radiation therapy. The difference between patients with stage II and stage III disease is not yet significant (p = 0.15). Numbers in parentheses indicate the number of patients at risk.

Of 6 patients with clinical recurrence, 1 has died. The locations of initial recurrence were skin (3 patients), lymph nodes (3 patients), and bone (1 patient). Local control has been possible with radiation therapy in 2 local recurrences and in 1 patient with symptomatic bone metastases. Relapsing patients have not experienced complete or partial responses with subsequent therapy, but metastatic disease has been stabilized in 4 patients with cyclophosphamide-methotrexate-5-fluorouracil (2 patients), androgens (1 patient), or estrogens (1 patient).

Adjuvant chemotherapy with A-C is quite well tolerated. In this evaluated group alopecia was the most common side effect. Myelosuppression was mild and manifested almost exclusively by leukopenia. Although 30 (50%) of the evaluated patients had some degree of leukopenia, dose reductions were required in only 14 patients (23%). There were no episodes of sepsis or bacterial infection. Moderate or severe thrombocytopenia did not occur in any of these patients. Nausea (or at least anorexia of some degree) was present in over half of the patients, usually in association with the oral cyclophosphamide treatment. Cessation of menses and/or hot flashes were described in 7 (64%) of the 11 premenopausal patients specifically questioned in this regard. Skin reactions were noted in 2 patients. The first of these patients was receiving concurrent irradiation, and the details have been reported elsewhere[7]. The second patient experienced recall of a radiation reaction when adriamycin was administered after irradiation. Neither of these skin reactions resulted in permanent disfigurement or required skin grafting. Five instances of apical fibrosis were noted on routine chest x-ray after local radiation therapy. These x-ray changes were either asymptomatic or associated with mild dyspnea (2 patients). On occasion this caused a diagnostic dilemma when the clinician was unaware of this particular side effect. Infrequently observed toxic effects included mucositis (1 patient), cystitis (2 patients), and conjunctivitis (1 patient). No deterioration of cardiac function has been detected to date by the serial studies of ventricular function. The major side effects of this adjuvant program are summarized in Table 5.

TABLE 5

SIDE EFFECTS OF ADJUVANT CHEMOTHERAPY

Side Effect	Number (%)
Bacterial infections	0
Overt cardiac toxicity	0
Myelosuppression	
Anemia (requiring transfusion)	0
Thrombocytopenia (platelets $< 100{,}000/mm^3$)	0
Leukopenia	
WBC $2500 - 4000/mm^3$	24 (40%)
WBC $< 2500/mm^3$	6 (10%)
Nausea	41 (67%)
Alopecia	60 (98%)
Cessation of menses/hot flashes	7 (64%)
Skin reactions	2 (3%)

DISCUSSION

This report describes the adjuvant treatment of breast cancer with the synergistic drug combination of adriamycin and cyclophosphamide[1,2]. These early results indicate an efficacy that is at least comparable to other on-going studies[11,12]. The toxicity, as shown, is acceptable to patients and easy to manage. Long-term toxicity is not yet known, but this is also true for the other current adjuvant programs throughout the world.

Potential (but not yet observed) disadvantages of this program include the use of a potentially cardiotoxic drug when some patients can be expected to survive many years, and the apparent difficulty in treating patients who subsequently recur.

Inherent advantages of our program include the theoretically kinetic superiority of a pulse (every 3-week) chemotherapy schedule employing synergistic agents,[3] ease of administration of the drugs requiring only 8 total office visits, and a total treatment time of about 6 months compared to 12-24 months for several other programs[11,12].

Although we have solved logistic and potential toxicity problems in combining adriamycin and irradiation in this program,[7] the exact role and need for regional and chest wall irradiation must be clarified with longer followup and further analysis.

ACKNOWLEDGEMENTS

The authors wish to thank John Gaines for assistance in preparing survival curves, Ellen Chase for editing and data collection, and many Tucson surgeons and medical oncologists for their participation in this program. This work was supported in part by a research grant (CA-17094) from the National Cancer Institute, National Institutes of Health, Department of Health, Education, and Welfare.

REFERENCES

1. Jones, S., Durie, B., Salmon, S. (1975) Combination chemotherapy with adriamycin and cyclophosphamide for advanced breast cancer, Cancer 36:90-97.
2. Corbett, T., Griswold, D., Mayo, J., et al (1975) Cyclophosphamide-adriamycin combination chemotherapy of transplantable murine tumors, Cancer Res. 35:1568-1573.
3. Salmon, S. (1977) Kinetic rationale for adjuvant chemotherapy of cancer. In Adjuvant Therapy of Cancer (Salmon, S., and Jones, S., eds.). Elsevier/North Holland Press (this volume).
4. Jones, S. (1974) Clinical Oncology in Arizona. Chemotherapy of breast cancer - investigational treatment, Arizona Med. 31:197-198.
5. Salmon, S. (1975) Clinical Oncology in Arizona. Progress in adjuvant chemotherapy of early breast cancer, Arizona Med. 32:108-109.
6. Ewy, G., Jones, S., Groves, B. (1976) Adriamycin heart disease, Arizona Med. 33:274-278.
7. Aristizabal, S., Miller, R., Schlichtemeier, A., et al (1977) Adriamycin-irradiation cutaneous complications, Int. J. Rad. Oncology (in press).
8. Hammond, N., Jones, S., Salmon, S., et al (1977) Bone scanning in an adjuvant breast cancer program, abstract, American Society of Clinical Oncology.
9. Kaplan, E. and Meier, P. (1958) Non-parametric estimations from incomplete observations, J. Amer. Stat. Assoc. 53:457-481.
10. Gehan, E. (1965) A generalized Wilcoxon test for comparing arbitrarily singly-censored samples, Biometrika 52:203-223.
11. Bonnadonna, G., Rossi, A., Vallagussa, P., et al (1977) The CMF program for operable breast cancer with positive axillary nodes, a report to the profession, Cancer (in press).

12. Fisher, B., Carbone, P., Economou, S., et al (1975) L-Phenylalanine mustard (L-PAM) in the management of primary breast cancer. A report of early findings, N. Engl. J. Med. 292:117-122.

Adjuvant Therapy of Cancer, S.E. Salmon and S.E. Jones eds.

RISK-BENEFIT CONSIDERATIONS FOR ADJUVANT L-PHENYLALANINE MUSTARD (L-PAM) CHEMOTHERAPY OF PATIENTS WITH BREAST CANCER AND NEGATIVE LYMPH NODES- A PRELIMINARY REPORT.

Richard S. Bornstein, M.D., Stanley N. Levick, M.D.
Leonard J. Levick, M.D., Sidney Sachs, M.D. Kenneth Algazy, M.D.
Mt. Sinai Hospital, University Circle
Cleveland Ohio, 44106
Albert Einstein Medical Center, Northern Division,
Philadelphia Pennsylvania, 19141

Breast cancer is the most frequent malignancy and the leading cause of cancer death in women. Traditional efforts based on eradicating the local disease and its regional extension have met with only limited success. According to Mueller & Jeffries (1), who studied the cause of death and rate of dying from several breast cancer populations, over 85% of women with breast cancer died of their disease. This fact, as well as other clinical and pathologic observations support the concept, to quote Baum (2) " breast cancer is a systemic process until proven otherwise".

As early as 1896, Beatson (3), who is remembered for reporting regression of breast cancer after oophorectomy, stated "the tumor in the breast is only a local manifestation of a blood affection". That breast cancer is a disseminated systemic process requires that the traditional therapeutic regimens be abandoned or augmented Local or extended surgery or radiation therapy given at the time of presentation have not and will not affect the systemic process; treatment techniques directed at both the local and systemic disease have the potential for being effective. One of the most exciting areas in cancer treatment involves the application of systemic treatment regimens, which have been shown efficacious in advanced disease, as adjunctive therapy in high risk patients who have little or no evidence of residual disease. The concepts upon which this systemic treatment of microscopic metastases are based, have been presented by previous speakers.

Who then are the "high risk" patients with breast cancer? Studies from the National Surgical Adjuvant Breast Project (NSABP) reported by Fisher have correlated recurrence rate and survival with pathologic nodal status. Patients with metastases in the regional lymph nodes have been referred to as "high risk" for recurrence, while those with negative lymph nodes have been called "low risk. The fc :r group have been the subject of several carefully controlled prospective clinical trials, previously reported at this meeting. The so-called "low risk" patients with negative nodes have not received similar trials. The recurrence rate in this group is 5% at 18 months, 18% at 5 years and 24% at 10 years.

While this is significantly better than the 76% recurrence rate in the positive node patients, this recurrence in one in four patients does not lend itself to the designation " low risk". Furthermore two other questions remain in regards to the nodal status of the individual patient. One involves the adequacy of the axillary dissection; are there nodes left behind which may be positive? The second involves the adequacy of the pathologic search for malignancy within the nodes which are resected; would serial sections yield a higher incidence of positive nodes?

Because of these questions and because of the feeling that patients with a one in four chance of recurrence have a significant risk, we began a prospective trial of patients with negative lymph nodes following surgical resection of their primary tumor and in whom no other evidence of disease was present. The drug l-phenylalanine mustard or L-Pam, known to be effective in advanced disease and for which encouraging preliminary results had been presented from the NSABP trial in patients with positive nodes, was selected. Furthermore L-Pam was associated with a relative lack of significant toxicity and offered the benefit of ease of administration. It is the purpose of this report to explore the risk-benefit considerations of L-Pam treatment in patients with breast cancer in whom the regional lymph nodes are uninvolved with tumors at the time of mastectomy.

In the first place, 70-75% of such patients are receiving unnecessary treatment, that is, they have been cured by the surgical resection alone. Short term toxicity consists of nausea and vomiting in some 20% to 30% and myelosuppression of some degree in all; in no patients did this become life threatening. This becomes a more significant problem when one utilizes multiple drug regimens.

While the immediate toxicity of L-Pam is minimal, there are certain long term theoretical problems to consider(4). Immunosuppression is a significant consequence of most cytoxic chemotherapeutic agents, including L-Pam. The data most often cited include the increased incidence of malignancy in patients with inherited immuno-deficiency diseases and the high incidence of de novo malignancy in organ homograft recipients. This latter frequency is about 100 times greater than would be expected in the normal population of similar age. This may represent a consequence of the immunosuppression or may be related to another potential risk of this type of therapy, carcinogenesis. Animal studies have amply documented the carcinogenic effect of most cytoxic agents; the data in humans, however, remains somewhat difficult to obtain. Penn (5) recently reported 166 malignancies in 160 patients who had previously been treated for cancer with chemotherapeutic agents. Most of the original cases of malignancy were of the hematologic variety and it has been speculated that the new malignancy, commonly a lymphoma or leukemia, might merely be the natural transition from one form of related malignancy to another, particularly in patients in whom the natural history had been altered by increased survival through the use of chemotherapy. It is also well known that persons with cancer have an increased incidence of second cancers. Thus it is still not clear whether drugs such as L-Pam increase the risk of second malignancy.

In view of these potential risk factors, what are the potential benefits which may accrue from the use of adjuvant L-Pam in patients with negative lymph nodes? As noted earlier many now consider that breast cancer is disseminated at the time of diagnosis. If this is true, then all attempts at purely localized management such as surgical resection of the primary tumor or post operative radiation therapy would be doomed to failure; in this circumstance, one must consider the use of adjunctive systemic treatment. The data of Schabel and others in animal tumor systems have shown a significant increase in the cure rate with the use of drug treatment following surgical removal of the primary tumor as compared to the use of surgery or chemotherapy alone. These principles of early systemic treatment have been shown to be valid in humans in regards to the treatment of osteogenic sarcomas and in the multimodality approach to the treatment of Wilm's tumor and embryonal rhabdomyosarcomas. More recently, the encouraging data of Fisher and Bonadonna in patients with breast carcinoma with positive lymph nodes have been presented. Very little comparable data exist in patients with negative nodes.

One study reported by Donegan (6) involved a series of 75 patients treated by surgery and 90 patients receiving similar surgery plus one year of chemotherapy with thiotepa. While there was no overall improvement in survival in the entire study, there was an interesting trend in patients with negative nodes. Although not statistically significant, the disease free survival appeared to be improved in those receiving adjuvant therapy and in whom axillary metastases was not present at the time of resection. More recently Donovan et al (7) reported on a 4-6 month course of cyclophosphamide following surgical resection of breast cancer. A significant increase in the ten year survival of treated patients as compared to historical controls was noted. When further analyzed, the improvement was due to a significant increase in survival of patients with histologically negative axillary lymph nodes. Among the treated patients with negative nodes, 16 of 20 (80%) survived 10 years as opposed to 33 of 78 (42%) of the untreated controls. While neither of these studies are definitive, they do lend some support to the concept of the treatment of patients with negative nodes.

Our trial was begun in January 1975, and to date, 54 patients have been entered; of these 21 have completed 18 months of treatment and an additional 8 have been followed over one year. Because of the small patient accrual expected in a single Medical Oncology practice, this pilot study was conducted in a non-randomized, non controlled fashion. L-Pam was given at a dose of 0.15 mg./kg. for 5 days and repeated at 6 week intervals for 18 months. Although this follow up period is quite short, there have been no recurrences in this group of patients. Furthermore, there have been no major toxic effects noted.

In conclusion, it appears that more questions have been raised than can answers be given. Although long term adjuvant chemotherapy may alter the natural history of breast cancer, it remains to be proven whether such improvement is out-weighed by the potential long term side effects. Will delayed recurrence result in significant long term improvement in survival and cure ? Will such an increase if it occurs fully justify the potential long term side effects of such a regimen ? Only time and adequately designed prospective randomized trials will give information in regards to these questions. On balance, it appears that such adjuvant studies are warranted in patients with breast cancer and negative lymph nodes.

REFERENCES

1. Mueller CB, Jeffries W: Cancer of the breast: its outcome as measured by the rate of dying and causes of death. Ann Surg 182:334-341, 1975.
2. Baum M: The curability of breast cancer. Br. Med J 1: 439-442, 1976.
3. Beatson GT: On the treatment of inoperable cases of carcinoma of the mammer: Suggestions for a new method of treatment, with illustrative cases, Lancet 2: 104-107, 1896.
4. Costanza ME: The problems of breast cancer prophylaxis. NEJM 293: 1095-1097, 1975.
5. Penn I: Second Malignant Neoplasms associated with immunosuppressive Medications, Cancer 37: 1024-1032, 1976.
6. Donegan WL: Extended surgical adjuvant thiotepa for mammary carcinoma. Arch Surg 109: 187-192, 1974.
7. Donovan IA et al: A prolonged course of cyclophosphamide as an adjunct to mastectomy in the primary treatment of breast carcinoma. Br J Surg 63: 817-818, 1976.

Adjuvant Therapy of Cancer, S.E. Salmon and S.E. Jones eds.

ADJUVANT CHEMOTHERAPY-RADIOTHERAPY IN BREAST CARCINOMA*

G. Ramirez,** F. J. Ansfield,+ W. H. Wolberg,++ H. L. Davis,**
A. Greenberg,** T. E. Davis,***, and E. C. Borden***
University of Wisconsin Center for Health Sciences
Madison, Wisconsin 53706

SUMMARY

Forty-two patients with breast carcinoma and positive axillary nodes who underwent a modified or a radical mastectomy were treated with 5-fluorouracil, radiation therapy to the chest wall, axillary, supraclavicular, and internal mammary areas and maintained on 5-fluorouracil for a period of one year. Over half of them have been followed for at least three years. Thirteen cases (31 percent) have recurred since the initiation of the study and five patients died as a result of their disease. The median time of appearance of recurrences was twenty months and the largest number of recurrences occurred in the premenopausal women with more than four positive nodes. The patients have been followed by periods ranging between twenty-four and 114 months.

Breast carcinoma presents as localized disease in over 70% of patients. Primary approaches to cure have been local therapies, i.e. surgery and radiotherapy. However, more than 50% of patients die with widespread metastases by ten years. Probably too much emphasis has been placed on local control although it is agreed that local control is necessary for cure. Extended radical mastectomy as proposed by Wangensteen[1] did not significantly alter the survival and Urban[2] concluded that extended radical mastectomy was especially indicated for Stage I infiltrating cancers that occur in the medial and central portions of the breast. However, when both the axillary and internal mammary nodes were involved, only 40% of his cases were free of disease at five years.[3] Irradiation therapy has been employed for many years as an adjuvant to surgery and some claim close to 100% control of local and regional disease is secured by combining surgery with 4,500-5,000 rads to the chest wall and peripheral lymphatics.[4] The results of the NSABP randomized trial using radiotherapy postoperatively as reported by Fisher et al[5] indicated that the use of postoperative irradiation decreased the number of local and

---

* This investigation was supported in part by Grant Number CA-14520, awarded by the National Cancer Institute, DHEW to the Wisconsin Clinical Cancer Center.

** Associate Professor of Human Oncology, University of Wisconsin, Madison, WI 53706

\+ Emeritus Professor of Human Oncology, University of Wisconsin, Madison, WI. Present address: 2315 No. Lake Dr., Milwaukee, WI 53211

++ Professor of Human Oncology and Surgery, University of Wisconsin, Madison, WI 53706

*** Assistant Professor of Human Oncology, University of Wisconsin, Madison, WI 53706

Address for reprints: Guillermo Ramirez, M.D., Department of Human Oncology, University Hospitals, 1300 University Avenue, Madison, Wisconsin 53706

regional recurrences. However, there was an apparent increase in failures due to distant metastases and no improvement in survival. Thus, it is difficult to advocate the use of irradiation alone as an effective adjuvant to surgery in the treatment of operable breast cancer. Several studies combining single agent chemotherapy and surgery were reviewed by Tormey.[6] Although no definitive conclusions could be drawn from the data, there were enough differences among the regimens to suggest that larger doses of a drug given over longer periods of time may be more effective and that long-term survival benefits may require more than perioperative therapy. Favorable results with 5-fluorouracil as an adjuvant to mastectomy, utilizing the "loading" course, were reported by Ansfield[7] but further follow up of the cases failed to prove that this approach influenced either the incidence of recurrence or the survival.[8]

In an effort to improve disease-free interval as well as the survival we decided to take advantage of the effectiveness of radiotherapy in controlling local disease and 5-fluorouracil as a systemic agent to avert the appearance of distant metastases.

MATERIALS AND METHODS

Patients with histologically proven positive nodes following modified or radical mastectomy were treated with 5-fluorouracil and irradiation. Each patient received a "loading course" of 5-FU, 12 mg/kg/day x 5 followed by 6 mg/kg/every other day to slight toxicity or a maximum of ten doses, was given to each patient. The patients were given 4,500-5,000 rads to the chest wall, supraclavicular, axillary, and internal mammary areas within two weeks of the end of the "loading" course.

Post-operative Co^{60} irradiation was delivered in a standardized technique. The chest wall, axilla, homolateral internal mammary nodes of the first five interspaces and the supraclavicular nodes were irradiated to a tissue dose of 5,000 rad in five weeks (five weekday treatments per week). Five treatment fields at a source-skin distance of 100 centimeters were used: (1) anterior supraclavicular-axillary field whose inferior border is at the second anterior costal cartilage; (2) internal mammary field which extends from the second anterior costal cartilage superiorly to the base of the xiphoid inferiorly, and from the midline of the sternum out laterally for a width of six centimeters; (3) medial tangential chest wall field; (4) lateral tangential chest wall field. (Fields 3 and 4 employ the M.D. Anderson tangential field applicator which blocks the inferior half of the treatment beam minimizing divergence into the underlying lung and provides penumbra trimmers for sharpening the superior and inferior treatment edges. Bolus is used on alternate treatment days to increase the surface dose.) (5) Posterior axillary field is used to bring the total mid-axillary depth dose to 5,000 rad in five weeks. To maximize homegeniety of dose distribution in each treatment session, the first four fields are treated daily and the posterior axillary field (Field number 5) is treated three times a week. During the course of irradiation and thereafter for a period of one year, the patients received weekly injections of 5-fluorouracil at the dose of 15 mg/kg/week, providing the white blood cell count was 3,800 mm^3 or higher, and no other signs of toxicity were present. The maximum single dose given was 1 gm. A total of forty-two patients were entered on the study; twenty-three were premenopausal and nineteen were postmenopausal. The age of the patients ranged between twenty-six and seventy years with the median of fifty years.

TABLE 1.

BREAST CARCINOMA

Adjuvant Combined Therapy

Patients' Distribution by # of Nodes

1-3 Nodes: 16	
Premenopausal:	9
Postmenopausal:	7
> 4 Nodes: 26	
Premenopausal:	14
Postmenopausal:	12

The distribution of patients is given in Table 1. Patients with more than four positive nodes formed the largest group; there were a total of twenty-three premenopausal patients and nineteen in the postmenopausal group. Toxic reactions included nausea and vomiting in about 50% of the patients, diarrhea, ulceration of the buccal mucosa and symptoms of esophagitis. Reactions in the irradiated areas included erythema, tenderness, occasional sloughing of the epidermis, and symptoms of esophagitis. Toxic symptoms were never severe enough to require discontinuation of therapy.

RESULTS

The patients have been followed for periods ranging between twenty-four and 114 months, with a median length of follow up of 36 months. To date, there are thirty-seven patients alive and five dead. One patient committed suicide eight months after she developed recurrences and is included as a failure. Twenty-nine patients are disease free. In some instances the drug was omitted for one or two weeks because of the skin reactions on the irradiated areas but the total amount of irradiation planned did not have to be altered because of toxicity. All of the patients completed one year of chemotherapy with 5-FU by weekly injection, as indicated above.

A total of thirteen patients have had recurrence (31%). The recurrences appeared between eight and ninety-seven months following surgery. The median time to recurrence is twenty months. In the group with recurrences, nine patients were premenopausal and four were postmenopausal. The sites of recurrences are shown on Table 2. One patient developed a recurrence on the chest wall and had a distinct separate carcinoma in the opposite breast as well, making it difficult to say whether this patient represented a failure of local control by irradiation or the chest wall lesions represent metastases from possibly a second primary. The largest proportion of failures occurred in premenopausal women with four or more positive nodes (Table 3), a pattern previously recognized by Fisher.[9] The overall survival for the patients on the

TABLE 2.

BREAST CARCINOMA

Adjuvant Combined Therapy

Sites of Recurrence

Supraclavicular Nodes:	
Ipsilateral	1
Contralateral	3
Lungs	2
Pleura	2
Bone	3
Liver	2
Breast	2
Chest Wall	1

TABLE 3.

BREAST CARCINOMA

Adjuvant Combined Therapy

Recurrences by # of Nodes

1-3 Nodes:	3
Premenopausal:	2
Postmenopausal:	1
> 4 Nodes:	10
Premenopausal:	7
Postmenopausal:	3

study is shown in Figure 1. When the survival is compared by menopausal status (Figure 2) not a great difference between the premenopausal and postmenopausal groups was observed. If the patient population was separated according to the number of positive nodes, the differences were too small to achieve statistical significance. (Figure 3)

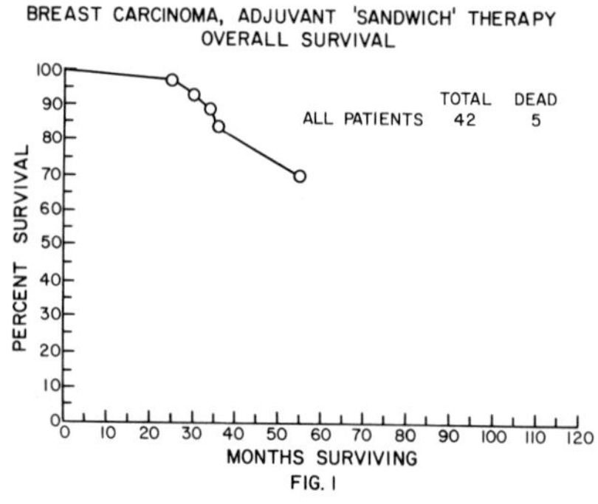

FIG. 1

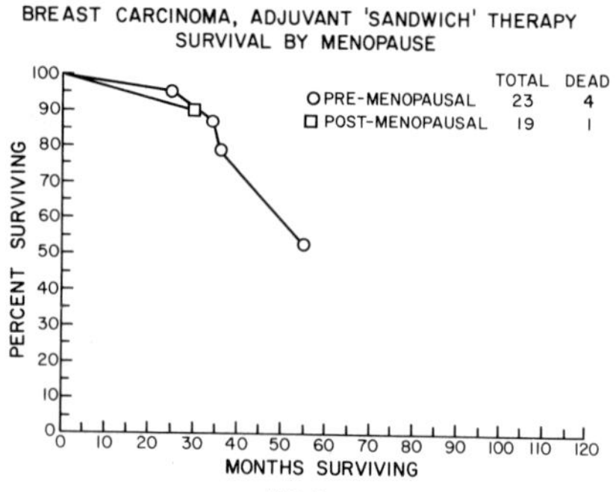

FIG. 2

The disease-free interval is shown in Figure 4. The median period of disease free for all patients is fifty-four months. When separated by menopausal status, the median disease-free interval is forty-two months for the premenopausal group and fifty-four months for the postmenopausal patients, again not statistically significant. No difference is observed when the groups are separated according to the number of positive nodes.

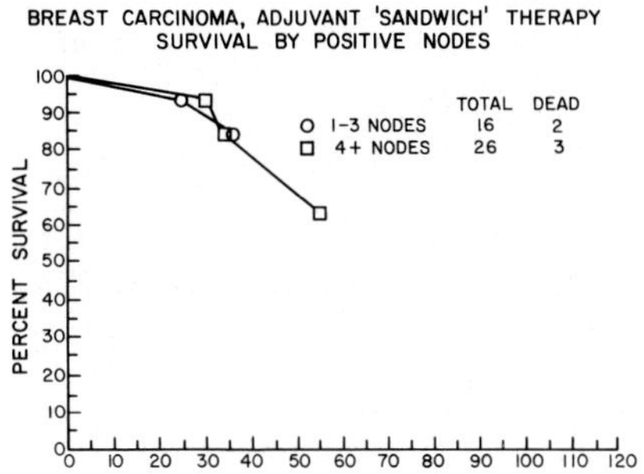

FIG. 3

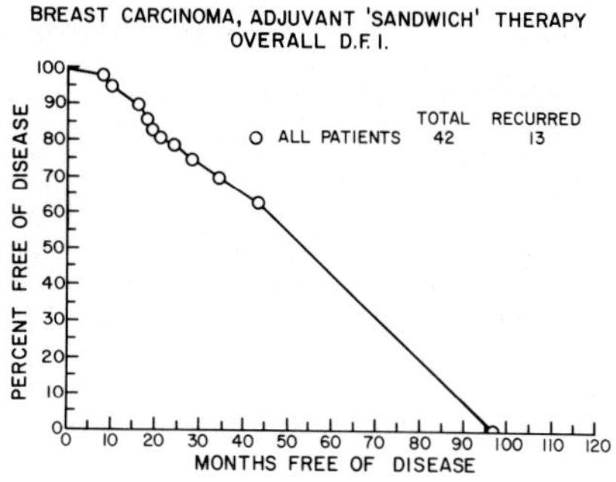

FIG. 4

DISCUSSION

In an attempt to increase the cure rates in breast carcinoma different therapeutic modalities have been proposed to improve the results obtained by surgery. Irradiation therapy has been used for many years. Techniques have varied considerably, but despite adequate local control obtained in most cases, the survival rates remain unchanged in the majority of published series. Since chemotherapy is capable of producing substantial temporary regressions in advanced disease, it has been proposed that these agents may increase the cure rate when given as adjuvants following surgery but most of the results have been disappointing, possibly because of doses employed were inadequate or the length of the treatment was insufficient. This study took advantage of the two modalities, chemotherapy and radiotherapy, in an attempt to decrease the number of recurrences as well as to improve the survival of the patients. The information obtained is somewhat encouraging in comparison with that of the NSABP study,[10] where the percentage of failures was greater than in this study, but we recognize that a longer follow up is needed to properly assess the benefit of the treatment and to determine whether there is a change in the overall survival As proposed by Carbone[11] we may have to learn to individualize treatment and utilize the modalities of chemotherapy, irradiation, hormonotherapy, and immunotherapy most effectively to achieve the maximum benefits.

REFERENCES

1. Wangensteen, O. H. (1952) Super-radical Operation for Breast Cancer in the Patients with Lymph Node Involvement. Proc. National Cancer Conf., Vol. 2, page 230.
2. Urban, J. A. (1963) Extended Radical Mastectomy for Breast Cancer. Am. J. of Surgery, Vol. 106, page 399.
3. Urban, J. A. (1968) Primary Operable Breast Cancer. Current Status of Treatment. Rocky Mountain Med. J., Vol. 65, page 39.
4. Fletcher, G. H. (1976) Reflections on Breast Cancer. Int. J. Radiation Oncology Biol. Phy., Vol. 1, pages 769-779.
5. Fisher, B., Slack, N. H. Cavanaugh, P. J., Gardner, B., and Ravdin, R. G. (October 1970) Postoperative Radiotherapy in the Treatment of Breast Cancer: Results of the NSABP Clinical Trial. Ann. of Surgery, pages 711-732.
6. Tormey, D. C. (1975) Combined Chemotherapy and Surgery in Breast Cancer: A Review. Cancer, Vol. 36, pages 881-892.
7. Ansfield, F. J. (1974) 5-FU as Adjuvant to Mastectomy in High Risk Patients. Am. Soc. of Clinical Onc. Abstracts, No. 772.
8. Ansfield, F. J. Personal Communication.
9. Fisher, B. (October 1970) The Surgical Dilemma in the Primary Therapy of Invasive Breast Cancer: A Critical Appraisal. Current Problems in Surgery, Vol. 1, page 53.
10. Fisher, B., Slack, N., Katrych, D., and Wolmark, N. (April 1975) Ten Year Follow-Up Results of Patients with Carcinoma of the Breast in a Cooperative Clinical Trial Evaluating Surgical Adjuvant Chemotherapy. Surgery, Gyn., and Obstetrics, Vol. 140, pages 528-534.
11. Carbone, P. P. (1975) Chemotherapy in the Treatment Strategy of Breast Cancer. Cancer, Vol 36, pages 633-637.

Adjuvant Therapy of Cancer, S.E. Salmon and S.E. Jones eds.
© 1977 Elsevier/North-Holland Biomedical Press, Amsterdam

ADJUVANT CHEMOTHERAPY WITH MELPHALAN, METHOTREXATE AND 5-FU IN BREAST CANCER - A PRELIMINARY REPORT

Shreyas Desai, Samuel Taylor, IV, John Merrill, Adrian Bianco
Howard Goldsweig, Tomas Kisielius, Janardhan Khandekar, William DeWys
Northwestern University
Chicago, Illinois 60611

INTRODUCTION

Combination chemotherapy with cyclophosphamide, methotrexate, and 5-Fluorouracil (CMF) given in the post-operative period may improve the disease-free interval more than single agent adjuvant chemotherapy.[1] This has been anticipated from a randomized trial comparing the two treatments demonstrating significant superiority of the drug combination in disseminated breast cancer.[4] A response rate of approximately 48% can be expected from CMF in stage IV breast cancer.[3] The major toxicities encountered with this combination were leukopenia, thrombocytopenia, alopecia, cystitis and mucositis.[1]

Many patients who are candidates for adjuvant chemotherapy are distressed about alopecia for cosmetic reasons. In our trial with melphalan, methotrexate and 5-Fluorouracil (MMF) in patients with advanced breast cancer, only 25% had appreciable hair loss and in most this was not cosmetically significant.[2] The response rate with MMF was 44% (CR 19%, PR 25%) in a population group that contained 59% of patients with visceral disease and 47% with performance status 2 or worse. This response rate is similar to that expected from CMF. This paper will report the efficacy and toxicities of the combination of melphalan, methotrexate and 5-Fluorouracil as adjuvant treatment for patients with stage II and III breast cancer.

METHODS

Thirty-three patients from Northwestern University Medical Center with stage II or III breast cancer were treated with a combination of melphalan, methotrexate and 5-Fluorouracil. Thirteen patients had 1-3 axillary lymph nodes positive for malignancy at the time of surgery, while 17 patients had $\geq$ 4 lymph nodes positive for malignancy at the time of surgery. Two patients did not have positive lymph nodes but since they had inflammatory carcinomas they were considered at a high risk for recurrence. One male patient had cancer infiltrating the pectoral muscles. In 30 patients the treatment was begun within 2 months of surgery. In two patients chemotherapy was started at 3 months and 18 months after the surgery. The median patient age was 52 years with a range from 28 to 73 years. All the patients had surgery prior to chemotherapy (23 patients had a modified radical mastectomy, 7 a radical mastectomy and 3 a simple mastectomy). Table 1 compares patient characteristics of this series with that of Bonadonna.[1]

TABLE 1

PATIENT CHARACTERISTICS ADJUVANT BREAST STUDY

A comparison with the treated patients reported by Bonadonna[1]

	MMF	CMF
Total No.	33	207
Age <49	12 (36)	95 (46)
Age ≥50	21 (64)	112 (54)
Pre-menopausal	12 (36)	95 (46)
Post-menopausal	20 (60)	112 (54)
Male	1	0
Mastectomy	33	207
Radical	6	148
Modified radical	23	0
Simple	4	0
Extended	0	59
Post-op radiation	17	0
Nodes		
1-3	13 (39)	139 (67)
≥ 4	17 (51)	68
Inflammatory carcinoma	2	0
Mean followup	12 mo.	13-7 mo.
Followup ≥12 months	18 (54)	118 (57)

Note: (Percentage in parentheses)

Seventeen patients received local radiation therapy after surgery. Prior to starting chemotherapy all patients had a complete history and physical examination, complete blood count, liver function tests, chest x-ray and a bone scan. Liver scan and biopsy were done in patients with abnormal physical or chemical findings. All patients had white counts $>4000/mm^3$, platelet counts $>100,000/mm^3$, BUN <25 mg%, and normal liver function tests.

Patients were treated with melphalan 3.5 mg/M^2 orally on Days 2-6, methotrexate 40 mg/M^2 intravenously on Days 1 and 8, and 5-Fluorouracil 600 mg/M^2 intravenously on Days 1 and 8. The cycle was repeated every 28 days. The doses of the drugs were adjusted based on the blood counts obtained prior to each treatment as well as inter-cycle toxicity (Table 2).

All the patients were followed by members of the medical oncology section and examined at monthly intervals. A complete blood count and platelet count were obtained prior to each visit. Liver functions were monitored at monthly intervals, carcino-embryonic antigen (CEA) every 2-3 months, chest x-rays every 3 months and bone scan every 6 months.

TABLE 2

DOSE MODIFICATION

Platelets	Percent of Full Dose WBC >4,000	WBC 4,000-2,500	WBC <2,500
>100,000	100	50	0
100,000-75,000	75	50	0
<75,000	0	0	0

RESULTS

The median duration of followup of these patients is 12 months (range 4 to 27 months). One patient has developed recurrence at 12 months. This patient, a 28 year old female, had inflammatory breast carcinoma with one positive axillary lymph node and a borderline CEA of 2.8 ng/ml at the start of treatment. After 6 months of treatment the CEA rose to 20 ng/ml. She developed right-sided pleural effusion at 12 months with class V cytology.

All other patients remain disease-free. None of 20 post-menopausal women has developed recurrence. The single recurrence was one of 12 pre-menopausal patients and one of 17 who had received local radiotherapy.

TOXICITY

Hematologic toxicity included moderate leukopenia (WBC 3999-2500/mm^3) in 20 patients (60%), and severe leukopenia in 3 patients (9%). Moderate thrombocytopenia (platelets 100,000-75,000/mm^3) was noted in 5 patients (15%) and more severe thrombocytopenia in 2 patients (6%). One patient required hospitalization because of bleeding and infection attributable to chemotherapy (WBC 400/mm^3, platelets 6,000/mm^3). Two patients developed herpes infection. Nausea and vomiting occurred in 16 patients (48%) but only one patient required dose adjustment because of this. Mucositis occurred in 7 patients (21%) and was avoidable by minor dose adjustments of methotrexate and 5-Fluorouracil. In none of the patients who developed mucositis was this severe enough to prevent oral intake. Three patients developed vertigo and ataxia thought to be due to 5-Fluorouracil requiring temporary dose reductions. At 43 instances the treatment was delayed because of hematologic or GI toxicities. Part of the treatment was discontinued in three patients. One patient developed progressive enlargement of the liver with a biopsy showing fatty infiltration thought to be due to methotrexate and she was then treated with melphalan and 5-Fluorouracil. One patient with scleroderma had severe skin reactions to methotrexate and required discontinuation of this drug. The third patient had progressive and severe nausea and vomiting with each injection and after 12 months of treatment she was continued on melphalan alone.

TABLE 3

TOXICITY

A comparison of MMF with that reported for adjuvant CMF[1]

	MMF	CMF
WBC 3,999-2,500	20 (60)	139 (67)
WBC <2,500	3 (9)	8 (4)
Platelets <75,000	2 (6)	29 (14)
Infection life-threatening	1	Not stated
Nausea and vomiting	20 (48)	"Majority"
Loss of hair	5 (15)	114 (55)
Mucositis	7 (21)	37 (18)
Cystitis	0	57 (28)
Ataxia	3 (9)	Not stated
Patients stopping treatment	0	17 (8)
No toxicity	5 (15)	8 (4)

Note: (Percentage in parentheses)

Only 2 patients had significant hair loss requiring a wig. An additional three patients noticed some hair loss but did not require a prosthesis. None of the patients developed cystitis. No drug related deaths were noticed. A comparison of drug toxicity with that reported with adjuvant CMF is given in Table 3.

DISCUSSION

The early findings from this trial of adjuvant chemotherapy of stage II, III and IV breast cancer patients indicate that prolonged administration of melphalan, methotrexate and 5-Fluorouracil may be effective in lengthening disease-free interval of pre-menopausal and post-menopausal women. With a median followup of 12 months there has been one recurrence. Considering the recurrence among 18 patients at risk at 12 months, this gives a 94% disease-free incidence at 12 months which is comparable to a 91% disease-free incidence at 12 months in Bonadonna's CMF series.[1]

Differences between our group of patients and Bonadonna's group of patients prevent any direct comparison. Our group consisted of stage II, III and IV breast cancer patients based on the 1976 classification of the American Joint Commission for Staging and End Results Reporting[5] and included patients with inflammatory carcinoma of the breast in the study. Also there is a difference in the prior treatment that the patients received. Approximately half of our patients received post-operative radiation therapy. The type of surgery that the patients had was also different. Whether these differences would lead to different recurrence patterns is not clear because of limited duration of followup.

The hematologic toxicity of the treatment is comparable to that reported with adjuvant CMF. The incidence of moderate leukopenia (3999-2500/mm^3) was 67% with CMF and with MMF it was 60%. The incidence of severe leukopenia was 4% with CMF while it was 9% in our study. We did note the occurrence of vertigo and ataxia in 3 patients requiring modification of the 5-Fluorouracil dosage. No drug related deaths occurred. One patient had a life-threatening episode of infection and bleeding attributable to the chemotherapy regimen.

The striking difference between the two studies is the lower incidence of alopecia in our study and the absence of cystitis. Only two patients had significant hair loss requiring a wig, while another three patients did notice increased hair loss while combing but did not think that they required a wig. As a result patient acceptance and cooperation was better. No patient discontinued treatment in our series but Bonadonna noted that 17 of 207 patients discontinued treatment for psychologic reasons. Also nausea and vomiting was usually mild occurring in 48% of the patients. Only one patient at 12 months required discontinuation of methotrexate and 5-Fluorouracil because of severe, progressive nausea and vomiting. With the reduced toxicity and better patient acceptance, this combination of chemotherapeutic agents offers an alternative to Bonadonna's CMF regimen especially when considering Phase IV use in the general hospital setting.

Our protocol offers patient convenience and ease of administration of drugs when compared to the N.S.A.B.P. protocol. That study also uses melphalan, 5-Fluorouracil and methotrexate but the 5-Fluorouracil is given as 5 daily injections and methotrexate is given on Days 1 and 5.

In view of the recent ECOG data[3] showing a higher response rate with the addition of prednisone to the combination of cyclophosphamide, methotrexate and 5-Fluorouracil in stage IV disease, a consideration should be given to addition of prednisone to the MMF regimen in the future.

In conclusion we feel that the combination of MMF may be superior to CMF because of reduced toxicity with comparable anti-neoplastic activity. This consideration is especially impórtant if therapy for longer than one year is planned. A randomized trial is needed to confirm these results.

ACKNOWLEDGEMENT

Supported in part by National Cancer Institute grants 2-RIO-CA-17145 and L-R25-CA-18004.

REFERENCES

1. Bonadonna, G., Brusamolino, E., et al.: Combination chemotherapy as an adjuvant treatment in operable breast cancer. NEJM 294:405-410, 1976.
2. Desai, S., Taylor, S.G., et al: Phase II study of melphalan, methotrexate and 5-Fluorouracil in breast cancer. ASCO 1976, Abstracts, 268.
3. ECOG, Minutes of Meeting. November 7-9, 1976, Chicago, Illinois.

4. Canellas, G.P., Pocock, S.J., et al.: Combination chemotherapy for metastatic breast carcinoma. Cancer 38:1882-1886, 1976.

5. Guy F. Robbins, et al.: Staging of the cancer of breast. American Joint Committee for Cancer Staging and End Result Reporting. Classification and Staging of Cancer by Site. Chapter ,18:215-228.

Adjuvant Therapy of Cancer, S.E. Salmon and S.E. Jones eds.
© 1977 Elsevier/North-Holland Biomedical Press, Amsterdam

MER CHEMOIMMUNOTHERAPY OF STAGE II BREAST CARCINOMA

Marjorie Perloff, M.D., James F. Holland, M.D.
Gerson J. Lesnick, M.D., and J. George Bekesi, Ph.D.
Mount Sinai School of Medicine
Department of Neoplastic Diseases
Fifth Avenue & 100th Street
New York, N.Y. 10029

Of 54 women treated with adjuvant chemotherapy for Stage II breast cancer, 17 have received MER in addition as the basis for chemoimmunotherapy. Thirty-eight patients received their treatment by random allocation. The patient characteristics of the two groups were not entirely similar, since the chemotherapy alone group had a somewhat more favorable prognosis. The mean number of positive axillary lymph nodes in the chemotherapy group was 6.9 (median 4, range 1-33) versus 10 in the chemoimmunotherapy group (median 9, range 4-33). Thirteen of 37 chemotherapy patients were premenopausal as opposed to 4 of 17 MER treated patients. Four chemotherapy and 3 chemoimmunotherapy patients refused further therapy at 3 to 11 months from the initiation of treatment.

Cyclophosphamide, methotrexate and 5-fluorouracil (CMF) was given to 13 patients non randomly in a fashion modelled after Bonadonna (1) with the exceptions of a slightly lower dose of 5FU (500mgm/m^2) and a longer duration of treatment. During the second year 6 cycles were given at 2 monthly intervals. A subset of 30 patients was treated according to Cancer and Leukemia Group B protocol #7581 in which patients were randomized to CMF, CMF vincristine and prednisone (VP), or CMF MER with all patients receiving intensification with 6 initial weekly treatments. Subsequently, monthly cycles were given for the duration of the first year and 6 cycles every two months during the second year. Observation times for these patients are somewhat shorter (2 patients more than 20 months) because the study was initiated in 1975 but the behavior of this group is similar to that of the whole. One chemotherapy and two chemoimmunotherapy patients have relapsed.

By life table analysis at 30 months 100% of 24 CMF patients and 88% of 13 CMF VP patients were disease free as opposed to 63% of 14 CMF MER and 66% of 3 CMF VP MER patients. Figure 1 describes the disease free interval of all chemotherapy versus all chemoimmunotherapy patients. With only one relapse among chemotherapy patients, 96% remain disease free at 30 months with 9 patients followed more than 20 months. Among the chemoimmunotherapy patients there are 4 relapses and 6 patients observed more than 20 months.

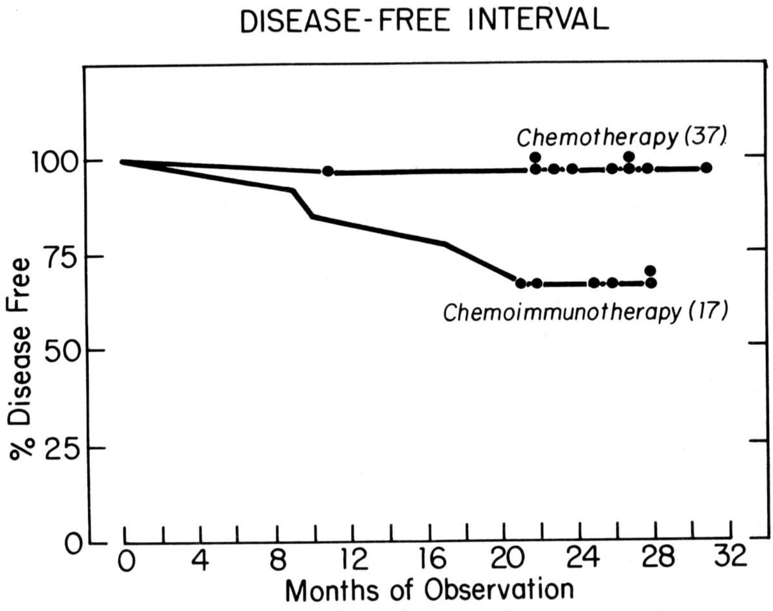

FIGURE I

Among 17 premenopausal patients in the entire study there have been no relapses versus 5 of 37 in the postmenopausal group. Among chemotherapy alone patients, no premenopausal patient has relapsed and one of 24 postmenopausal patients failed at 9 months (Figure 2). This is especially noteworthy because 18 of these 24 had 4 or more positive nodes.

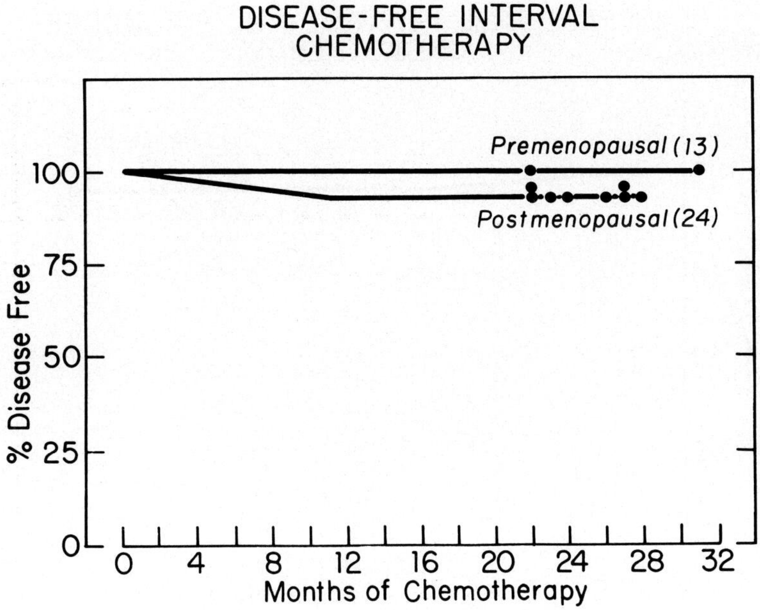

FIGURE 2

None of 12 patients with 1 to 3 positive lymph nodes (mean 2, median 2), has relapsed whereas 5 of 42 with 4 or more positive nodes (mean 10, median 6, range 4-33) have. Among chemotherapy patients the single relapse occurred in a patient with 4 or more positive nodes. (Figure 3).

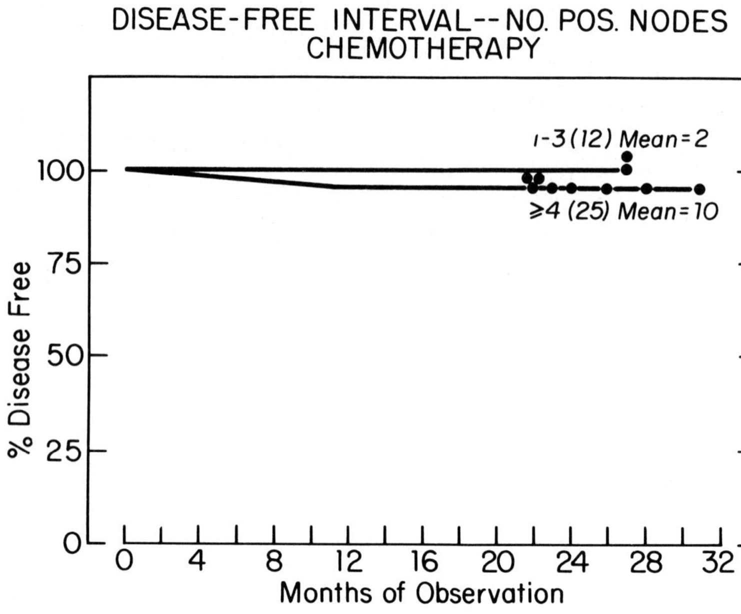

FIGURE 3

Drug toxicity was entirely tolerable and evenly distributed among all treatment groups. There were 21 episodes of leukopenia (WBC < 2500/mm^3). One patient was hospitalized twice with leukopenia and fever. There were no deaths and no other severe manifestations of toxicity.

All patients were staged with monthly SMA 12 blood chemistries and erythrocyte sedimentation rates as well as by chest x-ray, bone survey and bone scan every 6 months. Among the patients who relapsed, all were post-menopausal and had 6 or more positive nodes. The earliest failure was at 9 months. One relapsed patient developed a biopsy proven positive lymph node in her contralateral axilla and is disease free more than 2 years after completion of secondary treatment. One patient received 26 of 29 half doses of chemotherapy secondary to long-standing pancytopenia of unknown etiology (having met initial protocol requirements), one had postoperative radiotherapy, and one had only one year of treatment.

MER was initially given twice monthly at a dose of 200ug intradermally into each of 5 sites draining different lymph node bearing areas, excluding the infraclavicular area homolateral to the mastectomy. Because of the severity of the subsequent ulcerative lesions, dose titrations were ultimately carried out upon initial exposure to MER and then as often as lesion size indicated. Initial titrating doses decreased in log order from 100 to 0.01 ug. A trend towards increasing cutaneous sensitivity with time was apparent. Dose titrations were carried out 25 times in 13 of 17 MER treated patients. Thirteen patients developed at least 5 mm. induration to the 1 ug dose one to three weeks following titration. One patient responded with typical inflammatory lesions to a 10 picogram injection (10^{-11}gram). That dose which produced a 1 cm. inflammatory lesion with minimal central necrosis was adopted for subsequent administration into each of 5 sites. Ten patients were treated with doses of 1 ug or less per site following one or more titrations.

Serial skin tests with 5 recall antigens (PPD, mumps, candida, dermatophytin, varidase) and in vitro measurement of phytohemagglutinin and pokeweed mitogen stimulation in autologuous and allogeneic plasma, total lymphocyte count and quantification of T lymphocytes by E-binding rosettes at 4°C. were carried out in a subset of patients. No significant differences in immunologic parameters between patients receiving chemoimmunotherapy and the identical chemotherapy alone were observed.

In conclusion, the chemotherapy employed was tolerable, safe and effective. MER immunotherapy, as employed, led to no therapeutic advantage over chemotherapy alone and to no changes in a variety of immunologic parameters.

REFERENCES

1. Bonadonna, G., Brusamolino, E., Valagussa, P. et al.: Combination Chemotherapy as an Adjuvant Treatment in Operable Breast Cancer. NEJM 294:405410, 1976

Adjuvant Therapy of Cancer, S.E. Salmon and S.E. Jones eds.

FEASIBILITY OF ADJUVANT CHEMOTHERAPY OF BREAST CANCER IN A PRIVATE PRACTICE SETTING

Waisman, James: Ossorio, R. Clifford; Taub, Robert J.,
Avedon, Melvin, Van Scoy-Mosher, Michael B.
Cedars-Sinai Medical Center
8700 Beverly Blvd.,
Los Angeles, Calif. 90048

The demonstrated effectiveness of L-phenylalamine mustard (L-PAM) as an adjuvant to radical mastectomy in pre-menopausal women with positive axillary nodes[1] convinced us that the use of adjuvant chemotherapy for breast cancer should be initiated in our private practice setting. The known superiority of combination chemotherapy with cyclophosphamide, methotrexate and 5FU (CMF) over single agent chemotherapy[2] and the less favorable results with L-PAM in the post-menopausal age group directed our preference for CMF as adjuvant therapy.

This paper summarizes the results in 39 patients with Stage II & III breast cancer treated with adjuvant CMF, stressing the relatively unique implications of such therapy in a private practice setting.

Methods: Patient Population: 39 women post-modified radical mastectomy with disease confined to the breast and axilla are included. The median age is 55 with a range of 28-75. Criteria for inclusion are: the tumor not fixed to underlying muscle or chest wall, freely moveable axillary nodes, initial WBC greater than 4000, platelet count greater than 100,000 BUN less than 25, a normal bone scan, chest x-ray, skeletal survey and liver function tests. Patients with inflammatory cancinoma, skin ulceration, arm edema, nodes other than in axilla considered to contain disease or psychiatric disorders preventing informed consent are excluded. One woman is included with a T^2 medial quadrant lesion with negative axillary nodes who did not have an internal mammary node dissection. Two patients with simultaneous bilateral carcinomas of the breast with positive axillary nodes are included.

Treatment: All patients had had modified radical mastectomies consisting of removal of the breast, axillary contents, +/- the pectoralis minor muscle but excluding the pectoralis major. No patient had extended mastectomies with removal of the internal mammary nodes. Three patients had post mastectomy radiation therapy to the chest wall, internal mammary, supraclavicular and infraclavicular nodes.

Chemotherapy was started 2-4 weeks post mastectomy and in 3 patients, 1-2 weeks post radiation therapy, or 6-7 weeks post mastectomy. The dose of cyclophosphamide, methotrexate and 5FU was modified to allow for the maximum tolerated dose with the minimum interference in quality of life, in terms of such problems as fatique, weakness, nausea or vomiting. The mean dose of cyclophosphamide administered was 1.5 mgm./Kg./day p.o. on days 1-14, 5FU 10 mgm./Kg. IV on days 1&8 and methotrexate 0.6 mgm./Kg. IV on days 1&8. The course was repeated every 28 days. Therapy was continued for 12 cycles and then for 6 more courses given every 56 days, or ever other month during a second year of therapy. In 4 patients L-PAM was administered in place of cyclophosphamide at a mean dose of 0.08 mgm./Kg./D days 1-5 p.o. with otherwise no change in the methotrexate and 5FU schedule. The mean time on therapy is 12 months.

Follow-up: Chest x-ray, SGOT, SGPT, alkaline phosphotase, LDH and bilirubin were repeated every 3-4 months. Bone scan was done every 6 months. Liver scan was done in case of elevated liver function tests. Liver biopsy was performed in one patient with a suspicious liver scan. A skeletal survey was performed in the presence of bone pain or because of an abnormal bone scan.

Results: Table 1 presents the characteristics of the 32 patients who received CMF only. All recurrences occurred while patients were on therapy.

TABLE 1

CHARACTERISTICS OF 32 PATIENTS TREATED WITH CYCLOPHOSPHAMIDE, METHOTREXATE AND 5FU WITH FAILURE PROPORTIONS

Characteristics	#	%
Total with Recurrence	5/32	15.7
NODE		
0	0/1	-
1-3	1/16	6.3
greater than or equal to 4	4/15	26.7
STAGE		
T1	0/10	-
T2	3/20	15
T3	2/2	100
MENOPAUSAL STATUS		
PRE	1/9	11
POST	4/23	13
AGE		
greater than or equal to 50	4/21	19
less than or equal to 49	1/11	9

The difference in recurrence rate in patients having greater than or equal to 4 nodes vs. patient with 1-3 nodes (26.7% vs. 6.3%) is significant (P less than .05). The difference in recurrence rate in Stage $T^2 + T^3$ vs. Stage T^1 (15.9% vs. 0%) is significant (P less than .01). There is no statistical difference in the pre vs. the post-menopausal group (11% vs. 13%). There is no significant difference in the greater than or equal to 50 age group vs. those less than or equal to 49 (19% vs. 9%). Table 2 describes characteristics of all 39 patients which includes the 7 patients who had modifications in the standard protocal:

TABLE 2

CHARACTERISTICS OF 39 TREATED PATIENTS

(32 WITH CMF, 4 WITH AMF, 3 WITH RADIATION THERAPY AND CMF)

Characteristics	#	%
Total with Recurrence	5/39	12.9
NODE		
1-3	1/20	5
greater than or equal to 4	4/18	22.2
0	0/1	0
STAGE		
T1	0/12	0
T2	3/25	12
T3	2/2	100
MENOPAUSAL STATUS		
PRE	1/12	8.3
POST	4/27	14.8
AGE		
greater than or equal to 50	4/24	16.7
less than or equal to 49	1/15	6.7

In 4 cases L-PAM was substituted for cyclophosphamide (AMF) and in 3 radiation therapy post mastectomy was used. There were no recurrences in this sub-group. Again, patients with greater than or equal to 4 nodes vs. 1-3 nodes (22.2 vs. 5), Stage T2+T3 vs. T1 (15 vs. 0%) show a significant difference. Again, there is no significant difference in the greater than or equal to 50 vs. the less than or equal to 49 age group or in the pre vs. the post menopausal groups.

Table 3 describes the recurrences which occurred 5-14 months post-mastectomy.

TABLE 3

CHARACTERISTICS OF 5 RECURRENCES

Age	Menopausal Status	Stage	# Positive Nodes	Time Post Mastectomy in Months	Site of Recurrence
52	PRE	T3	3	14	liver
61	POST	T2	10	5	pulmonary modules
61	POST	T2	5	8	bone and local nodes
51	POST	T2	9	5	bone
49	POST	T3	11	7	bone and local skin

In 2 of the 3 patients with bony recurrence the bone scan and skeletal survey were concurrently positive; however, in one patient the bone scan alone was positive with simultaneous soft tissue recurrence. Two of the 5 patients had both regional and distant recurrence (neither had radiation therapy). No patient had local recurrence only. The one patient with hepatic metastasis expired 2 months after the first evidence of recurrence. All the other recurrences are alive but with progressive disease.

Table 4 presents the toxic manifestations in the 39 patients. There were no cases of infections requiring hospitalization because of granulocytopenia and no cases of bleeding secondary to thrombocytopenia. The 3 cases of stomatitis were self-limited and did not require a change in therapy. There were no cases of conjunctivitis. Hair loss was variable. There were no cases of total alopecia but emotional reaction was so severe in 3 pre-menopausal patients that L-PAM was substituted for cyclophosphamide. The one case of cystitis secondary to cyclophosphamide resolved with the temporary discontinuation of the drug and did not recur with reinstitution of therapy. 69% of the pre-menopausal patients had cessation of menses with variable periods of "hot flushes" in some patients. Nausea, with or without vomiting was variably associated with fatique, anorexia, weakness and there was no clear correlation to any specific drug except that protracted nausea in a few patients seemed to be more associated with cyclophosphamide.

TABLE 4

TOXIC MANIFESTATIONS

	#	%
<u>Bone Marrow Suppression</u>		
Leukopenia		
2500 - 3900	8/39	20.5
less than or equal to 2500	0/39	-
Thrombocytopenia		
75 - 125,000	5/39	12.8
less than or equal to 75,000	0/39	-
Mucositis	3/39	7.8
Loss of hair	25/39	64.1
Cystitis	1/39	2.6
Amenorrhea	9/13	69
<u>Gastrointestinal</u>		
Nausea only	30/39	77
Vomiting	5/39	12.8

These gastrointestinal and constitutional symptoms were successfully attenuated by dose modifications in most cases. One woman stopped therapy prematurely after 5 months.

Cost: The average cost for therapy was $175/month with a range of $155-225. This includes all scans, x-rays, laboratory work, chemotherapy and physician visits. 36 of our patients have private insurance and the rate of coverage was highly variable. Three had either federal (medicare) and/or state (medi-cal) assistance which paid 55-60% of the total cost.

Discussion: Our committment to adjuvant CMF was tempered both by the awareness that Bonnadonna's study was preliminary and unconfirmed and by our prior experience with higher dose CMF for more advanced breast cancer. The gastrointestinal and constitutional side effects seemed particularly unacceptable for the asymptomatic woman with no evidence of disease when the conclusive long term results were still pending. Nevertheless, it was our best judgement that combination chemotherapy did offer the best chance for increased survival and we were not restricted to protocals with either "no treatment" or inferior treatment arms. We were encouraged by evidence from Creech, et al[3] who showed that in advanced breast cancer low dose CMF was comparably effective to higher dose regimens. We were concerned that 17/207 (8.2%) of patients on CMF in Bonnadonna's series stopped therapy prematurely for psychological reasons and that one-third of his patients either discontinued treatment or decreased dose because of nausea or anorexia. Therefore, we embarked on a low dose CMF regimen. 1/39 or 2.6% of our patients stopped therapy with only rare instances of self-attentuation of dosage. The substitution of L-PAM for cyclophosphamide was supported by its efficacy in the pre-menopausal patients in Fisher's series and allowed for not only the amelioration of severe anxiety from hair loss but also allowed for ongoing compliance in 3 pre-menopausal women.

The emotional problems of therapy remain a dilemma. Although the physical side effects were, in general, well tolerated; many of the patients found the office visits themselves anxiety provoking, forcing a confrontation with the illness and the possibility of recurrence which the patient otherwise may have chosen to deny. The heightened anxiety described, starting 1-2 days prior to a course of chemotherapy, seemed more related to apprehension about what coming to us represented in general, rather than a specific fear of the chemotherapy itself. We have attempted various psychologically palliative measures with marginal success. In a few cases a nurse oncology specialist has given the treatment at home but because of the expense and the need to see us regularly this solution is inpractical. We have considered having all the adjuvant patients come on the same day to share their feelings and to limit exposure to some of our very ill patients but scheduling conflicts make this equally impractical. We have an ongoing weekly group-therapy session led by a clinical psychologist and the nurse oncologist, both specially trained to deal with cancer patients and with their families, but none of our patients on adjuvant therapy have availed themselves of this free service suggesting to us, in part, the desire not to focus on their disease any further. Ultimately, we have tried to change the women's basic orientation to therapy so instead of her viewing a visit as a constant reminder of her cancer and the threat of recurrence she would instead see the opportunity to exercise willful control of her destiny, previously not possible for similar women. Regretably, none of these approaches has significantly modified the emotional burdens for most patients.

Our results in these 39 patients indicate a successful limitation of toxicity with maintenance of near-normal functioning. We confirm the improved results in patients with stage T1 and with 1-3 positive nodes. We are concerned with the 15% overall recurrence rate reflecting poor results in the $T^2 + T^3$ lesions and in those with greater than four positive nodes. Whether this reflects a consequence of our lower dose schedule or is related to other factors is unclear. There was no significant difference in the dose of chemotherapy received by the recurrence group.

In one case, the use of the bone scan revealed recurrence not present on skeletal surveys which supports the routine use of bone scan for screening purposes.

We continue to have questions that need to be answered by the results from the large randomized trials. Specifically, we wonder about the treatment of the medial-quadrant lesion with negative axillary nodes who has not had an internal mammary node dissection. We also need to know the ideal duration of therapy. If the results from the randomized trials clearly establish a dose-response curve with definite prolonged survival we would have to reaccess the benefits of decreased recurrence rate vs. decreased toxicity. Finally, we are awaiting suggestions regarding the management of the emotional consequences of adjuvant therapy.

References:

1. Fisher, Bernard et al: L-Phenyl Alanine Mustard (L-PAM) in the Management of Primary Breast Cancer: N. Engl. J. Med: 292: 117-122, 1975
2. Bonnadonna, Gianni et al: Combination Chemotherapy as an Adjuvant Treatment in Operable Breast Cancer: N. Engl. J. Med. 292: 405-410, 1976
3. Creech, Richard et al: An Effective Low-Dose Intermittent Cyclophosphamide, Methotrexate, and 5-Fluorouracil Treatment Regimen for Metastatic Breast Cancer, Cancer 35: 1101-1107, 1975

Section III

LUNG CANCER

Adjuvant Therapy of Cancer, S.E. Salmon and S.E. Jones, eds.

COMBINED MODALITY APPROACHES IN LUNG CANCER

R. B. Livingston
Audie L. Murphy Memorial Veterans Hospital
7400 Merton Minter Boulevard
San Antonio, Texas

I. NON OAT CELL - RESULTS OF SURGICAL ADJUVANT APPROACHES

To appreciate the potential value of combined modality approaches in lung cancer, we must first consider the value of the major modality known to be curative: surgical resection. Using pathologic staging criteria based on the TNM classification, 5-year survival ranges from 44 to 53% for Stage I to 28-31% for Stage II and 0-8% for Stage III disease, if undifferentiated small cell carcinoma (only rarely a surgically curable disease) is excluded.[2,3,4,5,6] Patients with squamous carcinoma of a given stage have better survival in surgical series than those with adenocarcinoma or large cell undifferentiated tumors[2,3,6], probably related to the fact that squamous tumors tend to remain localized for longer periods: 46% of patients dying with squamous lung carcinoma in one large series[7] had autopsy evidence of disease still confined to the thorax.

Surgical "adjuvant" approaches to lung cancer began with the addition of radiotherapy, itself a modality of some curative potential[8]. Bloedorn et al[9] reported encouraging results with the use of pre-operative radiation, which led to the performance of large, prospective randomized trials reported by Shields[10] and by Warram[11]: neither demonstrated any advantage for the patients who received radiation, and the former trial suggested it was actually harmful. Controlled, prospective studies of post-operative radiation have also failed to demonstrate any benefit to the combined approach[12,13]. But there are problems with the interpretation of these trials: 1) the randomization was not stratified by stage or cell type; 2) pneumonectomy was the usual surgical procedure; and 3) radiation techniques may have been supoptimal.

Several pilot trials of post-operative radiotherapy suggest a real benefit from this approach in a defined subgroup of patients: those with gross nodal involvement by tumor. Kirsh et al[3] reported disease-free survival to 5 years in 11/32 squamous and 4/34 adenocarcinoma patients with Stage III disease who received 5000-5500r over 5-6 weeks after surgery. Green et al[14], employing a slightly lower radiation dose, found no advantage in Stage I disease to the combined treatment. But 23/66 patients with positive nodes survived 5 years after combined therapy, compared to a concurrent (non-randomized) control group, of whom 1/30 survived. It is possible that the negative results reported in earlier, randomized studies were related to increased morbidity (especially after pneumonectomy) in the Stage I majority, which canceled any benefit from radiation in the minority of resected patients with grossly positive nodes. Since the surgical mortality approaches or exceeds the long-term salvage rate from operative intervention alone in patients with Stage III disease, it appears likely that future efforts to attack this category of disease will involve the addition of radiation: a "surgery alone" control group, though theoretically desirable, is unlikely to find clinical acceptance.

Trials of chemotherapy in the surgical adjuvant setting have largely been focussed on 2 hypotheses which are now discredited: 1) that short-term exposure to drugs at the time of surgery might delay or prevent recurrence by killing tumor cells which were "seeded" by the operation, and 2) that alkylating agents are likely to be effective at killing micrometastatic lesions. Peri-operative trials of nitrogen mustard[15,16] and cyclophosphamide[15,17] failed to demonstrate any advantage in prospective, controlled studies. A frequently cited negative study by Brunner et al[18] actually showed significantly worse survival in patients randomly allocated to long-term, intermittent cyclophosphamide than in a concurrent control group undergoing surgery alone. However, there were more pneumonectomies in the drug-treated group and the cyclophosphamide schedule was an unusual one. In the VASAG study reported by Shields[19], neither high-dose intermittent cyclophosphamide alone nor its alternation with methotrexate, on an every 5 week schedule, showed an advantage or disadvantage relative to concurrent surgical controls. These were "poor risk" patients, while those treated by Brunner et al were in a "good risk" group at the time of operation. A problem in the VASAG study was that only one-third of the patients had "toxicity" recorded, and only 50% of the potential drug courses were given.

Long-term, low-dose continuous therapy with alkylating agents has been reported in several trials, most recently in a representative, large effort by the British Medical Research Council[19]: cyclophosphamide and busulfan were slightly inferior to no therapy.

Drug combinations in the setting of resected disease have received minimal trials. Karrer et al[20] reported "positive" early results with a combination of cyclophosphamide, 5FU, methotrexate and vinblastine vs. an untreated control, but there is no published long-term follow up. As yet unpublished results from the VASAG study of long-term, intermittent CCNU + hydroxyurea vs. surgical resection alone show no advantage. Katsuki et al[21] have reported a survival advantage for a large group of patients who have mitomycin C + chromycin A_3 on a long-term, intermittent basis, with or without radiation, compared to a group of historical controls. However, this advantage appeared to be primarily for the group of patients with "undifferentiated" tumors.

Remarkably, no surgical adjuvant studies have yet been reported with doxorubicin (adriamycin) alone or in combination, although it is probably the most active single drug against non oat cell lung cancer[22].

Probably the area of greatest interest today in combined modality approaches to lung cancer relates to surgery + immunotherapy. Elsewhere in this volume, McKneally et al describe their experience with intrapleural BCG, in which significant benefit to patients with Stage I, but not Stage II or III disease, has previously been reported in a randomized trial[23]. Takita, in another pioneering study[24], reported a very small, randomized series of patients with Stage III disease who underwent complete gross resection of tumor: 5 of 11 then were treated with autologous tumor cells and concanavalin A (or a diazotized protein extract) in Freund's adjuvant. This group had a median survival of 19 months, compared to 8.5 months for the controls. Stewart et al[25] recently reported preliminary analysis of another study in which a purified preparation of lung tumor antigen in Freund's adjuvant was given, with or without chemotherapy (high-dose methotrexate with citrovorum factor) and compared to a group of randomized, concurrently treated controls. The results appeared superior for the 2 groups receiving immunotherapy, although large, indolent skin ulcers at the infection site are a complication of this type of approach.

A provocative and controversial study is that carried out by Amery et al[26] with levamisole, an antihelminthic compound which has immunomodulatory properties, especially in the apparent restoration of T-cell function toward normal. In this randomized, prospective trial, patients were allocated before resection to receive placebo or levamisole, 150mg/day for 3 days, then 150mg/day for 3 days every 2 weeks (by mouth) to 2 years or recurrence of disease. With a median follow up of 24 months, the overall incidence of suspected or proven recurrence, and of deaths related to cancer, was no different in the 2 groups. But levamisole appears superior for all patients with squamous histology or more advanced (Stage II or III) tumors. That a dose-response effect may be involved is suggested by Amery's analysis, which shows that if the patient's initial weight was less than or equal to 70kg, levamisole treatment appears significantly superior to placebo in all respects. Specifically, its effect may be greatest on extrathoracic recurrence, in contrast to that of intrapleural BCG: only 1 of 25 patients under 70kg on levamisole developed extrathoracic recurrence at the time of the last analysis, compared to 13/36 on placebo.

II. NON OAT CELL - THERAPY OF REGIONAL, UNRESECTABLE DISEASE

Regional or limited unresectable disease is usually defined as that in which 1) clinical evidence of tumor is confined to the involved hemithorax ± ipsilateral supraclavicular nodes; 2) all the evident disease can be included within a single radiotherapy port; and 3) the tumor is either found to be unresectable at surgery or the patient is medically unfit for a procedure involving complete resection. Older series probably included a number of patients as "regional" who would now be staged as extensive, due to the more routine use of scans and other diagnostic procedures today. One such series, frequently cited, is that of the VA Lung Study

Group[27]: patients who received only supportive care had a median survival of 3.5-5.3 months, with somewhat better medians for those who were initially fully ambulatory (PS 8-10), around 6 months; at one year, overall survival regardless of histologic type was 10-13%. In a recent review of experience at M.D. Anderson Hospital, Lanzotti et al[28] cite new standards for survival in patients with regional disease who received "optimal management in a modern setting". As in most series, radiation therapy was the backbone of therapeutic management for these patients. Table 1 summarizes survival data from Lanzotti's series as it relates to cell type and to several prognostic factors which were found to be important after application of multifactorial regression analysis.

TABLE 1

REGIONAL DISEASE

"Optimal Management" - Lanzotti, 1972 (MDAH)

Factor	Median Survival Time (months) with or without factor	Comment	
Wt. loss > 12%	4.8 vs. 10.4	p=.003	important pre-Rx prognostic factors
PS: 2 vs. 0-1	3.7 vs. 8.7	p=.02	
Supraclavicular mets	5 vs. 8.8	p=.03	
Age ≥ 70	5.5 vs. 8.8	p=.05	
Cell type:			
Squamous	7.8	p>.6	
Adeno	7.8		
LCU	8.5		
SCU	9.7		

Treatment nearly always with XRT, ± chemo (varied).

PS 2 - In bed more than 50% of time during day

PS 0-1 - In bed less than 50% of time during day

LCU = large cell undifferentiated

SCU = small cell undifferentiated (oat cell)

From this analysis, it is apparent that weight loss, initial performance status, the presence or absence of supraclavicular metastases and age are all important pre-treatment variables within the category of "regional" disease, much more important than cell type. The Radiation Therapy Oncology Group (RTOG) has independently developed criteria for staging regional inoperable disease[29]. Basically, patients are considered Stage III if the lesion is T_3 and/or N_2; an effusion may be present if the cytology is negative; and there must be no superior vena caval obstruction or supraclavicular nodes. Patients are considered Stage IV if 1) the primary tumor is "T_4", extensive intrathoracically with involvement of non-pulmonary structures such as nerves, the heart or great vessels, vertebrae, or the chest wall; 2) an effusion is present with positive cytology; 3) superior vena caval obstruction exists; or 4) there are supraclavicular or biopsy-positive scalene nodes. Another prognostic factor which is not considered in either Lanzotti's paper or the RTOG classification relates to clinical inoperability vs. unresectability at thoracotomy: in an older series reported by Guttman[30], patients who were inoperable at thoracotomy, and who completed a full course of radiation therapy (5000r in 5 weeks, continuous fractionation) had better survival than patients similarly treated who were clinically inoperable: 58% and 40% at 1 year, 27% and 13% at 2 years, respectively. Much of the variability in reported results for the treatment of "regional" disease probably relates to variations in the "mix" of involved pre-treatment prognostic factors.

Split-course radiation therapy in regional disease is just as effective[31] as or superior[32] to continuous fractionation in terms of survival, better tolerated, and lends itself better to combined modality approaches. It is the standard against which such approaches should be measured. Salazar et al[29] reported an overall median survival of 6.5 months in a recent large series treated with the split-course approach, with response rates (>50% regression) of local tumor mass ranging from 32% for adenocarcinoma to 40% for squamous lesions and 55% for large cell undifferentiated tumors. Two striking facts emerge from this well-studied group: 1) Stage III patients (by RTOG criteria) had a higher local response rate (60%) and longer median survival (11.3 months) than did Stage IV (30% and 4.5 respectively); and 2) responders lived significantly longer than non-responders (13.3 vs. 7 months, $p < .05$). It should be noted that some patients with extensive disease (M_1) were included among the Stage IV group; the median survival of the "limited" Stage IV patients was about 5.5 months, identical to that in Selawry's collected and pooled series of 8504 patients treated with radiation[33], of whom 25% survived 1 year. Other recent series employing split course radiation cite 1 year survivals of 33%[34], 48% (Landgren et al[35] - "good risk" patients), and 38% (Abramson et al[36]).

The incidence of local recurrence as an isolated event is low among patients who receive modern radiation therapy: 9% in Salazar's series, while 65% manifested their first evidence of recurrence in a site outside the thorax (bone, liver or brain especially). Thus, the combination of radiation and chemotherapy is a logical one. Early studies[37,38] employed radiation in a continuous fractionation regimen and a short course or two of chemotherapy with a variety of agents. Neither a synergistic effort with radiation in terms of local control, nor a beneficial effect on long-term survival, were noted. Randomized, controlled trials which attempted to confirm reports of "radiosensitization" with 5FU and hydroxyurea also led to negative conclusions, as reported by Carr[39] and Landgren[35], respectively. There was, however, a higher response rate in patients with adenocarcinoma and large cell undifferentiated tumors among those receiving one or two courses of 5FU + radiation, compared to the radiation therapy alone group: 61 vs.

29%.

The use of chronic, low-dose chemotherapy, largely with alkylating agents, has been no more successful in conjunction with radiation among inoperable patients than it was when combined with resection in the operable group[40,41], the single exception being a small study with chlorambucil[42].

Based on the activity of bleomycin in squamous tumors[43] and its possible radiation-enhancing properties, Chan et al[44] performed a small, randomized study of split course radiation vs. radiation + bleomycin, 10 units/m^2 twice weekly for 6 weeks, given concurrently with the radiation. Only patients with squamous histology were studied, and the groups were balanced as to performance status. The median survival was 13 months for the combined group, with 4/15 surviving at 2 years, while those initially treated with radiation alone had a median survival of 6 months and 0/12 survived to 2 years.

There are few reported studies to date of radiation combined with long-term, intermittent high-dose chemotherapy. Petrovich has presented data from the VA Lung Study Group[45] which shows no advantage to added CCNU and hydroxyurea, given in conjunction with radiation and then alone: median survivals were in the range of 6 to 7 months and 1 year survival about 30% for both treatments and all non-oat cell subtypes. One randomized study[46] has shown some survival advantage over radiation alone (10.8 vs. 7.4 months, median) for patients treated with a "sandwich" approach involving cyclophosphamide, then radiation, and finally 4 or 8 more courses of cyclophosphamide. However, some patients with oat cell carcinoma were probably included in both treatment groups.

Samuels et al[47] reported a pilot study in 27 patients in which a "sandwich" approach was used, with combination chemotherapy given first: vincristine 2mg/wk, bleomycin 15 units twice weekly, and methotrexate 35-30mg twice weekly for 3 weeks. The patients then received 3000r in 2 weeks to the primary tumor, had a 4 week rest period, received another 3000r in 2 weeks, and resumed vincristine, bleomycin and methotrexate after a 2-4 week additional rest period. The median survival of all patients was 9.8 months, compared to 9 months for that of an immediate historical control of 58 patients who received split-course radiotherapy (no different). Among the 27 squamous patients, however, the median survival was greater than one year.

Hansen et al[48] also studied 27 patients with a "sandwich" approach. Cyclophosphamide 1.1gm/m^2 and methotrexate, 20mg/m^2 twice weekly, were given first, followed by radiation to the primary tumor, 5000r in 6 weeks by split-course, in conjunction with weekly actinomycin D and vincristine. The patients then resumed cyclophosphamide and methotrexate in the same dose schedule, with cyclophosphamide given every 3 weeks. Median survival of all patients was 13.2 months, with 11.5 months for 10 squamous and 15+ months for 12 adenocarcinoma and large cell undifferentiated patients. Six of 22 evaluable patients (27%) responded to the first course of chemotherapy.

The results of Samuels' and Hansen's pilot series suggest that there may be real benefit to a sequential combination of high-dose, intermittent chemotherapy and split-course radiation for non oat cell patients with regional disease. The combination of vincristine, bleomycin and methotrexate may be more effective for squamous, and that of cyclophosphamide and methotrexate for adenocarcinoma and large cell undifferentiated tumors. Our own pilot experience (Livingston, unpublished data) with split-course radiation and doxorubicin (adriamycin) in a "sandwich" has produced encouraging results in a small number of patients, as has that of Chan et al[49] with a program in which low-dose doxorubicin and radiation are given concurrently, followed by doxorubicin and cyclophosphamide in intermittent pulses. Neither of these programs yet involves enough patients or follow up time to assess adequately.

Pines has reported the results of a single study[50] combining radiation and immunotherapy. A total of 48 patients with regional, "advanced" squamous cell lung carcinoma who were able to complete 4000-6000r in 4-5 weeks were then randomized to receive BCG or no specific therapy. BCG (Glaxo) was given in a dose of 25-125 X 10^6 organisms by the Heaf gun technique, weekly or every 2 weeks, beginning 10-14 days after completion of the radiotherapy. At one year from the start of therapy, 20/25 BCG-treated patients were alive, compared to 11/23 controls ($p<.05$), with 3/25 still alive at 5 years in the BCG-treated group and none of the controls. The recurrence pattern was also different: 12/22 BCG-treated and 6/23 controls had local recurrence, while 2/22 on BCG and 12/23 controls had extrathoracic relapse, with or without local recurrence ($p<.02$).

In summary, results of combined modality ttudies to data in non oat cell carcinomas suggest the following: 1) local BCG (intrapleural) may prevent or delay recurrence in Stage I patients; 2) systemic levamisole or BCG may affect the occurrence of extrathoracic, distant metastases, in patients with resected or regional, inoperable tumors, especially those of squamous histology; 3) high dose, intermittent chemotherapy in conjunction with radiation (probably in a "sandwich" fashion) is feasible and deserves further trials in both node-positive resected and regional inoperable disease; 4) different drugs may be effective for different histologies (e.g., doxorubicin, bleomycin or methotrexate for squamous, cyclophosphamide or 5FU for adenocarcinoma); and 5) pre-treatment stratification by known prognostic factors of significance is important if future controlled studies are to be interpreted correctly. In resectable disease, stage and cell type are certainly important factors. In limited disease (inoperable) such factors as weight loss, performance status, age and the presence or absence of gross extrapulmonary disease are all important.

III. OAT CELL (SMALL CELL UNDIFFERENTIATED) - THERAPY OF LIMITED AND EXTENSIVE DISEASE

Oat cell carcinoma is rarely if ever a surgically curable tumor. Untreated, it is the most rapidly fatal of all forms of lung cancer, with median survivals of 6 weeks for extensive (beyond the hemithorax) and 3.5 months for limited disease[27]. It is the most sensitive to both radiation and chemotherapy, and has been the subject of intensive recent experimentation involving chemotherapy alone and chemotherapy plus radiation. In the scope of a brief review, the following facts are pertinent: 1) in limited disease radiation therapy alone can prolong median survival to about 6 months, with one-year survival of about 20%;[31,45,46,51,52] 2) in extensive disease, combination chemotherapy approaches can prolong median survival to about 6-8 months, with one-year survival of 10-25%[53,54,55]; and 3) at present, there is evidence for an advantage to the combined modality approach (chemotherapy + radiation) in limited, but not in extensive disease.

The best survival result yet reported with limited disease is that of Kent et al[56] from the National Cancer Institute: in 15 patients who receive simultaneous radiation and intensive, combination chemotherapy (doxorubicin 40mg/m^2, cyclophosphamide 1500mg/m^2, and vincristine 2mg, each repeated every 3 weeks for a total of 5 courses), median survival was prolonged beyond 20 months, and 70% survived a year. All 15 achieved complete remissions. But the toxicity from this regimen was formidable[57], including an unacceptably high treatment-related mortality (19% overall). In 16 patients with extensive disease who received the same treatment program, median survival was 11 months and 1 year survival 40%, in spite of clinical complete remissions in 87%. Another study of simultaneous radiation and chemotherapy for regional oat cell, reported by Petrovich et al, showed superiority of a combined program with CCNU and hydroxyurea to radiation alone: 8.8 vs. 5 months median survival. Yet by 1 year, only 30% were alive in each group[45].

Table 2 summarizes results reported by a variety of investigators in the treatment of oat cell carcinoma. The combined modality approaches seem clearly superior for patients presenting with regional disease, with survival at 1 year ranging from 38 to 50%, compared to 20% with radiation therapy alone; in addition, it appears that between 10 and 20% of these patients will be long-term (2 years or more) disease-free survivors. (It should be noted that 8 patients treated with combination chemotherapy alone had remarkably good survival). In extensive disease, however, the data shown (plus unpublished data from Maurer et al, Cancer and Acute Leukemia Group B) indicate no advantage, at least in terms of median or 1-year survival, for chemotherapy plus radiation over chemotherapy alone. The only study yet reported involving immunotherapy, that of Hornback et al[57], shows impressive survival in a small group which was predominantly extensive disease patients. This must be confirmed by other investigators.

TABLE 2

EFFECT OF SELECTED TREATMENT REGIMENS ON SURVIVAL, OAT CELL CARCINOMA (LIMITED AND EXTENSIVE DISEASE)

Stage	Regimen and Reference	No. Pts.	MST (wk)	1 Yr. Surv. (%)	Comment
Limited	Supportive care only[57]	31	14	7	
	Radiotherapy (XRT)[52]	73	30	22	Supervoltage
	XRT[51]	37	31	20	Supervoltage
	XRT[57]	53	15	9	Orthovoltage and supervoltage
	XRT[46]	14	21	20	Supervoltage
	XRT (split vs. continuous)[31]	58	~30	20	Supervoltage No difference
Combined modality approaches:	*CTX+XRT*[46]	27	31	38	"Sandwich"
	CTX+VCR+XRT[59]	23	50	50	"Sandwich"
	CTX+VCR+ADR+XRT[60]	17	38	--	Intermittent VCR; "Sandwich"
	CTX+VCR+ADR+XRT[61]	53	>41	>40	Weekly VCR+whole brain XRT: "Sandwich"
	CTX+MTX+CCNU (high dose)[62]	4	>52	75	
	HN_2+VLB+PROC+Prednisone[51]	31	13	<10	
	CTX+VCR+ADR+BLM[53]	4	>52	75	
Extensive	Supportive care only[27]	108	5	0	
	CTX (2 studies)[63,64]	>100	15-17	0	
	CTX+MTX[65]	29	25	9	
	CTX+MTX+CCNU (2 studies)[62,65]	80	27-34	7	
	CTX+MTX+CCNU (high dose)[62]	19	35	21	
	CTX+VCR+MCCNU+BLM[55]	14	30	--	
	CTX+VCR[59]	18	24	--	
	CTX+VCR+ADR[60]	27	27	--	
	CTX+CCNU[64]	83	19	--	
	CTX+ADR+VCR+BLM[53]	25	35	20	
	CTX+MTX+CCNU+VCR[54]	49	39	>25	
Combined modality approaches:	*CTX+VCR+MTX+XRT*[66]	18	39	44	
	CTX+VCR+ADR+XRT[61]	106	33	20-25	
Both	*CTX+VCR+ADR+XRT+BCG*[57]	29	>52	>50	8 limited/21 extensive

IV. CURRENT AND PLANNED APPROACHES WITH COMBINED MODALITIES

A. Non Oat Cell

In resectable disease, the major emphasis is on trials involving immunotherapy. McKneally has continued his trial of no therapy vs. intrapleural BCG for Stage I disease, and this may soon be tested on a nationwide basis under the aegis of the National Cancer Institute. Wright et al in Seattle, following McKneally's lead, are studying the effect of intrapleural BCG, with or without levamisole, vs. no treatment beyond surgery in patients with Stage I and II disease, and the Southwest Oncology Group will soon initiate a study limited to Stage I disease with the same program. The EORTC has implemented a program of post-operative radiation, followed by no further treatment, BCG alone, or a combination of CCNU, cyclophosphamide, methotrexate and BCG. In Stage II and III disease, the Southwest Oncology Group will attempt to examine the value of post-operative, split-course radiation alone vs. added intrapleural BCG + levamisole. Memorial Sloan-Kettering Cancer Center has a study in progress for Stage III patients involving radiotherapy followed by cyclophosphamide, with or without systemic _C. parvum_ administration, and a similar protocol without radiation for patients with earlier disease.

In regional, inoperable disease, the Southeastern Group is implementing a study of radiation, followed by observation vs. intravenous _C. parvum_ vs. levamisole. The EORTC has a study of radiation alone vs. added BCG, combination chemotherapy, or chemoimmunotherapy. In the Southwest Group, split-course radiation will be compared to added doxorubicin, levamisole, or a combination of the two. The RTOG has a dose-time study of radiation therapy schedules, with or without subsequent cyclophosphamide.

B. Oat Cell

"First generation" active studies in the Southwest Oncology Group (Livingston et al) and in the Acute Leukemia Group B (Maurer et al) both involved combination chemotherapy, with radiation to primary site ± CNS prophylaxis. In its current study, the Southwest Group has kept the "sandwich" principle and a combined modality approach, but in addition is testing the value of added BCG in a prospective, randomized fashion. The Southeast Group is about to implement a study in regional oat cell which will compare a "total" radiation therapy only approach to one with added chemotherapy (cyclophosphamide, doxorubicin, and DTIC). A study similar in design to this, but with different chemotherapy (CCNU and cyclophosphamide), has been active for some time as an RTOG/ECOG combined effort. The EORTC has a study which compares radiation therapy to the primary site + cyclophosphamide and vincristine, to vincristine and cyclophosphamide, to cyclophosphamide, vincristine, methyl CCNU and bleomycin, each with or without "prophylactic" whole brain radiation.

V. FUTURE DIRECTIONS

In resectable non oat cell disease, it appears likely that the major emphasis will be on incorporation of immunotherapeutic manipulations. Newer "immunoadjuvant" materials will certainly be tested as they become available, including thymosin, transfer factor, xenogeneic RNA, thiabendazole, interferon or its inducers, and especially tumor cell membrane extracts representing more purified, "specific" antigen. Already studies are being implemented in which different types of immunotherapy (local and systemic; "macrophage stimulant" and "T-cell stimulant") are combined: this trend will continue. In addition, the proper sequence of modalities should be tested: a recent animal model study of Pendergrast et al[67], in B_{16} melanoma, indicated that the most effective sequence was chemotherapy, followed by surgery, followed by immunotherapy.

For patients with regional, unresectable disease (non oat cell), a major thrust of future studies may be the exploration of new techniques which can, at least theoretically, increase the efficacy of radiation therapy. These are 1) the use of metronidazole or "second generation" hypoxic cell radiosensitizers; 2) the use of interstitial implants of radioactive materials at the time of thoracotomy; and 3) the use of "high LET" therapy (pi mesons or neutrons) which may allow for greater tumor doses and less damage to adjacent local tissues. It also seems likely that the role of "debulking" surgery, before or after chemotherapy and/or immunotherapy, followed by radiation and further systemic treatment, will be explored, again following positive leads from a number of experimental model approaches. Finally, the use of heat therapy, both "local" as by microwave application[68] and systemic, will be explored as an adjuvant to other modalities.

In oat cell carcinoma, different forms and combinations of immunotherapy will be examined. A trend is already apparent toward much more intensive, "acute leukemia style" induction chemotherapy[56,62], with or without subsequent or simultaneous radiation to the primary tumor, and toward the routine use of whole brain radiation as prophylaxis[57,61]. Newer approaches will include attempts to eradicate disease in the liver by similar radiation "prophylactically", and to explore possible benefits of half-body radiation therapy[69], probably after a remission has been achieved with chemotherapy and/or local radiation.

REFERENCES

1. American Joint Committee on Cancer Staging. (1972)
2. Naruke, J., et al. (1976) Surgical treatment for lung cancer with metastasis to mediastinal lymph nodes. J. Thorac. Cardiovasc. Surg. 71:279-285.
3. Kirsh, M., et al. (1976) Carcinoma of the lung: results of treatment over ten years. Ann. Thorac. Surg. 21:371-377.
4. Mountain, C., et al. (1974) A system for the clinical staging of lung cancer.

Amer. J. Roent. Rad. Ther. 120:130-138.

5. Paulson, D. and Reisch, J. (1976) Long-term survival after resection for bronchogenic carcinoma. Ann. Surg. 184:324-332.
6. Bergh, N. and Schersten, T. (1965) Bronchogenic carcinoma. Acta. Chir. Scand. Suppl. 347:1-42.
7. Matthews, Mary J. (1974) Morphology of lung cancer. Seminars in Oncology 1: 175-182.
8. Smart, J. (1966) Can lung cancer be curred by irradiation alone? JAMA 195: 1034-1037.
9. Bloedorn, F., et al. (1961) Combined therapy: irradiation and surgery in the treatment of bronchogenic carcinoma. Amer. J. Roent. 85:875-885.
10. Shields, T. (1972) Preoperative radiation therapy in the treatment of bronchogenic carcinoma. Cancer 30:1388-1394.
11. Warram, J. (1975) Preoperative irradiation of cancer of the lung: final report of a therapeutic trial. A collaborative study. Cancer 36:914-925.
12. Paterson, R., and Russell, M. (1962) Clinical trials in malignant disease. IV-lung cancer. Value of post-operative radiotherapy. Clin. Radiol. 13:141-145.
13. Bangma, P. and Tonkes, E. (1965) The value of postoperative radiotherapy of bronchogenic carcinoma. Nederl. T. Geneesk. 109:653.
14. Green, N., et al. (1975) Postresection irradiation for primary lung cancer. Radiology 116:405.
15. Shields, T., et al. (1974) Bronchial carcinoma treated by adjuvant cancer chemotherapy. Arch. Surg. 109:329-333.
16. Slack, N. (1970) Bronchogenic carcinoma: nitrogen mustard as a surgical adjuvant and factors influencing survival. Cancer 25:987-1002.
17. Higgins, T., et al. (1972) The use of chemotherapy as an adjuvant to surgery for bronchogenic carcinoma. Cancer 30:1383.
18. Brunner, K., et al. (1971) Unfavorable effects of long-term adjuvant chemotherapy with Endoxan in radically operated bronchogenic carcinoma. Europ. J. Cancer 7:285-294.
19. Stott, H., et al. (1976) Five-year follow up of cytotoxic chemotherapy as an adjuvant to surgery in carcinoma of the bronchus. Brit. J. Cancer 34:167-173.
20. Karrer, K., et al. (1973) Chemotherapeutic studies in bronchogenic carcinoma by the Austrian study group. Cancer Chemother. Rep. (Part 3) 4:207-213.
21. Katsuki, H., et al. (1975) Long-term intermittent adjuvant chemotherapy for primary resected lung cancer. J. Thorac. Cardiovasc. Surg.
22. Blum, R., and Carter, S. (1974) Adriamycin - a new anticancer drug with significant clinical activity. Ann. Intern. Med. 80:249-259.
23. McKneally, M., et al. (1976) Regional immunotherapy of lung cancer with intrapleural BCG. Lancet 1:377-379.

24. Takita, H. (1972) Adjuvant immunotherapy for lung carcinoma. Surg. Forum 23: 98.
25. Stewart, T., et al. (1976) Immunochemotherapy of lung cancer. Proc. AACR-ASCO 17:305.
26. Amery, W. (1976) Double-blind levamisole trial in resectable lung cancer. Ann. N. Y. Acad. Sci. 277:260-268.
27. Zelen, M. (1973) Keynote address on biostatistics and data retrieval. Cancer Chemother. Rep. (Part 3) 4:31-42.
28. Lanzotti, V., et al. (1977) New survival standards for inoperable lung cancer. Cancer 39:303-313.
29. Salazar, O., et al. (1976) Predictors of radiation response in lung cancer. A Clinico-pathological analysis. Cancer 37:2636-2650.
30. Guttman, R. (1965) Results of radiation therapy in patients with inoperable carcinoma of the lung whose status was established at exploratory thoracotomy. Am. J. Roent. Rad. Ther. 93:99-103.
31. Lee, R. et al. (1976) Comparison of split-course radiation therapy and continuous radiation therapy for unresectable bronchogenic carcinoma: 5 year results. Am. J. Roent. Rad. Ther. 126:116-122.
32. Abramson, N. and Cavanaugh, P. (1970) Short-course radiation therapy in carcinoma of the lung. Radiology 96:627.
33. Selawry, O. and Hansen, H. (1973) "Lung Cancer". <u>In</u> Cancer Medicine (Holland, J. and Frei, E., III, eds.) Lea and Febiger, Philadelphia, pp. 1473-1518.
34. Aristizabal, S. and Caldwell, W. (1976) Radical irradiation with the split-course technique in carcinoma of the lung. Cancer 37:2630-2635.
35. Landgren, R., et al. (1974) Split-course irradiation compared to split-course irradiation plus hydroxyurea in inoperable bronchogenic carcinoma - a randomized study of 53 patients. Cancer 34:1598-1601.
36. Abramson, N. and Cavanaugh, P. (1973) Short-course radiation therapy in carcinoma of the lung - a second look. Radiology 108:685-687.
37. Hall, T., et al. (1967) A clinical pharmacologic study of chemotherapy and X-ray therapy in lung cancer. Amer. J. Med. 43:186-193.
38. Krant, M., et al. (1963) Comparative trial of chemotherapy and radiotherapy in patients with nonresectable cancer of the lung. Amer. J. Med. 35:363-373.
39. Carr, D., et al. (1972) Radiotherapy plus 5FU compared to radiotherapy alone for inoperable and unresectable bronchogenic carcinoma. Cancer 29:375-380.
40. Kaung, D., et al. (1974) Preliminary report on the treatment of nonresectable cancer of the lung. Cancer Chemother. Rep. 58:359-364.
41. Hosley, H., et al. (1962) Combined radiation-chemotherapy for bronchogenic carcinoma. Cancer Chemother. Rep. 16:467.
42. Horwitz, H., et al. (1965)"Suppressive" chemotherapy in bronchogenic carcinoma. Amer. J. Roent. 93:615.

43. Blum, R., et al. (1975) Clinical review of bleomycin - a new antineoplastic agent. Cancer 31:903.

44. Chan, P., et al. (1976) Unresectable squamous cell carcinoma of the lung and its management by combined bleomycin and radiotherapy. Cancer 37:2671-2676.

45. Petrovich, Z., et al. (1976) Clinical report on the treatment of locally advanced lung cancer. Presented to American Society of Therapeutic Radiologists.

46. Bergsagel, D., et al. (1972) Lung cancer: clinical trial of radiotherapy alone vs. radiotherapy plus cyclophosphamide. Cancer 30:621-627.

47. Samuels, M., et al. (1975) Combination chemotherapy with bleomycin, vincristine, and methotrexate plus split-course radiotherapy in the treatment of non oat cell bronchogenic carcinoma. Cancer Chemother. Rep. 59:377-383.

48. Hansen, H., et al. (1972) Intensive combined chemotherapy and radiotherapy in patients with nonresectable bronchogenic carcinoma. Cancer 30:315-324.

49. Chan, P., et al. (1976) Coincident adriamycin and X-ray therapy in bronchogenic carcinoma: response and cardiotoxocity. Proc. ASCO-AACR 17:276.

50. Pines, A. (1976) A 5-year controlled study of BCG and radiotherapy for inoperable lung cancer. Lancet 1:380-381.

51. Laing, A. and Berry, R. (1975) Treatment of small-cell carcinoma of bronchus. Lancet 1:129-132.

52. Fox, W., and Scadding, J. (1973) Medical research council comparative trial of surgery and radiotherapy for primary treatment of small-celled or oat-celled carcinoma of bronchus. Lancet 2:63-65.

53. Einhorn, L., et al. (1976) Improved chemotherapy for small-cell undifferentiated lung cancer. JAMA 235:1225-1229.

54. Hansen, H. and Hansen, M. (1976) A comparison of 3 and 4 drug combination chemotherapy for advanced small cell anaplastic carcinoma of the lung. Proc. AACR-ASCO 17:129.

55. Livingston, R., et al. (1975) COMB: a four-drug combination in solid tumors. Cancer 36:327-332.

56. Kent, C. H. et al. (1976) "Total" therapy for oat cell carcinoma of the lung. Presented to the American Society of Therapeutic Radiologists.

57. Hornback, N., et al. (1976) Oat cell carcinoma. Early treatment results of combination radiation therapy and chemotherapy. Cancer 37:2658-2664.

58. Roswit, B., et al. (1968) The survival of patients with inoperable lung cancer: a large-scale randomized study of radiation therapy vs. placebo. Radiology 90:688-697.

59. Holoye, P. and Samuels, M. (1975) Cyclophosphamide, vincristine and sequential split-course radiotherapy in the treatment of small-cell lung cancer. Chest 67:675-679.

60. Holoye, P., et al. (1975) Cytoxan, adriamycin and vincristine combination

with radiation therapy in the treatment of small cell carcinoma of the lung. Proc. AACR 16:112.

61. Livingston, R., and Moore, T. (1976) Combined modality treatment of oat cell carcinoma of the lung. Proc. AACR-ASCO 17:152.

62. Cohen, M., et al. (1976) Intensive chemotherapy of small cell bronchogenic carcinoma. Proc. AACR-ASCO 17:273.

63. Green, R., et al. (1969) Alkylating agents in bronchogenic carcinoma. Am. J. Med. 46:516-524.

64. Edmonson, J. and Lagakos, S. (1976) Patterns of response and survival in small cell carcinoma of the lung. Proc. AACR-ASCO 17:145.

65. Selawry, O., et al. (1974) Improved chemotherapy for advanced bronchogenic carcinoma. Proc. AACR-ASCO 15:118.

66. Eagan, R., et al. (1973) Combination chemotherapy and radiation therapy in small cell carcinoma of the lung. Cancer 32:371-379.

67. Pendergrast, W., et al. (1976) A proper sequence for the treatment of B_{16} melanoma: chemotherapy, surgery and immunotherapy. J. Nat. Cancer Instit. 57:539-544.

68. LeVeen, H., et al. (1976) Tumor eradication by radiofrequency therapy. Response in 21 patients. JAMA 235:2198-2200.

Adjuvant Therapy of Cancer, S.E. Salmon and S.E. Jones eds.

REGIONAL IMMUNOTHERAPY USING INTRAPLEURAL BCG AND ISONIAZID FOR RESECTABLE LUNG CANCER: RESULTS IN THE FIRST 100 CASES.

M.F. McKneally and C. Maver

Albany Medical College, Albany, N.Y. 12208

SUMMARY

During the past 3 years we have entered 100 patients into a randomized prospective controlled trial of intrapleural immunotherapy using a single dose of 10^7 Tice BCG in the immediate postoperative period. The trial is based on the observation that postoperative empyema seems to improve the survival fraction after pulmonary resection. Median duration of observation is 640 days. The results suggest that intrapleural BCG therapy is effective in Stage I lung cancer but ineffective in more advanced disease.

INTRODUCTION

In 1972 we drew attention to the immunological significance of postoperative empyema following surgical resection for lung cancer.[1] This natural experiment in immunotherapy has been suspected by thoracic surgeons to be beneficial since the first successful pneumonectomy for lung cancer was performed in 1934.[2] That operation was complicated by empyema and the patient survived to complete a stage thoracoplasty and 30 more years of productive life, much of it in the practice of obstetrics. Several reports on the treatment of empyema contain data to support the view that its occurrence after lung cancer resection may have improved the survival rate[3,4,5,6] but Takita was the first to report that this complication was beneficial.[3] Cady and Clifton's earlier review of their experience at New York Memorial Hospital did not support this conclusion.[7] It is possible that a high immediate mortality from empyema in their series reversed the statistical correlation of empyema with prolonged survival. The biological question "does regional node stimulation in the field of lymphatic drainage improve the probability of long term survival?" can only be asked in patients who do not die in the immediate postoperative interval. In these patients, the natural history of the tumor and its alteration by chronic regional node stimulation can be recorded.

9 of our 18 patients who developed postoperative empyema survived more than 5 years in our experience at Albany Medical College. 22% of 411 lung cancer patients who underwent resection in the same interval survived. ($p = 0.0073$) This observation was extraordinarily stimulating, when viewed against the background of the low survival rate in lung cancer, and the body of experimental evidence then accumulated, which showed that cross protective immunity can be induced by microbial infection[8] and that infection with the BCG strain of Mycobacterium tuberculosis bovis can limit the growth of experimental[9] and certain human tumors[10] when locally injected in the region of the tumor. Reasoning that a similar protective tumor growth might be achieved with a controlled postoperative local infection, we set out to reproduce the natural experiment in a randomized, controlled clinical trial of intrapleural BCG infection after pulmonary resection for lung cancer.

Prior to the initiation of the study, we established in experimental animals:

1.) that intrapleural administration of this agent is safe when the dose is limited and antituberculous agents are administered.

2.) that the bronchial, vascular, and wound closures are not compromised by this agent after pulmonary resection.[11]

3.) that intrapleural BCG was efficient in reducing the growth of lung tumors in experimental animals.[12]

Preliminary studies in patients with malignant effusions had lead us to the conclusion that 10^7 colony forming units of BCG in the pleural space did not adversely effect the clinical course of cancer patients, and was often helpful in controlling the effusion.[13]

MATERIALS AND METHODS

In April, 1973, the first patients undergoing curative resection for lung cancer entered the study. This report summarizes our experience after 100 patients have been studied. All patients undergoing pulmonary resection for lung cancer were eligible for study. Preliminary evaluation included measurement of pulmonary function, routine blood chemical testing, and skin tests with PHA[14] and recall antigens (mumps, histoplasmin, old tuberculin, purified protein derivative, Candida, Trichophyton, Varidase). Uniform surgical criteria and techniques were used throughout.[15] Following resection the patients were stratified by cell type (anaplastic carcinoma, adenocarcinoma, and squamous carcinoma) and by stage. The staging followed the recommendations of the American Joint Committee on Cancer Staging.[16]

Following resection and before the chest drainage tubes were removed, the histologic diagnosis, tumor size, and lymph node status were recorded. The patients were then randomly assigned by a sealed envelope technique to receive BCG, or to enter the control group.

BCG treated patients were given a single intrapleural injection of 10^7 colony forming units of Tice strain BCG (one fiftieth of the vial supplied by the University of Illinois). The injection was given through the chest tube just prior to its removal in patients undergoing lobectomy and by thoracentesis in patients undergoing pneumonectomy (usually on postoperative day 4 to 6). The patients were treated with aspirin and benadryl for 48 hours to reduce the discomfort of the "influenzal" syndrome of fever and malaise which regularly occurred following BCG injection. They were discharged on approximately the fifth post-injection day. Fourteen days following injection of BCG, isoniazid 300mg./day was begun and continued for 12 weeks to prevent overgrowth of BCG organisms. Control patients began isoniazid 300mg./day on the 14th day following discharge from the hospital and continued this medication for 12 weeks. They did not receive a placebo injection intrapleurally. At 2,4,12,26 and 52 weeks and at 6 month intervals thereafter, all patients returned to the thoracic surgical outpatient office for followup by physical examination, chest x-rays, skin tests, blood chemical testing, and measurement of lymphocytotoxicity against lung tumor cells in vitro.

Patients who developed metastases or local recurrence were treated by x-irradiation, if appropriate, in the Division of Radiotherapy but continued to be followed in the Division of Thoracic Surgery. Any patient who was treated with adrenal cortical steroids for a subsequent brain metastasis was simultaneously treated with isoniazid if he received BCG in the postoperative interval.

Because temperature elevation to 102° - 104° was frequently observed following BCG treatment, patients whose cardiac or pulmonary performance was already compromised in the postoperative interval were excluded from randomization. Six such patients were excluded in the study interval. Two died of respiratory insufficiency and one died of a myocardial infarction in the immediate postoperative period. One excluded patient died of a second primary lung cancer which developed 18 months after his original surgery. Two excluded patients are well, one of whom required simultaneous myocardial revascularization at the time of pulmonary resection. Three additional patients were excluded because of a problem with BCG suspension. Flocculation of the organisms precluded adequate dilution.

The patients were regularly re-examined at 1,3,6,12,18,24 months and at 6 month intervals thereafter. Followup examinations included a physical examination, chest x-ray, complete blood count, and blood chemical profile, skin tests and a variety of in vitro immunological tests.

Time of Recurrence was defined as the first recorded observation in the chart of a sign or symptom which ultimately proved to be related to recurrent cancer. Statistical analysis was performed by Dr. Lloyd Lininger of the State University of New York at Albany. Survival curves were prepared by the method of Kaplan and Meier[17] and the significance of differences computed by the technique of Gehan.[18]

RESULTS

100 patients have been entered into the study. No patients have been lost to followup. The median duration of followup is 617 days and the longest followup on a BCG treated patient is 1400 days.

There was a significant reduction in the incidence of tumor recurrence in

Stage I patients treated with intrapleural BCG (p = 0.009) of thirty such patients, one has died of metastatic cancer, and a second one has developed a new lesion in another lobe which may be a recurrence or a second primary lung cancer. This lesion has been excised and the patient is well.

Of 33 Stage I control patients treated with INH, 11 have developed recurrent cancer. These results are illustrated graphically in Figure 1.

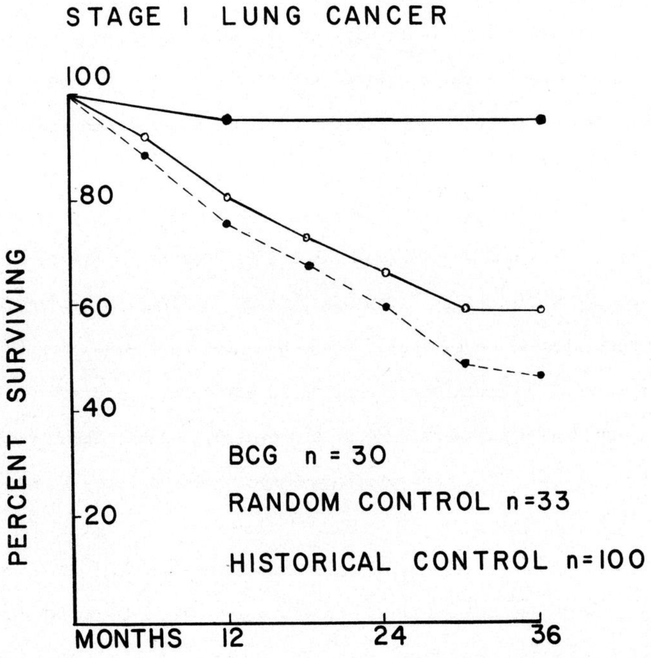

We compared the survival of our randomized INH treated control group with historial control patients and have concluded that they are representative of the usual survival pattern of resected, surgically staged lung cancer patients. There may be contamination of both the treated and control Stage I groups with unsuspected Stage III patients, inasmuch as the mediastinal lymph nodes were not biopsied by mediastinoscopy or mediastinal node dissection in every patient.

We have studied a smaller number of patients with more advanced but resectable disease. The results in these patients suggest that intrapleural BCG as administered in this program is not beneficial in Stage II and III lung cancer. There were 13 recurrences among 22 BCG treated patients in Stage II and III lung cancer, and 8 recurrences among 15 control patients. The pattern of recurrence among BCG treated patients was not unusual, following the pattern of persistence of lung cancer after curative resection described by Matthews.[19] The quality of life in surviving BCG treated patients was not impaired by the treatment.

Intrapleural BCG caused temperature elevation in most patients. The mean elevation was to 101.3°F and the maximum was 104°F. Febrile patients experienced malaise and, occasionally, chills. The usual fever subsided in 3 to 4 days, the longest fever persisted 43 days. Aspirin and benadryl were given for 48 hours to reduce these symptoms. Temperature elevation is not felt to warrant prolongation of the hospital stay, and patients were discharged while still febrile once their systemic symptoms abated. The mean prolongation of hospital stay in BCG treated patients was 5.3 ± 1.7 days.

A total of eleven complications occurred in the BCG treated group. One patient developed a non-mycobacterial empyema 6 months postoperatively which was drained surgically. A pleural biopsy taken at the time of open drainage showed no granuloma and grew no mycobacteria. *Escherichia coli* was cultured, and this patient was ultimately sterilized and closed by Clagett's technique.[20] He is well 3 years following resection. There was an apparent increase in minor wound or drain site infections, none of which required hospitalization. None of these infections were mycobacterial.

One patient in the INH treated control group developed a drug related neuropathy. This patient improved with vitamin supplements and an improved diet. The SGOT level was elevated above 100 units in 5 of 100 patients. No significant level of toxicity was evident clinically. The alkaline phosphatase was transiently elevated in all patients given intrapleural BCG. This was felt to be an asymptomatic controlled form of BCG induced granulomatous hepatitis.[21] We have been informed of three patients at other institutions who developed life threatening infections after intrapleural administration of an entire vial of Tice BCG (fifty times the recommended dose). It is clear that excessive doses of this agent do not improve its effectiveness and may do great harm.

The tuberculin test converted to positive (induration greater than 10 mm) in 30 of 32 BCG treated patients. The PHA skin test proved a vague predictor of prognosis, in that 14 of 23 patients with a negative PHA skin test (induration less than 10 mm) developed recurrent cancer, whereas cancer recurred in only 11 of 52 patients with a positive skin test. Skin test reactivity to recall antigens and lymphocytotoxicity against cultured tumor cells did not reflect or predict the clinical course.

DISCUSSION

The improvement recorded in the survival fraction of Stage I patients treated with intrapleural BCG is an encouraging lead in the treatment of this difficult disease. This observation requires independent confirmation in a larger series of patients. The treatment has the practical advantage of requiring only one application, and offering the patient little probability of morbidity. Once its efficacy is confirmed, it would be acceptable to apply intrapleural BCG even in those patients excluded in the present protocol because of hemodynamic or respiratory instability. The fact that two patients developed recurrent cancer in the subgroup on Stage I patients treated with BCG and INH suggests that additional treatment is appropriate.

It is clear that patients with more extensive cancer in Stage II and Stage III derive no detectable benefit from BCG and INH. It may be that the augmentation of the immune response which this treatment is presumed to invoke is insufficient to deal with the extent of disease present in these patients. Matthews has shown us the stark facts about the persistence of local and disseminated cancer in patients who undergo surgical resection.[19] She studied 216 patients who died within 30 days of curative resection for lung cancer, and found persistent cancer in 15% of patients with T1 lesions, and in 33% of patients with T2 lesions. 70% of patients with T3 lesions had local or disseminated cancer discoverable at autopsy.

There are few precedents in biology for cure of disseminated or locally advanced disease by immunotherapy. While human cancer is an unsolved biological problem, it seems unlikely that it will follow entirely new rules. Based on Matthews observations, we suspect that regional immunotherapy with surgical excision might be more efficiently coupled with other cytoreductive agencies, such as local x-irradiation and systemic chemotherapy for control of advanced or disseminated disease. The regional administration of BCG may serve to bring about first a local, and eventually a systemic specific immunization to tumor specific antigens co-resident in the lymphoid tissue undergoing BCG stimulation. If this mechanism is at work, then a systemic benefit from immunotherapy might be anticipated. If intrapleural BCG activates only a non specific response, its effect will be exerted only on locally persistent disease.

REFERENCES

1. Ruckdeschel, J.C., Codish, S.D., Stranahan, A. and McKneally, M.F. (1972) N. Engl. J. Med. 287, 1013-1017
2. Graham, E.A., Singer, J.J. (1933) J.A.M.A. 101, 1371-1374
3. Takita, H. (1970) J. Thorac. Cardiovasc. Surg. 59, 642-644
4. Sensenig, D.M., Rossi, N.P. and Ehrenhoft, J.L. (1963) Surg. Gynec. Obstet. 116, 279-284
5. Virkkula, L., Kostiainen, S. (1970) Scand. J. Thorac. Cardiovasc. Surg. 4, 267-270
6. leRoux, B.T. (1965) Brit. J. Surg. 52, 89-99
7. Cady, B., Cliffton, E.E. (1967) J. Thorac. Cardiovasc. Surg. 53, 102-108

8. MacKaness, G.B. (1969) J. Exp. Med. 129, 973-992

9. Bast, R.C., Zbar, B., Borsos, T. and Rapp, H.J. (1974) N. Engl. J. Med. 290, 1413-1420

10. Morton, D.L., Holmes, E.C., Eilber, F.R. and Wood, W.C. (1971) Ann. Intern. Med. 74, 587-604

11. Codish, S.D., McKneally, M.F. (1972) Fed. Proc. 31, 658

12. Codish, S.D., Ratnam, M. and McKneally, M.F. (1973) Fed. Proc. 32, 848

13. McKneally, M.F., Maver, C., Civerchia, L., Codish, S.D., Kausel, H.W. and Alley, R.D. (1975) Neoplasm Immunity:Theory and Application (Crispen, R.G., ed.) p. 153-159, ITR, Chicago

14. Bonforte, R.J., Topilsky, M., Siltzbach, L.E. and Glade, P.R. (1972) J. Pediatr. 81, 775-780

15. McKneally, M.F., Maver, C., Kausel, H.W. and Alley, R.D. (1976) J. Thor. Cardiovasc. Surg. 72, 333-338

16. Mountain, C.F., Carr, D.T. and Anderson, W.A.D. (1974) Am. J. Roentgenol. Radium Ther. Nucl. Med. 120, 130-138

17. Kaplan, E.L. and Meier, P. (1958) J. Am. Stat. Assoc. 53, 457-464

18. Gehan, E.A. (1965) Biometrika 52, 203-223

19. Matthews, M.J., Kanhouwa, S., Pickren, J. and Robinette, D. (1973) Cancer Chemotherapy Reports Part 3 (Vol. 4, No. 2) 63-67

20. Clagett, O.T. and Geraci, J.E. (1963) J. Thorac. Cardiovasc. Surg. 45, 141-145

21. Hunt, J.S., Silverstein, M.J., Sparks, F.C., Haskell, C.M., Pilch, Y.H. and Morton, D.L. (1973) Lancet 2, 820-821

(Supported in part by the New York State Kidney Disease Institute (Unit of NYS Dept. of Health) and NIH Grants RO1-CA-17346, MO1-RR00749 and NO1-CB-53940)

Adjuvant Therapy of Cancer, S.E. Salmon and S.E. Jones eds.

IMMUNOTHERAPY OF RESECTABLE NON-SMALL CELL CANCER OF THE LUNG: A PROSPECTIVE COMPARISON OF INTRAPLEURAL BCG + LEVAMISOLE VERSUS INTRAPLEURAL BCG VERSUS PLACEBO

Peter W. Wright, Lucius D. Hill, Richard P. Anderson, Samuel P. Hammar,
Irwin D. Bernstein, and Ross L. Prentice
Divisions of Tumor Immunology and Epidemiology & Biostatistics,
Fred Hutchinson Cancer Research Center;
Departments of Surgery and Pathology, The Mason Clinic; and
Departments of Medicine, Surgery, Pediatrics, and Biostatistics,
University of Washington, Seattle, Washington

INTRODUCTION

Despite improved methods of diagnosis and staging, the majority of patients still die following resection for primary cancer of the lung[1,2]. Several therapeutic modalities have been evaluated as possible adjuncts to surgical therapy in lung cancer patients. Pre- or post-operative radiotherapy and/or chemotherapy have been shown to be of limited or no value when compared to surgery alone[3-6]. Preliminary results of recent clinical trials utilizing intrapleural BCG or Levamisole have provided suggestive evidence for a benefit of adjunctive immunotherapy in patients with completely resected non-small cell cancer of the lung.

BCG has been extensively evaluated as a non-specific potentiator of cellular immunity. The administration of BCG has been shown to delay or prevent tumor induction, and to inhibit or enhance the growth of established tumors in selected animal model tumor systems[7]. Intrapleural and intravenous BCG have been shown to significantly lengthen survival in animals with pulmonary implants of tumor cells injected intravenously[8,9]. McKneally et al. have reported an increased disease-free remission duration in patients with stage I lung cancer receiving post-operative intrapleural BCG[10,11]. Current results of this trial are reported in greater detail elsewhere in this volume.

Levamisole, introduced as an antihelminthic, has recently been demonstrated to potentiate both humoral and cellular immune responses[12]. Preliminary studies in man have demonstrated that treatment with Levamisole may increase delayed cutaneous hypersensitivity reactions to DNCB in patients with lung cancer[13]. Amery et al. have evaluated Levamisole as a surgical adjuvant in patients with lung cancer[14]. They have reported that Levamisole-treated patients weighing less than 70 kg have an increased remission duration, decreased frequency of distant metastasis, and improved survival when compared to a concurrent control group receiving placebo[15].

The purpose of the present study is to evaluate the effects of intrapleural BCG alone and in combination with Levamisole. Since BCG and Levamisole are presumed to act by independent mechanisms (BCG to limit local tumor growth and Levamisole to limit distant metastases), the effect of these two agents in combination may be additive or synergistic.

MATERIALS AND METHODS

Patient eligibility and staging. Patients with histologically-proven epidermoid carcinoma, adenocarcinoma, or undifferentiated large cell carcinoma of the lung considered fully resectable and potentially curable by surgery alone, were eligible for study. Histological evaluation of the surgical specimen must have shown no evidence of mediastinal lymph node involvement or tumor at cut margins. Patients must have received no pre-operative chemotherapy, immunotherapy, or radiation therapy. Patients with serious concomitant disease, inadequate pulmonary function, or a history of active tuberculosis within five years were excluded.

Prior to surgery, a CBC, chemical screening battery, liver function studies, pulmonary function studies, and chest x-ray were obtained on all patients. Isotope scanning was done when indicated by symptoms or laboratory abnormalities. Mediastinoscopy or mediastinotomy, although not required, was generally performed on patients with large or centrally-located primary tumors. All patients were staged prior to surgery according to a clinical TNM classification[16,17].

Immunologic evaluation included skin tests with a defined battery of "recall" antigens and DNCB sensitization and challenge in all patients.

Randomization and therapy. Prior to surgery, patients were stratified according to the clinical TNM classification and assigned to one of three possible treatment groups using an unbalanced randomization scheme. Patients had a (1) 40% chance of being assigned to immunotherapy with intrapleural BCG and Levamisole; (2) a 40% chance of being assigned to immunotherapy with intrapleural BCG and Levamisole placebo; and (3) a 20% chance of being assigned to receive intrapleural BCG placebo and Levamisole placebo. Levamisole, 2.5 mg/kg (or its placebo) was given for three consecutive days prior to surgery and continued for two consecutive days of each week for 18 months or until relapse. Intrapleural BCG (Tice strain, 10^7 viable colony-forming units) was administered on the fourth post-operative day as described by McKneally et al.[10,11]. Two weeks following BCG administration, Isoniazid (INH), 300 mg/day, was given for 12 consecutive weeks. Patients receiving intrapleural BCG placebo received INH placebo. Patients were evaluated at six weeks and 12 weeks, and then at three monthly intervals following surgery.

RESULTS

One hundred and one patients were formally randomized between March 8, 1976 and January 10, 1977 when this analysis was conducted. On-study information on this patient population is shown (Table I).

TABLE I

ON STUDY INFORMATION

A.	Total number of patients randomized before surgery		101
B.	Number of patients failing to meet eligibility requirements after surgery		40
	Reasons for failure:		
		benign diagnosis	14
		metastatic cancer from non-lung primary	2
		lymphoma	1
		carcinoid	1
		small cell cancer of lung	4
		non-small cell cancer of lung + active TB	1
		non-small cell cancer of lung - unresectable	17
C.	Number of patients fulfilling all eligibility requirements after surgery		61
	Non-evaluable	post-operative complications	5
		refused further treatment	4
	Evaluable		52

Forty patients were excluded from further treatment on the study on the basis of findings at surgery. Sixty-one patients were found to fulfill all eligibility requirements of the protocol after surgery. Of these, five developed post-operative complications precluding the administration of intrapleural BCG, and four refused further treatment following surgery. Fifty-two patients were therefore considered evaluable for this analysis. The characteristics of this group are shown in Table II.

TABLE II

PATIENT CHARACTERISTICS (52 Evaluable Patients)

		Number
Male		37
Female		18
Median age (range)		65 (45-75)
Cell type	adenocarcinoma	30
	epidermoid carcinoma	15
	mixed	3
	large cell undifferentiated	6
	broncho-alveolar	1
Stage and TNM classification (Pathological)		
	$T_1N_0M_0$	18
I	$T_2N_0M_0$	19
	$T_1N_1M_0$	5
II	$T_2N_1M_0$	8
III	$T_3N_0M_0$	1
	$T_3N_1M_0$	1

Thirty-two patients have been followed six months or more. Two of eleven patients in an initial feasibility trial who received active Levamisole + intrapleural BCG following surgery in January and February 1976, and 4/52 patients in the randomized trial have developed tumor recurrence (Table III).

TABLE III

PATIENTS WITH RECURRENT CANCER

Patient Number	Stage	TNM Path.	Size 1° Tumor (cm)	Cell Type	Site Tumor Recurrence	Days to Objective Recurrence	Days to Death
Feasibility trial							
124	I	T_1N_1	2 x 1	adeno	liver	289	289
127	II	T_2N_1	4 x 4	adeno	contralateral lung	174	alive
Randomized trial							
4	I	T_2N_0	7 x 5	adeno	brain	182	203
11	I	T_2N_0	8 x12	epidermoid	local	144	248
68	I	T_2N_0	4 x 3	adeno	brain + bone	146	289
188	I	T_1N_1	3 x 3	undifferentiated	brain	106	alive

Since the number of patients with recurrence is small, it is impossible to make any statement concerning treatment effects at the present time. It is interesting to note that the first site of tumor recurrence was local in the one patient with epidermoid carcinoma, and distant in the remaining patients, all of whom had either adeno- or undifferentiated carcinomas.

Immunologic data. A high frequency of reactivity to both DNCB and a battery of "recall" antigens was observed in all patient groups pre-operatively (Table IV).

TABLE IV

SKIN TEST RESULTS

Patient Group	Initial DNCB Response: No. ≥ 2+ Response/ Total Patients	(%)	Mean Response	"Recall" Antigen Response: No. +/ Total Patients	(%)
Resectable	44/48	(92)	2.4	36/50	(72)
Unresectable	10/12	(83)	2.5	8/12	(67)
Benign diagnosis	7/7	(100)	2.6	7/9	(78)

The activity was somewhat (but not significantly) lower in patients with unresectable disease. Only one patient tested (a patient with resectable stage I disease) was unresponsive to both DNCB and to the recall battery. No difference in initial skin test reactivity is apparent in patients with tumor recurrence.

Complete pre- and post-operative skin test information for 41 of the 52 evaluable patients noted in Table II was available for analysis. Fifteen of these patients were reactive to PPD prior to surgery. In the remaining 26 PPD negative patients, it has been possible to evaluate the frequency of PPD conversion following the post-operative administration of intrapleural BCG (or its placebo). This data is summarized (Table V).

TABLE V

PPD CONVERSION[1]

Treatment Group	Yes	No	Total
Placebo	1	4	
BCG	5	3	
BCG + Levamisole	10	3	
TOTAL	16	10	26

[1] Patient's initial PPD negative, >10 mm induration after surgery.

Sixteen of the 26 (62%) of patients who were PPD negative prior to surgery, have shown conversion of their PPD response post-operatively. Conversion was specific for BCG immunotherapy, i.e., 15/16 conversions occurred in patients receiving Levamisole plus BCG. A higher incidence of conversion in patients receiving Levamisole plus BCG (5/8) is suggested when compared to patients receiving Levamisole placebo plus BCG (10/13), but the difference between these two treatment groups is not statistically significant. Converters and non-converters were also compared for their initial DNCB or recall antigen response, pathological TNM classification, cell type, stage, and primary tumor size. No dramatic differences between the two groups were apparent. Patients showing conversion tended to be a more advanced stage (25% were stage II or III), whereas patients failing to show conversion were all stage I.

A correlation between PPD conversion and clinical course has been observed. None of the 16 patients showing PPD conversion has yet shown tumor recurrence. By contrast, PPD conversion has not been observed in the two patients in the feasibility trial or in the four patients in the randomized trial with relapse. It should also be noted that five of eight patients showing PPD conversion at six weeks and followed for six months or more, have shown reversion to a negative PPD response. In 4/5 of these patients, the loss of PPD reactivity was specific, i.e., reactivity to other skin test antigens was retained. None of these patients has developed evidence of tumor recurrence during the period of observation.

Toxicity. The toxicity of the treatment regimens is shown (Table VI).

TABLE VI

TOXICITY

	Treatment		
	Placebo	BCG + LMS placebo	BCG + Levamisole
Total number of patients :	10	18	24
No. patients experiencing:			
Nausea	3	2	4
Anorexia	2	1	5
Change in taste or smell	1	1	5
Leukopenia	0	0	2
Fever (> 100°F) within 48 hours post intra-pleural inoculation	0	9	8

In general, the treatment has been well-tolerated with no medically serious complications observed. Mild to moderate G.I. disturbances have been the most common complaint. Nausea and anorexia have been observed in a significant number of patients receiving placebo. Alterations in taste or smell which have been previously reported for patients receiving Levamisole[18,19], appear to be relatively specific for this drug in our series. Reversible leukopenia has been previously reported in patients treated with Levamisole[18,19] and was also noted here in two patients. Post-operative fevers (> 100°F) were common in patients receiving intrapleural BCG, but generally of limited (less than 2-3 days) duration, and did not prolong the patients' hospital stay. Liver function test abnormalities have been previously noted in patients receiving intrapleural BCG and INH[11]. Although slight elevations of alkaline phosphatase levels were commonly observed, a transient increase in alkaline phosphatase as high as one and one-half to two times the upper limits of normal was noted in only one patient receiving intrapleural BCG. No case of disseminated BCG infection has been observed.

DISCUSSION

Only two of 11 patients in an initial feasibility trial and four of 52 patients in a prospective, randomized trial have shown tumor recurrence to date. Due to the small number of patient recurrences and limited follow-up time, no statement can be made concerning treatment effects at the present time.

Conversion of the PPD skin test response from negative to positive following intrapleural administration of BCG may prove to be of prognostic significance in our study. Although PPD conversions were noted in a high percentage (71%) of evaluable patients who received intrapleural BCG, conversion was not observed in the six patients with recurrent tumor. Moreover, none of the 16 patients with PPD conversion has yet shown tumor recurrence. The apparent higher conversion rate in our series in patients receiving Levamisole + intrapleural BCG, compared to patients receiving intrapleural BCG alone, suggests that Levamisole may augment the host response to BCG.

No clear relationship between PPD reactivity and clinical outcome has yet been described in other BCG immunotherapy studies. This lack of relationship is not altogether surprising, however, since previous studies have shown little or no clinical benefit from BCG immunotherapy. A more direct correlation between the response to PPD and treatment with BCG may be apparent in studies where BCG immunotherapy is more effective. For example, in McKneally's series, a high frequency of conversion to either PPD or old tuberculin (OT) skin test reactivity has been observed. In stage I disease, a significant correlation between skin test reactivity and tumor recurrence has been noted. In stage II disease, however, this correlation has been less exact. Some patients have developed tumor recurrence despite skin test conversion (C. Maver, Personal communication). These observations are consistent with the hypothesis that a host response to BCG is necessary, although not sufficient to derive clinical benefit from therapy.

Reports in animals have demonstrated that intact delayed hypersensitivity is required for the therapeutic effect of BCG[7]. Studies in the mouse have shown that an immune response to BCG (and not necessarily to tumor antigen) is required for suppression of local tumor growth following the administration of intralesional BCG[20]. Evaluation of the relationship of the immune response to intrapleural BCG and clinical outcome will provide a focus for our future study of lung cancer patients.

ACKNOWLEDGEMENTS

The authors gratefully acknowledge the participation of Drs. Phillip Jolly of the Mason Clinic, Roland Pinkham, Lloyd Johnson, Waldo Mills, William B. Hutchinson, Robert Coe, Lloyd King, and Howard Anderson of Swedish Hospital; George Thomas of Providence Hospital; Hubert Radke, Wesley Sikkema, Eugene Hessel, Tom Ivey, and Douglas Johnson of the University-affiliated hospitals, who have entered patients on this protocol; Drs. Terry Rogers, Leonard Hudson, Jon Huseby, Ed Morgan, and S. Laksminarayan, Pulmonary Disease consultants; Drs. Harold Hall, Bruce Kulander, Tom Norris, David Thorning, and Ed Barker, Pathology consultants; and the pharmacy staffs of the Mason Clinic, Swedish Hospital, Providence Hospital, and the University-affiliated hospitals in Seattle.

REFERENCES

1. Hyde, L., Wolf, J., McCracken, S., et al. (1973) Chest 64:309.
2. Benfield, J.R. (1975) Ann. Int. Med. 83:93.
3. Preoperative irradiation of cancer of the lung. Preliminary reports of a therapeutic trial: A collaborative study (1969) Cancer 23:419.
4. Shields, T.W., Higgins, G.A., Jr., Lawton, R., et al. (1970) J. Thorac. Card. Surg. 59:49.
5. Patterson, R., and Russell, M.H. (1962) Clin. Radiol. 13:141.
6. Carter, S.K. (1973) Cancer Chemother. Rep., Part 3, 4:109.
7. Bast, R.C., Jr., Zbar, B., Borsos, T., et al. (1974) N. Eng. J. Med. 290:1413.
8. McKneally, M.F., Maver, C., Civerchia, L., et al. (1975) In: Neoplasm Immunity, Theory and Application, R. Crispen (ed.), Inst. for Tuberculosis Research, Chicago, p. 153.
9. Baldwin, R.W., and Pimm, M.V. (1973) Int. J. Cancer 12:420.
10. McKneally, M.F., Maver, C., and Kausel, H.W. (1976) Lancet 1:377.
11. McKneally, M.F., Maver, C., Kausel, H.W., et al. (1976) J. Thorac. Card. Surg. 72:333.
12. Symoens, J. (1976) In: Control of Neoplasia by Modulation of the Immune System, M.A. Chirigos (ed.), Raven Press, New York.
13. Tripodi, D., Parks, L.C., and Brugmans (1973) N. Eng. J. Med. 289:354.
14. Study Group for Bronchogenic Carcinoma (1975) Br. Med. J. 3:461.
15. Amery, W.K., Proceedings, "Immunotherapy of Cancer: Present Status of Trials in Man" (NIH, Bethesda, Md., October 27-29, 1976).
16. Clinical staging system for carcinoma of the lung (1974) CA 24:87.
17. Mountain, C.F., Carr, D.T., and Anderson, W.A.D. (1974) Amer. J. Roentgenol., Radium Ther. Nucl. Med. 120:130.
18. Amery, W. (1975) Lancet 1:574.
19. Clara, R., and Germanes, J. (1977) Lancet 1:47.
20. Bartlett, G.L., Zbar, B., and Rapp, H.J. (1972) J. Nat. Cancer Inst. 48:245.

Adjuvant Therapy of Cancer, S.E. Salmon and S.E. Jones eds.

ATTEMPT AT IMMUNOTHERAPY WITH BCG OF PATIENTS WITH BRONCHUS CARCINOMA : PRELIMINARY RESULTS

P. POUILLART, T. PALANGIE, P. HUGUENIN, P. MORIN, H. GAUTIER, A. LEDEDENTE, A. BARON and G. MATHE

Institut de Cancérologie et d'Immunogénétique (INSERM), Hopital Paul-Brousse, 94800-Villejuif and Centre Medico-Chirurgical,Bligny, 91640,Briis-sous-Forges, France.

INTRODUCTION

Squamous cell carcinoma of the lung ranks as one of the most lethal of all malignancies. Bronchogenic carcinoma is poorly sensitive to chemotherapy (1, 3, 3) and radiotherapy seems unable to significantly increase the median life span of these patients (4, 5) and cure is anticipated only when complete surgical resection is possible. Under actual therapeutic conditions not more than 10 % of patients with squamous cell carcinoma of the lung can be cured (6). In some trials radiotherapy as an adjuvant to surgery appears to be as ineffective as chemotherapy (6, 7, 8).

The aim of the present work was to study the clinical role on survival of immunotherapy with BCG applied after surgical resection of squamous cell carcinoma of the lung.

PATIENTS AND METHODS

The trial, began in june 1973, included 43 patients operated on for squamous cell carcinoma of the bronchus. Twenty-two patients were selected at random for the group to be submitted to BCG application, and 21 patients received no further treatment after surgery. The distribution according to age and sex is shown in table 1 and figure 1.

TREATMENT

All these patients had undergone surgery at the time of randomization into the two groups for treatment. The distribution of the patients according the anatomical staging is presented in the table 2.

TABLE 1

SQUAMOUS CELL CARCINOMA OF THE BRONCHUS
PRESENTATION OF THE PATIENTS

SURGERY + BCG	SURGERY ALONE
22[x]	21

x- Only one woman entered this trial and was randomly allocated to BCG group.

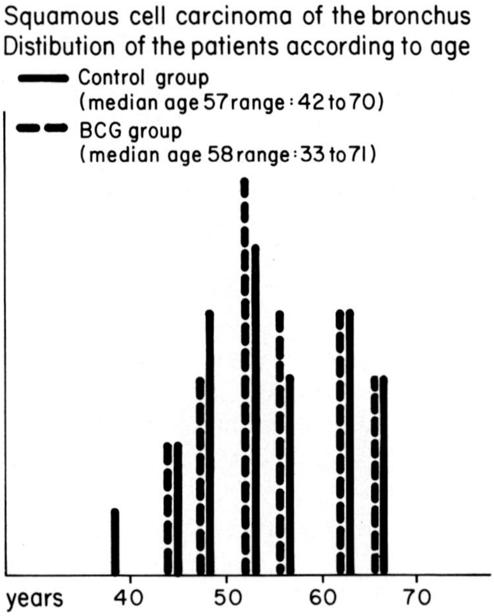

FIG. 1. : Squamous cellecarcinoma of the bronchus.
Distribution of the patients according to age

•—• Control group
•---• BCG group

TABLE 2

SQUAMOUS CELL CARCINOMA OF THE BRONCHUS
DISTRIBUTION OF THE PATIENTS
ACCORDING TO INITIAL STAGING

BCG GROUP		CONTROL GROUP	
Stage I	Stage II	Stage I	Stage II
10	12	10	11

The 22 patients submitted to immunotherapy received weekly applications of Pasteur Institute BCG on a scarification 1 m long made on the proximal extremity of each of the four limbs. The dose of live BCG applied was 75 mg, once a week (living Bacilli).

SURVEILLANCE OF THE PATIENTS

The conditions of the patients was followed in three ways : clinically, radiologically and immunologically.

The clinical examination of the patients was systematically repeated monthly : survey of the peripheral lymph node areas, of the liver, of the weight curve, of the neurological state was carried out.

Routine monthly radiological examinations of the lungs were associated with radiological survey of the skeleton ; every 3 months gamma-encephalography, examinations were made, or at the time of the appearance of neurological troubles. Finally the average survival time of both groups of patients were studied and presented actuarially. During evolution the cutaneous delayed hypersensitivity (DHS) to secondary antigens, the LIF activity of the sera and the mean lymphocyte count were checked every two months.

RESULTS

The application of BCG was well tolerated. Some patients manifested fever for 12 hours after applications of BCG. No other complications were observed in this group of patients.

Five patients out of 18 in the BCG group showed negative cutaneous DHS reactions at the time of their entry into this trial = 3 months after the beginning of BCG applications the skin tests for DHS became positive. Nine out of 21 non-treated patients initially had negative DHS reactions ; in three of them a spontaneous reversion to positive was noted in the three months following their entry into the trial (table 3).

TABLE 3

SQUAMOUS CELL CARCINOMA OF THE BRONCHUS
IMMUNOLOGICAL STATUS OF PATIENTS AT
TIME THEY ENTERED THE TRIAL

BCG GROUP		CONTROL GROUP	
I.S.	I.S.	I.S.	I.S.
(+)	(-)	(+)	(-)
13x	5xx	8xxx	9xxxx

x 2 patients died respectively at the 19th and 20th months
xx 1 patient died at the 11th month
xxx 1 patient died at the 15th month
xxxx 5 patients died respectively at the 4th, 5th, 6th, 13th and 22th months and 1 patient is in relapse at the 15th month

In the group treated with BCG, five patients (22, 7 %) died, respectively, at the 5th, 9th, 10th, 13th, 20th month and three others relapsed at the 11th, 13th, 15th months, but are still alive. In the non-treated group, 11 patients died respectively at the 4th, 6th, 7th, 8th, 11th, 12th, 13th, 18th, 20th, 23th, 35th months and two other patients relapsed at the 13th, 15th months (table 4).

TABLE 4

SQUAMOUS CELL CARCINOMA OF THE BRONCHUS
IMMUNOTHERAPY TRIAL - OVERALL RESULTS

	BCG GROUP	CONTROL GROUP
Nb of patients	22	21
Nb of dead patients	5 (5th,9th,10th,13th, 20th months)	11 (4th,6th,7th,8th,11th, 12th,13th,18th,20th, 35th months)
Nb of patients in relapse	3 (11th, 13th, 15th months)	2 (13th, 15th months)

The distribution of the patients according to anatomical stage showed that, in the BCG group, 10 patients were considered as stage I and 12 as stage II. In the control group, 10 patients were considered as stage I, and 11 patients as stage II.
The results presented in table 5 indicate that, in the BCG group, out of five dead patients, four of them were stage II, i.e, the histological study of the part operated on showed a mediastinal ganglionic extension.

TABLE 5

SQUAMOUS CELL CARCINOMA OF THE BRONCHUS
EVOLUTION ACCORDING TO INITIAL STAGING

	BCG GROUP		CONTROL GROUP	
	STAGE I	STAGE II	STAGE I	STAGE II
Alive free of disease	8	6	5	3
Alive in relapse	1	2	1	1
Dead	1	4	4	7

In the group left without treatment, four patients in stage I of the disease died and one is now in relapse ; seven patients in stage II died and another is now in relapse.

Comparison of the actuarial curves of survival revealed a difference at the 18th month in favour of the group submitted to immunotherapy (Fig. 2). Using the modified Wilcoxon test, the differences are significant at 7 %.

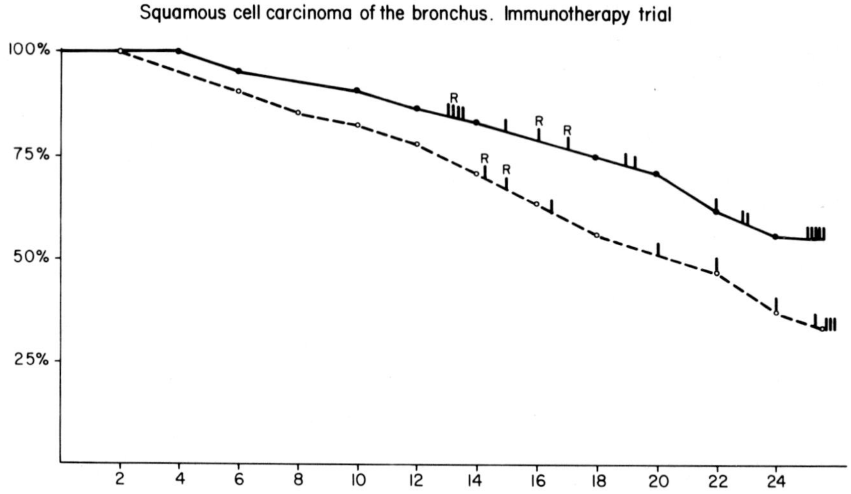

FIG. 2. : Squamous cell carcinoma of the bronchus. Immunotherapy trial

I alive patient

R I patient in relapse

In the immunotherapy group the chance of surviving for two years is over 60 % and is only 38 % in the non-treated group (Fig. 2, 3). Although the sample is small, the chance of surviving for two years, for patients at this stage of the disease, and who have been submitted to treatment with BCG, is of the order of 90 % against 58 % for the identical group of non-treated patients (Fig. 4).

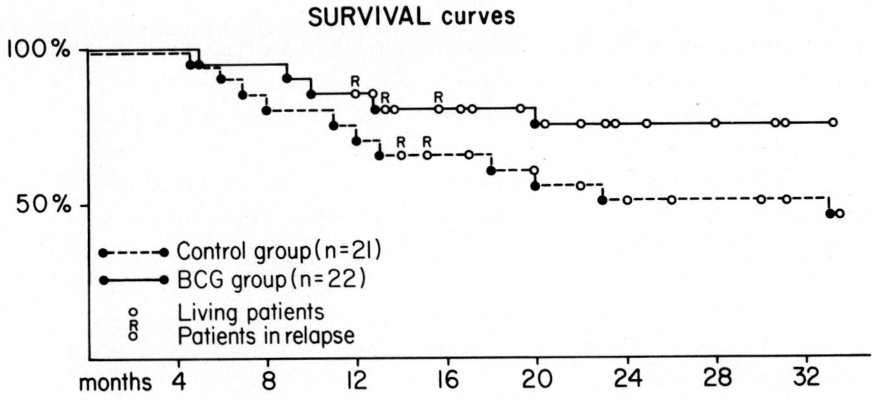

FIG. 3. : Survival curves. Present situation of patients in the two randomised groups of treatment

BCG group
Control group

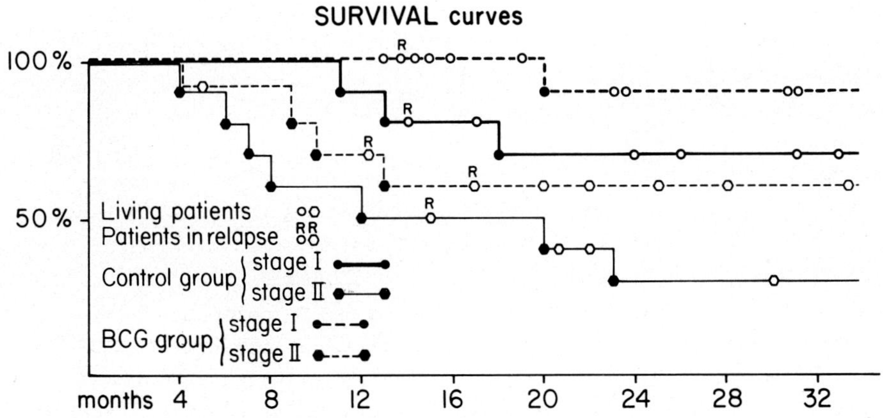

FIG. 4. : Present situation of patients. Distribution according to initial stage

Control group
BCG group

DISCUSSION

Radical surgery remains the only effective means of treatment for patients with squamous cell carcinoma of the bronchus. However, the small percentage of patients apparently cured five years after satisfactory surgery encourages one to investigate complementary therapeutic means liable to improve results already obtained. In this trial we have studied, in two randomised group of patients, the role of BCG applied systematically and regularly after surgery. The chance for surviving for two years is significantly higher for the treated patients than for the non-treated ones and the difference is much more apparent if one considers only the patients in stage I of their illness. The sample is too small for this difference to have anything but an indicative value, but the results we obtained confirm, once again, the great efficacy of BCG in cases where the tumour mass has been reduced as much as possible (9). In clinical conditions the efficacy of immunotherapy after application of cyto-reducing treatment has already been shown (10, 11). On the other hand, correlation between prognosis and the state of delayed hypersensitivity reactions of the primary type (12, 13) or of the secondary type in patients with resectable bronchus carcinoma (14), has been shown in patients initially treated by surgery or secondarily treated by chemotherapy (15). With regular administration of mycobacterium smegmatis, J. Decroix (16) obtained a significant increase of survival at three years, for patients with operated bronchus cancers over the recorded historical groups of non-treated patients. The results we obtained are at the limit of statistical significance. This study indicates some differences in behaviour of patients with (-) DHS reactions, since in the two groups, in spite of a reversion of reactivity to secondary antigens either spontaneously or under BCG, the prognostic significance remains disappointing in mid-term. The patients in stage II of the disease do not seem to benefit notably from immunotherapy in the first two years. It seems possible that BCG increases, at two years, the hope of survival of patients operated on for squamous cell carcinoma of the bronchus, but if we compare the slopes of the cumulative incidence of patients dead and relapsed in each of these groups, it appears that the curves of survival will not be different at the 3rd year of evolution (Fig. 5).

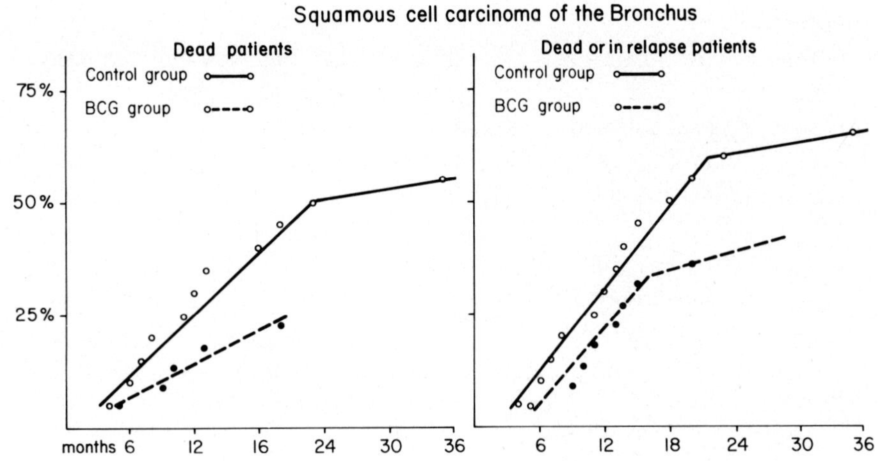

FIG. 5. : Cumulative incidence of death ; the comparison of the slope of the two curves demonstrates a significant improvment in the BCG group. Cumulative incidence of death and relapse ; there is no difference of the slope of the two curves. It seems that BCG is able to delay the time of relapse for more than 10 months.

This study is continuing along the same lines and it seems, as far as mid-term survival is concerned, that immunotherapy will be rapidly made part of the prescribed routine for the treatment of patients suffering from epidermal bronchus cancers.

CONCLUSION

Forty-three patients with resectable squamous cell carcinoma of the bronchus were randomised after surgery into two groups for treatment : 22 patients (group I) received weekly applications of BCG, 21 patients (group II) were considered as the control group and received no further treatment.

The comparison of the survival curves we obtained showed that the immunotherapy group presented an increased hope of survival time at two years. Four patients out of 22 of the BCG group have died and three are now in relapse, but alive ; eight patients out of 21 of the control group have died and two are now in relapse. The overall results indicate a better effect of BCG initially in stage I patients than stage II patients.

REFERENCES

1. EDMONSON J.H., LAGAKOS S.W., SELAWRY O.S., PERLIA C.P.,BENNETT J.M., MUGGIA F.M., WAMPLER G., BRODOVSKY H.S., HORTON J.H., COLSKY J, MANSOUR E.G., CREECH R., STOLBACH L., GREENSPAN E.M., LEVITT M., ISRAEL L., EZDINLI E.Z., CARBONE P.P. : Cancer Treatment Rep., 1976, 60, 925.

2. LIVINGSTON R.B., FEE W.H., EINHORN L.H., BURGESS M.A., FREIREICH E.J., GOTTLIEB J.A., FARBER M.O.: Cancer, 1976, 37, 1237.

3. VINCENT R.G., PICKREN J.W., FERGEN T.B., TAKITA H. : Cancer, 1975, 36, 873.

4. ROSWIT B., PATNO M.E., RAPP R., VEINBERG A., FEDER B., SUHLBARG J., REID C.B. : Radiology, 1968, 90, 688.

5. HANSEN H.H., MUGGIA F.M., ANDREWS R., SELAWRY O.S. : Cancer, 1972, 30, 315.

6. A collaborative study : Cancer, 1975, 36, 914.

7. STOTT H. : Brit. J. Cancer, 1976, 34, 167.

8. BRUNNER K.W., MARTHALER T.H., MULLER W. : Europ.J.Cancer, 1973, 7, 285.

9. MATHE G., POUILLART P., LAPEYRAQUE F.: Brit.J. Cancer, 1969, 23, 814.

10. MATHE G., AMIEL J.L., SCHWARZENBERG L., CATTAN A.,SCHLUMBERGER J.R., HAYAT M., DE VASSAL F.: Lancet, 1969, I, 697.

11. MATHE G., POUILLART P., SCHWARZENBERG L., AMIEL J.L., SCHNEIDER M., HAYAT M., DE VASSAL F., JASMIN C., ROSENFELD C., WEINER R., RAPPAPORT H.,: J.Nat.Cancer Inst., 1972, 35, 371.

12. EILBER F.R., MORTON D.L. : Cancer, 1970, 25, 362.

13. MORTON D.L., EILBER F.R., MARNGREN R.A., WOOD W. : Surgery, 1970, 68, 158.

14. ISRAEL L., MUGICA J., CHAMINIAN P. : Biomedicine,1973,19,68.

15. POUILLART P., BOTTO G., GAUTHIER H., HUGUENIN P., BARON A., LAPARRE C., HOANG THY HUONG T., PARROT R., MATHE G. : Nouv. Presse Med., 1976, 5, 1037.

16. DECROIX J. : Personal communication

Adjuvant Therapy of Cancer, S.E. Salmon and S.E. Jones eds.

TREATMENT OF OAT CELL CARCINOMA OF THE LUNG STANFORD EXPERIENCE 1972-1976

C.J. Williams[*†], M. Alexander[*], E. Glatstein[**], J.R. Daniels[*]
Stanford University School of Medicine
Stanford, California 94305[††]

SUMMARY

Trials conducted at Stanford during the past 4 years have explored combined modality therapy of oat cell carcinoma. Initial comparisons (Oat 2/3) suggested the marginal superiority of a 4-drug combination (POCC) over a 3-drug combination (COM) but called into question the efficacy of involved field radiation therapy and spotlighted the high incidence of brain extension. A subsequent study (Oat 4/5) did demonstrate effective prevention of brain extension by prophylactic whole brain irradiation. However, involved field irradiation (3000 rads in 2 weeks) failed to prevent local relapse or to improve survival in the setting of concurrent vigorous combination chemotherapy.

INTRODUCTION

Oat cell carcinoma of the lung, despite its grim reputation, is the one area in lung cancer where most gains in survival and possibly cure are likely to occur. Despite the short survival[1,2], oat cell carcinoma is the most responsive type of lung cancer to both radiation therapy[3] and chemotherapy[4].

The previous dismal results with surgery[2] are a reflection of the high incidence of disseminated disease at diagnosis[5,6,7,8]. Though radiation therapy proved to be marginally better than surgery, it is also a local therapy; relapse with metastatic disease was common and survival was little changed[9]. The recognition of the extent of dissemination at diagnosis led to the use of systemic therapy. Initially single agents[10] improved survival and then combination chemotherapy was shown to be superior to single agents[11]. Combined modality therapy then evolved using both combination chemotherapy and radiation therapy[12,13].

MATERIALS AND METHODS

Oat 1: A phase II study (Oat 1) of a 4-drug combination of procarbazine, vincristine, cyclophosphamide and CCNU (POCC, Table 1) was begun at Stanford in late 1972.

---

* Division of Oncology
** Division of Radiation Therapy
† Fellow supported by Cancer Research Campaign, London, England
†† Study supported by Cancer Center Support Grant (specialized) CA 05838-15

TABLE 1

CHEMOTHERAPY SCHEDULES

POCC - cycle repeated every 28-35 days		COM - cycle repeated every 21 days	
Procarbazine	100mg/m^2 p.o. d 2-15	Cyclophosphamide	2 gm/m^2 I.V. d 1
Vincristine	2.0mg I.V. d 1 & 8	Vincristine	2.0mg I.V. d 1
Cyclophosphamide	600mg/m^2 I.V. d 1 & 8	Methotrexate	30mg/m^2 I.V. d 15
CCNU	60mg/m^2 p.o. d 1		

Oat 2/3: In 1973, Eagan et al[14] reported encouraging results with COM (Table 1) and a randomized comparison between POCC and COM was begun at Stanford in 1973 (Oat 2/3). Twenty-three previously untreated patients with a proven diagnosis of oat cell cancer of the lung entered the study. Initial staging included chest x-ray, bone survey and scan, bone marrow biopsy, liver scan, brain scan or brain computerized-axial tomogram (CAT), serum chemistries and full blood count and platelets. Staging was based on the International Union Against Cancer (IUCC) system as modified by the Radiation Therapy Oncology Group (RTOG)[15]. Twelve patients were randomized to receive POCC and eleven to receive COM. All patients received involved field radiation (IF-XRT) (Table 2) after 2 to 3 cycles of chemotherapy.

TABLE 2

INVOLVED FIELD RADIATION IN OAT 2/3 AND 4/5

Stage	Field and Techniques	Dosimetry
I and II	Primary tumor, hilar, mediastinal and supraclavicular port, first 3000 rads by A-P opposed technique, remainder by A-P oblique technique	5000-5500 rads over 5 weeks in 20-25 fractions
III and IV	Thorax--primary tumor, hilar, mediastinal and supraclavicular port, A-P opposed technique	3000 rads over 2 weeks in 10 fractions
	Liver--A-P opposed technique	2500 rads over 3 weeks in 15 fractions
	Pleura--Hemithorax	1500-2500 rads over 2-3 weeks in 10-15 fractions

Following radiation therapy chemotherapy was planned until tumor progression or until two years' disease free survival from the initiation of treatment.

Responses were scored as complete (CR - disappearance of all known disease); partial (PR - $\geq$50% regression of all measurable lesions and no new lesions). All lesser responses were called no response (NR). One month's duration of response was required for CR or PR.

RESULTS

Patient characteristics at entry were similar for POCC and COM (Table 3).

TABLE 3

PATIENT CHARACTERISTICS: OAT 2/3 AND OAT 4/5

	OAT 2/3		OAT 4/5	
	POCC + IF-XRT	COM + IF-XRT	POCC + WB	POCC + IF-XRT + WB
N	12	11	12	13
Mean age (yrs.)	58.5 (46-74)	59.6 (52-67)	54.8 (31-65)	56.2 (46-68)
Sex	9 ♂: 3 ♀	8 ♂: 3 ♀	♂ 5: ♀ 7	♂ 9: ♀ 4
Stage				
I and II	1	1	0	0
III and IV	11	10	12	13
Karnofsky status (mean)	70 (30-100)	66.3 (30-100)	65.8 (20-100)	69.1 (30-90)

The median survival of all patients was 11 months. For those receiving POCC it was 14 months compared with 10 months for those receiving COM (P = 0.055). The actuarial survival curves are shown in Figure 1.

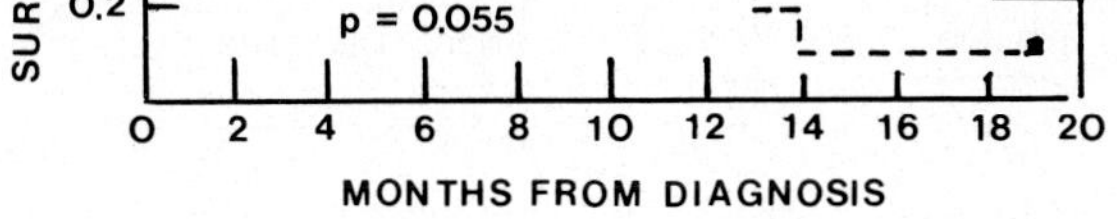

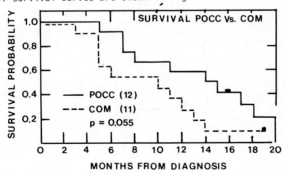

Fig. 1. Actuarial survival: POCC vs. COM

The response rates for POCC and COM (Table 4) were equivalent with 15 of 22 evaluable patients having an objective response. One patient had no followable disease after thoracotomy and was not evaluable. The proportion of patients with an objective response was not improved by IF-XRT compared to the initial chemotherapy responses (70% vs. 68% respectively). However, 8 of 20 evaluable patients had further local disease regression after radiotherapy, while 3 progressed. Of the patients who progressed during IF-XRT, one did so in bone, one progressed in the chest while receiving liver and whole brain irradiation and the other progressed in the chest immediately after thoracic radiation. Three patients received hepatic irradiation and none had a clinical relapse, though hepatic disease was present at the one autopsy performed on these patients.

TABLE 4

RESPONSES TO CHEMOTHERAPY: OAT 2/3

Chemotherapy	CR	PR	NR	Not evaluable
POCC (12)	3	5	4	0
COM (11)	2	5	3	1

Initial sites of relapse: The initial site of relapse was not evaluable in 8 patients due to lack of initial response or specific site of relapse. Eight of 15 relapses (Table 5) occurred in the thorax, 5 in patients who had received thoracic radiation. Of these, 2 had received 5000 rads; 2, 4000 rads and 1, 3000 rads. Of the 3 who did not receive thoracic radiation, 2 initially responded to COM but relapsed before radiation and the third relapsed in the thorax while receiving liver and CNS radiation.

TABLE 5

INITIAL SITE OF RELAPSE: OAT 2/3 AND OAT 4/5

	OAT 2/3*		OAT 4/5*	
Site	POCC + IF-XRT	COM + IF-XRT	POCC + WB	POCC + IF-XRT + WB
Chest	2	6	7	8
Bone	3	1	3	3
CNS	2	1	0	0
Liver	0	1	0	1

* Several patients relapsed simultaneously in more than one site.

Three patients had an initial CNS relapse and three others had CNS extension following relapse at another site. The CNS failures were equally divided between POCC and COM groups.

Toxicity: Leukopenia was common in both regimes but thrombocytopenia was more prominent in the POCC patients and was the primary cause of dose modification. There were two episodes of bacteremia, both in the COM arm; one was associated with shock. There were no drug related deaths. The conclusions for the study were: a) Combination chemotherapy produced a markedly increased survival but no cures. b) POCC and COM were not markedly different in remission rates or survival but POCC was probably superior. c) Thoracic relapses continued despite IF-XRT to the chest; this includes 2 patients with localized disease receiving

5000 rads. d) Brain extension was a frequent complication (6/19 patients).

Having observed 6 CNS relapses in the first 19 patients the last 4 patients in this study received prophylactic whole brain irradiation (WB), 3000 rads mid plane dose being given by an opposed lateral field technique over 14 days in 10 fractions.

Oat 4/5: The subsequent randomization (Oat 4/5) was designed to test the role of IF-XRT and prophylactic WB irradiation. Patient selection and staging was as in Oat 2/3. Only patients with advanced disease (Stage III and IV) were entered into this study; all patients received 2-3 cycles of POCC and half were then randomized to receive IF-XRT (as delivered to the advanced patients in Oat 2/3). All patients received prophylactic whole brain irradiation at this time. POCC chemotherapy was resumed following radiotherapy as in Oat 2/3.

Twenty-seven patients were admitted to this study (14 POCC + IF-XRT + WB and 13 POCC + WB). One patient in each group was not evaluable for improper omission or use of IF-XRT and was excluded from analysis. Patient characteristics were similar (Table 3) apart from a predominance of women in the POCC + WB group.

Survival: The median survival of the entire group was 10 months. For the POCC + WB group it was 11 months compared with 9 months for the POCC + IF-XRT + WB group. Actuarial survival curves are shown in Figure 2.

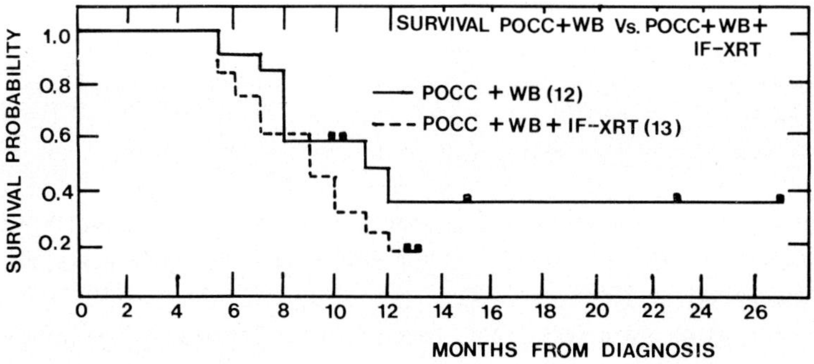

Fig. 2. Actuarial survival: Oat 4/5

Responses: Prior to IF-XRT there were 5 CR, 4 PR and 4 NR in the POCC + IF-XRT + WB group. In the POCC + WB arm there were 2 CR, 7 PR and 3 NR after 3 cycles of chemotherapy. As in Oat 2/3 no patients improved their overall remission status following IF-XRT though local regression continued. In the POCC + WB arm 3 PR's became CR and 2 NR's became PR with continued POCC.

The initial sites of relapse were similar in both arms (Table 5) and it was evident that IF-XRT, as given in this study, did not prevent relapse in an irradiated site. In addition, 2 patients with no objective response progressed during IF-XRT. One patient in the POCC + WB group received 5000 rads emergency mediastinal radiation for superior vena cava syndrome and is the only long term survivor off chemotherapy (27+ months, 13 months off chemotherapy).

Hematologic suppression following IF-XRT resulted in delay of reinstitution of the chemotherapy. The mean time interval between the end of the cycle prior to IF-XRT and the start of the cycle after IF-XRT was 66 days (28-92 days) compared with 30 days (18-70 days) between equivalent cycles in the POCC + WB group.

Dose reductions were similar in both arms (Table 4) and the incidence of leukopenia and thrombocytopenia was similar to that in Oat 2/3. There was 1 toxic death in the entire study and 1 hospitalization for infection in each group.

TABLE 6

DOSE REDUCTIONS: OAT 4/5

Drug		% of calculated dose given POCC + WB	% of calculated dose given POCC + IF-XRT + WB
Procarbazine	Prior to XRT*	64%	65%
	Post XRT**	41%	55%
Vincristine	Prior to XRT	72%	77%
	Post XRT	56%	41%
CCNU	Prior to XRT	85%	92%
	Post XRT	60%	80%
Cytoxan	Prior to XRT	72%	73%
	Post XRT	45%	61%

* Prior to XRT POCC cycles 1-3

** Post XRT POCC cycles 4-9

Eight of 13 patients in the IF-XRT arm had progression of disease within the first 2 cycles of POCC after IF-XRT. In the POCC + WB arm 4 of 12 relapsed during an equivalent period.

Prophylactic whole brain radiation: None of the 27 patients who received CNS prophylaxis in this study had a CNS extension. However, the median survival (11.4 months) of these patients and the 4 patients in Oat 2/3 who received prophylactic WB radiation was not increased when compared with the historical control of the 19 patients (mean survival 10.5 months) who did not receive CNS prophylaxis.

CONCLUSIONS

The use of involved field irradiation of 3000 rads in 2 weeks in the setting of combination chemotherapy failed to demonstrate an improved survival and did not alter the pattern of relapse. The IF-XRT dose used in this study has been employed in many previous trials. Although it is efficient at producing prompt regression of oat cell cancer, it now seems unlikely that it is capable of sterilizing residual tumor even in the face of an apparently satisfactory chemotherapy response. The high incidence of local relapse undoubtedly reflects improved control of disseminated microscopic disease with combination chemotherapy. Previously the death of these patients occurred so quickly that local recurrence rates were underestimated. It remains for further trials to study the efficacy of IF-XRT when given at higher doses and to patients receiving more effective chemotherapy. It may be significant that many of the patients in the IF-XRT group relapsed soon after their irradiation. Due to the time required for administration of IF-XRT and recovery of the bone marrow, there was a substantial period (mean 66 days) when no chemotherapy was given.

Oat cell carcinoma frequently extends to the brain[13,16]. In 31 consecutive patients who received CNS prophylaxis there were no cases of CNS extension. This contrasts strongly with 6 CNS relapses in the first 19 patients of Oat 2/3 who did not receive CNS prophylaxis. Survival was not affected, presumably because current chemotherapy cannot provide long term control of the systemic disease.

New trials in the management of oat cell cancer of the lung must focus on providing more effective chemotherapy. Radiation to involved sites of disease may be further explored with higher doses of radiotherapy, but the optimal timing for such treatment is unclear. The demonstration of effective CNS prophylaxis suggests that the amount of residual tumor may be critical. We feel that the morbidity associated with CNS extension justifies prophylaxis despite our inability to demonstrate improved survival using current chemotherapy programs.

REFERENCES

1. Hyde, L., et al (1969) Natural course of inoperable lung cancer. Chest 64:309-312.
2. Mountain, C.F., et al (1974) A system for the clinical staging of lung cancer. Am. J. Roent. Ther. Nuc. Med. 120:130-138.
3. Carr, D.J., et al (1972) Radiotherapy plus 5 FU compared with radiotherapy alone for inoperable and unresectable bronchogenic carcinoma. Cancer 29:375-380.
4. Selawry, O.S. (1974) The role of chemotherapy in the treatment of lung cancer. Sem. in Onc. 1:259-272.
5. Muggia, F.M. and Lakshman, R.C. (1974) Lung cancer: diagnosis in metastatic sites. Sem. in Onc. 1:217-228.
6. Hansen, H.H. and Muggia, F.M. (1971) Early detection of bone marrow invasion in oat cell carcinoma of the lung. New Engl. J. Med. 284:962-963.
7. Sarin, C.L. and Nohl-Oser, H.C. (1969) Mediastinoscopy: a clinical evaluation of 400 consecutive cases. Thorax 24:585-588.

8. Hansen, H.H. and Muggia, F.M. (1972) Staging of inoperable patients with bronchogenic carcinoma with special reference to bone marrow examination and peritonoscopy. Cancer 30:1395-1401.
9. Fox, W. and Scadding, J.G. (1973) Medical Research Council comparative trial of surgery and radiotherapy for primary treatment of small-celled or oat celled carcinoma of the bronchus. Lancet 11:63-65.
10. Bergsagel, D.E., et al (1972) Lung cancer: clinical trial of radiotherapy vs. radiotherapy plus cyclophosphamide. Cancer 30:621-627.
11. Maurer, L.M. and Tulloch, M. (1974) Combination chemotherapy vs. single agent chemotherapy in treatment of small cell carcinoma of the lung. Proc. AACR 15:125.
12. Maurer, L.M., et al (1973) Combination chemotherapy and radiation therapy for small cell carcinoma of the lung. Cancer Chemother. Rep. 4:171-176.
13. Holoye, P.Y. and Samuels, M.L. (1975) Cyclophosphamide, vincristine and sequential split-course radiotherapy in the treatment of small cell lung cancer. Chest 67:675-678.
14. Eagan, R.T., et al (1973) Combination chemotherapy and radiation therapy in small cell carcinoma of the lung. Cancer 32:371-378.
15. Rubin, P. (1973) Panel report--radiotherapy for lung cancer. Cancer Chemother. Rep. 4:311-315.
16. Skarin, A., et al (1975) Combined intensive chemotherapy and radiotherapy in oat cell carcinoma of the lung. Proc. ASCO 16:264.

Adjuvant Therapy of Cancer, S.E. Salmon and S.E. Jones eds.
© 1977 Elsevier/North-Holland Biomedical Press, Amsterdam

TREATMENT OF SMALL CELL CARCINOMA OF THE LUNG WITH CYCLOPHOSPHAMIDE, ADRIAMYCIN, AND VP16-213 WITH OR WITHOUT MER

Joseph Aisner, M.D.
Peter H. Wiernik, M.D.
and Robert J. Esterhay, Jr., M.D.
Clinical Oncology Branch, National Cancer Institute,
Baltimore Cancer Research Center
22 S. Greene Street
Baltimore, MD 21201, U.S.A.

INTRODUCTION

Small cell carcinoma of the lung is a rapidly fatal disease, with a mean duration of survival of <8 weeks in untreated patients[1]. Surgery is not beneficial for survival or palliation and most surgeons consider surgery with curative intent not indicated for this disease[2]. Radiation therapy produces responses but the median duration of survival is rarely >5 months and nearly all patients die of metastases, suggesting that this is a disseminated disease at presentation[3]. The combination of radiotherapy with chemotherapy has improved the short term survival[4]. Many physicians, however, feel that initial therapy should include combination chemotherapy to control the foci of disseminated disease[5,6].

Cyclophosphamide and adriamycin are both active single agents in the therapy of small cell carcinoma[7], and the combination of these agents is synergistic in animals[8]. VP16-213 has also been reported to be a highly active single agent[9]. MER, the methanol extracted residue of BCG, is a broad and non-specific immune modulator and is capable of increasing immunologic defense against a wide variety of tumors in animals[10]. Since many investigators have advocated initiating treatment with chemotherapy[5,6], we undertook to study the use of only intensive combination chemotherapy using cyclophosphamide, adriamycin, and VP16-213. In addition, we undertook to evaluate the role of MER as adjuvant immunotherapy.

MATERIALS AND METHODS

All patients with documented small cell carcinoma of the lung who had not received prior chemotherapy were eligible for this study and 31 have been started on treatment since August, 1975. All patients, who received one full course of therapy were considered evaluable and one patient who received less therapy was excluded from analysis for early death. Patients were stratified according to whether they had received prior radiation therapy (6 patients) or no prior therapy (24 patients). Pretreatment evaluation included: history and physical examination, chest roentgenograms, skeletal survey, SGOT, SGPT, alkaline phosphatase, total bilirubin, white blood cell count and differential, platelet count, serum Ca^{++}, serum electrolytes, serum creatinine, BSP retention, bone, brain and liver scans, and bilateral iliac crest aspirations and biopsies. Patients were staged as limited disease, which was defined as disease confined to one hemithorax ± mediastinal involvement, or extensive disease. According to these criteria 9 patients (30%) had limited disease, and 21 (70%) had extensive disease (Table 1). Prior to initiating therapy, patients were randomized to receive or not receive MER.

Table 1

Sites of Extrapulmonary Disease in 21 Patients

Bone	13
Liver	6
Marrow	5
Skin and Soft Tissue	4
Pleura	3
Brain	2
GI	1

Chemotherapy schedule: All medications were administered intravenously on a 21 day cycle: cyclophosphamide 1000 mg/m^2 given on day 1, adriamycin 45 mg/m^2 given on day 1 and VP16-213, 50 mg/m^2 given on days 1-5. Initial adriamycin doses were modified according to the results of liver function tests and BSP retention. Doses of chemotherapy for subsequent courses were modified according to hematologic nadir counts. Adriamycin was continued to a maximal cumulative dose of 540 mg/m^2 or its equivalent based on cumulative totals of the modified dosages (e.g. a modified dose of 50% would give a maximal cumulative dose of 270 mg/m^2). Methotrexate 40 mg/m^2 IV day 1 was then substituted for adriamycin, and subsequent dosage modifications were made for hematologic nadir counts. MER, 1 mg divided into 5 sites on the trunk, was given intradermally on days 1 and 11. Dosage modification with serial 10 fold dilutions to the lowest reacting concentration were used once local reactions became intolerable. Central nervous system irradiation was given only when patients developed evidence of intracranial metastases.

Table 2

STRATIFICATION ACCORDING TO PRIOR RADIOTHERAPY

	No Prior RT	Prior RT
CR	11	0
PR	10	0
OR	1	2
NMD	2	1
NR	0	3
TOTALS	24	6

Complete response (CR) was defined as the complete resolution of all signs and symptoms, disappearance of all measurable disease, and the normalization of biological markers, if present, lasting a minimum of 30 days. Partial response (PR) represented a decrease of 50% or greater in the product of the greatest perpendicular dimensions of all measurable lesions lasting a minimum of 30 days. Objective response (OR) represented a measurable decrease in tumor dimensions but < PR. Three patients had non-measurable disease (NMD), and were followed for survival. Survival data was calculated from the day of diagnosis.

RESULTS

Overall there were 11 CR (37%), 10 PR (33%), 3 OR (10%) and the 3 patients with NMD (10%) are surviving at 512+ days (d), 437 + d, and 329 + d respectively. Three patients (10%) failed to respond. Twenty-seven of the 30 evaluable patients had measurable disease. Stratification according to prior therapy (Table 2) revealed that all patients without prior radiotherapy had at least an OR and 21 of 22 (95%) such patients with measurable disease had either CR (11-50%) or PR (10-45%). There were equal responses among those treated with or without MER (CR 6 and 5, respectively, PR 5 and 5, respectively). The median duration of response for all responders was 112+ d (range 4-450 + d) and the median duration of survival for all patients was 189 + d (range 19-512 + d). The median survival of 6 patients with prior radiotherapy was 135 d (range 19-437+ d). The median response duration for patients without prior therapy was 138+ d (range 30+ - 450+ d), and the median duration of survival for these patients was 189 + d (range 59 - 512+). The median durations

Table 3

Response and Survival Duration

Response	Response* Duration (days)	Survival Duration (days)	Day of Relapse
CR (11)	168+ (30+ - 450+)	201+ (65+ - 504+)	92, 153, 350++
PR (10)	76+ (30+ - 261)	115+ (60+ - 374)	35**, 83**, 197++, 261

*Median (range)

**2 patients died while responding (cardiac deaths)

++ relapsed in site of primary

of response and survival of patients with CR or PR are given in Table 3, and the median response and survival data for patients with CRor PR according to the use of MER are given in Table 4. There are no appreciable differences in response rates, response durations or survival durations with the use of MER. Stratification according to the extent of disease revealed no significant differences in response rates (Table 5). The median response duration for patients with limited disease was 98+ d (range 30+ - 168+ d) and median survival was 152+ d (range 60+ - 512+ d). Median response duration for patients with extensive disease was 150+ d (range 4-450+ d) and the median survival was 207+ d (range 19 - 504+ d). There was also no difference in response rate, response duration, or survival if these groups were analyzed with respect to treatment or no treatment with MER.

Table 4

Influence of MER on Response and Survival Duration

		Response* Duration (days)	Survival Duration (Days)	Day Relapse
CR	MER (6)	126+ (30+ - 450+)	154+ (65+ - 504+)	153, 350
	no MER (5)	168+ (92-372+)	207+ (195+ - 383+)	92
PR	MER (5)	83+ (35 - 261)	150+ (93+ - 374)	35, 83, 261
	no MER (5)	69+ (30+ - 197)	109+ (60+ - 289)	197

*median (range)

Table 5

INFLUENCE OF EXTENT OF DISEASE ON RESPONSE

	Limited Disease	Extensive Disease
CR	4	7
PR	3	7
OR	0	3
NMD	2	1
NR	0	3
TOTALS	9	21

Toxicity

Toxicity was moderately severe and included alopecia, nausea and vomiting, and blood count suppression. Two patients with prior radiotherapy died of bacteremia while severely myelosuppressed. Both patients were responding to therapy. In addition, 2 patients died of myocardial infarction from pre-existing arteriosclerotic cardiovascular disease. Neither patient was receiving chemotherapy at the time, and neither patient was myelosuppressed at the time of death. There were no other drug related deaths and most patients received all therapy as out-patients. Count suppression eventually required some dosage modification in every case (Table 6).

The percentage of planned drug to be administered was high. Some dose modifications were required early, but usually dose modifications for severe count suppression were not necessary until far into therapy. The use of MER made no difference in percentage of dose modification or number of patients requiring such modifications.

Table 6

Mean Percent Dose Administered Per Course

	1	2	3	4	5	6	7	8	9	10
CTX	99.8	89.7	86.5	85.4	80.2	81.0	77.4	67.0	65.2	59.2
AMN	89.2	89.5	89.3	86.5	82.9	82.1	79.6	82.0	82.4	74.6
VP16	99.8	98.2	98.4	99.4	98.2	94.8	93.9	87.4	90.0	86.7

MER toxicity included fever, chills, local pain, and less frequently, weeping ulcer formation. An allergic dermatitis necessitating discontinuation of MER occurred in one patient, and two other patients refused further MER injections after the sixth and thirteenth courses respectively. Fever secondary to MER administration was seen during periods of drug induced granulocytopenia on 7 occasions in 4 patients. This necessitated hospitalization for observation to determine if an infection were present.

DISCUSSION

Many observers feel that small cell carcinoma of the lung is a disseminated disease at the time of presentation, and therefore warrants aggressive systemic therapy[5,6]. In the present study we have combined 3 active agents (cyclophosphamide, adriamycin and VP16-213) (CAVp16) to produce an excellent response rate among all treated patients in this small series. All patients without prior treatment responded to therapy, and the CR + PR rate for patients without prior treatment and measurable disease was 95%. The response rate and survival duration were better for patients treated with this combination from the onset than for patients treated first with radiotherapy. This was true even though the latter patients were initially believed to have "localized disease" and then developed signs of extensive disease. Among patients without prior treatment, there was no difference in response rate, response duration, or survival between patients with limited or extensive disease. These data suggest that this intensive chemotherapy regimen is an effective treatment regimen for all patients, with oat cell carcinoma of the lung regardless of extent of disease.

The results of therapy with CAVp16 in previously untreated patients are superior to the results obtained by radiotherapy alone, and at least as good as other published reports using radiotherapy followed by chemotherapy, or chemotherapy alone. In the present study 6 of the 10 patients with PR are still improving and may yet achieve CR. Regardless of how the treatment groups were subdivided (i.e. CR, limited disease, etc.) MER as used in the present study did not alter the response rate, response duration, or the survival. MER also had no appreciable effect on drug toxicity. It did, however, add morbidity in the form of local pain, inflammation, and ulcer formation and in several instances confused the management of neutropenic patients. Thus, at the present time MER does not appear to have a beneficial effect in the management of this disease.

The data in this study suggest that the combination chemotherapy regimen of CAVp16 is a highly effective treatment program for all patients with small cell anaplastic carcinoma of the lung. The current data further suggest that this combination can be used for total therapy of this disease. Further studies using this combination chemotherapy regimen are warranted.

REFERENCES

1. Green, R.A., et al. (1969) Alkylating agents in bronchogenic carcinoma. Am J Med 46:516.
2. Mountain, C.R. (1974) Surgical therapy in lung cancer: Biologic, physiologic, and technical determinants. Seminars in Oncol 1:253.
3. Fox, W. and Scadding, J.G. (1973) Medical Research Council comparative trial of surgery and radiotherapy for the primary treatment of small celled or oat celled carcinoma of the bronchus. Lancet II:63.
4. Eagen, R.T., et al. (1973) Combination chemotherapy and radiotherapy in small cell carcinoma of the lung. Cancer 32:371.
5. Hansen, H.H. (1973) Should initial treatment of small cell carcinoma include systemic chemotherapy and brain irradiation? Cancer Chemother Rep III 4:239.
6. Johnson, R.E., et al. (1976) Small cell carcinoma of the lung: attempt to remedy causes of past therapeutic failure. Lancet II: 289.
7. Selawry, O.S. (1973) Monochemotherapy of bronchogenic carcinoma with special reference to cell type. Cancer Chemother Rep III 4:177.
8. Tobias, S.K., et al. (1975) Adriamycin and cyclophosphamide therapy for L1210 leukemia. Clin Res 23:344A.
9. Jungi, W.F., and Senn, H.J. (1975) Clinical study of the new podophyllotoxin derivative 4' Demethylepipodophyllotoxin 9-(4, 6-o-ethylidene-p-D-glucopyranoside) (NSC 141540-VP16-213), in solid tumors in man. Cancer Chemother Rep 59:737.
10. Weiss, D.W. (1976) MER and other mycobacterial fractions in the immunotherapy of cancer. Med Clin North Amer 60:473.

Adjuvant Therapy of Cancer, S.E. Salmon and S.E. Jones eds.

IMMUNOTHERAPY FOR ADVANCED LUNG CANCER

R. Crispen, S. Warren, B. Nika
University of Illinois, Chicago and
Lutheran General Hospital, Park Ridge, Illinois

Introduction

Therapy by immunological modification for bronchiogenic carcinoma using BCG vaccine was reported in 1969 by Hadziev[1] in Bulgaria. That report of a controlled study showed an increase survival from three to fourteen months for the treated patients as compared to the controls. McNeally[2] has recently reported that the intrapleural injection of BCG followed 14 days later with isoniazid therapy has resulted in a significant increase in the disease-free interval for patients with Stage I disease but is much less effective in patients with disease in the later stages. Pouillant and Mathe[3] reported longer survival in Stage I and II squamous cell carcinoma after systemic BCG vaccination by scarification. Pines[4] demonstrated that BCG vaccination combined with radical radiotherapy for squamous cell cancer was beneficial.

Methods and Materials

In the present study, patients with advanced lung cancer in which lymph nodes or invasion of adjacent structure were involved were entered into the protocol. The entrance into the study was designed for restricted randomization. Under this procedure blocks of 20 patients were assigned to either experimental or conventional treatment by random numbers. This method was chosen to insure that a sufficient number of patients would be available in each group for analysis at the end of two years. Life table analysis was used to allow each patient to contribute to the results according to the length of time in the study. A parallel analysis for historical controls was performed on the patients entered into the tumor registry at Lutheran General Hospital to compare whether the concurrent controls were a representative sample of the statistical population and whether there was any new factors evident in the type of patient or methods of treatment.

Survival time was used as the criterion of determining the effect of the immunotherapy, although other means of measuring differences between the two groups were recorded.

The BCG vaccine used was the TICE strain made at the University of Illinois in the high dose percutaneous concentration. Application was by the multi-puncture technique on the arms using double strength vaccine and applied at two adjacent sites. This resulted in a dose of approximately 2 x 10^8 CFU (colony forming units) spread over 72 punctures by the double application of the 36-point vaccination disc.

Fifty-five patients were entered into the study of which 32 were vaccinated and 23 were conventionally treated controls. The vaccination was performed once a week for 5 weeks, then every two weeks for 4 weeks and then finally monthly for 10 months resulting in 17 vaccinations in the first year. After completion of the first year the patients were skin tested with tuberculin at three-month intervals and revaccinated if the induration was less than 15mm or the quality of the reaction had decreased substantially.

Side effects of the therapy ranged from fever to 38.5°C for 24 hours beginning 24 hours after vaccination and occasionally mild flu-like symptoms occurring between the first and third months of therapy. No patient developed evidence of systemic disease or required hospitalization because of the vaccinations; anti-tuberculosis drugs were not required and none of the patients withdrew from the protocol because of the therapy.

Patients were initially tuberculin tested with Purified Protein Derivative (PPD) at 5TU. Readings were done at 48 hours and only induration was recorded. A measurement of 10mm was considered positive.

Sex differences were 22 males and 10 females for the vaccinated group and 17 males and 6 females in the control group. The average age of the vaccinated group was 61.4 years and 60.0 years for the controls. Statistically, there was no difference between the two groups.

Results

Histological grouping and staging of the patients are shown in Table I. The groups are comparable, and it should be noted that the patients were predominantly of Stages III and IV (19/23 control, 24/32 vaccinated).

Table I

Histological Classification and Stages

Histology	Stage 2		3		4	
	Control	BCG	Control	BCG	Control	BCG
Squamous	2	6	4	5	2	4
Adenocarcinoma	1	1	2	5	2	1
Undifferentiated	1	1	2	2	3	3
Small cell	0	0	3	3	1	1
	4	8	11	15	8	9

The major prognostic indicator is the tuberculin pre-test; the results of which are shown in Table II.

Table II

Tuberculin Pre-Test

Tuberculin (5TU)	Controls	BCG
PPD + (10mm)	40% (8/20)	25% (8/32)
PPD -	60% (12/20)	75% (24/32)

Comparison of the historical controls with concurrent controls demonstrates that the concurrent control sample was a true representation of the population of patients with bronchiogenic carcinoma in Lutheran General Hospital. There has been no major changes in the modes of treatment or changes in the characteristics of the patients entering the hospital for the period of the study as compared to the historical controls for the period from 1970 through 1975. The comparison of the BCG treated group with both of the control groups showed a consistently longer survival time.

The effect on survival by BCG vaccination is more clearly seen in Table III.

Table III

Observed Percent Survival of Patients with

Stages II, III and IV Bronchiogenic Carcinoma

Week	Concurrent Control	BCG
13	75%	84%
31	50%	51%
47	25%	44%

The data demonstrates that at the time when 75, 50 and 25% of the controls are expected to be surviving that the treated group has 84%, 51% and 44% surviving respectively. Although the number of treated and control patients surviving at the 50% point are nearly equal, this may be antifactual due to the number of patients currently being studied. The most important fact is the larger number of patients surviving longer after BCG treatment at the end of the year. This relationship is still valid at the end of 2 years (104 weeks) with 14% of the controls surviving compared to 24% of the treated patients ($p < .01$).

When the survival data is plotted as a function of time, the resulting curve fits an exponential distribution (r^2=.91) and allows an estimate to be made of the median survival time remaining after six months of therapy. For the historical controls, this estimate is 25 weeks; for concurrent controls, it is 26 weeks but for BCG-treated patients, it is 38 weeks. This is more easily compared in Table IV.

Table IV

Median Remaining Survival Time (weeks) After

Six Months of Treatment

Historical Controls	Concurrent Controls	BCG
24.7	26.2	38.2

Discussion

It has been the observation in this study as well as observed by others that a portion of the patients entered into a protocol will die early irrespective of the treatment given - both conventional and experimental. Immunotherapy is a cumulative process and sufficient time must be available for the treatment to stimulate the host's defenses for the maximum effect to be realized. These observations suggest that some patients with inadequate immune response or extensive spread of the disease do not have the time or the ability to develop an adequate response and, therefore, quickly succumb to overwhelming disease. A positive tuberculin response indicated an intact functioning cell mediated immune response. Although a negative tuberculin test could mean that the person has not been exposed to mycobacteria naturally, it is more likely in this older aged population that it is an indicator that the cell mediated immunity has been depressed by the disease.

In this study, the effect of BCG vaccination is to extend survival of the patients. The Eastern Cooperative Oncology Group (ECOG) activity rating scale (4-0) averaged 1.91 for the controls and 1.47 for the vaccinated group, and the average Karnoski score (0-100) for the control group was 66 and for the vaccinated was 74 over an observation period of 75% of the survival time of both groups of patients which indicates that the vaccinated did have a better quality of life during their longer survival. The treatments were well tolerated by the patients and acceptance of the program was high. Few patients refused to participate and those who did refused because of difficulties in returning for the scheduled vaccinations.

In summary, BCG vaccination appears to be effective adjuvant therapy for advanced bronchiogenic carcinoma.

REFERENCES

1. Hadziev, S., Kavaklieve-Dimitrova, J. (1969) Application du BCG dans le cancer chez l'homme. Folia Med Neerl II 8-14.

2. McNeally, M., Maver, C., Kausel, H. (1976) Regional immunotherapy of lung cancer with intrapleural BCG. Lancet I 377-379.

3. Pouillant, P., Mathe, G., Palangie, T., Schwarzenberg, L., Huguein, P., Marin, P., Goutier, M., Parrot, R. (1976) Trial of BCG immunotherapy in the treatment of resectable squamous cell carcinoma of the bronchus (Stage I and II). Cancer Immunology and Immunotherapy I 271-273.

4. Pines, A. (1976) A 5-year controlled study of BCG and radiotherapy for inoperable lung cancer. Lancet <u>I</u> 380-381.

Section IV

GASTROINTESTINAL CANCER

Adjuvant Therapy of Cancer, S.E. Salmon and S.E. Jones eds.

THE ROLE OF 5-FLUOROURACIL AS AN ADJUVANT TO THE SURGICAL TREATMENT OF LARGE BOWEL CANCER[1]

Theodor B. Grage,[2] Gerald E. Metter,[3] George N. Cornell,[4]
Joseph Strawitz,[5] George J. Hill,III,[6] Robert W. Frelick,[7]
and Scot E. Moss[8]

INTRODUCTION

Resection of colo-rectal carcinoma continues to be the primary form of treatment, though survival rates following treatment for this disease have plateaued during the last 20 years. It is becoming increasingly attractive to combine surgical resection with long-term adjuvant chemotherapy for a variety of solid tumors. Significant improvement in salvage rates appears to be forthcoming in osteogenic sarcoma, Wilm's tumor and carcinoma of the breast. No such advances have been reported for carcinoma of the lung, stomach, pancreas or colo-rectum. The first major cooperative trial combining chemotherapy and surgery for the treatment of bowel cancer was reported by Holden in 1967 using the agent thiotepa in the immediate postoperative period, involving some 693 patients. This study revealed no significant improvement in survival in those patients receiving chemotherapy.[1] The Veterans Administration Surgical Adjuvant Group has studied over 1500 patients in a variety of programs using FUDR and 5-Fluorouracil (5-FU) in the form of brief postoperative courses and subsequently prolonged trials of intermittent postoperative systemic 5-FU. In the most recent trial survival was consistently better in the treated group than in the control group, although the difference was statistically not significant.[2,3,4]

In another prospectively controlled trial of 156 patients randomized to receive intravenous 5-FU during the intra-operative period and oral 5-FU in the postoperative period revealed no significant treatment benefit in terms of survival or disease free interval for the group of patients receiving 5-FU.[5]

DESCRIPTION OF STUDY

Beginning in 1971 the Central Oncology Group (COG) studied the effect of adjuvant chemotherapy with 5-FU upon survival and recurrence rate in 394 patients with colo-rectal carcinoma, who either underwent a curative or a palliative resection.[6] Chemotherapy was started within 30 days after operation and consisted of intravenous 5-FU, 12 mg/kg/day x 4 and then 6 mg/kg on alternate days x 5, followed by 12 mg/kg/week for one year. In 289 evaluable patients follow-up ranged from three

---

1. Supported by Central Oncology Group Grants CA 12282 and CA 12271 from the National Cancer Institute, Public Health Service.
2. University of Minnesota, Minneapolis, Minnesota.
3. University of Wisconsin, Madison, Wisconsin.
4. Cornell Medical Center, New York, New York.
5. American Oncologic Hospital, Philadelphia, Pennsylvania.
6. Marshall University, Huntington, West Virginia.
7. Wilmington Medical Center, Wilmington, Delaware.
8. University of Wisconsin, Madison, Wisconsin.

months to 65 months with a median follow-up of 30 months. Patients were found to be unacceptable for the following reasons: 16 were ineligible and did not meet study requirements for entry, 35 were invalid due to improper drug dosage or being on study for insufficient period of time, 24 patients were inadequately followed and the protocol requirements were not adhered to, and in 7 patients insufficient information was available to evaluate the patients.

Seven patients assigned to the 5-FU arm were removed from study because of intolerance to the drug. Of the 282 remaining patients 204 patients underwent curative resections and 78 patients underwent palliative resection. To provide an unbiased treatment comparison patients were allocated, at random, to treatment or control groups, on the basis of a centralized randomization procedure. To insure even distribution of assignment to the treatment and to the control group the patients were further stratified as to primary site, whether in the colon or rectum, presence or absence of lymph node involvement, and presence or absence of obstruction at the time of operation.

RESULTS

Of 199 patients randomized to chemotherapy, drug toxicity was severe in seven patients, however, there have been no drug related deaths. Other toxicities included nausea and vomiting 46%, diarrhea 45%, stomatitis 21%, leukopenia 57% and thrombocytopenia 32%.

Table I summarizes the status of the patients undergoing curative resection, of which 97 patients were classified as Dukes' B (tumor penetrated full-thickness of bowel) and 104 patients classified as Dukes' C (lymph nodal metastases).

Curative Resections

Treatment	Alive				Dead		Total	
	NED		*Recurrence*					
	#	%	#	%	#	%	#	%
A	60	65	13	14	20	22	93	101
B	68	61	18	16	25	23	111	100
Total	128	63	31	15	45	22	204	100

Table 1 - Summary status of 204 patients undergoing curative resection for colorectal carcinoma, Dukes' B & C only.
Note: Treatment A - 5-FU Group
Treatment B - Control Group
NED - No evidence of disease

The survival curves and duration of disease free interval curves were calculated using the Kaplan-Meier life table method and the differences in the survival and disease free interval curves between the control and chemotherapy group were evaluated statistically using Gehan's modification of the Wilcoxon test.

Figures 1 and 2 show the overall survival rates and disease free intervals in the curative group. Survival continues to be moderately more favorable in the treatment group although the difference is not significant (p = .09). However, the treatment group does have a significantly better disease free interval (p = .045).

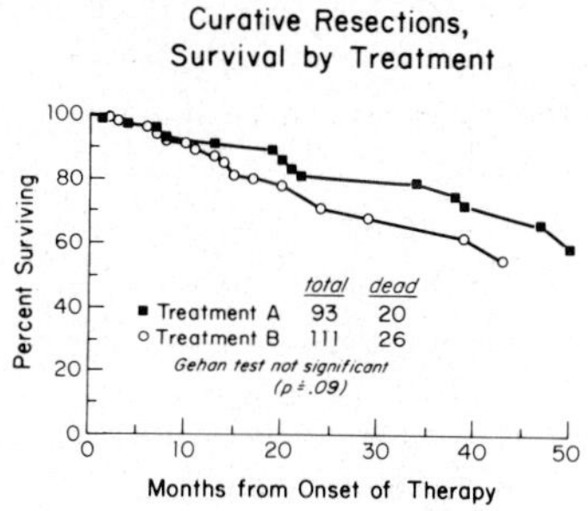

Figure 1. Survival curves of 204 patients following curative resection. Treatment A - 5-FU group, Treatment B - control group.

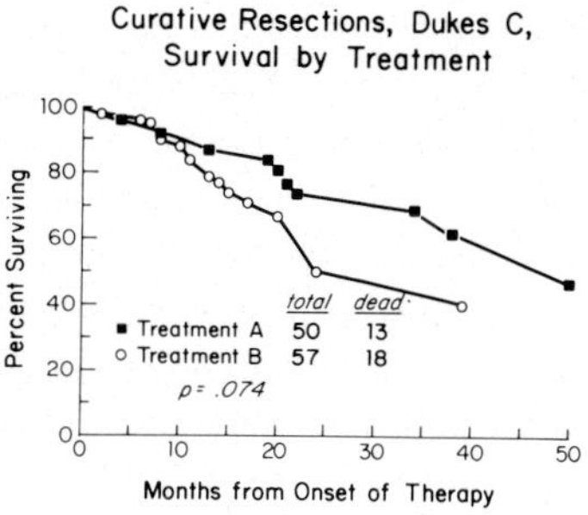

Figure 2. Survival curve of patients following curative resection. The 5-FU group did better, however, p-value is only .07.

Two variables had a significant influence on survival, site and stage of disease. The survival and disease free interval was significantly better for patients with carcinoma of the colon vs rectum (p = .038 and .027 respectively). Comparing the treatment arms within sites, the difference in treatment is primarily in the rectal group. The chemotherapy arm is significantly better than the control arm for both survival (p = .024, Figure 3) and disease free interval (p = .037) in patients with carcinoma of the rectum.

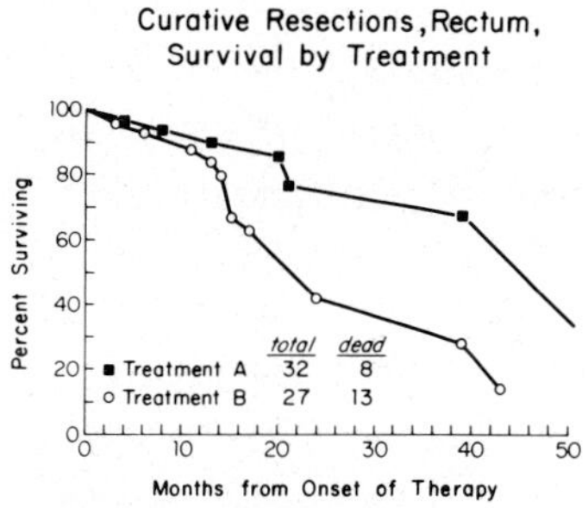

Figure 3. Survival curves of patients with carcinoma of the rectum. The 5-FU group did significantly better compared to the control group (p = .024).

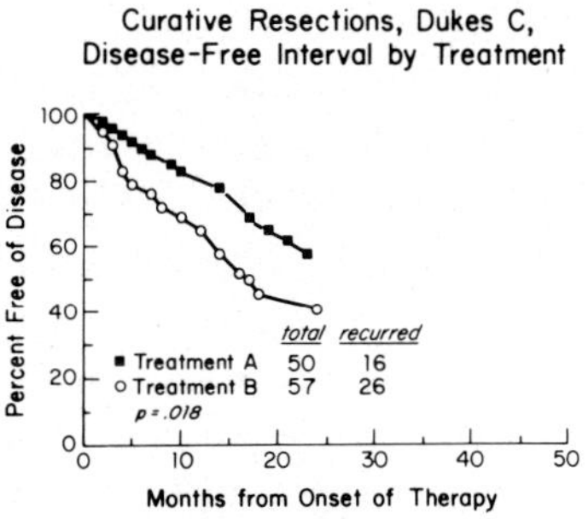

Figure 4. Disease free interval curve in Dukes' C patients. The 5-FU group did significantly better than the control group (p = .018).

The other variable examined was Dukes' Stage. Dukes' B patients obviously do better than Dukes' C patients. The disease free interval for patients with

Dukes' C lesions is significantly longer for those on chemotherapy (p = .018). (See Figure 4). With respect to survival, the treatment arms do not differ significantly.

The small but consistent benefit in the 5-FU treated arm favors prolongation of disease free interval more than survival and is significant in only two of many variables examined, namely, patients with rectal carcinoma and patients with Dukes' C lesions.

Table II summaries the results of the palliative resections. There is no significant difference in survival between the two treatment arms, however, the asymptomatic interval in the chemotherapy group is slightly longer. (p = .027) (See Figure 5).

Palliative Resections

Treatment	Alive				Dead		Total	
	Asymptomatic		*Symptomatic*					
	#	%	#	%	#	%	#	%
A	8	21	6	15	25	64	39	100
B	2	5	11	28	26	67	39	100
Total	10	13	17	22	51	65	78	100

Table II. Summary status of 78 patients undergoing palliative resection for colo-rectal carcinoma.
Note: Treatment A - 5-FU group
Treatment B - Control group

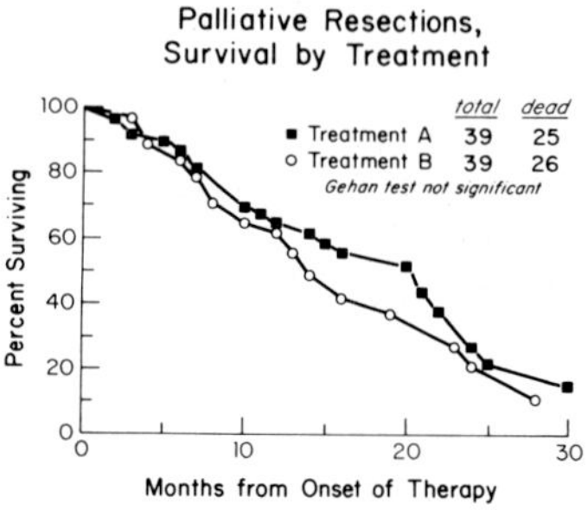

Figure 5. Survival curves after palliative resection reveals no significant improvement in the patients treated with 5-FU. (Treatment A).

We conclude that the treatment benefit following the administration of 5-FU as an adjuvant to the surgical treatment of colo-rectal cancer is small, mainly seen in prolongation of disease free interval and confined to patients with either Dukes' C lesions or patients with carcinoma of the rectum.

REFERENCES

1. Dixon, W.J., Longmire, W.P., Jr. and Holden, W.D.: Use of Triethylenethiophosphoramide as an adjuvant to the surgical treatment of gastric and colo-rectal carcinoma: Ten-year follow-up. Ann. Surg., 173:26, 1971.
2. Dwight, R.W., Humphrey, D.W., Higgins, G.A. and Keehn, R.J.: FUDR as an adjuvant to surgery in cancer of the large bowel. J. Surg. Oncol., 5:243, 1973.
3. Higgins, G.A., Dwight, R.W., Smith, J.V., Keehn, R.J.: Fluorouracil as an adjuvant to surgery in carcinoma of the colon. Arch. Surg., 102:339, 1971.

4. Higgins, G.A.: Chemotherapy, adjuvant to surgery, for gastrointestinal cancer. Clinics in Gastroent., 5:795, 1976.

5. Lawrence, W.,Jr., Terz, J.J., Horsley, J.S.,III, King, R.E., Lovett, W.L., Brown, P.W., Ruffner, B.W., Regelson, W.: Chemotherapy as an adjuvant to surgery for colorectal cancer. Ann. Surg., 181:616, 1975.

6. Grage, T.B., Metter, G.E., Cornell, G.N., Strawitz, J.G., Hill, G.J., Frelick, R.W. and Moss, S.E.: Adjuvant chemotherapy with 5-fluorouracil after surgical resection of colo-rectal carcinoma (COG Protocol 7041). A preliminary report. Am. J. Surg., 133:59, 1977.

Adjuvant Therapy of Cancer, S.E. Salmon and S.E. Jones eds.

ADJUVANT CHEMOTHERAPY AND CHEMOIMMUNOTHERAPY FOR LOCALLY ADVANCED LARGE BOWEL ADENOCARCINOMA

Preliminary Report of a Continuing Southwest Oncology Group Study

Frank J. Panettiere, M.D.
University of Texas Medical Branch, MW408
Galveston, Texas 77550, U.S.A.

BACKGROUND

When colon adenocarcinoma penetrates fully through the muscularis, even if all known disease is resected, surgery fails to cure 2/3 of patients. Fifty percent of those treated with so called curative surgery alone will die of recurrent cancer within three years. To try to improve upon this dismal situation, in August 1975, the Southwest Oncology Group decided to institute an adjuvant drug therapy program.

For chemotherapy, we decided to select a regimen which is most effective for disseminated disease and today, combination chemotherapy with Methyl CCNU plus 5-FU seems to be the most effective program to cause regressions of far advanced large bowel adenocarcinoma. Microscopic tumor such as is treated in an adjuvant setting should, compared to gross tumor, contain a higher proportion of cells near blood vessels and in active proliferation. Because of these two features, chemotherapy drugs should be far more effective in an adjuvant setting than when they are used to treat obvious metastatic tumor.

Although the place of chemotherapy, at least against gross disseminated tumors, is well documented, what role, if any, immunotherapy might play in the management of localized or disseminated large bowel cancer is much less certain. The immunotherapy about which we have the most information is BCG by scarification. We elected not to use BCG by this route for several reasons. We were concerned about patient acceptability of this procedure with its discomfort and inconvenience. We felt that patients who were without any clinical evidence of disease would not

---

Supported in Part by SWOG Grant, DHEW CA 03096

long adhere to a program which would require repeated scarifications. Our other main objection to BCG scarification was that the maximal effect would occur in lymphocytes far away from any drainage from the gastrointestinal tract. Mavligit and his group[1] have shown that in colon cancer, regional nodes are deficient in reactivity to tumor antigens. BCG has been given by mouth to patients with metastatic tumors and reported side effects are very minimal. Moreover, conversion of skin tests as well as prolongation of survival have been reported.[2] We elected to give BCG by the oral route for patient acceptability as well as to attempt to stimulate the appropriate lymphoid tissues.

Because without adjuvant therapy the prognosis of these patients is so poor, and because a number of studies suggest that adjuvant chemotherapy or immunotherapy may well be beneficial,[3,4] we felt that we could not justify a no-treatment control arm. Although the effectiveness of chemotherapy in large bowel cancer, at least when it is disseminated, is well documented, what benefit, if any, oral BCG might offer is far less certain. Therefore, we felt we could not justify treating patients with it alone. For these reasons, we designed a randomized program wherein 1/2 of patients receive systemic chemotherapy composed of 5-FU combined with Methyl CCNU and the other half receive the identical chemotherapy plus oral BCG immunotherapy.

We could not justify continuing therapy for an indefinite period in a situation where 1/3 of patients had been cured surgically prior to entry on the program. Moreover, both chemotherapy and immunotherapy are most likely to be effective initially when the tumor burden is small. Therefore, if a cure is not effected early, further therapy is likely to result in nothing other than unnecessary toxicity and inconvenience. For such reasons, we decided that all active adjuvant therapy should be discontinued after one year.

TREATMENT PROGRAM

To qualify for entrance on this study, it is required that a patient must have adenocarcinoma of the large bowel which has penetrated through the entire muscularis and/or has involved regional lymphnodes. All known disease must have been removed surgically. Before any patient is deemed eligible, both the surgeon's operative report and the pathology report must have been submitted to and reviewed by this author. No prior chemotherapy or radiotherapy is permitted. Randomization is to be accomplished and protocol therapy begun between two and six weeks of the definitive surgical resection.

The chemotherapy program consists of courses begun every eight weeks or as soon thereafter as recovery from myelosuppression permits. A single course consists of Methyl CCNU given orally on day 1 plus 5-Fluorouracil given intravenously on days 1, 8, and 15. The initial dose of Methyl CCNU is 175 mg/M^2. The three initial 5-FU doses are 400 mg/M^2 each. Subsequent doses are adjusted upwards or downwards based on the white count and platelet nadirs of the previous course.

Those randomized to receive immunotherapy receive the identical chemotherapy plus Connaught strain BCG, one vial (6 x 10^8 organisms), by mouth every two weeks for the year of therapy.

THERAPEUTIC EFFECTS

Although, as of February 14, 1977, 191 patients had been entered on this study, the longest followup was 22 months, and only 15 had been on study for one year or more. We have at least 5 months followup on 86 patients. One of the 86, a patient on both chemotherapy and immunotherapy, died due to tumor progression at the 5 month point. As of the present, no other patient has died. Therefore, the current survival curve shows 100% alive up to 5 months, and 98.8% chance of being alive from 5 months to the longest followup point of 22+ months. The graph shows how this <u>very preliminary</u> curve compares with four representive "historical control" series. These include data from a large cancer institute (M.D. Anderson)[5], a university medical center (LSU)[6], all 88 U.S. Air Force Hospitals, large and small, worldwide (as yet unpublished data) and a representative European study (Sweden)[7].

At this time, two clinical relapses (including the only death), have occurred in the group receiving chemotherapy with oral BCG. The projected chance of patients so treated being clinically disease free at 12 months is 89%. The chemotherapy alone group has had three relapses and currently shows an 82% chance of being clinically disease free at 12 months.

The development of clinical relapse after exposure to this therapy does not seem to impair response to future therapy. One who relapsed at 4 months died at 5. However, one each relapsed at 6, 8, and 10 months and each of these is alive, at 18+, 10+, and 14+ months respectively. The other patient has just relapsed at 12 months.

TOXICITY

Because of the demonstrated effectiveness of Methyl CCNU plus 5-FU in advanced cancer, in many centers this combination is being employed as an approach to post operative adjuvant therapy. Therefore, our toxicity experience is important to help guide others who might choose to follow such a program.

Superficially, toxicity does not seem to be cummulative. The mean leukocyte count nadir was 4,067 after the first course. The means for the next 4 courses

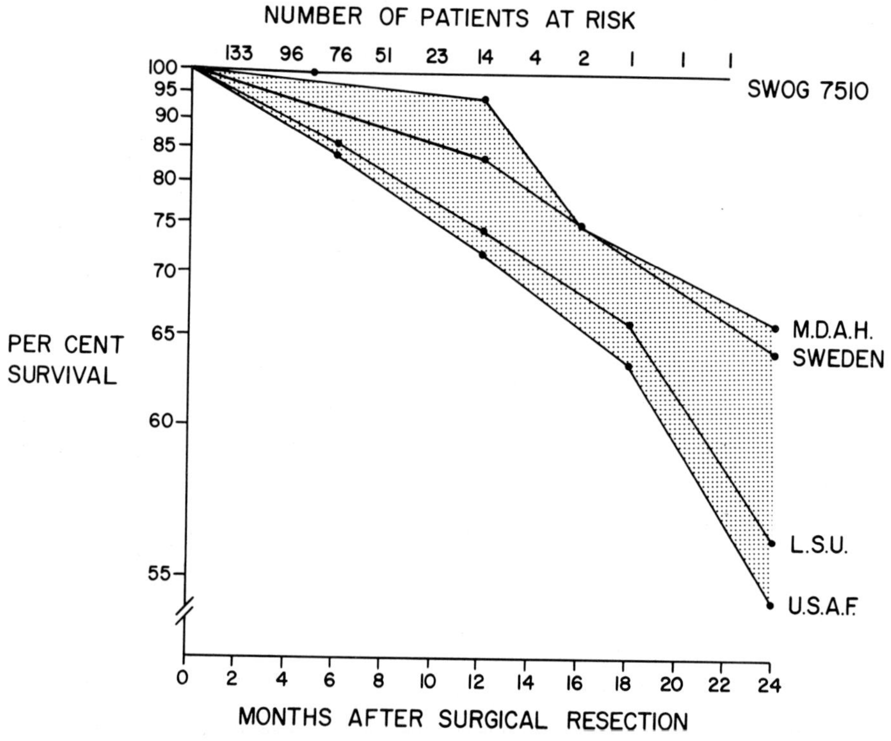

CURRENT SURVIVAL CURVE COMPARED TO HISTORICAL EXPERIENCE

were 3959, 4229, 4084 and 4041 respectively. Serial platelet count nadirs for the first five courses are 148392, 131584, 139405, 146965 and 153250. (At this time, we have data on less than 12 patients for courses after the fifth and therefore have not calculated such information.)

The observation that myelosuppression does not seem to increase with subsequent courses can be explained by studying the amount of chemotherapy drug given each course. If we consider the dose given in course one as 100%, the means for the second through sixth courses respectively are as follows: for Methyl CCNU, 94%, 88%, 80%, 65%, 53%; for 5-FU, 95%, 94%, 90%, 88%, and 82%.

Even more important may be our observations concerning the effects of oral BCG. We have discovered nothing we could attribute as indicative of toxicity from this agent. However, we did find data suggestive that this substance may ameliorate bone marrow toxicity. Table I displays the mean nadirs for each course. In parentheses are the numbers of individuals whose data are incorporated in each mean.

TABLE I

MEAN NADIRS WITH AND WITHOUT BCG

Course	*Leukocyte Nadir*		*Platelet Nadir* ($x10^3$)	
	BCG (-)	*BCG (+)*	*BCG (-)*	*BCG (+)*
1	*3850 (38)*	*4303 (35)*	*138 (38)*	*161 (34)*
2	*3930 (30)*	*3987 (31)*	*139 (30)*	*124 (30)*
3	*4114 (21)*	*4343 (21)*	*115 (21)*	*163 (21)*
4	*3747 (15)*	*4420 (15)*	*140 (15)*	*155 (14)*
5	*3750 (6)*	*4333 (6)*	*151 (6)*	*156 (6)*

Moreover, 37% of patients who received BCG, and 31% of those who did not, never had the white count fall below 4000. The platelet count never fell below 100,000 in 59% of the BCG treated patients and 36% of those who did not receive BCG.

The apparent effect of BCG on the amount of myelosuppressive drug received for each course after the first is displayed on Table II. We defined for each patient the amount given for his first course as 100 and calculated what proportion thereof was given in subsequent courses and tabulated the means of these observations. Again, the number of determinations is given in parentheses.

TABLE II

MEAN AMOUNTS OF DRUG GIVEN

Course	Methyl CCNU		5-Fluorouracil	
	BCG (-)	BCG (+)	BCG (-)	BCG (+)
1	100	100	100	100
2	93.7 (36)	95.1 (37)	91.1 (35)	99.7 (35)
3	86.1 (26)	88.8 (31)	94.3 (30)	93.7 (28)
4	79.2 (24)	81.4 (24)	84.8 (16)	90.2 (20)
5	58.0 (15)	72.1 (15)	84.5 (10)	90.5 (11)

The fact that very often those receiving oral BCG have higher blood counts despite their having received higher amounts of myelosuppressive drugs is certainly suggestive that oral BCG may ameliorate bone marrow toxicity. However, due to relatively small numbers and relatively large standard errors, only one of these pairs of data is statistically significant at this time. Therefore, until we accumulate more data, we can only say that such an effect is only an intriguing possibility.

The toxicity of the chemotherapy regimen is adequate to assure that enough is given to cause a definite biologic effect. On the other hand, toxicity does not appear too excessive for an adjuvant program. (There has been no fatal toxicity. The lowest white count for any patient was 1,200. However, four patients did experience transient thrombocytopenia to levels below 25,000.)

FUTURE PLANS

Entry on this SWOG study is being actively continued for a number of reasons: (1) In the absence of a no-further-therapy concurrent control group, we are seeking large numbers of patients so as to determine the effectiveness of these programs within relatively narrow limits of certainty. (2) Larger numbers of individuals will help make more certain whether oral BCG does ameliorate bone marrow toxicity. (3) We are seeking large numbers of patients to help us determine the prognostic significance of a large number of pretreatment characteristics. These should help us learn whether, in relatively uniformly treated patients, prognosis may be affected by such features as whether the patient had been operated upon at a major medical center or at a community hospital, whether he had had a prior bowel perforation and abscess formation, his reactions to various skin tests, determinations of immunoglobulin levels, absolute lymphocyte counts, and prechemotherapy CEA levels, and other factors. Although these pretreatment characteristics are currently being coded, with such a short followup duration and with only five relapses and one death to date, we have not yet analysed for prognostic significance. Eventually, such a prognostic factor analysis, based on a large patient population, is likely to help predict duration of survival. In this way, it should prove useful to assure comparability of future groups of patients treated for this tumor.

CONCLUSIONS

Although at this time it appears that the chemotherapy program we used may be effective in delaying relapses and in prolonging survival, it is far too early to make any such conclusion. Given by mouth, BCG has not had any demonstrable toxicity and there is suggestive evidence that it may have an effect in ameliorating bone marrow toxicity and allowing higher doses of myelosuppressive drugs to be administered.

REFERENCES

1. *Mavligit, G.M., et al: Immune Reactivity of Lymphoid Tissues Adjacent to Carcinoma of the Ascending Colon. Surg Gynec Obstet 139:490-412, 1974.*
2. *Falk, R.E., et al: Use of Oral and Intraperitoneal BCG in Treatment of Metastatic Melanoma and Adenocarcinoma. Pages 169-178 in R.G. Crispen, ed. Neoplasm Immunity: Theory and Application. ITR, Chicago 1975.*
3. *Higgins, G.A., et al: Fluorouracil as an Adjuvant to Surgery in Carcinoma of the Colon. Arch Surg 102:339-343, 1971.*
4. *Mavligit, G.M., et al: Immunotherapy--Its possible application in the Management of Large Bowel Cancer. Amer J Digest Dis 19:1047-1053, 1974.*

5. Mavligit, G.M., et al: *Prolongation of Postoperative Disease-Free Interval and Survival in Human Colorectal Cancer by BCG or BCG plus 5-Fluorouracil.* Lancet 871-876, April 24, 1976.

6. Falterman, K.W., et al: *Cancer of the Colon, Rectum and Anus: A Review of 2313 Cases.* Cancer 34:951-959, 1974.

7. Berge, T., et al: *Carcinoma of the Colon and Rectum in a Defined Population.* Acta Chiur Scand Suppl 438, 1973.

Adjuvant Therapy of Cancer, S.E. Salmon and S.E. Jones eds.
© 1977 Elsevier/North-Holland Biomedical Press, Amsterdam

CHEMOPROPHYLAXIS FOR PATIENTS WITH POSTOPERATIVE HIGH RISK COLORECTAL CANCER

Min C. Li*, M.D., Stuart T. Ross, M.D.
Nassau Hospital, Mineola, N.Y.

SUMMARY

The effectiveness of a short-term fluorouracil chemoprophylaxis regimen commencing four to six weeks after "curative" surgery was evaluated in a homogenous group of 183 patients with colorectal cancer. In Duke's class C disease five-year survival with no evidence of disease (NED) was 24.3% when treated by surgery alone, but was 56.7% when a prophylactic regimen of fluorouracil was added ($P < .01$), an increase of 33.2%; in Duke's class B disease, five-year survival NED was raised from 58.5% to 81.6%, an increase of 23.1% ($P < .02$). More striking are the one-two-three-year NED survivals in Duke's class C disease. The one-two-three-year NED survivals for the chemoprophylaxis group are 100%, 96% and 75% respectively, in contrast to 70.7%, 48.8% and 34.1% in the group with surgery alone. The present data indicate that fluorouracil chemoprophylaxis offers a significant improvement of five-year cure rate of patients with Duke's class B and C disease, an overall increase of 28.1% ($P < .01$).

INTRODUCTION

The five-year survival rate following curative surgery for colon-rectal cancer has reached a plateau. In the past 20 years there is no significant change in the statistics according to the reports of the American Cancer Society, various cooperative clinical groups and the National Institutes of Health. Table I illustrates the summary of these data as analyzed by Carter[1].

Table I

Historical Controls

National Statistics [1] Duke's Class	5-year Survival Rate	Nassau Hospital Statistics [2] Duke's Class	5-year Survival Rate	
A	80%	A	93%	(1960-1970)
B	50%	B	58.5%	(1960-1965)
C	25%	C	24.3%	(1960-1965)
D	2%	D	--	

In the beginning of 1965 we attempted to design a different study using fluorouracil after curative surgery for colorectal carcinoma[2]. The time to initiate,

---

* Present address: Scripps Memorial Hospital, P.O. Box 28, La Jolla, Ca. 92038

the dosage and the duration of fluorouracil therapy were predicated on the following principles: 1) Dealing with the viable cell numbers of 1 X 10^6 or less in each site of micrometastases. 2) Viable cells are entering the proliferative cycle when fluorouracil is being administered. 3) Minimal supression of host defense following fluorouracil therapy. 4) Uniformity of surgical techniques, staging of disease, supportive medical care and follow-up.

MATERIAL AND METHODS

Patients who had curative surgery from the beginning of 1960 until the begining of 1965 were used as controls. Patients with Duke's class B & C disease who had curative surgery from 1965 to the beginning of 1970 were treated with fluorouracil. No fluorouracil therapy was given to Duke's class A disease after surgery. The principles of curative surgery included wide resection of tumor, removal of lymphatic drainage systems and measures to avoid cancer cell contamination and venous embolism. In order to keep strict uniformity with our controls in factors such as surgical techniques, staging of disease, preoperative and postoperative care, the entire series of operations was performed by one surgeon in one community hospital. Fluorouracil was given by one medical oncologist.

The staging of disease has been determined according to Duke's Classification. Cases in which cancer had spread to the adjacent peritoneal surface, the omentum, or tumor adhering to other parts of the bowel or pelvic organs and ascites were considered advanced and were excluded, as were cancers not originating in the mucosa. Table II shows the relative compatibility of age, location, histological diagnosis and number of regional lymph node involvement in Duke's class C disease in both treated and control groups.

Table II

Age, location, histological diagnosis & nodal involvement*

	Surgery Alone %	Surgery Plus Chemoprophylaxis %
Age, Yr		
31-40	4.1	3.1
41-50	10.7	6.2
51-60	23.1	23.4
61-70	33.9	29.1
71-80	19.8	25.0
81-90	6.6	3.1
90	1.7	0
Location		
Rectum	30.9	50
Recto sigmoid	33.3	10.9
Sigmoid	19.8	26.6
Other	15.9	12

	Surgery Alone %	Surgery Plus Chemoprophylaxis
Histopathologic diagnosis		
Infiltrating adenocarcinoma	57.1	62.5
Adenocarcinoma	41.3	35.9
Anaplastic carcinoma	1.6	1.6
Regional lymph node involvement (Stage III), No.		
Four or more	66	60
Three or less	34	40

* Based on the original entry of 228 patients.

with surgery alone, but was 57.7% when a prophylactic fluorouracil therapy was added ($P < .01$). In Duke's class B disease the 5-year survival was raised from 58.8% to 81.6 ($P < .02$). More striking are the differences in one, two and three-year survivals in Duke's class C disease. The difference in the two groups for class B disease is not statistically significant until the fifth year.

Figure I

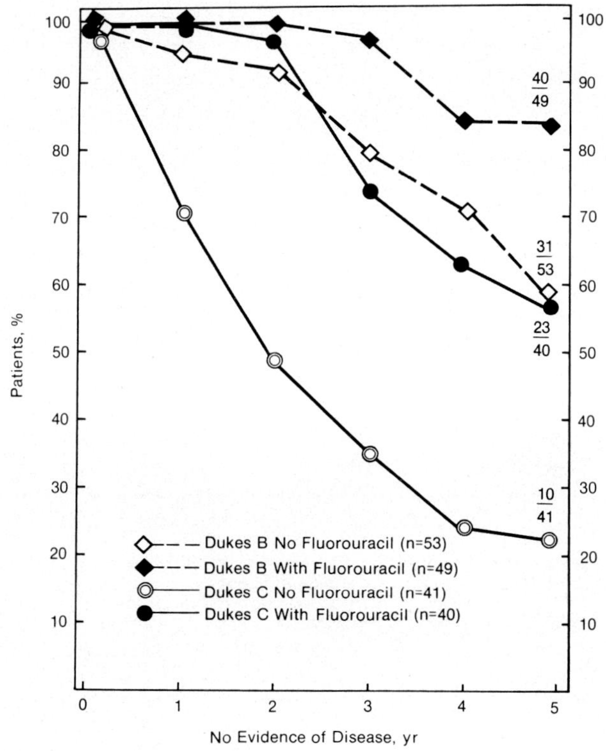

Comparison of results of surgery alone vs surgery plus chemoprophylaxis in patients with colorectal cancer.

Follow-up consisted of a thorough physical and endoscopic examination at least every 6 months by the surgeon. Questions were aimed at the status and degree of well being and any symptoms that would suggest recurrence or metastatic disease. In addition, other immediate medical problems were taken care of by the primary physicians as frequently as needed. Roentgenographic examination of the colon, chest x-rays, complete blood count and alkaline phosphatase determination were done yearly. Determination of CEA was not available at the time of the study.

Originally, there were 228 patients entering the study. One patient died of postoperative complications, 11 patients died of unrelated disease, but showed no evidence of cancer. Three patients were lost to follow-up, thirty patients had Duke's class A disease and were not treated with fluorouracil. They were excluded from evaluation. Thus, only 183 patients are included in the study.

Fluorouracil was administered to all patients in the study group with Duke's class B & C disease, beginning four to six weeks after surgery. We determined the dosage of drug according to the clinical and nutritional status, body weight and age of patient in contradistinction to the conventional method of mg/Kg body weight or mg/sqM. Chemotherapy was given in an office or clinic setting. Table III shows the drug regimens.

Table III

Drug Regimens

Regimen I for Patients:		
< 65 of age	FU	1,000 mg I.V. Push on day 1
or		↓
> 60 Kg/B.wt	FU	500 mg I.V. daily X 4
or		↓
Nutrition good		Repeat once after 4 weeks
Regimen II for Patients:		
> 65 of age	FU	500 mg I.V. Push daily X 5
or		↓
< 60 Kg/B.wt		Repeat once after 4 weeks
or		
Undernourished		

The drug toxicity after therapy usually included leukopenia of 2-3000 WBC/cu mm and thrombocytopenia of 100-150,000 platelets cu mm. Most patients had tolerable stomatitis and occasionally bouts of diarrhea for 1-3 days. There has been no mortality.

RESULTS

Figure I compares the results of surgery alone Vs surgery plus postoperative fluorouracil therapy in a total of 183 patients. The data are for disease free survival. In Duke's Class C disease, five year survival was 24.3% when treated

DISCUSSION AND CONCLUSION:

Our data indicate that fluorouracil chemoprophylaxis offers a statistically significant improvement of 5-year disease free survival of patients with Duke's class B or C disease, in contrast with our own historical controls and with comparable national statistics. We feel that the unique features of our study given in Table IV may be responsible for the results. A prospective repeat study, with these features, by other investigators utilizing concurrent randomized controls may be worthwhile.

Table IV

Unique Features of Study

1.	Surgical techniques, staging, supporting care	Uniform
2.	Fluorouracil therapy	Uniform initiation and dosage
3.	Short-term therapy	Little or no immunosuppression
4.	Follow-up	Over 5 years
5.	Loss in follow-up	1.5%

REFERENCES

1. Carter, S.K. (1976) Seminars in Oncology, Colon Carcinoma, Vol. III, No4, pp 433-447, Grune & Stratton, N.Y.

2. Li, M.C., Ross, S.T. (1976) Chemoprophylaxis for Patients with Colorectal Cancer, Prospective study with five-year follow-up. JAMA Vol.235, No 26, 2825-2828.

Adjuvant Therapy of Cancer, S.E. Salmon and S.E. Jones eds.

SYSTEMIC ADJUVANT IMMUNOTHERAPY AND CHEMOIMMUNOTHERAPY IN PATIENTS WITH COLORECTAL CANCER (DUKES' C CLASS): PROLONGATION OF DISEASE FREE INTERVAL AND SURVIVAL

Giora M. Mavligit, Jordan U. Gutterman, Mary Anne Malahy
Michael A. Burgess, Charles M. McBride, Andre Jubert*,
and Evan M. Hersh.

The Departments of Developmental Therapeutics, National Large Bowel Cancer Project and Surgery, University of Texas System Cancer Center, M.D. Anderson Hospital and Tumor Institute, 6723 Bertner Avenue, Houston, Texas 77030, U.S.A.

*Present address: St Mary's Hospital, Grand Rapids, Michigan

SUMMARY:

The poor post-surgical prognosis in patients with colorectal cancer of the Dukes' C classification has prompted a clinical trial of adjuvant immunotherapy versus chemoimmunotherapy intended to prolong either the disease-free interval or the overall survival or both. One hundred and twenty-one patients have been entered on this study. Fifty-two patients received BCG alone and 69 patients received the combination of 5-FU and BCG. The disease-free interval and the overall survival were compared with similar parameters in a group of historical controls with similar prognostic characteristics who were operated on in our institution prior to the initiation of the current study. There was no difference as yet between BCG alone and the combination of 5-FU + BCG in terms of both the disease-free interval and the survival. Both treatments, however, were significantly better than the controls. Adjuvant therapy, especially with BCG is advocated for patients with colorectal carcinoma, Dukes' C class, following potentially curative surgery.

INTRODUCTION:

Since the results from surgical treatment of colorectal cancer seem to have reached a plateau [1], the administration of surgical adjuvant therapy appears to be the rational approach in order to achieve further improvement in the prognosis of these patients [2]. The need for systemic adjuvant therapy is particularly urgent in patients with Dukes' C lesions, i.e. those in whom the primary tumor has involved the regional mesenteric lymph nodes. The natural history of this group of patients, with approximately 70-75% chance for surgical failure and recurrent tumor, strongly indicates that foci of micrometastasis were present in adjacent structures or in distant organs already at the time of surgery. Systemic adjuvant therapy should therefore be directed against those foci of micrometastasis with the hope to increase the surgical cure rate or to prolong the tumor-free interval and/or the overall survival.

MATERIALS AND METHODS:

From April 1973 to October 1976, a total of 121 patients with carcinoma of the large bowel - Dukes' C classification (involvment of regional lymph nodes without invasion of adjacent structure or distant organs) were entered onto a clinical trial of adjuvant therapy. The latter consisted of immunotherapy with BCG by scarification or the combination of immunochemotherapy with BCG plus oral 5-Fluorouracil as previously described [3,4]. Treatment evaluation in terms of disease-free interval and overall survival was compared with the same clinical parameters in a consecutive series of comparable (by the above definition of Dukes' C lesion and by the major prognostic criteria) historical surgical control patients with Dukes' C lesions, operated on at M. D. Anderson Hospital in 1963 - 1973. Control patients who died in the immediate postoperative period (60 days) and a few who died of causes other than cancer (when this could definitely be established) were purposely excluded for valid comparison to the study group. Control patients not operated on at the M. D. Anderson Hospital were also left out for the following reason: In general, patients are not being referred to M. D. Anderson unless a relapse has occurred, i.e. the vast majority of the post-operative outside referrals were patients who have already relapsed and subsequently expired. In other words, we could not consider the outside patients as a homogenous and representative group in the absence of those who were apparently cured by surgery and had never been sent to M. D. Anderson Hospital. Furthermore, in order to answer the question: Is surgery at M. D. Anderson equal to surgery elsewhere in terms of postoperative disease-free interval and survival, we compared those parameters considering only the patients who had a tumor relapse after surgery with the exclusion of those who remained free of disease both at the M. D. Anderson Hospital and in the population of patients who were referred to M. D. Anderson after having had the primary surgery elsewhere. We found virtually no difference in either the disease-free interval or the survival between M. D. Anderson patients and those operated on elsewhere. This has allowed us to consider the patients who received adjuvant therapy regardless of their place of surgery. Further details of the randomization to treatment arms, criteria for exclusion from this study and the statistical methods for data analysis have been discussed at length in our previous publications on this study [3,4].

RESULTS AND COMMENTS:

Fifty-two patients received BCG alone and 69 patients received the combination of BCG + 5-FU. With the longest follow-up being 42 months, 15 and 19 patients, respectively, have relapsed (Figure I). The disease-free interval for each adjuvant treatment group is estimated to be significantly prolonged compared to the surgical controls ($P=0.02$, $P<0.01$, respectively). No difference was noted (as yet) between the two adjuvant treatment arms ($P=0.95$).

The overall survival for each treatment group (Figure II) is estimated to be significantly prolonged as compared to the surgical controls ($P=0.02$, $P<0.01$, respectively) while no difference was noted (as yet) between the two adjuvant treatment arms ($P=0.58$).

Since both adjuvant treatment regimens seem to be equally beneficial at this time, all 121 patients on adjuvant therapy were lumped together for further analysis and comparison with surgical controls of Dukes' B class (negative regional nodes). The disease-free interval (Figure III) for all 121 Dukes' C patients receiving adjuvant therapy, although significantly prolonged when compared to surgical Dukes' C controls ($P=0.002$), still falls significantly short of the disease-free interval of surgically-treated patients with Dukes' B lesions ($P=0.01$). Nevertheless, the overall survival (Figure IV) for all 121 Dukes' C patients receiving adjuvant therapy, was not only significantly prolonged when compared to surgical Dukes' C control patients ($P=0.001$), but the survival curve almost overlaps that of surgically-treated Dukes' B patients ($P=0.41$). We have therefore not only achieved a statistically significant prolongation in both the disease-free interval and the overall survival by administration of adjuvant therapy (especially BCG), but furthermore, we were able to show a marked shift in the prognosis of adjuvant-treated Dukes' C patients mostly toward that of surgically-treated Dukes' B patients in whom an approximately 60% 5-year survival can be anticipated, as compared to 35% for surgically-treated Dukes' C patients.

To further reassure that the natural history of patients with Dukes' C lesions did not change in time (by the quality of surgery and other unknown factors) and to substantiate their comparability to the patients receiving adjuvant therapy, we have divided the group of Dukes' C surgical controls into two subgroups, namely those who were operated on between 1963 - 1967 and those who were operated on between 1968 - 1972. The disease-free interval and overall survival curves for both subgroups of patients were almost identical (Figures V and VI) with $P=0.42$, $P=0.31$

Figure I

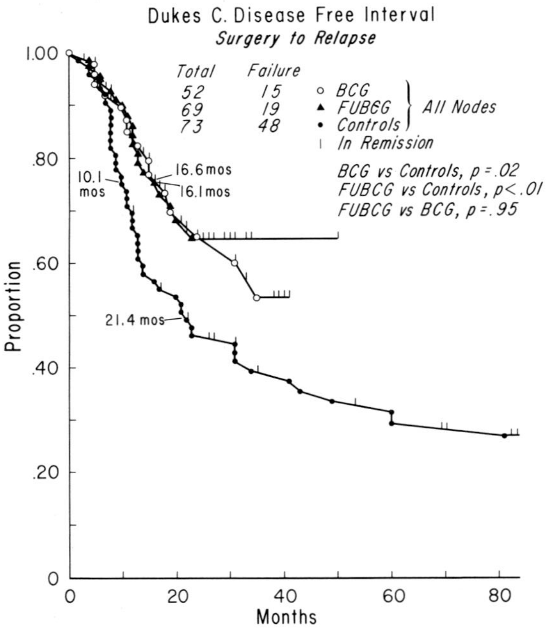

Figure II

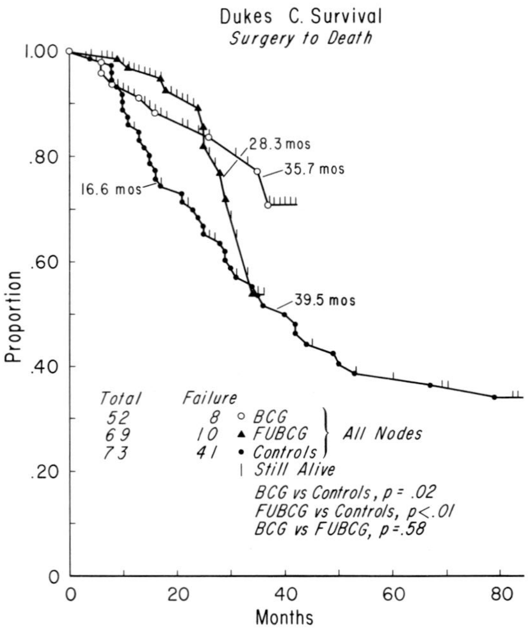

Figure III

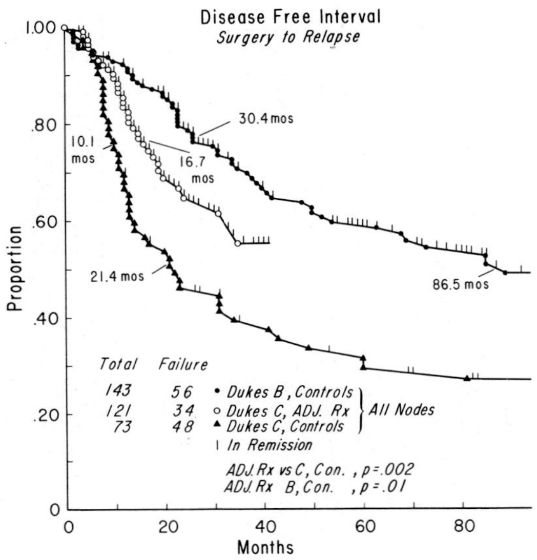

Figure IV

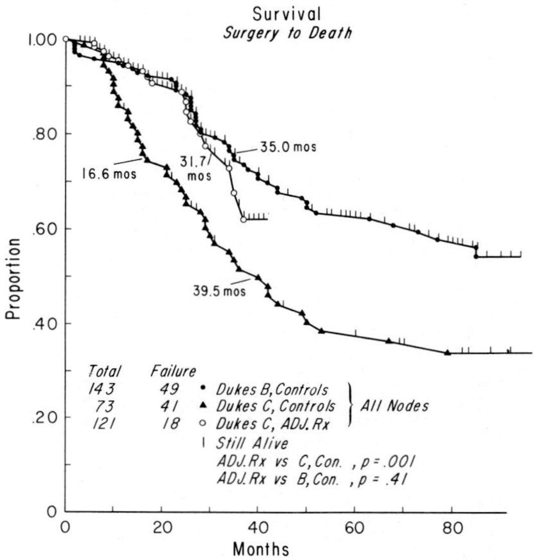

Figure V

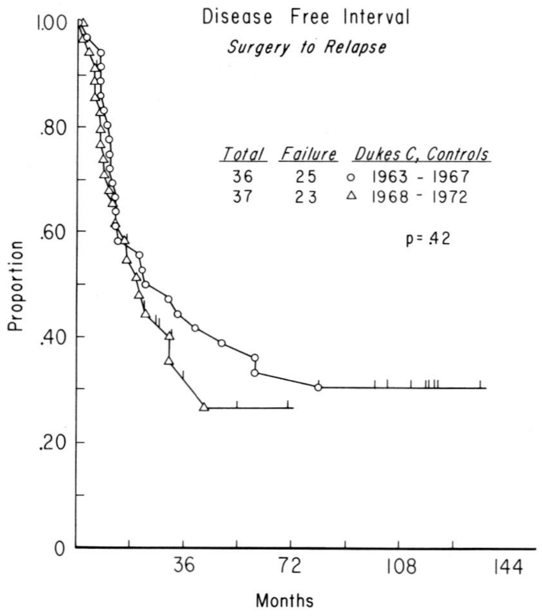

Figure VI

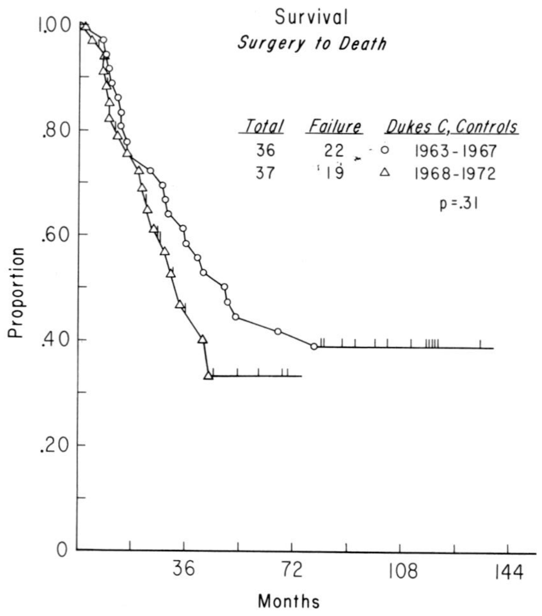

respectively. Furthermore, the nodal status of surgical Dukes' C controls was not different from that of the patients treated with adjuvant therapy (Table I). The mean number of lymph nodes examined in the surgical specimen was similar, and the mean number of nodes involved with tumor was slightly increased among the patients receiving adjuvant therapy. This should, if anything, confer upon the latter a slightly poorer prognosis as compared to the surgical controls.

TABLE I

COMPARISON OF NODAL STATUS IN PATIENTS WITH DUKES' C LESIONS

	Historical (Surgical) Controls		Adjuvant Rx
	1963 - 1967	1968 - 1972	1973 - 1976
No. of Patients	36	37	121
No. of Nodes Examined (Mean)	14.9	15.2	13.7
No. of Nodes with Tumor (Mean)	3.6	3.4	4.4

The pattern of relapse among patients receiving adjuvant therapy is shown in Table II. Among 84 patients with primary carcinoma of the rectosigmoid portion of the large bowel, there were 26 relapses of which 18 occurred locally. In contrast, there were 8 relapses among 37 patients with primary carcinoma arising proximal to the rectosigmoid, of which only 2 occurred locally (P=0.07). The occurrence of distal metastasis was equally distributed between the primary sites mentioned above.

TABLE II

FAILURE ON ADJUVANT THERAPY ACCORDING TO SITE OF PRIMARY TUMOR

Primary Site	No. of Pts. Entered	No. with Recurrence			
		Local	Distal	Both	All
Rectosigmoid	84	8*	8	10*	26
Proximal to Rectosigmoid	37	2*	6	0	8

*P=0.07 for Local Recurrence

This pattern of relapse indicates the urgent need to bolster the resistance and augment the protection against local recurrence, perhaps by the administration of post-operative radiotherapy to suitable patients with rectal and rectosigmoid primary. The protection against the development of distant metastasis, especially in the liver and the lungs, may be improved by giving the 5-FU intravenously rather than orally and perhaps by additional administration of intravenous C. parvum - a potent immune stimulant which tends to localize in these organs and hopefully cause a regression of foci of micrometastasis. These modifications in the treatment regimen have already been made and the new study is presently under way.

REFERENCES:

1. Silverberg, E., et al. 1975, Major Trends in Cancer: 25 Year Survey, Ca, 25:2-7.
2. Burchenal, J.H., 1976, Adjuvant Therapy - Theory, Practice, and Potential. Cancer, 37:46-57.
3. Mavligit, G.M., et al. 1975, Adjuvant Immunotherapy and Chemoimmunotherapy in Colorectal Cancer of the Dukes' C Classification. Cancer, 36:2421-2427.
4. Mavligit, G.M., et al. 1976, Prolongation of Postoperative Disease-Free Interval and Survival in Human Colorectal Cancer by BCG or BCG Plus 5-Fluorouracil. Lancet, 1:871-876.

ACKNOWLEDGMENTS:

This work was supported by P.H.S. grant 1 R26 CA 15458-01 and in part by Hoffman-LaRoche grant 169196. Giora M. Mavligit and Jordan U. Gutterman are the recipients of career development awards CA 1 KO 4 CA 00130-02 and CA 71007-03, respectively, from the National Institutes of Health. The contribution of patients from Ferguson Hospital, Grand Rapids, Michigan, is acknowledged.

Adjuvant Therapy of Cancer, S.E. Salmon and S.E. Jones eds.

GASTRIC CARCINOMA--SURVIVAL WITH ADJUVANT CHEMOTHERAPY: A PILOT STUDY AT THE PENNSYLVANIA HOSPITAL

Harvey J. Lerner, M. D.
Pennsylvania Hospital
Eighth and Spruce Streets
Philadelphia, Pennsylvania 19107 U. S. A.

An overview of the treatment of stomach cancer throughout the world since the pioneering resections done by Bilroth[1] and Schlatter[2] at the end of the 19th century confirm the belief that this is a difficult and resistant disease form. Although the incidence of stomach cancer is on the decline in this country, it still remains the seventh leading cause of death by cancer in the United States; in other countries the decline is less marked, and gastric carcinoma accounts for more than half of all male cancer deaths in Japan.

The decline in incidence of gastric cancer has been described as gratifying but puzzling, and to date no one reason has been advanced and accepted for the small but steady downward trend observed in the last 30 years. As recently as 1930, gastric cancer was the leading cause of cancer death in this country. It is acknowledged, however, that the decrease in mortality reflects a declining incidence rate rather than any breakthrough in treatment of diagnosis. The resectability rate, which was very low in 1900, is now reported to be between 30% and 40%.[3]

Moreover, although incidence figures continue to show some improvement, the five-year survival rate following diagnosis of cancer of the stomach is still dismally low. The American Cancer Society estimates 22, 900 new cases in 1976 with an associated high death rate.

Adenocarcinoma of the stomach is known to be a rapidly progressing disease form. The widely accepted 5 year survival rate of 5% to 15% in resected patients falls when metastases are present or when the disease has progressed beyond the resectable stage.

MATERIALS AND METHODS

In the decade from January, 1964, to December, 1974, we recorded the following experience with patients diagnosed and treated for adenocarcinoma of the stomach at the Pennsylvania Hospital.

Over this period a total of 122 adults were admitted with a confirmed diagnosis of gastric cancer. Thirteen were lost to follow up and we report the outcome of the remaining 109 patients. None of these 109 patients received any chemotherapy.

Although the patients ranged in age from 22 to 92, most were elderly with an average age of 65.9 years and a median of 67. We saw approximately the same number of men and women, and sex or age at the time of diagnosis had no apparent effect on survival.

Patients presented with symptoms of bleeding, belching, bloating, vomiting, rapid satiety, pain and weight loss. The diagnosis was confirmed by upper gastrointestinal studies, gastroscopy with or without biopsy, and cytologic examination of gastric secretions.

A second and separate patient population received chemotherapy with and without surgical resection. This group totaled 33 patients. All were known to have adenocarcinoma of the stomach, with the diagnosis confirmed by laparotomy or gastroscopy and biopsy. Of this group, eleven patients had non-resectable disease, while 22 had either partial or total gastric resections.

All patients in this group were placed on a chemotherapeutic regimen of one half gram of 5-FU intravenously on day 4, 11, 18, and so on. In addition to the 5-FU, these patients received hydroxyurea, 80 mg/kg as a single oral dose on day 1, 8, 15, and so on. This chemotherapy was continued indefinitely, or until there was progression of the cancer.

Side effects were minimal. Some nausea, probably as a result of the hydroxyurea was reported but was controlled by the usual means. A transient leukopenia, with a white blood cell count lower than 3000, appeared infrequently, but omitting one week of chemotherapy allowed the white count to rise to an acceptable level. Mild leukopenia was the only instance that required even temporary discontinuation of drug therapy.

RESULTS OF THE SURGERY WITH NO CHEMOTHERAPY

Our experience with eleven patients whose disease was so far advanced that surgery was not possible showed, as might be expected, their survival rate was extremely poor, ranging from 0. 1 month to 6 months, with a median survival of one month.

Twenty-four patients underwent laparotomy and biopsy but were not resected because of the extensive nature of the disease. Their survival rate was no better than the non-operative group, ranging from 0. 1 month to 7. 5 months, with a median survival of 1. 2 months.

The remaining 74 patients were resected with the intention of possible cure. Sub-total gastrectomies were performed on 60 patients.

Survival ranged from 0 to 80 months, with an average survival of 15. 5 months and a median survival of 8 months.

Among the fourteen patients who had total gastrectomies, survival ranged from 0. 1 month to 72 months, with an average survival of 17. 7 months and a median survival of 5. 5 months.

As would be expected, the patients who were found to have metastases at operation proved to have an even more limited survival rate. Thirty-two patients had tumor metastases to one-half the total lymph nodes examined for

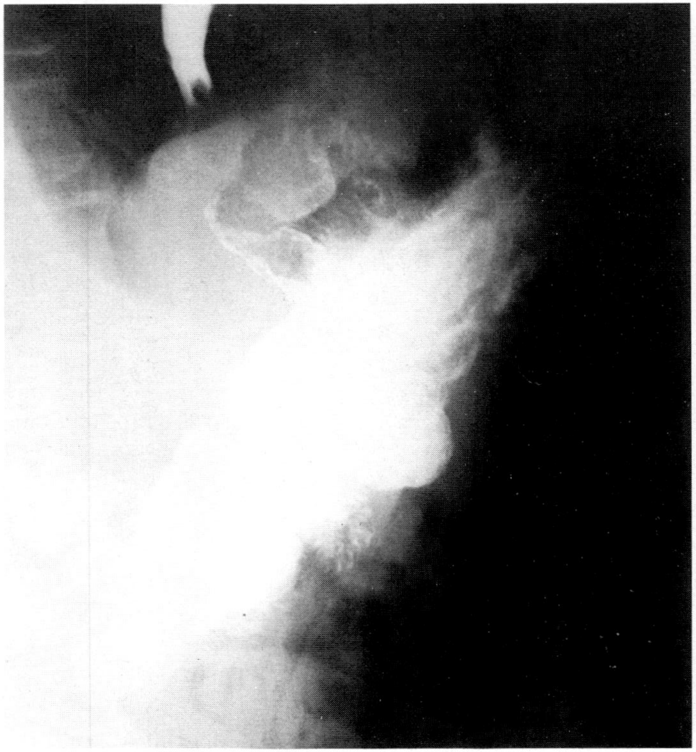

Patient A. K. Pre Treatment--non-resectable lesion at esophago-gastric junction.

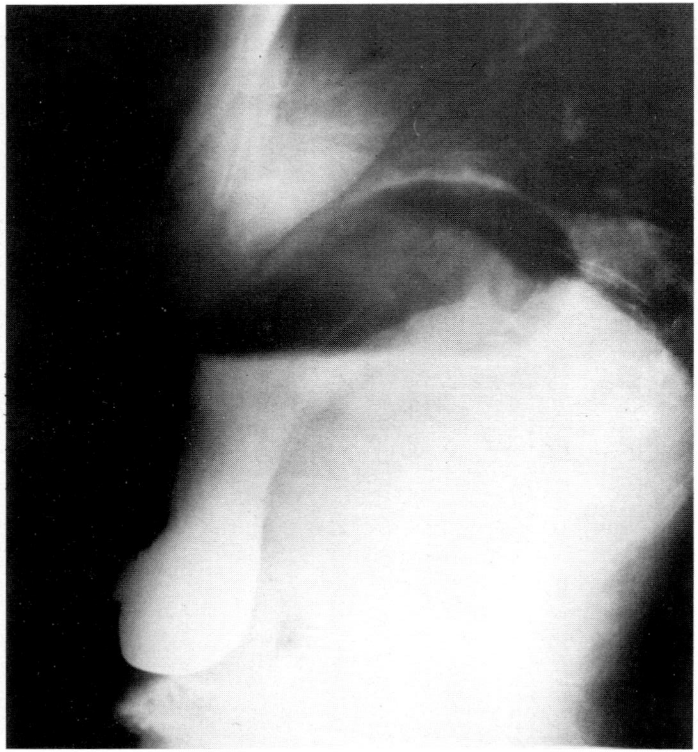

Patient A. K. after 8 months of treatment with HU-FU demonstrates marked regression.

that particular patient. Survival ranged from 0.1 month to 16 months, with a median survival of only 0.5 months for this group of patients.

Only six patients who were resected did not demonstrate lymph node metastasis. Survival ranged in this group from 4 to 36 months, with an average of 18.5 months.

There were eleven operative deaths in this series.

RESULTS WITH CHEMOTHERAPY--HU-FU

Survival of the eleven non-resected patients, 9 males and 2 females ranging in age from 48 to 82 years with an average of 65 years, ranged from two to 29 months, with a median of 4 months. Although the gastric carcinoma was advanced in these 11 patients, we noted a significant objective response in 5 patients. One patient experienced a complete remission and died 29 months following diagnosis of a CVA.

In the group of 22 patients receiving partial or total gastrectomy for possible cure, there were 15 males and 7 females. Ages ranged from 32 to 88, with an average age of 62.5 years. In several patients of this group, metastatic adenocarcinoma was observed at the time of surgery. Of these patients who underwent partial or total resection, the median survival was 25 months. One patient is still alive at 142 months, and two others lived 65 and 80 months respectively following diagnosis and operation.

DISCUSSION

Despite major improvements in diagnosis, anesthesia, surgical techniques and post-operative care, the survival rate for adenocarcinoma of the stomach remains a dismal one. In our series of 109 patients, almost all patients seen were diagnosed too late to effect any kind of surgical care. Among those resected, the five year survival rate was extremely low suggesting that other modalities of therapy will be needed to control gastric cancer. The poor survival rate in gastric cancer was the reason for adjuvant chemotherapy. A recent experimental study demonstrated the advantage of using the combination of HU-FU. In 1973, Oscar Frankfurt, of Moscow's Laboratory of Experimental Oncology, treated murine Ehrligh ascites tumor with 5-FU in combination with other drugs. He counted the tumor cells present following injection and reported a significant enhancement of the anti-tumor activity of 5-FU by hydroxyurea.[4]

SUMMARY

In the period from January, 1964, to December, 1974, 122 patients were admitted to Pennsylvania Hospital with a diagnosis of gastric adenocarcinoma. Of the 109 patients followed to their death, only seven survived 5 years; the longest survival was 80 months.

Among the 35 patients not resected, median survival was only one month. Of the 74 patients who had surgical resections survival ranged from a median of 5.5 months for those who had total gastrectomy to a median of 8 months for those receiving sub-total gastrectomy.

In the 11 non-resectable patients who received chemotherapy with HU-FU, the median survival increased from 1 month to 4 months, with 3 patients still alive at 4, 6, and 7 months. Objective regression was observed in 5 of these 11 patients.

In the 22 resected patients who received adjuvant HU-FU, the median survival increased to 25 months with several patients alive at 41, 51, and 142 months.

The use of HU-FU as an adjuvant is well tolerated and appears to significantly increase the median survival time in both resected and non-resectable gastric cancers.

BIBLIOGRAPHY

1 Bilroth, T.: Uber einem neuen Fall von Gelungener Resektion des carcinomatosen Pylorus. Wien Med Wochenschr 31:1427-1429, 1881.

2 Schlatter, C: Uiber Ernahrung und Vendauung nach vollstandiger Entfernung des Magens. Chirurg 19:757-761, 1897.

3 Gilbertsen, V.A.: Results of treatment of stomach cancer: An appraisal of efforts for more extensive surgery and a report of 1,983 cases. Cancer 23: 1305-1308, 1969.

4 Frankfurt, Oscar S.: Enhancement of the Antitumor Activity of 5-Fluorouracil by Drug Combinations. Cancer Research 33, 1043-1047, May, 1973.

Supported by the Memorial Fund for Cancer Research and in part by Grant CA13613 from the National Cancer Institute.

Adjuvant Therapy of Cancer, S.E. Salmon and S.E. Jones eds.

ADJUVANT RADIOTHERAPY FOR CARCINOMA OF THE SIGMOID COLON AND RECTUM

Marvin M. Romsdahl, M.D., Ph.D. and H. Rodney Withers, M.D., Ph.D.
The University of Texas System Cancer Center
M. D. Anderson Hospital and Tumor Institute
6723 Bertner Avenue
Houston, Texas

INTRODUCTION

Adenocarcinoma of the colon and rectum contributes a highly important health problem inasmuch as 99,000 individuals were expected to develop this disease in 1976[1]. Occurring almost equally in men and women, it is second in incidence only to skin cancer. Its impact is reflected in the fact that 49,000 will die of colon-rectum cancer annually, or approximately 50% of the number newly diagnosed. Five-year survival statistics suggest an even lesser prognosis for the evaluable period 1965-1969, with 71% surviving when disease is localized and 43% when associated with regional spread. Efforts directed toward earlier diagnosis, public education, improved operative management of patients, and implementation of adjunctive measures have not changed survival to a measureable extent during the past 35 years. Since surgery represents the only known means for potential cure of colon-rectal carcinoma, it appears rationale that improvements in survival and clinical management of this disease will come from measures combined with operative treatment. Recognizing that achieving an improvement in survival represents a seemingly formidable goal, we have directed our efforts toward one of the severe manifestations confronting many patients. This problem concerns local recurrence of sigmoid colon-rectal cancer in the pelvic and perineal areas following definitive surgery.

The logic for a regional approach in dealing with sigmoid colon-rectal carcinoma is based on certain clinical features. First, approximately 50% of these tumors are in the rectum and 65-70% in the combined sigmoid colon-rectal region. Secondly, separate reports agree that local recurrence is greater for neoplasms arising below the peritoneal reflection than above this level[2]. Thirdly, it has been confirmed that local recurrence increases progressively in the sigmoid colon-rectal segment with closer proximity to the anus.

Colon cancer is more favorably treated when found proximal to the sigmoid colon, partially due to the feasibility of performing a wider surgical excision and more complete regional lymphadenectomy. Local recurrences are thought to be higher in the sigmoid colon and rectum because of the rich plexuses of veins and nerves of this region, lack of a protective peritoneal wall below the peritoneal reflection, and the common finding of a large tumor confined to a rigid pelvis with attendant difficult in performing a wide surgical resection.

The problem of local recurrence is reported to be as high as 23% to 34% for neoplasms below the peritoneal reflection and 3.6% to 10.8% for those above this level, but confined to the sigmoid colon or rectum[3]. While some of these patients also have distant disease not amendable to regional treatment measures, others have only recurrence of local disease and its associated symptoms of pain, urinary bladder dysfunction, and bowel obstruction.

Radiotherapy as an adjunct to the surgical management of sigmoid colon-rectal carcinoma dates back approximately 60 years, although most experience in this approach has been in the past two decades. Combining radiotherapy with surgery became feasible with improved utilization of high-dose techniques in radiotherapy. Allen and Fletcher found no recurrences in 50 patients treated preoperatively with 5000 rads[4]. A study using 2000-2500 rads prior to abdominoperineal resection showed an improvement in local recurrences from 40% to 27%[5]. Small amounts of subclinical disease, considered to be present but not apparent in wounds following definitive surgical treatment, require 4500-5000 rads delivered in 5 weeks for eradication[6]. We have employed this in the postoperative period as a means to reduce the potential for local recurrence of sigmoid colon-rectal carcinoma.

MATERIALS AND METHODS

Patients were selected for adjunctive radiotherapy based on having resectable lesions penetrating the entire bowel wall and/or metastatic disease to regional lymph nodes (Withers, H.R. and Romsdahl, M.M., unpublished). Individuals with evidence of distant metastases at the time of surgery and residual local disease were not included in this program. Control subjects forming a comparison group were patients formerly treated at The University of Texas System Cancer Center since 1969 and receiving surgery alone or surgery with adjunctive chemotherapy or chemoimmunotherapy.

Patients: Fifty patients were treated by radiotherapy in the postoperative period, beginning 3-8 weeks following the operative procedure. Abdominoperineal resection and anterior resection of the sigmoid colon-rectum were the most commonly employed surgical procedures. A Hartman Procedure (leaving a short distal rectal segment), local excision, and posterior exenteration were utilized in a small number of patients.

The extent of disease in this patient population is further appreciated by analyses of the resected surgical specimens. Twenty-seven or 49 specimens showed metastatic disease in regional lymph nodes while 40 of 49 subjects had disease extending into the pericolic fat or adventical tissue. One patient had a solitary metastatic nodule in the liver which was resected and another metastatic disease to the skin in the perianal region.

While this study included primarily patients receiving their initial treatment at The University of Texas System Cancer Center M. D. Anderson Hospital, two were managed for local recurrence after primary surgical treatment outside our institution. Another patient received radiotherapy after abdominoperineal resection was performed in another hospital, leaving residual tumor in the pelvis. The remaining 47 patients received their initial surgical treatment at M. D. Anderson Hospital.

Radiotherapy: Following abdominoperineal resection, the usual radiotherapy was 4500 rads central midline in 25 fractions through anterior-posterior fields using 25 MV x-rays. The upper margin was mid L5 with the lower margin to include the perineum. Subsequently, 1000 rads in 4 fractions was given using a perineal field and the ^{60}Co unit.

After anterior resection procedures, 4500 rads central midline dose in 25 fractions was given through anterior-posterior fields using 25 MV x-rays. The upper margin was mid L5 and the lower margin the inferior aspect of the obturator foramen. Thereupon 600 rads was delivered as a central midline dose in 4 fractions using a reduced posterior field and the ^{60}Co unit. Some patients with substantially large, but resectable, tumors had surgical clips applied to areas deemed most suspect for recurrence of disease. These areas were then considered in the radiotherapy delivered to a reduced field (Plate 1).

This technique varied in certain circumstances although it was the method employed for most patients. During the initial period of this program, 12 patients were treated with extended fields, 8 extending to include L4 and 4 extending to the level of L2. The remaining patients were treated to the pelvis only and this is our current policy.

RESULTS

The patients in this analysis have been entered regularly over a period of 2 to 60 months with a median follow-up period of approximately 28 months.

Local Recurrence: During the period of this program, disease in the pelvis has been controlled in 48 of 50 patients for a local recurrence rate of 4% at this point in time. Recurrence of carcinoma in the treated volume occurred only in 2 patients, both with penetrating lesions extending into adjacent fibroadipose tissue and metastatic disease in regional lymph nodes. Patients in the comparison group, during this same period of observation and as determined by Kaplan-Meier plots of local control as a function of time since curative surgery, showed 20% local recurrence for penetrating lesions without involved lymph nodes, 45% recurrence for penetrating lesions with tumor involved lymph nodes, and a 50%

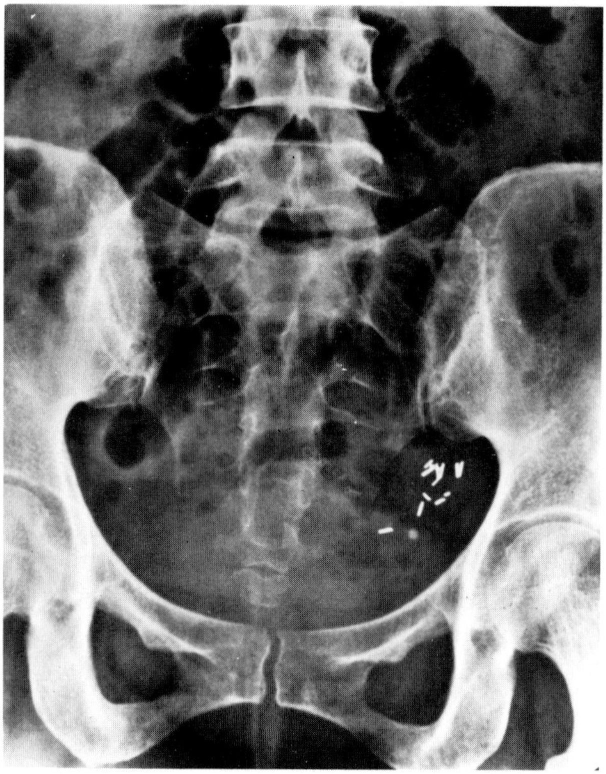

Plate 1. Following resection of a large pelvic tumor, the area in closest proximity to the pelvic wall of this patient was identified with metallic clips. These serve to insure inclusion of this area in the treatment field and planning boosts to reduced fields.

local recurrence rate for lesions involving adjacent organs such as the vagina, uterus, urinary bladder, or prostate—with or without involved regional lymph nodes.

Metastatic Disease and Survival: Eight of the 50 treated patients have developed metastatic disease. Of these 8 subjects, 7 did not develop symptoms characteristic of pelvic recurrence nor was pelvic disease a prominent feature in 3 autopsies performed. The remaining patient developed pain in the pelvis during postoperative radiotherapy which continue until he expired with abdominal carcinomatosis 6 months following abdominoperineal resection.

Six of the 50 individuals included in this adjunctive radiotherapy series have expired at the time of this analysis. One individual succumbed due to severe radiation enteritis and consequent bowel obstruction, perforation, and sepsis. No evidence of carcinoma was found on autopsy. Four patients died from problems arising from metastatic disease, but with local regional control of sigmoid colon-rectal carcinoma. The remaining patient died primarily of metastatic disease and carcinomatosis, but without control of pain in the pelvic region.

TABLE I

PRELIMINARY OBSERVATIONS FOLLOWING SURGERY AND ADJUNCTIVE RADIOTHERAPY FOR SIGMOID COLON-RECTAL CARCINOMA

Number of patients	50	
Current clinical status*		
No evident disease		40
Pelvic area controlled		48
Metastatic disease		8
Radiation enteritis		4
Expired		6

* Median follow-up period: 28 months.

Complications of Treatment: The major problem associated with adjunctive postoperative radiotherapy has been radiation enteritis and associated small bowel obstruction. The use of radiotherapy, being a regional therapeutic measure, is expected to affect small intestine which characteristically occupies the pelvis (Plate 2). Five patients developed this complication with 4 requiring a surgical procedure as part of their management. Of these 4, 3 received central midline doses of 4000-4600 rads utilizing fields extending cephalad to the top of L4 in addition to a boost dose to the pelvis through anterior-posterior or perineal portals. The remaining fourth patient requiring surgery for radiation enteritis and bowel obstruction received 4450 rads central midline dose to a field with a superior border near the top of L2, followed by a pelvic boost dose of 1000 rads. While these 4 patients were found to be free of

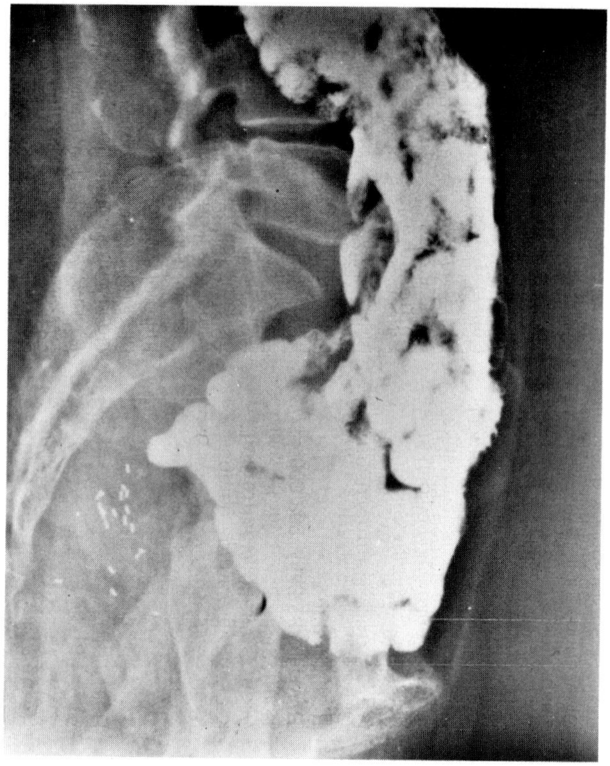

Plate 2. Metallic clips in the presacral region indicate the area in closest proximity to rectal carcinoma surgically treated by abdominoperineal resection. A study of the small bowel, using barium, demonstrates its position in relation to the pelvis.

metastatic disease at the time of surgery for radiation enteritis, one subsequently developed a recurrence in the pelvis. One patient, whose treatment field extended to the top of L2, became obstructed with inelastic and friable bowel unsuitable for intestinal by-pass procedures and died of perforation and peritonitis. These 4 patients developing radiation enteritis and bowel obstruction were included in the 12 patients treated through extended fields. Consequently, we have elected to discontinue radiation therapy at these doses outside the pelvis.

Three patients developed radiation cystitis and associated hematuria which was of a transient nature and requiring no specific measures.

There were no cutaneous or perineal complications arising from the employment of radiotherapy.

DISCUSSION

The results of this preliminary study suggest that the combined modalities of surgery and radiotherapy may result in a decrease in local or regional recurrence of sigmoid colon-rectal carcinoma in the pelvis. The follow-up periods are somewhat short to make an accurate assessment of the value of this approach in management. Local recurrence of carcinoma in the pelvis, when it occurs, is a substantial problem both for the patient and the physician. Discomfort and pain preclude carrying out normal activities of daily living and the physician has great difficulty in eliminating symptoms by the usual measures available for this purpose. Prophylactic measures to avoid this problem appear highly desirable; however, further follow-up observations will be needed to assess the true value of this measure for advanced sigmoid colon-rectal carcinoma. Moreover, it is necessary that the advantages of preventing potential pelvic recurrences in patients undergoing 'curative' surgery are not substituted for radiation enteritis and related complications.

Experience arising from this program suggests that it is probably necessary to deliver approximately 5000 rads in 25-30 fractions to obtain high probability of control for subclinical colon carcinoma following 'curative' surgery. Intestinal complications appear to increase when larger fields are treated and the dose is greater than 4500-5000 rads in 25-30 fracticns. Consequently, the margin between therapeutic effective doses and doses leading to complications appear very narrow. Further evaluation of treated patients and optimal implementation of radiotherapy techniques will help determine the value of this adjunctive measure for sigmoid colon-rectal carcinoma.

REFERENCES

1. American Cancer Society (1975) Cancer Facts and Figures '76, 8-14
2. Gilchrist, R.K. and David, V.C. (1947) Ann. Surg. 126, 421-439
3. Southwick, H.W. and Cole, W.H. (1955) S. Chn. North America 35, 1363-1372
4. Allen, C.V. and Fletcher, W.S. (1972) Am. J. Roentgenol. 114, 504-508
5. Higgins, G.A., Conn, J.H., Jordan, P.H., Humphrey, E.W., Roswit, B., and Keehn, R.J. (1975) Ann. Surg., 181, 624-631
6. Fletcher, G.H., Lindberg, R.D., Tapley, N.duV., Guillamondegul, O.M., Byers, R.M., Perez, C.A., and Gunderson, L.L. (1976) Current Problems in Cancer 1(5), 3-4

Section V

GENITOURINARY AND GYNECOLOGIC CANCER

Adjuvant Therapy of Cancer, S.E. Salmon and S.E. Jones eds.

THE MULTIMODALITY MANAGEMENT OF TESTICULAR TERATOMAS

M.J. Peckham, W. Hendry, T.J. McElwain, F.M.M. Calman
Royal Marsden Hospital and
Institute of Cancer Research
Sutton, Surrey (England)

INTRODUCTION

In attempting to define a rational basis for combining chemotherapy, radiotherapy and surgery in the management of malignant disease it is relevant to pose three questions:

1. In what circumstances should combined therapy be considered?
2. What form should chemotherapy, radiotherapy and surgery take?
3. How best should these three treatment methods be integrated?

The objective of this paper is to consider the range of clinical and biological problems posed by teratomas of the testis and to outline an integrated policy of management. Although the data discussed in this report relate to patients managed by orchidectomy and radiotherapy, the concepts discussed are equally relevant to patients treated by orchidectomy and node dissection with or without subsequent irradiation. It is not proposed to attempt to review the extensive literature in this field which is referred to in more detail in two recent reviews (Peckham & McElwain, 1975[1] and Peckham, 1976[2]).

PATIENTS AND METHODS

Histology

The histological classification employed is that described by Pugh (1976)[3]. The corresponding histological categories of Dixon and Moore (1952)[4] are indicated in parenthesis.

Teratoma differentiated (excluded from this analysis)

Malignant teratoma, intermediate (MTI) (Teratocarcinoma)

Malignant teratoma, undifferentiated (MTU) (Embryonal carcinoma)

Malignant teratoma, trophoblastic (MTT) (Choriocarcinoma)

Staging classification

Stage I	Negative lymphogram, no metastases detected elsewhere	
Stage IIA	Positive lymphogram, with small volume node metastases ($\leqslant$2 cm maximum diameter). No metastases elsewhere	
Stage IIB	Positive lymphogram, bulky metastases ($>$ 2 cm maximum diameter). No metastases elsewhere	
Stage III	Nodes involved above and below diaphragm	A small volume B bulky disease
Stage IV	Minimal lung ($\leqslant$ 4 metastases)	A small volume nodal metastases B large volume nodal metastases
Stage IV	Advanced lung ($>$ 4 metastases)	
Stage IV	Extrathoracic (liver, bone, brain, etc.)	

Staging protocol

Staging includes lymphography, ultrasonic scanning of liver and para-aortic region, CT scanning of liver and para-aortic region (in selected patients), intravenous pyelography, whole lung tomography and measurement of serum alphafoeto protein (AFP) and human chorionic gonadotrophin (HCG) levels. Laparoscopy is performed in selected patients.

Radiotherapy

Radiotherapy to ipsilateral pelvic and para-aortic nodes using 6 or 8 MeV photons is routinely employed in Stage I patients. In Stage IIA patients the mediastinal and supraclavicular nodes are irradiated subsequently. In Stages IIB, III and IV a flexible and individualized radiotherapeutic approach is essential (*vide infra*). A minimum tumour dose of 4,000 rads is employed in Stage I patients and, using multiple fields and progressive reduction of target volume, 5,000 rads to involved nodes in Stage IIA. Irradiation is given at a rhythm of 800 - 1,000 rads/week.

Chemotherapy

Between 1962 and 1971 actinomycin D as a single agent was employed for Stage IV or relapsed patients. Since 1972 a variety of regimes have been investigated including vinblastine, actinomycin D and methotrexate (McElwain & Peckham, 1974[5]). Imidazole carboxamide and adriamycin (DTIC 70 mgm/m^2 days 1 - 5 IV, adriamycin 40 mgm/m^2 day 1, repeated 3 - 4 weeks), high dose cyclophosphamide (Buckner et al, 1974[6]), vinblastine and bleomycin, using the VB-3 regime of Samuels et al (1976)[7] and Cis-platinum diammino dichloride (50 - 130 mgm/m^2 IV with 24 hour forced diuresis).

Surgery

Radical node dissection as a primary procedure has not been performed on patients in this series. Surgical exploration with excision of residual disease after radiotherapy and chemotherapy is being employed to an increasing extent.

Patients

Details on 275 patients treated for testicular teratoma at the Royal Marsden Hospital between 1962 and 1975 form the basis for this report. The breakdown according to stage and histology is shown in Table 1.

TABLE 1

Stage		Histology		
		MTI	MTU	MTT
I	110	57	51	2
II	44	20	23	1
III	16	6	9	1
IV	105	26	73	6
	275	109	156	10

RESULTS OF TREATMENT AND IMPLICATIONS FOR FUTURE MANAGEMENT

In attempting to define in what circumstances combined therapy should be considered it is necessary to categorize the deficiencies of more classical approaches to treatment which involve orchidectomy followed by either nodal irradiation, surgical extirpation or both.

Of the entire group 132 (48%) are alive. Figure 1 shows survival according to stage. The majority of deaths occurred within the first two years and approximately 20% of Stage I, 40% of Stage II and 80% of Stage III and IV patients have died of their disease.

Examination of the survival of Stage I patients in relation to histology (Figure 2) shows that93% of MTI patients are alive compared with 67% of MTU patients (the difference is significant $p = < .01$). No significant differences in survival in relation to histology are present in Stages II, III and IV.

SURVIVAL OF PATIENTS WITH TESTICULAR TERATOMA
ROYAL MARSDEN HOSPITAL (1962-1975)

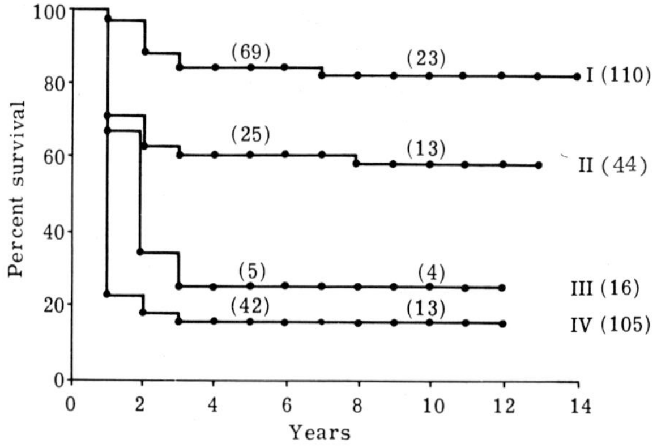

Fig. 1.

SURVIVAL OF PATIENTS TREATED WITH ORCHIDECTOMY AND NODAL IRRADIATION FOR STAGE I MALIGNANT TESTICULAR TERATOMA
ROYAL MARSDEN HOSPITAL (1962-1975)

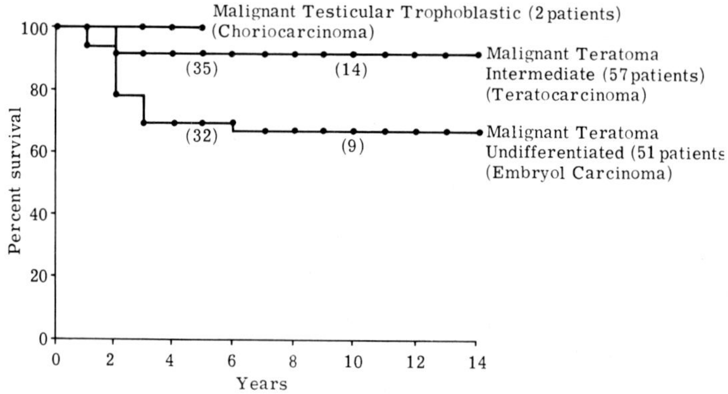

Fig. 2.

Figure 3 shows the survival of Stage II patients subdivided into A and B according to tumour volume. Stage IIA survival results are comparable to Stage I whereas the prognosis for IIB is significantly worse ($p < .01$). The poor prognosis in the latter group, most of whom have palpable bulky tumour producing ureteric displacement, can be correlated with a high local recurrence rate after irradiation. We have previously shown that metastatic volume is an important determinant of radiation control probability, an observation which has important implications for clinical management (Tyrrell & Peckham, 1976[8]).

The pattern of relapse in Stages I and IIA patients is shown in Figure 4. Of 42 relapses only one patient had an abdominal node recurrence. In 32 instances (76%) metastases were present in mediastinal or neck nodes and/or lungs. There were four scrotal relapses, one in liver and brain and three in bone. Figure 5 shows that 80% of relapses had occurred by one year.

From these observations we can conclude that approximately 20% of Stages I and IIA patients harbour occult metastases outside the retroperitoneal area *ab initio* and that in most cases these become apparent in supradiaphragmatic nodes and lung.

The prospective identification of the 'occult Stage IV' patient

Histology is an inadequate prognostic indicator and as yet there are no available pathological staging data (cord and tunica infiltration, vascular and lymphatic permeation) in adequately clinically staged patients. Two tumour markers AFP and HCG are available. Figure 6 shows post-orchidectomy pre-irradiation AFP levels in Stages I and II patients. 9/33 (27%) Stage I patients, 3/8 (38%) Stage IIA and 9/12 (75%) Stage IIB patients had elevated titres. Ideally more than one measurement should be made before and after orchidectomy, since an elevated titre due to the primary tumour falls within a half time of six days following orchidectomy (Figure 7). From these limited observations there is no clear correlation between an initially elevated titre and subsequent prognosis (Figure 8). Limited experience with an immunoperoxidase technique for demonstrating β-HCG in the primary tumour sections has shown no clear correlation with subsequent clinical behaviour.

SURVIVAL OF STAGE II TESTICULAR TERATOMA PATIENTS
ROYAL MARSDEN HOSPITAL (1964-1975)

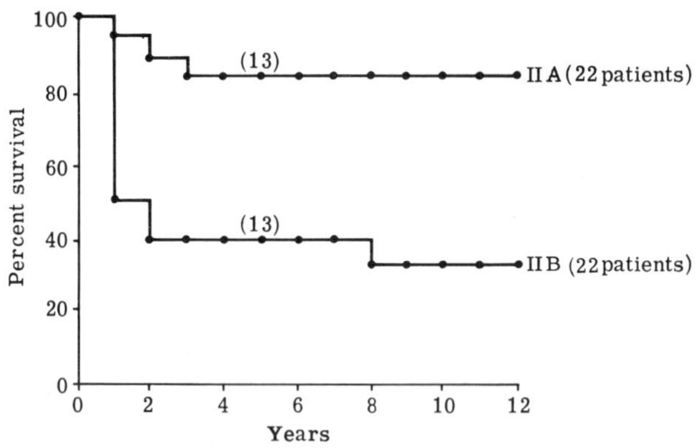

Fig. 3.

SITES OF RELAPSE IN STAGE I AND IIA TESTICULAR
TERATOMA PATIENTS TREATED BY ORCHIDECTOMY
AND NODAL IRRADIATION

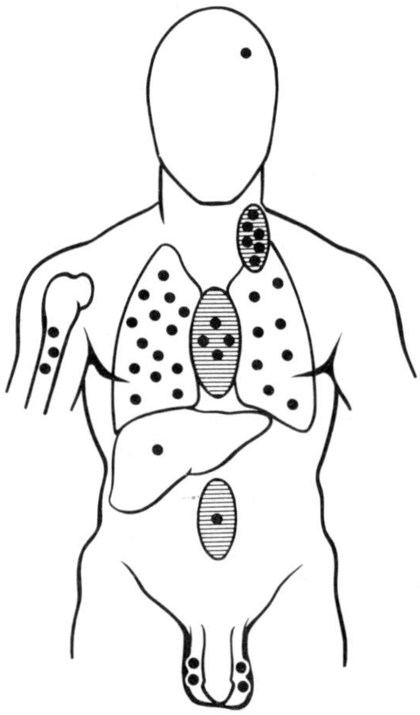

Fig. 4.

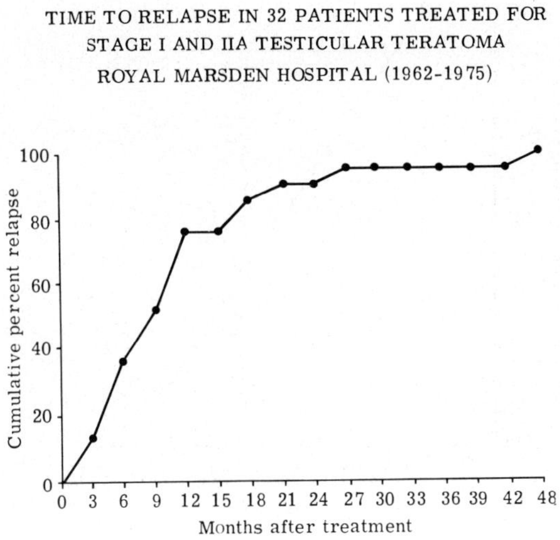
TIME TO RELAPSE IN 32 PATIENTS TREATED FOR
STAGE I AND IIA TESTICULAR TERATOMA
ROYAL MARSDEN HOSPITAL (1962-1975)
Cumulative percent relapse
100
80
60
40
20
0
0 3 6 9 12 15 18 21 24 27 30 33 36 39 42 48
Months after treatment

Fig. 5.

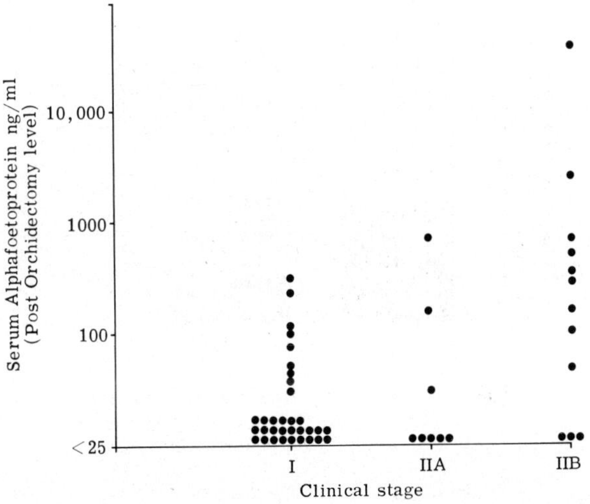
Serum Alphafoetoprotein ng/ml
(Post Orchidectomy level)
10,000
1000
100
<25
I
IIA
IIB
Clinical stage

Fig. 6.

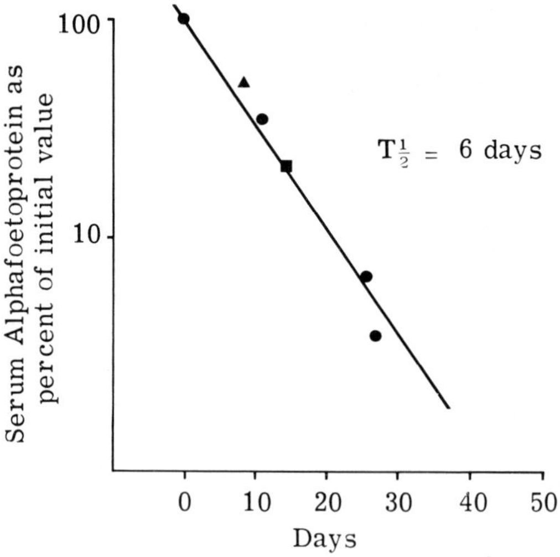

Fig. 7. Serum alphafoeto protein levels (as % of initial titre) in three patients following orchidectomy

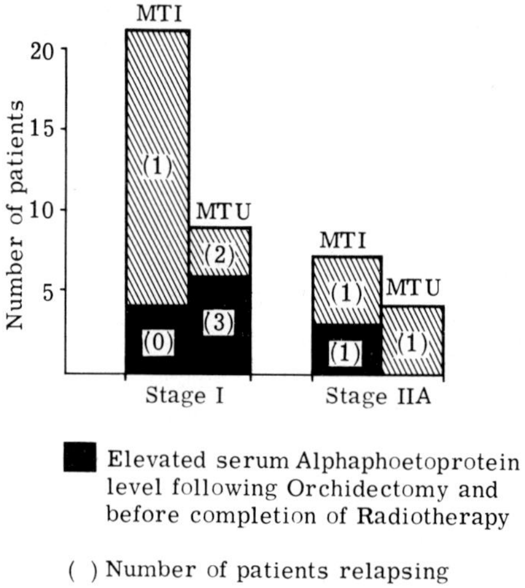

Fig. 8.

AN INTEGRATED APPROACH

In our experience complete responses with combination chemotherapy have been low; (vinblastine, actinomycin D and methotrexate 7/42 patients (17%); DTIC/adriamycin 3/13 patients (23%); vinblastine, bleomycin 3/20 (15%) and Cis-platinum diammino dichloride 3/14 (21%)). Samuels et al (1976)[7] have reported complete responses in 45/107 patients (42%) treated with vinblastine and bleomycin.

Thus, despite intensive efforts to eradicate disease in Stage IV patients only 13 patients of a total of 105 treated between 1962 and 1975 are surviving. Of this small group two had surgery, three pulmonary irradiation, five combined chemotherapy and pulmonary irradiation and one actinomycin D, one vinblastine/bleomycin and one vinblastine, actinomycin D and methotrexate. However, despite the disappointing results in terms of survival, impressive tumour regression can be achieved with combination chemotherapy. Samuels et al (1976)[7] have reached similar conclusions regarding the definition of at-risk categories. In their experience with the vinblastine/bleomycin combination the complete response rates in patients with minimal lung disease were excellent (9/11 patients) whereas in patients with bulky abdominal nodal metastases results were poor (3/17). It appears essential on the basis of the clinical evidence to hand to integrate drugs, radiation and surgery in selected categories of patients.

Stages I and IIA

The classical treatment comprising orchidectomy and nodal irradiation cures 80% of patients with minimal morbidity, preservation of potency and (in many men) of fertility. Limited data on the energetic treatment of patients detected clinically or with tumour markers early in relapse suggests that at least half may be reclaimed. Patients relapsing with cervical nodes are treated by excisional biopsy, vinblastine/bleomycin, using the Samuels' regime and Cis-platinum diammino dichloride. If supradiaphragmatic irradiation has not been given this is employed subsequently and electively when the patient is in complete clinical and marker remission. If there is minimal lung disease ($\leqslant$ 4 metastases) the metastatic sites are irradiated after chemotherapy. Whole lung irradiation has not so far been given when bleomycin is used.

Conclusions in Stages I and IIA

Although approximately 1/5 patients in these stage categories are in 'occult stage' III or IV, there is no clear way of identifying this group at the outset. All Stage I MTU and Stage IIA patients should be seen monthly for the first year, have lung tomography on alternate visits and monthly AFP and β-HCG titres. Vigorous therapy (*vide infra*) in early relapse offers the best chance for tumour eradication.

Stages IIB, III and IV patients

Survival results are poor, with 24/143 (16.7%) patients currently alive. A multimodality approach must be considered in all these categories.

(a) Infradiaphragmatic bulky nodal metastases

Irradiation as a primary or sole treatment method should be abandoned. These patients are usually beyond the scope of surgical resection and a drug/radiation/surgery policy is advocated.

(b) Bulky supradiaphragmatic nodal metastases pose similar problems treatment necessarily placing more reliance on drugs and radiation, particularly with mediastinal adenopathy.

(c) Minimal lung disease

Approximately 40% of selected patients with limited lung metastases have been reported curable with radiotherapy (Van der Werf Messing, 1976[9]). An occasional patient is curable by resection. In this category of patient it is appropriate to consider chemotherapy combined with radiotherapy and possibly surgery.

(d) Multiple lung metastases

This is essentially a chemotherapeutic problem. However, the following points may be noted:

1. Bulky metastases (nodal or lung) will pose the same problem as shown for Stage IIB and require surgery and/or irradiation.

2. Brain metastases may eventually prove to be a problem as chemotherapy control rates improve.

3. In a small group of MTI patients we have had encouraging results with chemotherapy and pulmonary irradiation (*vide infra*).

(e) Stage IV, liver, bone or brain

These patients have a very poor prognosis and it is doubtful whether the multimodality approach has more than a palliative role.

Stage IIB

As much information as possible about the extent and position of the tumour mass is acquired using ultrasonography, intravenous pyelography, lymphography and CT scanning. Laparoscopy is performed if there is any suspicion of liver metastases.

Serum markers are measured and in this and other advanced categories a pilot study of AFP levels in the cerebrospinal fluid is being carried out. Treatment is initiated with chemotherapy (vinblastine, bleomycin followed by Cis-platinum diammino dichloride). If regression is not achieved the drug approach may be switched to an alternative regime (DTIC/adriamycin (MTI), vinblastine, actinomycin D, methotrexate (MTU)) if the mass is considered too large for radiation therapy. Following chemotherapy radiotherapy is given to the para-aortic and pelvic nodes and an elective surgical exploration performed four to six weeks later. This is shown schematically in Figure 9 and Figure 10 summarizes results in a small group of eight patients with extensive abdominal node metastases who have undergone surgical resection after irradiation ± chemotherapy. A similar approach is adopted in Stage III although abdominal surgery is clearly not indicated if there is uncontrolled bulky supradiaphragmatic, particularly mediastinal, nodal involvement.

Stage IV

In the minimal lung group associated with small volume nodal metastases, chemotherapy is employed initially and followed by nodal and lung metastatic irradiation. In patients with pulmonary metastases radiotherapy planning is carried out before chemotherapy is initiated so that subsequent irradiation can be delivered accurately.

When multiple metastases are present whole lung irradiation is not worth-while unless chemotherapy achieves complete radiological clearance. Thus of 16 patients irradiated after partial remission only one patient remains alive, whereas of six patients achieving complete remission four are alive and disease-free. All four patients had MTI tumours, three received DTIC and adriamycin and the fourth one course of DTIC alone. The latter patient developed an endobronchial deposit 12 months later which was treated with further irradiation and DTIC. He remains disease-free at 34 months. Two patients are disease-free at 32 months and the fourth at eight months. The survival of patients with minimal lung disease treated

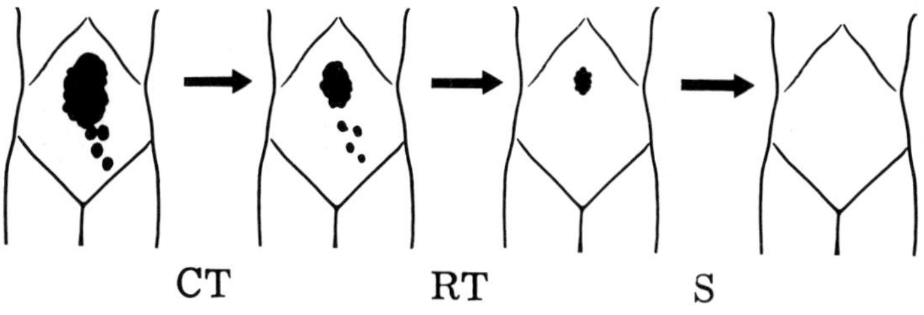

Fig. 9. Schema of combined chemotherapy (CT) radiotherapy (RT) and surgical (S) approach for Stage IIB teratomas

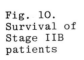

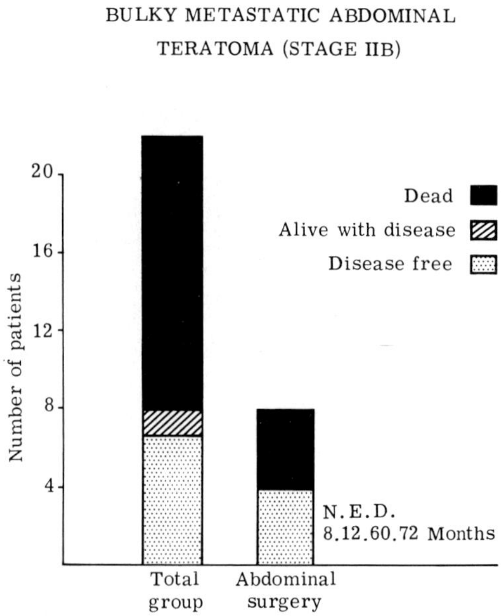

Fig. 10. Survival of Stage IIB patients

(NED = no evidence of disease)

with lung irradiation with or without chemotherapy and of patients with multiple metastases treated after chemotherapeutic complete remission is shown in Figure 11. Sequential pulmonary function studies have been carried out on all patients receiving pulmonary irradiation and chemotherapy and the results will form the subject of a separate publication. However, it can be said that an enhanced response of the lung to radiation was observed in three patients receiving drugs with or immediately before irradiation (cyclophosphamide, actinomycin D, DTIC and adriamycin) whereas there was no evidence that a variety of drugs (including actinomycin D) exerted an influence upon the response of the lung to radiation if a gap of 30 days or more elapsed between chemotherapy and radiotherapy. The schematic approach is illustrated in Figure 12.

CONCLUSIONS

1. Small volume nodal metastases from testicular teratoma are readily eradicated by moderate doses of radiation (4,000 to 5,000 rads). Patient selection, careful treatment planning and close monitoring on follow-up result in a good prognosis for Stages I and IIA patients.

2. There is a volume related tumour control probability with radiation and almost certainly with chemotherapy. For bulky nodal disease whether alone or in association with disease at other sites a policy of chemotherapy followed by irradiation and finally by surgical exploration and excision of residual tumour appears logical and is being explored.

3. In the lung it appears highly likely that metastatic volume is an important determinant of response to therapy both with drugs and radiation. This argues for early detection of relapse and immediate initiation of therapy. Limited data suggest that volume reduction with chemotherapy followed by pulmonary irradiation can be curative in situations where either modality alone would not be expected to eradicate tumour. Although tumour markers are useful in follow-up for the detection of relapse they have not so far proved to be of value for the identification of patients harbouring occult metastases at the time of primary treatment.

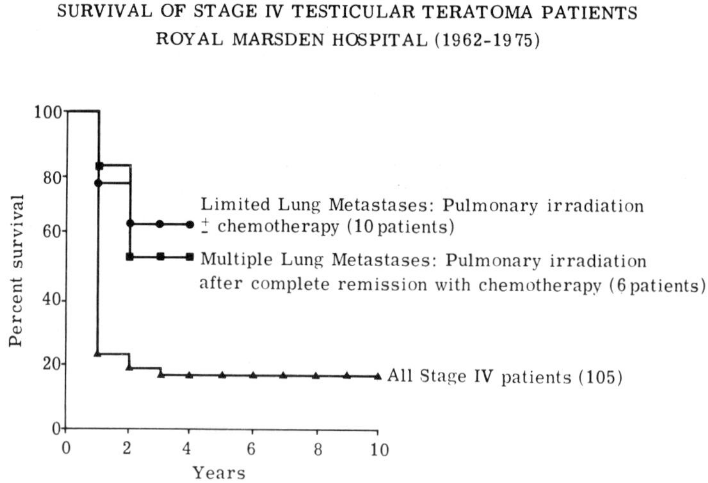

Fig. 11.

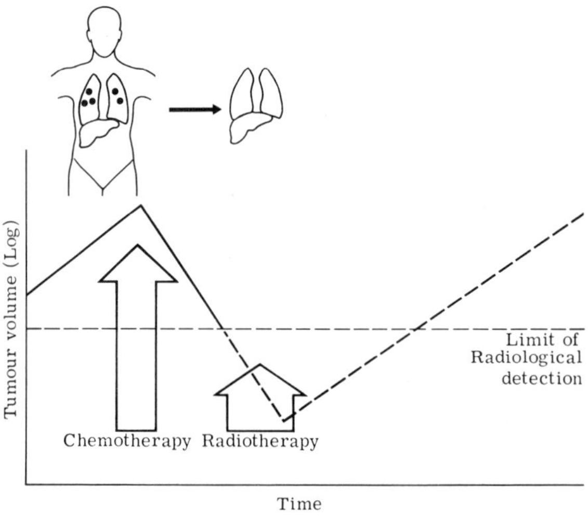

Fig. 12. Schema of combined drug/radiation approach for Stage IV (lung) teratoma

ACKNOWLEDGEMENTS

We are grateful to the many surgeons and radiotherapists who have referred patients to the Testicular Tumour Unit. We are also grateful to Miss Marion Anderson for preparing the manuscript.

REFERENCES

1. Peckham, M.J. and McElwain, T.J. (1975)
Testicular tumours.
Clinics in Endocrinology and Metabolism 4, 665-692

2. Peckham, M.J. (1976)
Testicular tumour response to irradiation and chemotherapy.
In Scientific Foundations of Urology II. Ed. D. Innes Williams and G.D. Chisholm. Publ. William Heinemann, London. pp 400-409

3. Pugh, R.C.B. (1976)
Testicular tumours - The panel classification
In Pathology of the Testis. Ed. R.C.B. Pugh. Publ. Blackwell Scientific Publications, London. pp 144-146

4. Dixon, F.J. and Moore, R.A. (1952)
Tumours of the male sex organs.
In Atlas of Tumor Pathology. Armed Forces Institute of Pathology, Washington, D.C., 8 fasc. 31b & 32

5. McElwain, T.J. and Peckham, M.J. (1974)
Combination chemotherapy for testicular tumours.
Proceedings of the Royal Society of Medicine 67, 297-300

6. Buckner, C.D., Clift, R.A., Fefer, A., Funk, D.D., Glucksberg,H., Neiman, P.E., Paulsen, A., Storb, R. and Thomas, E.D. (1974)
High-dose cyclophosphamide (NSC-26271) for the treatment of metastatic testicular neoplasms.
Cancer Chemotherapy Reports 58, 709-714

7. Samuels, M.L., Lanzotti, V.J., Holoye, P.Y., Boyle, L.E., Smith, T.L. and Johnson, D.E. (1976)
Combination chemotherapy in germinal cell tumors.
Cancer Treatment Reviews 3, 185-204

8. Tyrrell, C.J. and Peckham, M.J. (1976)
The response of lymph node metastases of testicular teratoma to radiation therapy.
British Journal of Urology 48, 363-370

9. Van der Werf Messing, B. (1976)
Radiotherapeutic treatment of testicular tumors.
International Journal of Radiation Oncology, Biology, Physics 1, 235-248

Adjuvant Therapy of Cancer, S.E. Salmon and S.E. Jones eds.
© 1977 Elsevier/North-Holland Biomedical Press, Amsterdam

TRIPLE THERAPY AS AN ADJUVANT TO TESTICULAR CANCER SURGERY[+]

Fred J. Ansfield, M.D.* and Guillermo Ramirez, M.D.**

SUMMARY

We observed salutary responses in advanced testicular cancers other than seminoma with the use of the Li et al regimen consisting of actinomycin D, chlorambucil, and methotrexate. As a result beginning 14 years ago all patients who had testicular cancer surgery were given this combination as an adjuvant. Of the 32 patients who received this adjuvant therapy, 78% are alive with no evidence of disease for periods of more than 4 to 12 years. This includes 4/4 patients who had choriocarcinoma, 11/17 embryonal cell cancer, and 10/11 teratocarcinoma. No patient received post-operative radiotherapy.

INTRODUCTION

In 1960 our first publication [1] on the preliminary therapeutic results with Mithramycin reported two dramatic regressions in patients with advanced embryonal cell testis cancer and one minor response in a case of choriocarcinoma. Because the following 12 cases of testicular cancer failed on this drug and the severe toxicity that resulted with our dosage regimen, a switch was made to triple therapy as published by Li et al [2], also in 1960. About two years after observing salutary results with this combination in advanced testicular cancer, a decision was made to offer it as adjuvant therapy to all patients following testicular cancer surgery other than those with seminoma.

MATERIALS AND METHODS

The dosage schedule we used in both groups, those with advanced disease and those with no known remaining disease was similar to that given by Li et al with several exceptions. Instead of a standard actinomycin D dose of 0.5 mg daily used by the latter, we employed 10γ/kg/day which in almost all cases exceeded the 0.5 mg dose. More recently instead of administering 10 mg chlorambucil daily, 8 mg were given most patients except large men who still received 10 mg daily.

In patients who did not have a lymphadenectomy after the diagnosis was established, triple therapy was initiated about 7-10 days after resection of the testicle and spermatic cord If the patient had a lymph node dissection, two to three weeks and sometimes longer elapsed before

+ This investigation was supported in part by Grant Number CA-14520, awarded by the National Cancer Institute, DHEW to the Wisconsin Clinical Cancer Center

* Emeritus Professor in the Department of Human Oncology, University of Wisconsin, Madison, WI. Present address: 2315 No. Lake Dr., Milwaukee, WI 53211

** Associate Professor in the Department of Human Oncology, University of Wisconsin, Madison, WI 53706

Address for reprints: Guillermo Ramirez, M.D., Department of Human Oncology, University Hospitals, 1300 University Avenue, Madison, WI 53706

healing was sufficiently advanced for aggressive chemotherapy to be initiated. Post-operative radiotherapy, although frequently requested by the referring physician, was always interdicted, as this would reduce the bone marrow potential to a level where strongly myelosuppressive chemotherapy could not be employed without hazard.

The planned dosage schedule was as follows: chlorambucil, 8 to 10 mg daily for 27 days; methotrexate, 5 mg daily for 27 days; actinomycin D, 10 γ/kg/day from days 3 through 7, 13 through 17, and 23 through 27. This was then followed by a rest period of two weeks and then by one week of chlorambucil and methotrexate, adding the actinomycin D on the last 5 days. Thereafter, this week of triple therapy was repeated with 21 to 30 day intervals between the seven days of treatment and this schedule was continued for one to two and one-half years.

The majority of patients in both groups, those with advanced disease and the adjuvant group, were unable to tolerate the 27-initial days of therapy without interruption because of the development of severe toxicity. If more than moderately severe nausea, vomiting, stomatitis, diarrhea, bleeding, or leukopenia under 2,500/mm^3 or thrombocytopenia under 60,000/mm^3 developed the course was temporarily halted until the blood counts recovered to the above levels or the other moderately severe reactions abated somewhat. It was felt important not to wait until the WBC count recovered to 3,500/mm^3, for example, or the platelet count to 100,000/mm^3 or for the stomatitis to heal significantly before resuming the aggressive chemotherapy. It was observed that a WBC count which may have dropped to 1,000/mm^3 or under or a platelet count to 20,000/mm^3 or under at the peak of toxicity that return of the WBC count to a level of 2,500/mm^3 or the platelet count to 60,000/mm^3 were signals to immediately resume the chemotherapy. In these cases the recovery proceeded further despite reinstituting the 3-drug combination. It was observed fairly early in our experience in treating patients with disseminated testicular cancer that complete regressions that persisted occurred more frequently in patients treated very aggressively. A partial regression over a period of several months without continued further reductions in tumor size was, with rare exception, of little value as early reactivation was almost invariably the rule.

Despite the intentional production of moderately severe reactions which in a few instances progressed to severe or almost life-threatening toxicity, of the 76 patients in both groups so treated there were no toxic or drug-related deaths. Appropriate supportive therapy was administered as needed but these young vigorous adults, especially the group on adjuvant therapy, weathered the toxicity with minimal supportive requirements other than chlorpromazine orally or parenterally to control nausea and vomiting so that fluids and nourishment could be retained.

Patients were informed before therapy was initiated that unpleasant reactions would result from the chemotherapy but when the average patient recognized that the goal was hopefully a cure there were only three drop-outs as treatment was continued.

Early in our treatment of testicular cancer a number of patients were referred that did not have a node dissection. Chemotherapy was not postponed as delaying it for the time consumed in a lymphadenectomy may have outweighed any benefit that might have resulted from this major surgical procedure. Sufficient morbidity has occurred as a result of a lymph node dissection as wound dehiscence and internal ejaculation to question the net benefit from this surgery, especially since not all the nodes are found and removed. Moreover, Patton et al[3] in a series of 389 military personell whom they treated found that 24% of patients with embryonal cell carcinoma with negative nodes at lymphadenectomy and 26% with teratocarcinoma also with negative nodes died of their testicular cancers. Since 1964, however, all patients referred to us for adjuvant chemotherapy received node dissections by their surgeons. If a node dissection was not done, in more recent years we did lymphangiography. If no suspicious nodes were discernible, lymphadenectomy was by-passed and chemotherapy initiated.

As to the duration of administration of triple therapy, for patients with recurrent disseminated testicular cancer, other than seminoma, an effort was made to treat them for 2 1/2 years. After the first 27 days of therapy followed by a two-week rest period, then one week of treatment, patients thereafter were given three to four week rest periods between each one week of treatment during the first year providing a complete regression occurred. For the younger more stoic men who tolerated the week of treatment without serious discomfort, the three-week interval was selected, and in the others the four-week rest period. During the next 1 1/2 years, the interval between the one week courses of treatment was increased to five and later six weeks. If in two to three months continued regression did not occur a switch to other chemotherapy was made as a static condition was not considered useful.

The duration of treatment for patients given triple therapy as an adjuvant to surgery depended upon whether a node dissection was performed and the results. If none was done and the lymphangiograms were negative treatment was arbitrarily given for one year. If a lymphadenectomy yielded no positive nodes treatment was give for one year but if nodes were positive treatment was given for two years.

CLINICAL RESULTS

Forty-four patients with accurately measurable disseminated lesions were given triple therapy as above. Their tumor type, response, the number with less than 6 months improvement, survival and present status are shown in Table 1. Overall there was an 80% regression rate with a decrease in tumor size of at least 50%. Unfortunately far too many had reactivation in six months. Under survival, if two years did not elapse with a no evidence of disease (NED) status the likelihood of recurrence is still high.

Choriocarcinoma was the most responsive with 9/10 showing objective regressions but only two for longer than five years. Similarly although 18 of 22 patients with embryonal cell cancer improved, only two achieved a NED status for at least five years. In teratocarcinoma only one of eight remained tumor-free for longer than five years. Although these five patients have now survived over five years with no evidence of disease, this is only an 11% "cure" rate. This tends to confirm the observation that if a patient with testicular cancer is free of disease at two years following surgery, with rare exception, he can be considered "cured".

TABLE 1

CLINICAL RESULTS OF TRIPLE THERAPY IN DISSEMINATED TESTICULAR CANCER

Cell Type and No. Pts.	Objective Regressions	No. Pts. With < 6 Mos. Improvement	Survival - Mos. N.E.D.
Choriocarcinoma 10	9	4	158, 66, 19*, 13, 13, 7
Embryonal 22	18	8	106, 65, 17, 11, 10*, 9*, 8, 7*, 7, 2*
Teratocarcinoma 12	8	5	78, 21*, 9*
Totals	35/44 (80% response rate)		

* living, with tumor

Thirty-two patients were given triple therapy as an adjuvant to surgery (Table 2). Four had choriocarcinoma and all are alive NED for over 4 to 12 years. This is extremely significant as prior to triple therapy this disease was almost invariably fatal. Of 17 patients with embryonal cell cancer, 12 had node dissections, 7 of which were positive. Eleven of the 17 are tumor-free for more than 3 years. Of 11 with teratocarcinoma, 4 had positive nodes and 10 are alive NED for more than 3 years. This is in sharp contrast to 1/12 patients with disseminated teratocarcinoma that is in the NED status.

Twenty-seven patients with disseminated testicular cancer were treated at our institution by staff other than the authors and it was established at the outset that those patients were not to be included in this series. The treatment approach was entirely unlike that used in this study in terms of lack of aggressiveness. Treatment was withheld in these 27 patients if early visible stomatitis appeared or if the WBC count dropped to 3,500 or the platelet count to 80,000. Then retreatment was postponed until almost complete recovery from all of the toxic reactions.

TABLE 2

TRIPLE THERAPY AS AN ADJUVANT TO TESTICULAR CANCER SURGERY

Cell Type and No. Pts.	Node Dissection Done? And If So, Findings	Tumor-Free Duration	Present Status
Choriocarcinoma 4	No - 2 1 neg.; 1 pos.	38 mos. to 11 yrs.	All 4 living tumor free
Embryonal 17	No - 5 5 neg.; 7 pos.	10 pts. 2 to 10 yrs. 7 pts. < 2 yrs.	13 living 11 tumor free
Teratocarcinoma 11	No - 2 5 neg.; 4 pos.	8 pts. 2 to 10 yrs. 3 pts. < 2 yrs.	10 living tumor free

DISCUSSION

This concept of using a combination of drugs against solid tumors was the first and served as a forerunner in the newer attack against hematologic as well as solid tumor neoplastic malignancies. Today this combination is considered old-fashioned in sophisticated oncology circles. There is no question that the combination used by Samuels et al[4] with bleomycin plus vinblastine or their 5-drug combination of bleomycin, cyclophosphamide, vincristine, methotrexate and 5-fluorouracil produced a higher incidence of complete regressions than triple therapy as we used it, but not much higher and less than half of their patients reached the 2 year mark for follow-up. Also it was at a high price with 4 drug-related deaths in the 83 patients they treated. The median nadir of the leukocyte count in their series was 700/mm^3 but a number of their patients had prior chemo- or radiotherapy.

Cvitkovic et al[5] using a combination of potent compounds including Adriamycin and cis-platinum achieved 18/27 complete responses but the longest follow-up was only 6 months.

Vechinski et al[6] reported a 51% 5-year survival in a review article of a number of series totalling 699 patients with embryonal cell and teratocarcinoma of the testis treated with retroperitoneal node dissection and postoperative radiotherapy. Patients with choriocarcinoma were excluded but with their zero prognosis the 51% 5-year survival would be significantly reduced had they been included.

Several adjuvant studies with combination chemotherapy in testicular cancer have recently been instituted. However, until an approach is found that yields a higher salvage rate than the 78% obtained with the Li et al regimen used aggressively and for as long a period of follow-up, we see no indication to alter our course.

REFERENCES

1. Curreri, A. and Ansfield, F. (1960) Mithramycin--Human Toxicology and Preliminary Therapeutic Investigation. Cancer Chemotherapy Rep, 8:18-22.
2. Li, M., Whitmore, W. Jr., Golbey, R., and Grabstald, H. (1960) Effects of Combined Drug Therapy on Metastatic Cancer of the Testis. JAMA, 174:145-153.
3. Patton, J. and Mallis, N. (1959) Tumors of Testis. J. Urol., 81:457-461.
4. Samuels, M., Holoye, P., and Johnson, D. (1975) Bleomycin Combination Chemotherapy in the Management of Testicular Neoplasia. Cancer, 36:318-326.
5. Cvitkovic, E., Hayes, D., and Golbey, R. (1976) Primary Combination Chemotherapy (VAB III) for Metastatic or Unresectable Germ Cell Tumors. ASCO Abstracts No. C-237, page 296.
6. Vechinski, T., Jaeschke, W., and Vermund, H. (1965) Testicular Tumors: An Analysis of 112 Consecutive Cases. Am J of Roentgenology, Radium Therapy and Nuclear Medicine, 95:494-514.

Adjuvant Therapy of Cancer, S.E. Salmon and S.E. Jones eds.

ADJUVANT IMMUNOTHERAPY WITH BCG OF ADVANCED OVARIAN CANCER: A PRELIMINARY REPORT

David S. Alberts, M.D.
Section of Hematology & Oncology
University of Arizona College of Medicine
Tucson, Arizona 85724
For the Southwest Oncology Group

INTRODUCTION

The greater than 10,000 deaths per year from ovarian cancer makes it the most common gynecologic cancer killer. Despite improved surgical and radiotherapeutic methods, there appears to have been no change in overall survival patterns during the last three decades. The majority of patients with ovarian cancer of epithelial type (approximately 55%) have regional (i.e., stage III disease) or distant (i.e., stage IV) disease at the time of initial evaluation. The 5-year survival rate for these advanced cancer patients averages 7% (range, 6-16%) following surgery and radiation therapy or surgery and chemotherapy (range, 0-9%). Clearly, there is a need for new multimodality therapeutic approaches for this unfortunate group of patients.

While ovarian carcinomas of epithelial type are sensitive to a number of chemotherapeutic agents, treatment has not markedly prolonged median survival[1,2]. The combination of adriamycin and cyclophosphamide has been reported to induce a high percentage of partial remissions in patients with stages III and IV disease[2,3]. Unfortunately, remission duration is relatively short and it is still too early to determine whether this combination therapy will prolong survival.

One new direction for the therapy of ovarian carcinoma is the use of nonspecific immunostimulants, such as BCG or C. parvum, added to conventional chemotherapy regimens. The evidence for tumor associated antigens in ovarian cancer, the recognized relationship of immunocompetence to survival in this disease, and the positive experimental evidence for curative immunotherapy in mouse ovarian tumor models suggests that ovarian cancer may be amenable to the use of immunotherapeutic approaches[4-8].

The few published trials of immunotherapy in ovarian cancer patients include small numbers of patients and have not been randomized. Recently, Hudson et al. innoculated 10 patients with ovarian tumor cells mixed with BCG[9]. Patients selected had advanced ovarian cancers which had at least stabilized after a minimum of 3 months of conventional chemotherapy. Survival from the time of surgery was superior for the chemoimmunotherapy group compared to "matched" historical controls.

Wanebo et al. have carried out a randomized study of combination chemotherapy plus C. parvum versus combination chemotherapy alone in patients with alkylator resistant stage III and IV ovarian cancer[10]. Debulking surgery was attempted in 19 and radiation therapy in 12 of 38 patients entered into the study. Twenty patients were treated with a cyclophosphamide-adriamycin-5-fluorouracil (CAF) plus C. parvum regimen and 18 received only CAF. There was only 1 patient in complete remission for 53 weeks following the start of therapy in the CAF + C. parvum group versus 1 complete remission at 47 weeks and 2 partial remissions for 28 and 33 weeks in the CAF group of patients. At the time of evaluation (December, 1976), 9 patients had died in each group (median survival of 8 and 11 weeks for CAF + C. parvum and CAF, respectively). The addition of intravenous C. parvum to CAF did not improve the response rate, duration of remission, or short-term survival in alkylator resistant ovarian cancer patients.

Approximately 15 months ago the Southwest Oncology Group initiated a randomized study for the evaluation of BCG as an immune adjuvant to adriamycin-cyclophosphamide (AC) chemotherapy for patients with advanced ovarian cancers of epithelial type. The preliminary results of this study will be the focus of this paper.

PATIENTS AND METHODS

Starting in January, 1976 patients with recurrent (e.g. radiation therapy failures) or stages III and IV ovarian cancer of epithelial type who had measurable disease and had received no prior chemotherapy were entered into the Southwest Oncology Group Study 7524 (Figure 1, schema).

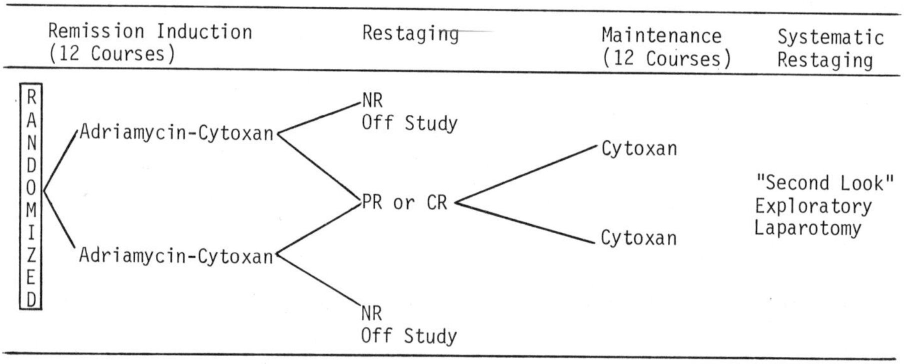

Figure 1. Treatment schema for Southwest Oncology Group Study 7524. See text for details.

Histopathologic review is conducted for all study cases. Patients with adequate bone marrow reserve (i.e. normal blood counts, no prior radiation therapy to the pelvis within the prior year, and age below 65) receive adriamycin (40 mg/M^2 intravenously) and cyclophosphamide (200 mg/M^2 daily for 4 days, orally) beginning two days after adriamycin administration. Patients with impaired bone marrow reserve (i.e. WBC less than 4,000/mm^3 or platelet count less than 125,000/mm^3, history of prior hematologic intolerance to radiation therapy, history of extensive pelvic or abdominal radiation therapy, or age over 65 years) receive adriamycin and cyclophosphamide at one half the usual dosage with gradual escalation of dosages on subsequent therapy courses as tolerated. At the time of registration, half the patients are assigned to receive Pasteur Institute BCG, 6 x 10^8 viable organisms by scarification to rotating upper and lower extremity sites on days 8 and 15 of each course of adriamycin-cyclophosphamide (AC) therapy. Courses of therapy are repeated at 3-4 week intervals depending upon tolerance to the myelosuppression caused by chemotherapy.

The adriamycin dosage is not to exceed a total of 500 mg/M^2 BSA but the cyclophosphamide or cyclophosphamide plus BCG therapy continues for a total of 2 years for those patients showing complete or partial response, improvement or stabilization of disease. In the case of severe skin reactivity or systemic symptoms (e.g. fever, chills, and weakness) related to BCG administration, immunotherapy is reduced to one scarification (day 15) in each course followed by reduction in individual BCG dose until it is tolerated. Patients continuing to experience significant systemic BCG toxicity are placed on daily isoniazid and pyridoxine therapy.

The prestudy evaluation includes routine hematologic tests and serum chemistries as well as chest x-ray, sigmoidoscopy, barium enema, intravenous pyelography and pericentesis and/or thoracentesis with cytologic evaluation as indicated. Where available, laparoscopy, abdominal and pelvic sonography, computerized axial tomography and whole-body radionuclide scanning are recommended for initial tumor localization and followup evaluation.

No patient is determined to be in complete remission unless a "second look" exploratory laparotomy shows no evidence of residual disease. Patients classified as having a partial remission must have at least a 50% or greater decrease in tumor mass and/or complete disappearance of proven malignant effusions for greater than one month. Patients who are classified as "improved" must have at least a 25%-49% reduction in tumor mass for at least one month.

RESULTS

At this time available results are only preliminary. Fifty-six patients from 13 Southwest Oncology Group institutions have been entered in the first year of the study of which 37 are currently evaluable (i.e. two or more therapy courses) for response (Table 1).

TABLE 1
THERAPY OF ADVANCED OVARIAN CARCINOMA
SOUTHWEST ONCOLOGY GROUP STUDY 7524
PATIENT ENTRIES BY INSTITUTION*

Institution Name	No. Evaluable Patients Entered On-Study
University of Arizona College of Medicine	6
Ohio State University Hospitals	5
University of Kansas Medical Center	4
Cleveland Clinic	4
University of Utah Medical Center	4
University of Oklahoma Medical Center	3
Henry Ford Hospital	3
Wilford Hall USAF Medical Center	1
Brooke Army Hospital	1
Providence Hospital, Detroit	1
Las Vegas - Tulane University	1
Scott & White Clinic	1
Kuakini Medical Center, Hawaii	1

* Only evaluable patient entries included (i.e. at least two courses of therapy).

Staging and prior surgery and radiation therapy data for the 37 evaluable patients are included in Table 2. Note that despite subrandomization, more patients in the AC group have histories of "recurrent" disease and prior radiation therapy.

TABLE 2

THERAPY OF ADVANCED OVARIAN CARCINOMA

STAGING AND PRIOR THERAPY HISTORY

SOUTHWEST ONCOLOGY GROUP STUDY 7524

	Adriamycin Cytoxan	Adriamycin Cytoxan + BCG
Number Evaluable *	22	15
Stage III	8	9
Stage IV	8	5
Recurrent	6	1
Oophorectomy	4	4
Hysterectomy & Oophorectomy	8	6
Biopsy Only	9	5
Cytology Only	1	0
Prior Radiation	5	1

* Evaluable - at least two courses of therapy administered.

Of the 22 patients on AC alone, only 5 have had documented partial remissions, whereas 5 additional patients have shown improvement (Table 3). There have been 10 partial remissions out of the 15 patients entered on the AC + BCG arm of the study. Of the 5 other patients, 2 have shown improvement.

TABLE 3

THERAPY OF ADVANCED OVARIAN CARCINOMA: PRELIMINARY RESULTS OF A RANDOMIZED STUDY

SOUTHWEST ONCOLOGY GROUP STUDY 7524 (February, 1977)

	Adriamycin Cytoxan	Adriamycin Cytoxan + BCG	p Value
Number of Evaluable Patients	22	15	
Number of Partial Responders*	5	10	$< .02$
Number of Improved Patients†	5	2	
Number Dead	9	1	$< .05$
Mean WBC Nadir x $10^3/mm^3$	2.6 ± 1.66	3.22 ± 1.75	$> .05$
Mean Platelet Nadir x $10^3/mm^3$	197 ± 103	225 ± 57.5	$> .05$

* Partial Remission - 50% or greater decrease in tumor size for at least 1 month.
† Improved - 25%-49% decrease in tumor size for at least 1 month.

The partial remission rate for AC + BCG patients of 66.7% is at this time statistically different ($p < .02$, chi square test) from the 22.2% partial remission rate observed for the AC group. The median duration of partial remission for both groups of patients has not been reached. With respect to survival, of the evaluable patients, 9 of 22 receiving AC have died compared to only 1 of the 15 receiving AC + BCG. Survival for the AC + BCG patients is at this early point statistically better than for those receiving only AC (Figure 2). A two-tailed Wilcoxon test was used to compare differences between the two survival curves and the calculated Z value of -2.117 is significant ($p < .05$).

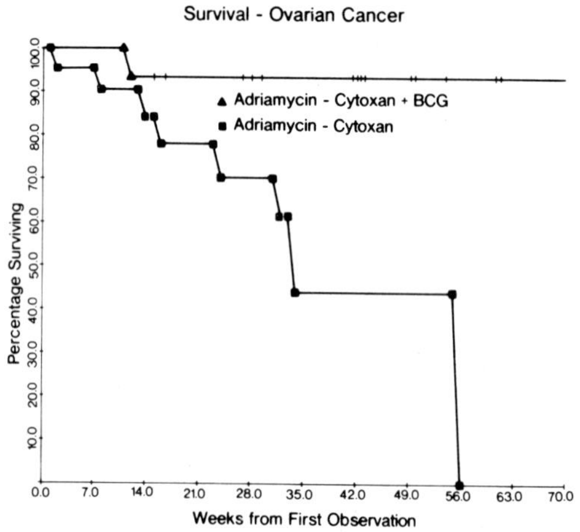

Figure 2. Survival curves for AC vs. AC + BCG patients with advanced ovarian cancer.

Myelosuppression from both combinations was well tolerated (Table 3). Life-threatening leukopenia was not observed. The mean nadir WBC for patients receiving AC was $2{,}600/mm^3$ and for AC + BCG, $3{,}200/mm^3$ ($p > .05$). Only 2 patients on AC and 1 on AC + BCG developed a WBC of less than $1000/mm^3$. One patient on the AC therapy developed a pneumonia from which she recovered. Its onset was not related to severe leukopenia. As seen in Table 3, thrombocytopenia was not observed in either arm of this study. BCG toxicity was minor with only 4 patients experiencing severe skin reactions and 2 patients having fever and chills which responded promptly to isoniazid. There were no instances of liver dysfunction related to BCG immunotherapy.

DISCUSSION

These preliminary results of this Southwest Oncology Group Study (7524) of chemotherapy vs. chemotherapy plus adjuvant BCG immunotherapy in advanced ovarian cancer patients suggest advantage for the AC + BCG treatment both with respect to partial response rate and survival. The larger number of "recurrent" patients who had received prior radiation therapy in the AC arm of the study is of uncertain importance. These patients have had their disease for a longer period prior to AC chemotherapy; however, only 2 of these 6 "recurrent" patients have died. Since randomization has been substratified with respect to prior radiation therapy, the numbers of patients in the "recurrent" and radiation therapy groups should eventually distribute evenly into the two therapy arms of the study.

It will take between 1 and 2 more years of patient accrual and followup before we can be certain of these preliminary results. If this study remains positive it will provide an important new approach to the treatment of patients with recurrent or stages III and IV disease. Nonspecific immunostimulant therapy added to an effective combination chemotherapy regimen will hopefully offer the possibility of improved 5 year survival rates. Obviously, this relatively well tolerated chemo-immunotherapy regimen could be used to treat earlier stage disease where there is a high risk of relapse despite aggressive surgery and adjuvant radiation therapy and/or single agent chemotherapy (e.g. melphalan).

Although all patients in this study are being followed for changes in both cellular and humoral immunity with routine recall antigen skin testing, total lymphocyte counts and quantitative immunoglobulins, it is still too early to determine whether the BCG therapy will have an important effect on these immunologic parameters.

ACKNOWLEDGEMENTS

I would like to thank Drs. Sydney E. Salmon and Stephen E. Jones for their advice in the design of this study and John Gaines and Cole Thies of the University of Arizona College of Medicine, Biostatistics Department for their analysis of study results. This work was supported in part by CA-13612, CA-17049, and by the respective institutional and administrative grants of the Southwest Oncology Group (see Table 1).

REFERENCES

1. Young, R.C. and DeVita, V.T. (1974) The design of clinical trials in the therapy of ovarian carcinoma. Am. J. Obstet. Gynecol. 120:1012-1024.
2. Lloyd, R.E., Jones, S.E., et al. (1976) Combination chemotherapy with adriamycin (NSC-123127) and cyclophosphamide (NSC-26271) for solid tumors: a phase II trial. Cancer Treat. Rep. 60:77-83.
3. Parker, L.M., Lokich, J.J., et al. (1975) Adriamycin-cyclophosphamide therapy in ovarian cancer. Proc. AACR and ASCO 16:263.
4. Gall, S.A., Walling, J., et al. (1973) Demonstration of tumor-associated antigens in human gynecologic malignancies. Am. J. Obstet. Gynecol. 115:387-393.
5. Order, S.E., Donahue, V., et al. (1973) Immunotherapy of ovarian carcinoma, an experimental model. Cancer 32:573-579.

6. Khoo, S.K., and MccKay, E.V. (1974) Immunologic reactivity of female patients with genital cancer: status in preinvasive, locally invasive, and disseminated disease. Am. J. Obstet. Gynecol. 119:1018-1025.
7. Di Saia, P.J. (1976) Overview of tumor immunology in gynecologic oncology. Cancer 38:566-580.
8. Wolff, J.P., and De Oliveira, C.F. (1974) Lymphocytes in patients with ovarian cancer. Obstet. Gynecol. 45:656-658.
9. Hudson, C.N., McHardy, J.E., et al. (1976) Active specific immunotherapy for ovarian cancer. Lancet 2:877-879.
10. Wanebo, H.J., Ochoa, M. et al. (1977) Randomized chemoimmunotherapy trial of CAF and intravenous C. parvum for resistant ovarian cancer-preliminary results. Proc. AACR (in press).

Adjuvant Therapy of Cancer, S.E. Salmon and S.E. Jones eds.

ADJUVANT PREOPERATIVE EXTERNAL IRRADIATION WITH OR WITHOUT INTRACAVITARY RADIUM IN THE MANAGEMENT OF ENDOMETRIAL CARCINOMA

Anam Sudarsanam, Komanduri Charyulu
Brace Hintz, Hervy Averette, and Jerome Belinson
University of Miami
P.O. Box 520875 Biscayne Annex
Miami, Florida 33152

SUMMARY

Preoperative external irradiation with or without intracavitary radium was given to 38 patients. Retrospective analysis of this group of patients contrasted with 18 patients given post-operative external irradiation is presented. There was, 1) distinct downgrading of pathological stage, 2) significantly better local disease-free status, and 3) a trend for higher survival rate in the preoperative radiotherapy group.

INTRODUCTION

Preoperative external irradiation has been shown to be effective in the management of endometrial carcinoma (1). The published data on the subject is based on techniques of external radiation therapy directed to pelvis. Such a method delivers a homogeneous dose to the primary and its echelons of spread in the pelvis. However, pelvic external irradiation does not eradicate the possible presence of micrometastases in the para-aortic nodes that drain the lymphatics from the fundus of the uterus. Hence, this technique would be applicable only to Stage I cases of endometrial carcinoma where such metastases are less likely.

Preoperative intracavitary radium has been reported to improve the five-year survival rates among patients with Stage I disease (2). Controversy exists whether such intracavitary radium therapy accomplishes the objective of providing free margins of resection when the carcinoma may have spread subclinically to tissues adjacent to the corpus.

In 1970 we undertook a pilot study in which patients would receive preoperative en bloc external irradiation to pelvis and para-aortic areas with possible additional intracavitary radium. This report presents the analysis of patients in this preoperative radiation study as well as a group of patients given post-operative radiation therapy at our institution.

METHODS AND MATERIALS

From January 1970 to December 1974, the total population of patients with endometrial carcinoma referred for radiotherapy was 79 of whom 23 received various palliative therapies. Thirty-eight patients with clinical Stage I and II were enrolled in the preoperative en bloc external irradiation to pelvis and para-aortic areas with or without intracavitary radium. Only 6 patients among this group could not have para-aortic external irradiation due to extreme obesity or advanced age. Twenty patients did and 18 did not receive additional intracavitary radium (Table 1).

TABLE 1

ENDOMETRIAL CARCINOMA STUDY GROUP

	External Radiation only	External Radiation + radium	Total
Pre-operative radiotherapy	18	20	38
Post-operative radiotherapy	10	8	18
Total patients:			56

The remaining 18 patients had prior total abdominal hysterectomy and were referred for post-operative irradiation. Half of these received en bloc pelvic and para-aortic radiation and the other half had pelvic external irradiation. Eight of these patients had intracavitary vaginal radium, whereas, 10 patients did not. In both groups the external radiation was given to pelvic and para-aortic areas en bloc if such therapy was given. The dose was 4000 rads in

20 fractions in 28 days in thin patients and 4320 in 24 fractions in 32 days to obese patients. Similar dose regimens were given to the pelvis if para-aortic regions were not irradiated.

The intracavitary radium therapy in the preoperative series was given in the afterloading manner using a central tandem in the uterus and vagina with a plastic cylinder in the vagina surrounding the tandem. The number of radium sources placed in the tandem was chosen so as to irradiate the fundus, corpus, and upper two-thirds of the vagina. The intracavitary dose to point A was 3600 rads.

In the post-operative patients, intracavitary radium application was given by vaginal cylinder; the dose to the vaginal surface by this method was 4000 rads.

In the preoperative patients, hysterectomy was performed one to three months after radiation therapy.

RESULTS

The preoperative radiation category consisted of 24 clinical Stage (CS) I patients and 14 CS II patients. In comparison, the post-operative series had 15 CS I patients and only 3 CS II patients (Table 2).

TABLE 2

CLINICAL STAGE OF DISEASE IN PRE AND POST-OPERATIVE RADIOTHERAPY GROUPS

	Stage I	Stage II
Pre-operative group	24	14
Post-operative group	15	3

Preoperative irradiation eradicated the carcinoma in the corpus in 17 of the 38 patients. Additional therapy with intracavitary radium resulted in 10 of 20 patients without residual tumor in the hysterectomy specimen compared to 7 of 18 not given radium therapy (Table 3).

TABLE 3

PRE-OPERATIVE EXTERNAL RADIATION WITH OR WITHOUT ADDITIONAL INTRACAVITARY RADIUM

Proportion of hysterectomy specimen with no residual tumor

Clinical stage	Intracavitary radium		
	Yes	No	Total
I	5/10	6/14	11/24
II	5/10	1/4	6/14
Totals:	10/20	7/18	17/38

The operative findings and the histology of the hysterectomy specimens permits assignment of pathological stage (PS) to all patients in both the preoperative and post-operative subsets. Such staging is shown in Table 4 assigning PS 00 to hysterectomy specimens with no residual tumor after preoperative irradiation.

TABLE 4

CORRELATION OF CLINICAL STAGE VS. PATHOLOGICAL OR SURGICAL STAGE

Stage	Pre-operative group	Post-operative group
Clinical	I(24) II(14)	I(15) II(3)
Pathological or Surgical	00*(17) I(19) II(1) III(1)	I(12) II(3) III(2) IV(1)

Number in parenthesis indicate number of patients
* No residual tumor in hysterectomy specimen

There is distinct downgrading of disease stage after preoperative external irradiation even though an initial preponderance of CS II disease existed in the preoperative radiation patients compared to the post-operative radiotherapy group. The single case of extension and all the deaths in the post-operative radiotherapy patients were PS II or higher. Deaths in the preoperative category did not correlate with PS.

The local disease-free status is shown in Table 5, and Figure 1.

TABLE 5

LOCAL DISEASE-FREE STATUS* FOLLOWING EXTERNAL RADIATION WITH OR WITHOUT ADDITIONAL INTRACAVITARY RADIUM

	Intracavitary radium		
	Yes	No	Totals
Pre-operative group	20/20	17/18	37/38
Post-operative group	7/8	7/10	14/18

* Minimum two-year follow-up

One out of 38 patients given preoperative external radiation had local failure in contrast to 4 out of 18 patients in the postoperative series ($p < 0.05$). The single patient with local failure in the preoperative series was among the 18 patients who did not receive intracavitary radium. In the post-operative patients, 3 out of 10 with no radium failed locally, whereas, 1 of 8 with additional radium had local failure.

Fig. 1

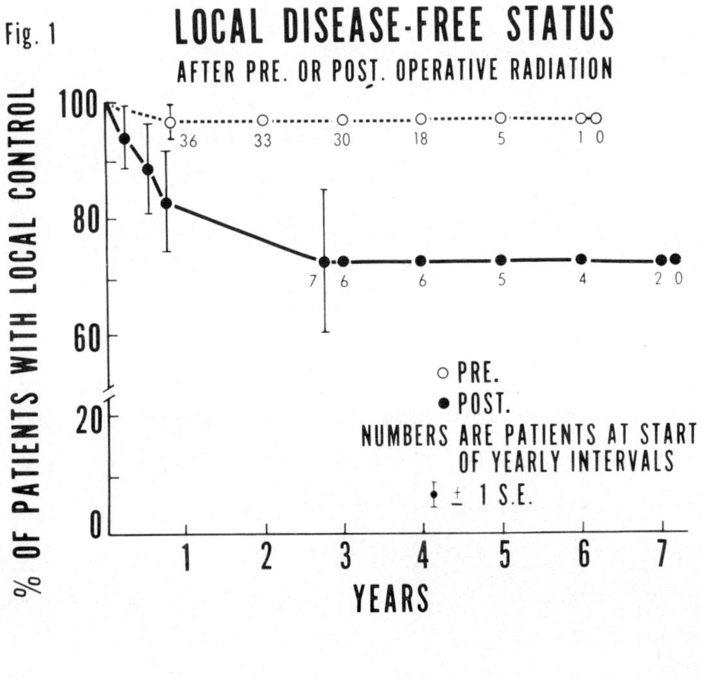

The five-year actuarial survival rates were 89% and 78% in the pre and post-operative radiation groups, respectively (Figure 2). Interpretation of these figures should perhaps take into account the relative preponderance of CS II cases in the preoperative category.

In the group of preoperative patients, 3 out of 21 with residual tumor in the hysterectomy specimen died of disseminated neoplasm whereas, 1 out of 17 without residual tumor died of upper abdominal metastases. This latter patient did not receive para-aortic irradiation, but the three former patients did.

Fig. 2

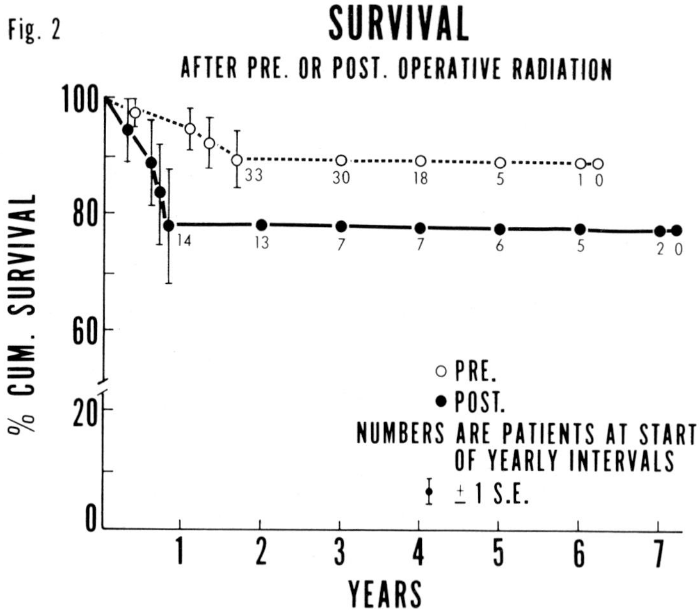

The complications of therapy are shown in Table 6. Two patients in the preoperative radiotherapy subset had severe toxicity requiring surgical intervention. The five other patients had mild toxicity. Of the 5 patients exhibiting toxicity in the post-operative radiotherapy group, one died from enteritis. All of the patients who developed proctitis, cystitis, or vaginal stenosis had received intracavitary radium applications.

TABLE 6

INCIDENCE OF RADIATION COMPLICATIONS

Complication	Pre-operative group(38)	Post-operative group(18)
Cystitis	1	0
Vaginal stenosis	1	2
Proctitis	4*	1
Enteritis	1**	2***

Numbers in parentheses are patients treated
* One patient required colostomy
** Required small bowel resection
*** One patient died (clinical Stage II)

DISCUSSION

The results of this study suggest that preoperative radiation has several benefits compared to post-operative irradiation. There is a statistically better local control rate in the preoperative radiotherapy series. Due to small numbers, it is difficult to identify the role of additional therapy with intracavitary radium in eradication of tumor at the primary site. The downgrading of pathological Stage (PS) is another distinct trend in the preoperative patients in this study. Out of 14 clinical Stage (CS) II in the preoperative radiation patients, there remained only one patient with PS II and PS III at subsequent surgery. The five-year actuarial survival of 89% in the preoperative radiotherapy group appears to be higher than 78% in the post-operative radiotherapy group. One should note that there is a difference in the composition of CS I and II in the two subsets of patients. In the preoperative series, there were 14 CS II patients out of 38 and in the post-operative there were 3 out of 18 patients in CS II. One might anticipate, therefore, lesser survivals in the preoperative category rather than higher as seen in the study. However, a larger sample of patients with randomization is necessary to determine the statistical significance of these survival differences and the role of additional intracavitary radium.

Keller and others (3) report that hysterectomy alone may suffice for surgically selected Stage I endometrial carcinoma. We would question whether primary hysterectomy even in CS I patients could jeopardize the survivals of patients with higher PS detected at surgery. Analysis of deaths in our post-operative radiotherapy group indicates poor survival in patients with PS II and above. In contrast preoperative radiation seems to diminish the percentage of higher pathological stages.

The beneficial effect of para-aortic radiation could not be ascertained. Since no complications could be attributed to its use, we suggest further prospective trials.

The complications in our study may in part be attributed to the additional intracavitary radium. A lesser intracavitary radium dose may minimize these complications while preserving the theoretical benefit of local boost.

Acknowlegement: Our sincere thanks to Miss Iris Kiem, biostatistician for statistical analysis; Doctor Pavel Houdek, physicist for dosimetry; Mrs. Jean Postlewaite, and Mrs. Bess Rosen for compiling the data and preparation of the manuscript.

REFERENCES

1. del Regato, J.A., and Chahbazian, C.M. (1972), External Pelvic Irradiation as a Preoperative Surgical Adjuvant in Treatment of Carcinoma of Endometrium. Am J Roentgenol Rad Ther and Nuc Med 114; 106.
2. Weigensberg, I.J., (1976), Preoperative Radiation Therapy in Endometrial Carcinoma. Preliminary Report of Clinical Trial. Am J Roentgenol Rad Ther and Nucl Med 127; 319.
3. Keller D. et al. (1974), Management of Patient with Early Endometrial Carcinoma. Cancer; 1108.

Section VI

PEDIATRIC CANCER

Adjuvant Therapy of Cancer, S.E. Salmon and S.E. Jones eds.

ADJUVANT THERAPY IN WILMS' TUMOR, RHABDOMYOSARCOMA, OSTEOSARCOMA, AND OTHER CHILDHOOD NEOPLASMS -- AN OVERVIEW

Wataru W. Sutow, M. D.
The University of Texas System Cancer Center
M.D. Anderson Hospital and Tumor Institute
Houston, Texas.

INTRODUCTION

Over a period of many years, current techniques of multidisciplinary and adjuvant therapy have been developed, field-tested, and, refined in childhood cancer, particularly in such malignant solid neoplasms as Wilms' tumor, rhabdomyosarcoma and osteosarcoma.[1] Given optimal clinical circumstances and with the application of coordinated maximal therapy, children with Wilms' tumor, for example, can anticipate better than 90% probability of long-term disease free survival.[2] Even when there has been potential or actual spread of tumor intra-abdominally, there exists a greater than 80% probability of overall survival.[2] Such performance results, already achieved, have led Zubrod[3] to observe that "pediatric medicine is ten years ahead of adult medicine in effective utilization of combined modalities". While this recognition is encouraging to the pediatric oncologists, the data themselves permit assessment of the progressive steps by which the present high success rates have been attained and provide perspectives for continuing efforts to control other tumors.[1,4]

WILMS' TUMOR

A highly effective composite program for the management of patients with Wilms' tumor has evolved from the systematic development of each treatment component (surgery, radiotherapy and chemotherapy) and the integration of the various modalities. Published data provide some retrospective information regarding the capability of surgery alone (nephrectomy) or surgery combined with radiotherapy to achieve cures in children with Wilms' tumor.

A compilation of data from six clinical reports covering 1018 patients treated with surgery alone (without radiotherapy and without chemotherapy) indicated a survival rate of only 18%.[5] Data from 2449 patients treated from 1914 to 1969 with surgery combined with radiotherapy (but no chemotherapy) showed a survival rate of 31%.[5] In comparison, the cure rates recently reported from the prospective National Wilms' Tumor Study[2] are summarized in Table 1.

TABLE 1

RESULTS - NATIONAL WILMS' TUMOR STUDY [2]

Patient Group	Number of Patients	Actuarial Proportion of Patients	
		Disease-Free At 2 Years	Alive At 2 years
Group I (with XRT)*			
Under 2 yrs. of age	38	90%	97%
Over 2 yrs. of age	39	83%	97%
Group I (no XRT)			
Under 2 yrs. of age	36	88%	94%
Over 2 yrs. of age	41	71%	92%
Group II & III			
Both drugs	59	81%	86%

* XRT = Radiotherapy

The type of multimodal therapy that has brought about the control of Wilms' tumor is exemplified (see Figure 1) by the two drug combination therapy (actinomycin D and vincristine) in patients with actual or potential residual tumor intra-abdominally (Group II and III patients).[2] All of these patients will have had nephrectomy and radiotherapy to the tumor bed.

A comparison of these various statistics documents a progressive and significant improvement in the survival rates which have reached the remarkable level of 97% for certain categories of patients with Wilms' tumor.[2] The aspects of the treatment programs that appear to have contributed meaningfully to the attainment of such survival data include the following:

1. Improvement of surgical techniques, of anesthesia and of postoperative care.
2. Improvement in the administration of radiation therapy.
3. Meaningful collaboration of the surgeon, radiotherapist and chemotherapist for the structuring of an optimal therapeutic program.
4. More precise determination of the extent of the tumor in the patient utilizing the skills of the pediatric oncologist, the diagnostic radiologist, the surgeon and the pathologist.
5. Combination of drugs and of treatment modalities.
6. Recognition of the presence or absence of certain prognostic factors, (such as the age of the patient and the histopathology of the tumor) and the utilization of those factors in the stratification of the treatment decisions.

7. Intensive multimodal therapy of metastatic disease.

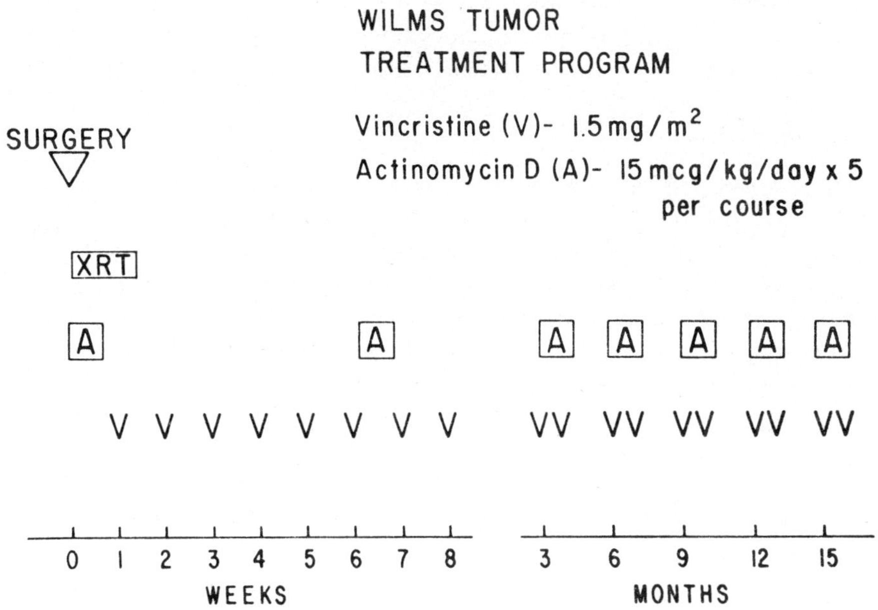

Fig. 1. Schema showing multimodal, multidrug treatment regimen for Wilms' tumor. XRT = radiation therapy A = actinomycin D V = vincristine

The improving prognosis has now emphasized the need to include several other important considerations, such as :[6]

1. Reduction in the ultimate cost of survival. High survival rates necessitate a continuing and meticulous examination of the cost of survival in the patient. Particularly, the late consequences of therapy must be identified and measured.[7-10] Efforts to prevent, minimize or correct these therapy-related problems constitute an essential component of the treatment plan when cure becomes routine. One of the most serious late effects of therapy is the development of a histologically different second malignant neoplasm.[7-11]
2. Surviving children eventually will reach reproductive age. Thus, the knowledge of the genetic risks that offsprings of the survivors face must be determined as precisely as possible.[12] Genetic counseling, therefore, is another essential component of any comprehensive treatment program.

3. The concept of cure itself may require thoughtful deliberation and redefinition. In a broad sense, the mere eradication of tumor, however complete, does not always provide the quality of life that may be considered normal. Therefore, psychosocial rehabilitation as well as physical rehabilitation become important aspects of treatment planning.[6]

RHABDOMYOSARCOMA

Integrated, multidisciplinary treatment, particularly the coordination of radiotherapy and chemotherapy, has resulted in a substantial increase in the rate of survival among children with rhabdomyosarcoma. Even in high-risk clinical situations (such as the location of the primary lesions in the nasopharynx, maxillary antrum or peritonsillar areas -- anatomical regions where complete surgical extirpation is not possible) the disease-free survival rate exceeds 80% and the local control rate (of primary tumor) is above 90%.[13] (See Figure 2)

The schematic presentation of two treatment programs (regimens E and F) used in the Intergroup Rhabdomyosarcoma Study[14] (see Figure 3) illustrates the manner in which multidrug chemotherapy and irradiation are integrated. In regimen E, three drugs (vincristine, actinomycin D and cyclophosphamide in the combination acronymically designated VAC) and in regimen F, four drugs (adriamycin added) are administered on a schedule that assimilates the traditional VAC administration[15] with the intermittent high-dose cyclophosphamide pulses.[16]

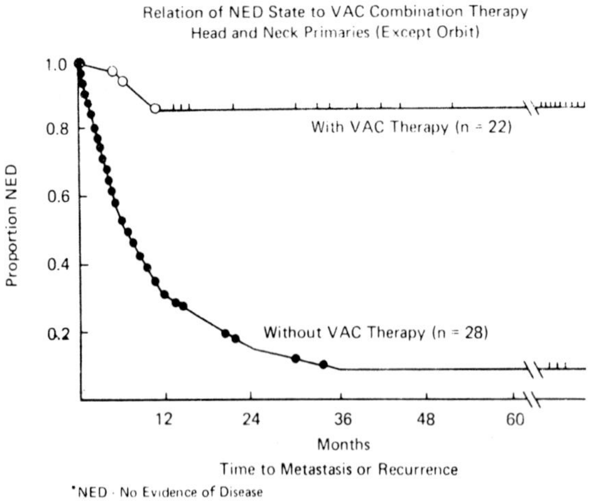

Fig. 2. Disease-free survival curve in patients with rhabdomyosarcoma primary in the head and neck (except orbit). VAC = vincristine, actinomycin D and cyclophosphamide.

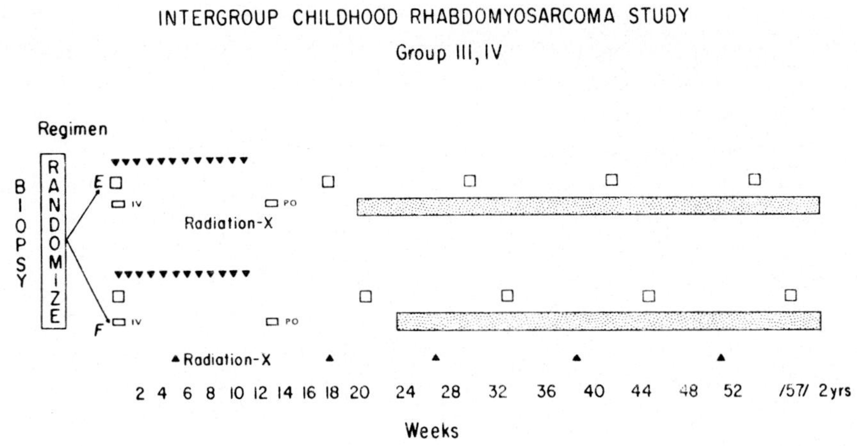

Fig. 3. Multidisciplinary, multidrug treatment regimens E and F used for Group III and IV patients in the Intergroup Rhabdomyosarcoma Study. Vincristine = inverted solid triangle. Actinomycin D = open squares. Cyclophosphamide pulses = open rectangle. Cyclophosphamide daily dose schedule = stippled bar. Adriamycin = upright solid triangle.

The schema shows still another potential of adjuvant therapy. Drugs only are administered for the initial 5 weeks. In almost all cases, rhabdomyosarcoma will respond with rapid shrinkage of tumor. As a result, the radiotherapist will have a smaller volume of tumor to treat and the surgeon may be able to re-evaluate operability or in some cases be able to perform satisfactory surgery utilizing less extensive and less mutilating approaches.[7,18]

OSTEOSARCOMA

Osteosarcoma is the third malignant solid tumor in which adjuvant therapy has brought about significant changes in treatment attitudes and results. This was a tumor that was considered to be chemoresistant and radioresistant. The cure rate had remained constant, between 5% and 20%, regardless of the type of therapy, for decades.[19] In recent years, several types of adjuvant chemotherapy programs have been developed. This has resulted in a marked increase in survival rate to levels now consistently above 50%.[20]

Currently the adjuvant programs may be divided into three general types: the use of adriamycin alone as single-agent therapy,[21] the administration of high-dose methotrexate with citrovorum factor[22,23] and the use of different drugs in combination.[20,24] COMPADRI-III is one such combination chemotherapy adjuvant regimen and is illustrated in Figure 4.

The effectiveness of adjuvant chemotherapy in this tumor is indicated by a 79% survival at 3 years in a group of patients treated at M. D. Anderson Hospital.[25] (see Figure 5) These patients were under 20 years of age at diagnosis, had primary tumors involving extremity bones, underwent amputation, and had no metastases at time of amputation. Chemotherapy for the treated subgroup consisted of COMPADRI-I and COMPADRI-II regimens.[20] The comparison subgroup received no adjuvant chemotherapy. The high proportion surviving indicates that, in addition to improving the primary control rate, multimodal therapy extends the time of survival for patients with metastases and also produces cures in some patients who fail on primary therapy.

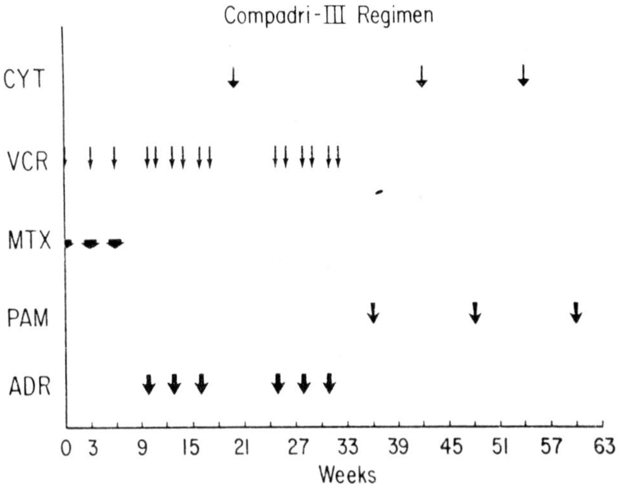

Fig. 4 Schematic outline for COMPADRI-III regimen. CYT = cyclophosphamide, 10 mg/kg/dayx7. VCR = vincristine, 1.5 mg/M^2. MTX = methotrexate 75-200 mg/kg. PAM = phenylalanine mustard, 0.3 mg/kg. ADR = adriamycin, 60 mg/M^2

As the therapeutic effectiveness of chemotherapy became established, its potential usefulness in the treatment of other aspects of osteosarcoma has been explored. One such investigation involves efforts to control the primary tumor by local resection with prosthetic manoeuvers to avoid amputation and save the limb.[23,26] Another area of clinical activity is the continuing multimodal attempts to achieve cures in patients who have developed metastases.[23,27,28]

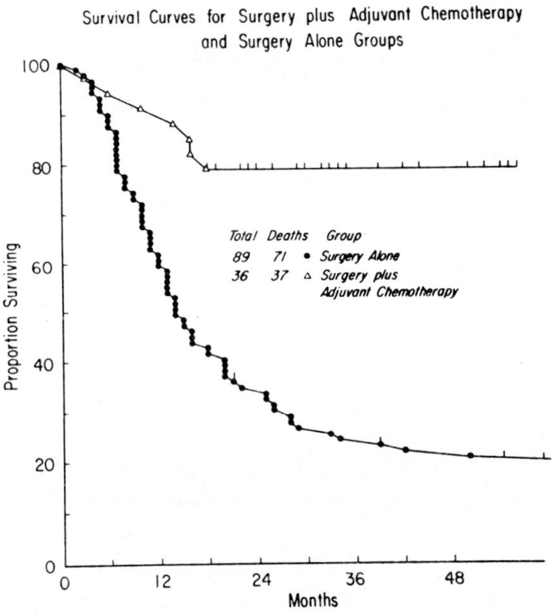

Fig. 5. Comparison of survival curves in osteosarcoma of extremities treated with amputation alone versus amputation plus adjuvant chemotherapy.

OTHER PEDIATRIC SOLID TUMORS

Adjuvant therapy has been investigated in other childhood solid tumors. However, the infrequency of occurrence of specific tumors in the pediatric population or the relative ineffectiveness of treatment programs currently available preclude the meaningful analysis of success rates in tumors other than those already discussed. Among the tumors for which progress appears to be occurring but with sufficient inconsistencies to prevent precise quantitative assessment of the treatment potential are Ewing's sarcoma,[24,29,30] neuroblastoma,[31-33] gynecologic tumors and testicular tumors. Still unestablished is the degree of effectiveness of any adjuvant chemotherapy programs in hepatoma, brain tumors, and, retinoblastoma.

CONCEPTUAL ASPECTS

The concept of adjuvant therapy[34] makes at least three basic assumptions. First, there must be more than one form of treatment, each of which is capable by itself of eradicating the tumor to variable degrees. Second, the need to consider additional therapy implies that the tumor may not be completely eradicated by one form of therapy, such as, for example, the failure of target-limited treatment with surgery and irradiation to affect distant micrometastases. And, third, cure is the goal of therapy.

The logical base for the evaluation of any therapeutic technique is the tabulation of adequate quantity of treatment results with satisfactory follow-up times. Such exist for Wilms' tumor, rhabdomyosarcoma and osteosarcoma. The data permit an assessment of the tactics that have been successfully utilized, delineation of the patterns of failures that still exist, and definition of the principles involved in the structuring of optimal therapy for solid tumors.

Some of the requirements for multidisciplinary therapy can be paraphrased from the requirements that are commonly outlined for multidrug chemotherapy: there should be a minimum of overlap of treatment-limiting toxicities; each modality can be utilized at optimal intensity; the modalities preferably should have different mechanisms of action; and there should be no cross-resistance among the modalities.

The technical objectives of adjuvant therapy might be classified as efforts (a) to modify the extent, intensity and/or the duration of other modalities, (b) to increase the effectiveness of other modalities, and (c) to decrease the toxicity of other modalities. The clinical objectives of adjuvant therapy can likewise be enumerated: (a) to eradicate residual tumor at site of primary lesion, (b) to eradicate micrometastases at distant sites and (c) to eradicate existing macrometastases. Successful attainment of the various objectives should result in prevention of clinical metastases and improvement of cure rates.

The factors that limit the effectiveness of multidisciplinary therapy or any component thereof will include: the mass (size or volume) of the tumor, the extent of the tumor, the sensitivity of the tumor, and the tolerance of the treatment by the patient.

Evans[4] has succinctly enumerated the lessons emerging from pediatric oncology as follows:

A. The importance of the team approach to cancer treatment.

B. Early weighting of all available forms of treatment.

C. Skilled and vigorous application of treatment.

D. Consideration of the biology and natural history of the tumor in treatment planning.

E. Recognition of toxicities of all forms of treatment.

Burchenal,[34] from the vantage point of a veteran chemotherapist with unparalleled clinical experience has also addressed the theory, practice and potential of adjuvant therapy. He emphasized several considerations in addition to those already discussed. Adjuvant chemotherapy should be started as soon as possible after surgery when the body burden of tumor cells is theoretically minimal. Drug or drug combinations should be given at maximum tolerated doses; reduction in doses may be associated with significant decrease in antitumor activity. Burchenal urges that the "pride of discipline" be put aside for complete collaboration. Intensive adjuvant therapy is best given by a physician of great expertise and experience. Adjuvant therapy should be especially considered in patients with high risk of becoming a treatment failure.[34]

At this writing, the role of immunotherapy as an adjunctive measure has not been established even in neuroblastoma[35,36] which was one of the first human tumors shown to have tumor-associated immune reactions.

SUMMARY

Concepts and methodology of adjuvant multidisciplinary therapy of malignant solid tumors have been effectively field tested in pediatric cancer, specifically in Wilms' tumor, rhabdomyosarcoma and osteosarcoma. These programs have utilized, in sequence or concomitantly, the surgical removal of the primary lesion in most cases, radiation therapy to the tumor bed and/or residual tumor, and, administration of systemic chemotherapy over a long period of time.

Cure rates, under favorable clinical circumstances, exceed 90% in Wilms' tumor, 65% in rhabdomyosarcoma, and 50% in osteosarcoma. The significant improvements in cure rates have permitted major modifications in the therapeutic approaches to these tumors.

The current data permit a review of the tactics that have been successfully utilized, delineation of the patterns of failure that still exist and definition of principles involved in the structuring of optimal strategy for solid tumors.

REFERENCES

1. Sutow, W.W. and Sullivan, M.P.: Childhood cancer - the improving prognosis.

Postgraduate Medicine 59:131-137, February 1976.

2. D'Angio, G. J., Evans, A. E., Breslow, N., Beckwith, B., Bishop, H., Feigl, P., Goodwin, W., Leape, L. L., Sinks, L. F., Sutow, W., Tefft, M. and Wolff, J.: The treatment of Wilms' tumor - results of the National Wilms' Tumor Study. Cancer 38:633-646, October 1976.
3. Zubrod, C.G.: Contribution of chemotherapy to the control of cancer. Heath Memorial Award Lecture. In: Cancer Chemotherapy - Fundamental Concepts and Recent Advances. Chicago, Year Book Medical Publishers, Inc. 1975, pp 7-17.
4. Evans, A. E.: Pediatric cancer treatment: a model for oncology. Am. J. Roentgenol., Radium Therapy and Nuclear Medicine 127: 891-895, 1976.
5. Sutow, W.W.: Wilms' Tumor. Methods in Cancer Research 13:31-65, 1976.
6. van Eys, J., Sullivan, M.P., Sutow, W.W., Fernandez, C.H., Ayala, A.G., Strong, L.C., Tapley, N. duV., Young, S.E. and Cangir, A.: Childhood tumors. In: Clark, R.L. and Howe, C.D.: Cancer Patient Care at M. D. Anderson Hospital and Tumor Institute. Chicago, Year Book Medical Publishers, Inc., 1976, pp 309-360.
7. Meadows, A.T., D'Angio, G.J., Evans, A.E., Harris, C.C., Miller, R.W. and Mike, V.: Oncogenesis and other late effects of cancer treatment in children Radiology 114:175-180, January 1975.
8. Li, F.P. and Stone, R.: Survivors of cancer in childhood. Annals of Internal Medicine 84:551-553, May 1976.
9. Jaffe, N.: Late side effects of treatment: skeletal, genetic, central nervous system and oncogenic. Pediatric Clinics of North America 23:233-244, February 1976.
10. Everson, R.B.: Late mortality in Wilms' tumor (letter). Lancet 1:810, April 5, 1975.
11. Li, F.P., Cassady, J.R. and Jaffe, N.: Risk of second tumors in survivors of childhood cancer. Cancer 35:1230-1235, April 1975.
12. Strong, L.C.: Genetic and teratogenic aspects of Wilms' tumor. In: Pochedly, C. and Miller, D. (editors): Wilms' Tumor, New York, John Wiley & Sons, 1976, pp 65-77.
13. Fernandez, C.H., Sutow, W.W., Merino, O.R. and George, S.L.: Childhood rhabdomyosarcoma: analysis of coordinated therapy and results. Am. J. Roentgenology Radium Therapy and Nuclear Medicine 123:588-597, March, 1975.
14. Maurer, H.M.: The Intergroup Rhabdomyosarcoma Study (NIH): Objectives and clinical staging classification. J. Pediat. Surg. 10:977-978, December 1975.
15. Sutow, W.W.: Chemotherapeutic management of childhood rhabdomyosarcoma. In: Neoplasia in Childhood. Year Book Medical Publishers. Chicago, 1969, pp 201-217.
16. Finklestein, J.Z., Hittle, R.E. and Hammond, G.D.: Evaluation of a high dose cyclophosphamide regimen in childhood tumors. Cancer 23:1239-1242, May 1969.

17. Rivard, G., Ortega, J., Hittle, R., Nitschke, R. and Karon, M.: Intensive chemotherapy as primary treatment for rhabdomyosarcoma of the pelvis. Cancer 36:1593-1597, November 1975.

18. Kumar, A.P.M., Wrenn, Jr., E.L., Fleming, I.D., Hustu, H.O. and Pratt, C.B.: Combined therapy to prevent complete pelvic exenteration for rhabdomyosarcoma of the vagina or uterus. Cancer 37:118-122, January 1976.

19. Friedman, M.A. and Carter, S.K.: The therapy of osteogenic sarcoma: current status and thoughts for the future. J. Surg. Oncology 4:482-510, 1972.

20. Sutow, W.W., Gehan, E.A., Vietti, T.J., Frias, A.E. and Dyment, P.G.: Multi-drug chemotherapy in primary treatment of osteosarcoma. J. Bone & Joint Surg. 58-A:629-633, July 1976.

21. Cortes, E.P., Holland, J.F., Wang, J. J. and Glidewell, O.: Adriamycin (NSC-123127) in 87 patients with osteosarcoma. Cancer Chemotherapy Reports (Part 3) 6:305-313, October 1975.

22. Jaffe, N., Frei, III, E., Traggis, D. and Bishop, Y.: Adjuvant methotrexate and citrovorum-factor treatment of osteogenic sarcoma. New Eng. J. Med. 291: 994-997, November 7, 1974.

23. Jaffe, N., Frei, III, E., Traggis, D. and Watts, H.: Weekly high-dose methotrexate-citrovorum factor in osteogenic sarcoma: pre-surgical treatment of primary tumor and of overt pulmonary metastases. Cancer 39:45-50, January 1977.

24. Rosen, G.: Management of malignant bone tumors in children and adolescents. Pediatric Clinics North America 23:183-213, February 1976.

25. Gehan, E.A., Sutow, W.W., Uribe-Botero, G., Romsdahl, M. and Smith, T.L.: Osteosarcoma: the M. D. Anderson Hospital Experience, 1950-1974. In: Immuno-therapy of Cancer: present status of trials in man. (in press)

26. Rosen, G., Murphy, M.L., Huvos, A.G., Gutierrez, M., and Marcove, R.C.: Chemotherapy, en bloc resection, and prosthetic bone replacement in the treatment of osteogenic sarcoma. Cancer 37:1-11, January 1976.

27. Rosen, G., Tefft, M., Martinez, A., Cham, W. and Murphy, M.L.: Combination chemotherapy and radiation therapy in the treatment of metastatic osteogenic sarcoma. Cancer 35:622-630, March 1975.

28. Jaffe, N., Traggis, D., Cassady, J.R., Filler, R.M., Watts, H. and Frei, E.: Multidisciplinary treatment for macrometastatic osteosarcoma. British Medical Journal 2:1039-1041, 1976.

29. Fernandez, C.H., Lindberg, R.D., Sutow, W.W. and Samuels, M.L.: Localized Ewing's sarcoma - treatment and results. Cancer 34:143-148, July 1974.

30. Jaffe, N., Traggis, D., Sallan, S. and Cassady, J.R.: Improved outlook for Ewing's sarcoma with combination chemotherapy (vincristine, actinomycin D and cyclophosphamide) and radiation therapy. Cancer 38:1925-1930, November 1976.

31. Helson, L.: Management of disseminated neuroblastoma. Ca 25:264-277, September/October 1975.

32. Jaffe, N.: Neuroblastoma: review of the literature and an examination of factors contributing to its enigmatic character. Cancer Treatment Reviews 3:61-82, June 1976.

33. Evans, A. E., Albo, V., D'Angio, G.J., Finklestein, J.Z., Leiken, S., Santulli, T., Weiner, J. and Hammond, G.D.: Cyclophosphamide treatment of patients with localized and regional neuroblastoma. A randomized study. Cancer 38:655-660, August 1976.

34. Burchenal, J.H.: Adjuvant therapy - theory, practice, and potential. Cancer 37:46-57, January 1976.

35. Bernstein, I., Hellstrom, I., Hellstrom, K.E. and Wright, P.W.: Immunity to tumor antigens: potential implications in human neuroblastoma. J. Nat. Cancer Inst. 57:711-715, September 1976.

36. Nesbit, M.E., Kersey, J., Finklestein, J., Weiner, J. and Simmons, R.: Immunotherapy and chemotherapy in children with neuroblastoma. J. Nat. Cancer Inst. 57:717-720, September 1976.

Adjuvant Therapy of Cancer, S.E. Salmon and S.E. Jones eds.

RESULTS IN CHILDREN OF ACUTE LYMPHOID LEUKAEMIA PROTOCOL ICIG-ALL 9 CONSISTING OF CHEMOTHERAPY FOR ONLY NINE MONTHS FOLLOWED BY ACTIVE IMMUNOTHERAPY

Comparison with the results of more prolonged chemotherapy protocols. Recognition of two groups of acute lymphoid leukaemias from prognostic parameters.

G. Mathé, F. De Vassal, L. Schwarzenberg, M. Delgado, J. Pena-Angulo, D. Belpomme, P. Pouillart, D. Machover, J.L. Misset, J.L. Pico, C. Jasmin, M. Hayat, M. Schneider, A. Cattan, J.L. Amiel, M. Musset and C. Rosenfeld.
Institut de Cancérologie et d'Immunogénétique (INSERM), Unité Fred-Siguier de l'Hôpital Paul-Brousse et Service d'Hématologie de l'Institut Gustave-Roussy, 94800-Villejuif, France.

INTRODUCTION

In 1962, we started a controlled study (the principle of which was based on our experimental data[1]) to compare active systemic immunotherapy (AI) with no treatment for patients with acute lymphoid leukaemia (ALL) after stopping their remission chemotherapy. The difference in remission duration and survival in favour of AI became significant so rapidly[2] that, for obvious ethical and juridical reasons, we were not authorized to introduce more patients than the 30 already in the trial, nor to perform another trial with controls left without treatment. We recently published two critical discussions of this trial[3,4].

Since then, we have conducted several trials on AI, the overall results[1] of which indicate: a) the absence of late relapse, the remission curve forming a plateau of cure expectancy after 4 years; b) the absence of lethal toxicity of immunotherapy, in contrast to the high lethality in remission due to maintenance chemotherapy (4 to 28%)[see 5]; and c) the possibility of making a prognosis at the beginning of the disease on three parameters: the WHO Reference Center cytologic type[6,7], the immune (T or null) cell type[8,9], and the volume of the neoplasia[10].

In 1970, we established a protocol, ICIG-ALL 9, with a short duration of remission chemotherapy (9 months) followed by AI; the results after 3 to 5 years are now available. We can thus:a) compare these results with those of other protocols conducted by us with

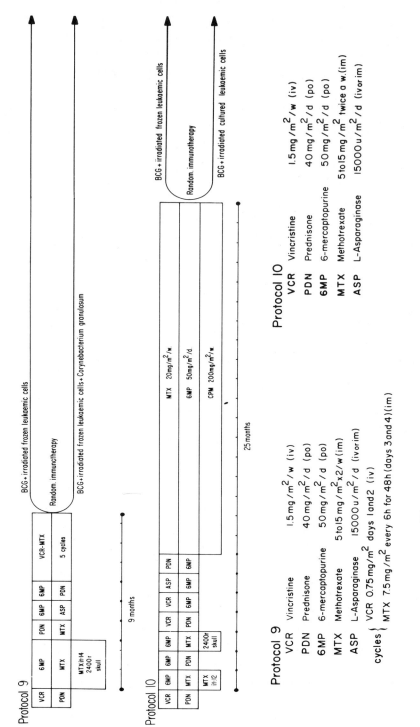

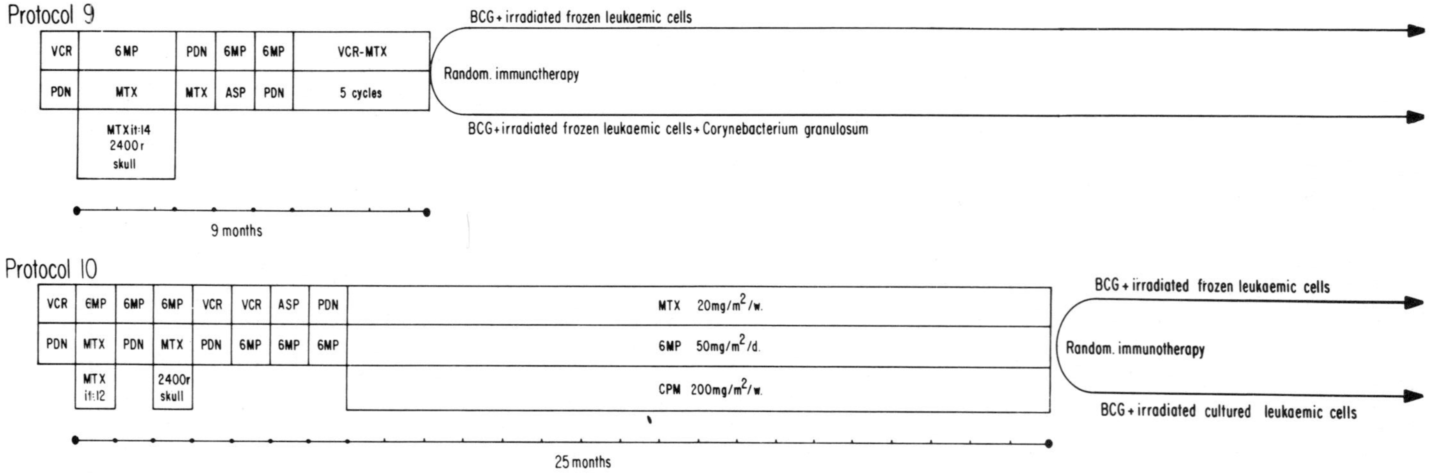

Protocol 9

VCR	Vincristine	$1.5\ mg/m^2/w$ (iv)
PDN	Prednisone	$40\ mg/m^2/d$ (po)
6MP	6-mercaptopurine	$50\ mg/m^2/d$ (po)
MTX	Methotrexate	5 to 15 $mg/m^2 x 2/w$ (im)
ASP	L-Asparaginase	$15000\ u/m^2/d$ (iv or im)

cycles { VCR $0.75\ mg/m^2$ days 1 and 2 (iv)
MTX $7.5\ mg/m^2$ every 6h for 48h (days 3 and 4) (im)

Protocol 10

VCR	Vincristine	$1.5\ mg/m^2/w$ (iv)
PDN	Prednisone	$40\ mg/m^2/d$ (po)
6MP	6-mercaptopurine	$50\ mg/m^2/d$ (po)
MTX	Methotrexate	5 to 15 mg/m^2 twice a w. (im)
ASP	L-Asparaginase	$15000\ u/m^2/d$ (iv or im)

Fig. 1 Scheme of protocols 9 and 10.

more prolonged remission chemotherapy given before the AI, or studies conducted by other groups applying only prolonged maintenance chemotherapy[11,12,13,14,15,16,17] and b) estimate the value of the prognostic parameters mentioned above.

PATIENTS AND METHODS

Protocol ICIG-ALL 9 is described in Fig. 1 along with protocol 10, for comparison. This figure shows that protocol 9 comprises only nine months of remission chemotherapy before immunotherapy, while protocol 10 has a much longer maintenance chemotherapy for 25 months including a combination of 6-mercaptopurine (6-MP), methotrexate (MTX) and cyclophosphamide (CPM) for the latter 18 months of this period.

Thus we can compare the effect of AI applied between the 9th and the 25th months in protocol 9, with one of the best maintenance chemotherapy programmes applied during this period in protocol 10. This is a valid comparison as the age and sex ratio and the proportions of children with the two poor prognostic parameters (the incidence of the prolymphoblastic types and the incidence of the V+ forms[6,10]) do not differ in these two studies (see Table 1) (see significance of V+ and V- below).

Partial results of the comparison of these protocols in patients of all ages have recently been published[5].

Other conditions allowing this comparison are the absence of differences in the present results between the two branches of AI of the respective protocols: a) in protocol 9 the addition of C. granulosum to BCG and leukaemic cells does not improve their effect[5]; b) in protocol 10, the results of the groups receiving BCG and pooled leukaemic cells taken from the patients at the beginning of their diseases and preserved at -196° do not differ from those of the group receiving BCG and leukaemic cells of the cultured "Reh" line[18], the cells of which present three markers [including the tumour associated antigen(s)] characteristic of the fresh leukaemic cells used for initiating the culture of this line[19].

Comparison of the toxicities of immunotherapy and complementary chemotherapy will be confined to deaths other than from leukaemia. A comparison of the results of sperm, lymphocyte chromosome and bone marrow stem cell investigations carried out on patients submitted to short chemotherapy protocols or to long chemotherapy protocols is under study[20].

TABLE I

REPARTITION OF THE PATIENTS IN PROTOCOLS ICIG-ALL 9 AND 10 ACCORDING TO AGE, SEX, PROGNOSTIC PARAMETERS AND CYTOLOGIC TYPES

PROTOCOLS	NUMBER OF CASES	A G E	SEX		CYTOLOGIC TYPES					PROGNOSTIC FACTORS		
			F	M	PLb^{+}	PLc^{++}	MLb^{+++}	mLb^{++++}	Unclassified	mLb & V- MLb & PLc	PLb & V+ MLb & PLc	Unclassified
9	31	2 to 13 years <5 years : 12 (39%)) 84% 5 to 10y: 14 (45%)) >10 y : 5 (16%)	9 29%	22 71%	7 23%	13 42%	4 13%	2 6%	5 16%	10 32%	16 52%	5 16%
10	14	1 to 13 years <5 years : 8 (57%)) 86% 5 to 10y: 4 (29%)) >10 y : 2 (14%)	5 36%	9 64%	3 21%	3 21%	5 36%	1 7%	2 14%	4 29%	7 50%	3 21%

$^{+}$PLb Prolymphoblastic

$^{++}$PLc Prolymphocytic

$^{+++}$MLb Macrolymphoblastic

$^{++++}$mLb Microlymphoblastic

We attempted to make a prognosis at the beginning of the disease based on the two parameters mentioned above: (a) the cytological types of the WHO International Reference Center for the Histological and Cytological Classification of the Neoplastic Diseases of the Haematopoietic and Lymphoid Tissues[7] (prolymphoblastic, macrolymphoblastic, microlymphoblastic and prolymphocytic); and b) the volume of the neoplasia (we call V+, the cases in which the number of leukaemic cells in the blood is $\geqslant$10,000/mm3 and/or with spleno-adenomegaly, and V-, the cases in which the number of leukaemic cells is $\leqslant$10,000/mm3 and/or without spleno-adenomegaly. From our previous work[1,10], we considered the microlymphoblastic and the V-macrolymphoblastic and prolymphocytic types were of good prognosis, and that the prolymphoblastic and V+ macrolymphoblastic and prolymphocytic types of poor prognosis. In 1970, when we started protocol 9, the immune marker study[8,9] was not yet operational for all patients.

RESULTS

1.- Overall results of protocol ICIG-ALL 9

Of the 31 children under the age of 15 years introduced into the trial, 29 (94%) entered so-called "complete remission" (the two failures were two patients whose disease was of the prolymphoblastic type). 22 children were submitted to immunotherapy and randomized between AI with *C. granulosum* (10 patients) and AI without *C. granulosum* (12 patients).

Fig. 2 gives a curve made according to the direct method[21] of the cumulative duration of first remission. One observes that this curve is broken to form a plateau at the second year for 14 patients out of 29; 13 subjects out of 25, the follow-up of whom is now 50 months, are still in first remission.

Fig. 3 gives the "direct method" curve[21] of the cumulative survival. One sees that 18 out of 30 patients were alive at the 36th month, 17 out of 27 at the 50th month (no deaths occurred between these two dates).

2.- Comparison of the results of protocol ICIG-ALL 9, with short pre-immunotherapy chemotherapy, with the results of protocol ICIG-ALL 10, with long pre-immunotherapy chemotherapy

The comparison of the results of protocol 9 comprising a short post-remission chemotherapy (9 months) followed by AI, with those of protocol 10, comprising a 25 month chemotherapy, does not show any significant difference in the proportion of patients belonging to the plateaux of the cumulative remission duration curves (Fig. 2)

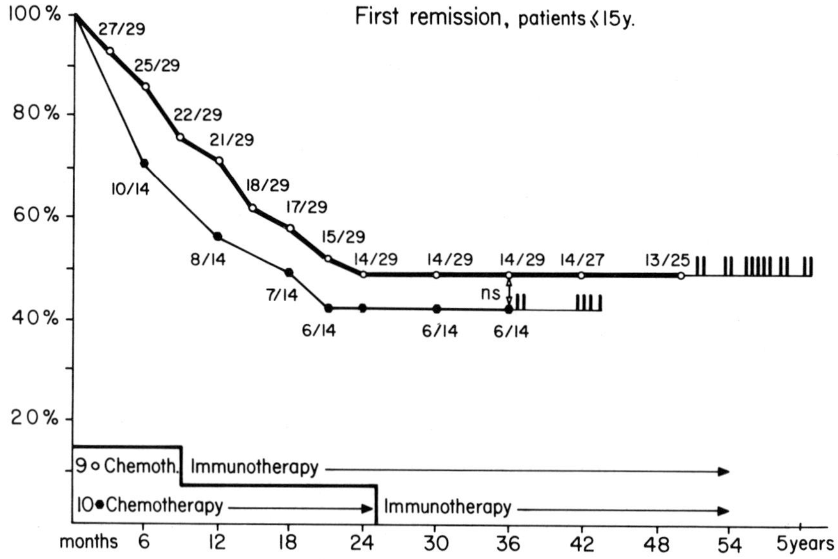

Fig. 2 Curves (established according to the "direct" method) of the cumulative duration of the first remission of children submitted respectively to protocols 9 and 10.

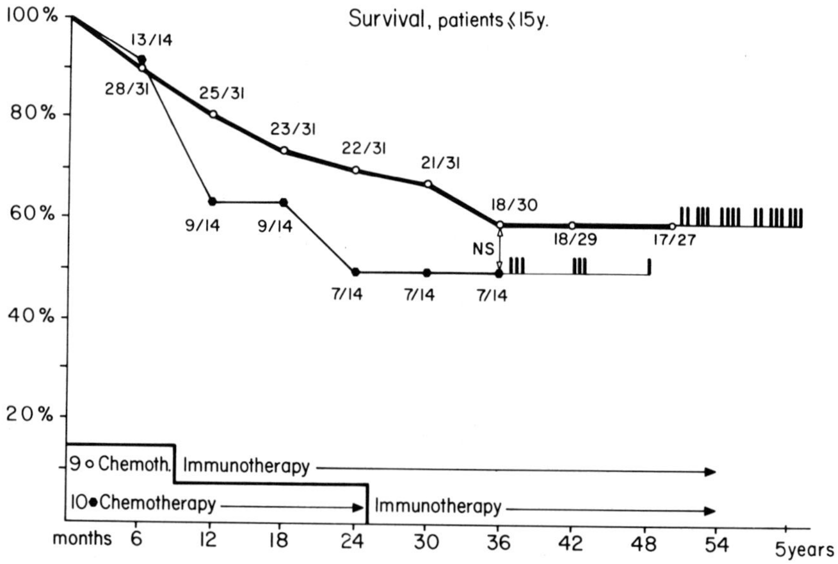

Fig. 3 Curves (established according to the "direct" method) of the cumulative duration of survival of children submitted respectively to protocols 9 and 10.

and the cumulative survival curves (Fig. 3).

3.- Results according to the classification of the patients on the prognostic parameters available in 1970.

Fig. 4 shows a very significant difference between the cumulative remission duration curves of the "good prognostic group" (all micro-lymphoblastic and V-macrolymphoblastic and prolymphocytic types), and the "poor prognostic group" (V+ macrolymphoblastic and prolymphocytic and all prolymphoblastic types) of protocol 9: the curve of the first group forms a plateau, expressing cure expectancy, for 8 out of 10 patients between the 20th and the 50th month, while the curve of the other group only forms a plateau for 2 out of 14 patients (the difference is significant $p < 10^{-4}$).

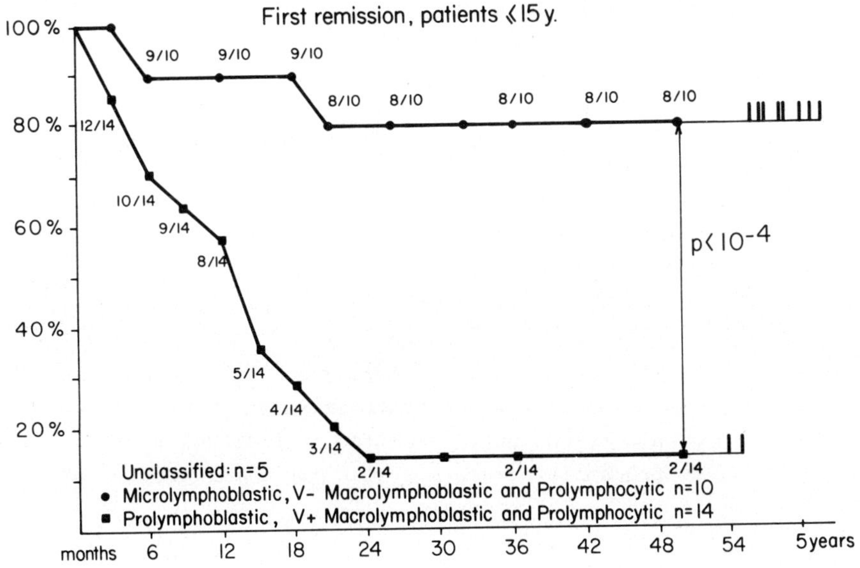

Fig. 4 Curves (established according to the "direct" method) of the cumulative duration of the first remission of the two groups of patients submitted to protocol 9, according to prognosis parameters. See the signification of V+ and V- in the text.

Fig. 5 shows a similar difference, significant at $p < 0.01$, between the respective curves of cumulative survival of these two groups: the curve of the good prognostic group forms a plateau for 9 out of 10 patients between the 6th and the 50th month, while the curve of the poor prognostic group forms a plateau for only 5 out of 15 patients and only between the 42nd and the 50th month.

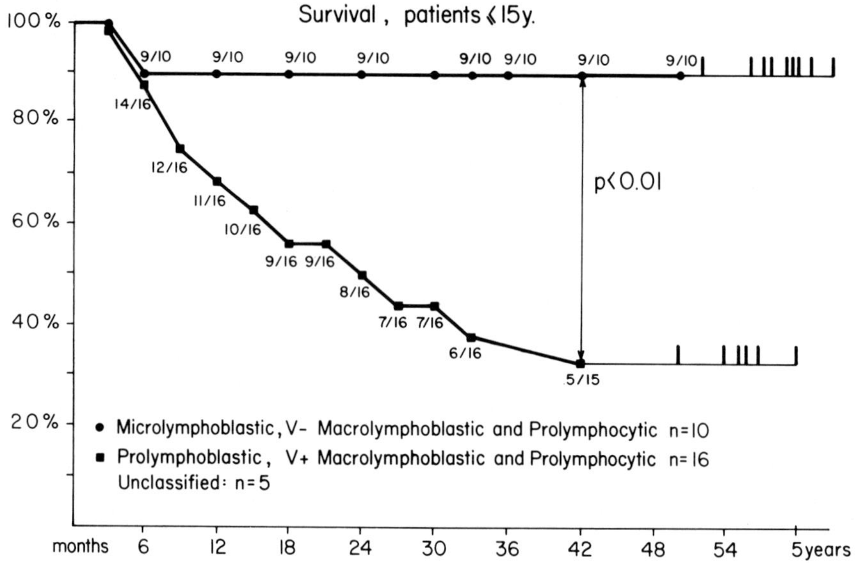

Fig. 5 Curves (established according to the "direct" method) of the cumulative duration of survival of the two groups of patients submitted to protocol 9, according to prognosis parameters. See the signification of V+ and V- in the texte.

4.- Comparison of active immunotherapy toxicity with post-remission chemotherapy toxicity.

We regret that there were 6 deaths during protocols 9 and 10 during the 611 months' chemotherapy, in contrast to no deaths during the same length of AI. These 6 deaths, during chemotherapy, were due to chest infections in 5 cases, and to a gastrointestinal haemorrhage in one case.

No side effects of AI for protocol 9 have been noted except a slight fever < 38°C the day of BCG application. We do not consider this to be a manifestation of toxicity, but an expression of the BCG bacteriemia which, from our experimental data[22,23], we regard as necessary for immunotherapy efficacy[24], and which is, therefore, an indication of the correct BCG application.

The comparison of the data on sperm, lymphocyte chromosome and bone marrow stem cell investigations of the patients submitted, respectively, to short and long chemotherapies will be published later[20].

DISCUSSION

1. Overall results. Cure expectancy

The results in children <15 years of age for the ICIG-ALL protocol 9 are remarkable for three features: a) the break in the curve of first remissions to form a plateau between the second and the 5th year, a plateau which, from other studies, can be considered as a high probability of cure expectancy; b) the high percentage of all patients treated who are in this plateau of first remission: about 50% of all children submitted to the trial; and c) the still higher proportion (about 60%) of patients who are in the plateau of survivors, with no death between the 3rd and the 5th year.

2. Comparison of the results of protocol 9 with short pre-immunotherapy chemotherapy, with those of protocols with long pre-immunotherapy chemotherapy and those published in the literature with long maintenance chemotherapy

a) Protocol 9 versus protocol 10

First remission and cure expectancy. Fig. 2 shows that for protocols 9 and 10, the children of which are strikingly comparable as regards age, sex and prognostic factors, there is no difference in the percentage of children belonging to each of the remission curve plateaux; in other words, both have a high probability of cure expectancy.

From this comparison, we can deduce that from the 9th to the 25th month, active immunotherapy is as efficient as one of the best maintenance chemotherapies (6-MP, MTX and CPM).

Survival. Fig. 3 shows that, while the median survival time for protocol 10 patients is 2 years, this median has still to be attained for protocol 9 patients between the 4th and the 5th year. However, the respective proportions of patients belonging to each of the plateaux between the 4th and 5th year are not significantly different.

b) Protocol 9 results versus results of another protocol (ICIG-ALL 11) with long pre-immunotherapy chemotherapy

We have conducted another protocol, ICIG-ALL 11, with long pre-immunotherapy chemotherapy (19 months of 6-MP, MTX and CPM), but without an initial post-remission chemotherapy similar to that of protocols 9 and 10[25,26]. Because of this difference, we did not include it in the above comparison. However, it should be mentioned that the proportions of the patients belonging to the first remission and survival plateaux (being 54% and 71%, respectively) are not significantly different from those in protocol 9.

c) Protocol 9 results versus results of long maintenance chemotherapy protocols obtained from the literature

Efficiency. We have also compared the results of protocol 9, comprising short chemotherapy followed by AI, with those of protocols composed of only long maintenance chemotherapy, which are already published or are under publication, and have a follow-up > 4 years[11,12,13,14,15,16,17].

From this comparison, it seems reasonable to conclude that a protocol comprising a short complementary cell-reducing chemotherapy followed by active-immunotherapy (AI) is as effective as the most efficient branch of the comparable Memphis protocol called "total therapy study VII-1970-1971", comprising a 3 year maintenance chemotherapy[15]: in this branch, 43% of the patients are on the plateau (which is less than for protocol 9, but not significantly different), while the proportions are 32%, 23% and 18% for the other branches. It is superior to the other maintenance chemotherapy protocols or branches of protocols published in the literature[11,12,13,14,15].

With regard to the Acute Leukemia Group B results[16,17], we were only able to obtain survival curves, but not first remission curves: from Holland's[16] presentation, it appeared that, among the very numerous branches of protocols 6307-6311, 6313, 6601, 6801 and 7111, only two present a survival plateau after 6 years; one branch of protocol 6601 has a plateau for 25% of the patients and one branch of protocol 6801 has a plateau for 65% of the patients, which is no different to the plateau of survival of protocol 9 patients.

The EORTC Haemopathy Working Party[27] has compared maintenance chemotherapy and AI between the 12th and the 24th month after first remission in a randomized trial. They observed no significant difference between the maintenance chemotherapy and immunotherapy branches for remission and survival durations. This observation supports our observation on the comparison of the results of protocol 9 with those of protocols 10 and 11, and allows us to conclude that AI is as active as the best maintenance chemotherapy between the first and the second year after remission induction, a period during which no chemotherapist would leave an ALL patient without maintenance chemotherapy.

This conclusion, as well as the results of the study by Ekert et al.[28,29] showing that chemo-immunotherapy is much more active than chemotherapy, can be added to the result of our first pilot trial[2,3,4] and to the data presented in this paper, to argue in favour of the efficiency of AI in ALL.

We will only comment briefly on the negative results of three attempts at AI of ALL[30,31,32]; these have been discussed more fully elsewhere[3,4]. Briefly, a negative result does not prove that the method is not effective, but that its application in the given trial was not efficient. Negative results have been registered in immunotherapy trials of other diseases on which the results of most trials have shown the efficiency of this therapeutic weapon[33], and furthermore, negative results have been reported in chemotherapy trials on diseases in which its efficiency has been demonstrated by many other trials[see 34].

Considering the absolute, as well as the comparative results of protocol 9, we can conclude not only that a protocol comprising a short cell-reducing complementary chemotherapy followed by AI is of great efficiency, but also that immunotherapy of acute lymphoid leukaemia is indicated on both scientific and ethical bases.

Toxicity. The above recommendation is not only justified by the efficiency of AI, but also by the differences in the toxicities of AI and maintenance chemotherapy. In over 300 patients who have been submitted to it[1,35], immunotherapy has not induced a single death in protocols 9,10 or 11, whereas the lethal toxicity of maintenance chemotherapy varies from 4 to 28% in the literature[see 5].

The EORTC Haemopathy Working Party[27] has confirmed this important fact, registering 4 deaths out of 29 randomized maintenance chemotherapy patients and 0 out of 29 immunotherapy patients.

In addition, one must inquire about late side-effects and, to this end, we are conducting an investigation on sperm, lymphocyte chromosomes and bone-marrow stem cells.

3. Correlations between early prognosis typing and disease evolution

The very marked differences observed between patients submitted to protocol 9 and distinguished at the beginning of their disease on the W.H.O. Reference Center cytological typing[6,7] and the volume of the neoplasia[10], as belonging to either the "good prognosis group" (microlymphoblastic and V-macrolymphoblastic and prolymphocytic types) or the "poor prognosis group" (prolymphoblastic and V+ macrolymphoblastic and prolymphocytic types) (Figs. 4 and 5) confirm our previous observations[1,4].

The value of these parameters for prognosis have been confirmed by some research groups treating patients by maintenance chemotherapy only[17,36], but not by others[37,38].

Similarly, whereas Brouet et al.[39] do not find any prognostic difference between the T and null cell types of Jean Bernard ALL patients submitted to maintenance chemotherapy, we find that, in the immunotherapy patients, the T-type leukaemias relapse rapidly, while the null cell leukaemias have a high cure expectancy[8,9].

Hence, the discrepancies between the different research groups as to the value of prognostic parameters, whether they be due to differences in the populations of treated patients or to differences in the diagnostic criteria used on identical patients in different treatment centers, may also be due to differences in treatments: cytological and immune parameters do not permit the prognostic groups to be distinguished in Jean Bernard's patients who were submitted to maintenance chemotherapy[37,39], whereas they do in our patients who were submitted to immunotherapy[6,8,9,10].

This leads us to search for new drugs, treatment combinations and modalities of applications in order to treat the poor prognosis patients with a more intensive therapy, even if this treatment involves a certain risk. Taking such a risk for the good prognosis patients (with a cure expectancy of 80%) is obviously unethical. Treating the poor prognosis patients with a more intensive therapy than the good prognosis ones has already improved the overall prognosis for patients in our protocol ICIG-ALL 12 compared to protocols 9, 10 and 11.

SUMMARY

Protocol ICIG-ALL 9 with only nine months' remission chemotherapy followed by active immunotherapy has given a cure expectancy (the proportion of the patients on a plateau of first remission) of about 50%, while 60% of the children are on the plateau of survival.

These results do not differ from those of another protocol (ICIG-ALL 10) conducted on an identical population of patients and comprising a 25 month remission chemotherapy before immunotherapy.

This observation, confirmed by a randomized trial of the EORTC Haemopathy Working Party, indicates that between the 9th and the 25th month, active immunotherapy is as efficient as maintenance chemotherapy.

The overall results of this protocol with short chemotherapy followed by active immunotherapy have been compared with those of another prolonged maintenance chemotherapy before immunotherapy protocol (ICIC-ALL 11), and with published protocols comprising only long maintenance chemotherapy: protocol 9 is, as far as the first remission plateau (cure expectancy) and the survival plateau are concerned, superior to most of these protocols (or their branches).

Lethal toxicity of active immunotherapy is nil, in contrast to the proportion of deaths (4 to 28%) occurring during remission in the patients submitted to maintenance chemotherapy.

Thus active immunotherapy is scientifically and ethically indicated in acute lymphoid leukaemia treatment.

However, not all patients with so-called acute lymphoid leukaemias should be treated identically: our early prognosis parameters (WHO cytological types and volume of the tumour, in this study) allow us to distinguish a good prognosis group in which protocol 9 gave an 80% cure expectancy.

The patients with a poor prognosis should be the object of further research for a more efficient therapy. Even if this should be more intensive, the risk is justified in this group, while it is not so for the good prognosis group. Research in this direction has already led to improved prognosis for acute lymphoid leukaemia patients submitted to the protocol we apply at present.

ACKNOWLEDGEMENT

The authors would like to thank Dr R. Powles for his valuable assistance in the preparation of the text.

REFERENCES

1. Mathé G. Active immunotherapy of cancer: its immunoprophylaxis and immunorestoration. An introduction. Heidelberg-New York, 1976, Springer Verlag.
2. Mathé G., Amiel J.L., Schwarzenberg L., Schneider M., Cattan A., Schlumberger J.R., Hayat M., De Vassal F. Lancet 1969, i, 697.
3. Mathé G. Biomedicine, 1977, 26, (in press).
4. Mathé G., Amiel J.L., Schwarzenberg L., Schneider M., Cattan A., Schlumberger J.R., Hayat M., De Vassal F. Biomedicine 1977, 26 (in press).

5. Mathé G., Schwarzenberg L., De Vassal F., Delgado M., Pena-Angulo J., Belpomme D., Pouillart P., Machover D., Misset J.L., Pico J.L. Jasmin C., Hayat M., Schneider M., Cattan A., Amiel J.L., Musset M., Rosenfeld C. in Symposium on "Immunotherapy of cancer: present status of trials in man", 27-29th October 1976, Bethesda. New York, 1977, Raven Press (in press).
6. Mathé G., Pouillart P., Sterescu M., Amiel J.L., Schwarzenberg L., Schneider M., Hayat M., De Vassal F., Jasmin C., Lafleur M. Europ. J. Clin. Biol. Res., 1971, 16, 554.
7. Mathé G., Rappaport H. Histological and cytological typing of neoplastic diseases of haematopoietic and lymphoid tissues. Geneva, 1976, World Health Organization.
8. Belpomme D., Dantchev D., Du Rusquec E., Grandjon D., Huchet R., Pouillart P., Schwarzenberg L., Amiel J.L., Mathé G. Biomedicine 1974, 20, 109.
9. Belpomme D., Mathé G., Davies A.J.S. Submitted to The Lancet.
10. Mathé G., De Vassal F., Delgado M., Pouillart P., Belpomme D., Joseph R., Schwarzenberg L., Amiel J.L., Schneider M., Cattan A., Musset M., Misset J.L., Jasmin C. Cancer Immunol. Immunoth., 1976, 1, 77.
11. Bernard J., Weil M., Jacquillat C. Wadley Medical Bulletin 1975, 5, 1.
12. Clarkson B.D., Dowling M.D., Gee T.S., Cunningham I.B., Burchenal J.H. Cancer 1975, 36, 775.
13. Fernbach D.J., George S.L., Sutow W.W., Ragab A.H., Lane D.M., Haggard M.E., Lonsdale D. Cancer 1975, 36, 1552.
14. Lonsdale D., Gehan E.A., Fernbach D.J., Sullivan M.P., Lane D.M., Ragab A.H. Cancer 1975, 36, 341.
15. Simone J.V. Personal communication.
16. Acute Leukemia Group B. James Holland, in Symposium on "Immunotherapy of cancer: present status of trials in man". 27-29th October 1976, Bethesda. New York, 1977, Raven Press (in press).
17. Lee S.L., Kopel S., Glidewell O. Seminars in Oncology 1976, 3, 209.
18. Mathé G., Rosenfeld C., in preparation.
19. Rosenfeld C., Venuat A.M., Goutner A., Guegand J., Choquet C., Tron F., Pico J.L. Proc. Amer. Cancer Res., 1975, 16, 29.
20. Mathé G., Venuat A.M., Rosenfeld C., Pouillart P. in preparation.
21. Schwartz D., Flamant R., Lellouch J. L'essai thérapeutique chez l'Homme. 1 vol., Paris, 1970, Editions Médicales Flammarion.

22.Khalil A., Rappaport H., Bourut C., Halle-Pannenko O., Mathé G. Biomedicine 1975, 22, 121.

23.Rappaport H., Khalil A. Cancer Immunol. Immunoth., 1976, 1, 45.

24.Mathé G. Cancer Immunol. Immunoth., 1976, 1, 3.

25.Mathé G., De Vassal F., Schwarzenberg L., Delgado M., Pena-Angulo J., Belpomme D., Pouillart P., Machover D., Misset J.L., Pico J.L. Jasmin C., Hayat M., Schneider M., Cattan A., Amiel J.L., Musset M., Rosenfeld C. in preparation.

26.Mathé G., De Vassal F., Schwarzenberg L., Delgado M., Pena-Angulo J., Belpomme D., Pouillart P., Machover D., Misset J.L., Pico J.L. Jasmin C., Hayat M., Schneider M., Cattan A., Amiel J.L., Musset M., Rosenfeld C. Biomedicine 1977, 26 (in press).

27.E.O.R.T.C. Hemopathies Working Party, in Symposium on "Immunotherapy of cancer: present status of trials in man". 27-29th October 1976, Bethesda. New York, 1977, Raven Press (in press).

28.Ekert H., Jose D.G. Lancet 1975, ii, 713.

29.Ekert H., Jose D.G., Waters K.D., Smith P.J., Mathews R.N. in Symposium on "Immunotherapy of cancer: present status of trials in man". 27-29th October 1976, Bethesda. New York, 1977, Raven Press (in press).

30.Heyn R., Joo P., Karon M., Nesbit M., Shore N., Breslow N., Weiner R., Reed A., Sather H., Hammond D. in Symposium on "Immunotherapy of Cancer: present status of trials in man". 27-29th October 1976, Bethesda. New York, 1977, Raven Press (in press).

31.Leventhal B.G. in Symposium on "Immunotherapy of cancer: present status of trials in man". 27-29th October 1976, Bethesda. New York, 1977, Raven Press (in press).

32.Medical Research Council. Brit. Med. J. 1971, 4, 189.

33.Symposium on "Immunotherapy of cancer: present status of trials in man", 27-29th October 1976, Bethesda. New York, 1977, Raven Press (in press).

34.Clarysse A., Kenis Y., Mathé G. Cancer chemotherapy. Its role in the treatment strategy of hematologic malignancies and solid tumors. 1 vol., Heidelberg-New York, 1976, Springer Verlag.

35.Schwarzenberg L., Simmler M.C., Pico J.L. Cancer Immunol. Immunoth., 1976, 1, 69.

36.Necheles T.F., Brenner J.F., Bonacossa I., Fristensky R., Neurath P.W. Biomedicine 1976, 25, 241.

37.Jacquillat C., Weil M., Gemon M.F., Boiron M., Bernard J. P. 113 in "Therapy of acute leukamias" (F. Mandelli, S. Amadori, G. Mariani, eds). 1 vol., Rome, 1975, Minerva Medica.

38.Murphy S.B., Borella L., Sen L., Mauer A. Brit. J. Haemat., 1975, 31, 95.

39.Brouet J.C., Valensi F., Daniel M.T., Flandrin G., Preud'homme J.L., Seligmann M. Brit. J. Haemat., 1976, 33, 319.

Adjuvant Therapy of Cancer, S.E. Salmon and S.E. Jones eds.

ADRIAMYCIN, CYTOXAN AND VINCRISTINE IN THE ADJUVANT TREATMENT OF LOCALIZED EWING'S SARCOMA

Franca Fossati Bellani, Sandro Barni, Marco Gasparini,
Fabrizio Lombardi, Angelo Lattuada, Gianni Bonadonna.
Istituto Nazionale Tumori, Milano
Italy

INTRODUCTION

During the past 15 years high-energy radiotherapy represented the treatment of choice for clinically localized Ewing's sarcoma and replaced with comparable results surgical resection or amputation[1]. However, there is ample evidence that even optimal radiotherapy is followed by a limited long-term disease-free survival[2]. A number of studies have reported that chemotherapy can induce tumor regression of clinically advanced Ewing's sarcomas[3]. Recently, single and multiple drug chemotherapy were combined with radiotherapy in the primary management of localized tumor[4-8]. The intent of the new combined modality approach was to eradicate the foci of micrometastases which in the large majority of patients, are responsible for the failure of local radiotherapy. There is initial evidence that this new strategy has improved the disease-free survival in different series of patients[4-8].

From 1970 to 1973, 6 patients with clinically localized Ewing's sarcoma were treated at the Istituto Nazionale Tumori of Milan with local radiotherapy and sequential combination chemotherapy according to a protocol designed for childhood soft tissue sarcomas. The drugs employed were adriamycin (ADM), vincristine (VCR), methotrexate (MTX) and cyclophosphamide (CTX). The updated disease-free survival is 66% (4 of 6 patients) after a minimum follow up observation of 4.5 years[9]. The favourable results obtained in this small series of patients prompted us to design in 1974 a new treatment protocol for localized Ewing's sarcoma. This report presents the preliminary evaluation of the combined protocol study.

PATIENTS AND METHODS

From January 1974 to August 1976, 19 consecutive patients with biopsy proven diagnosis of Ewing's sarcoma were admitted to the combined modality study. Nine patients were males and 10 were females. The age ranged from 2.9 to 21 years (mean 12.8). The sites of primary tumor are outlined in Figure 1.

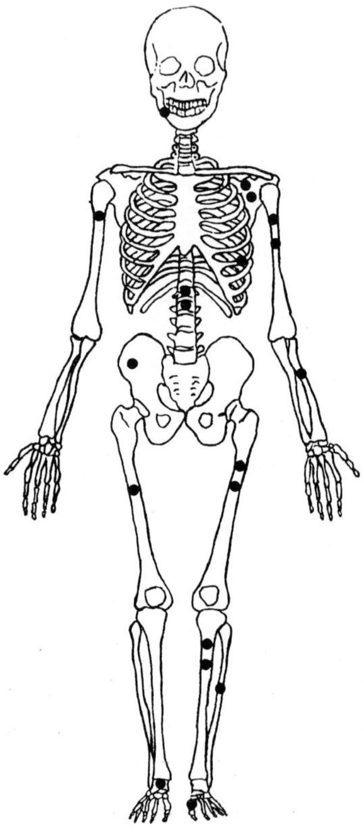

Fig. 1: Primary sites in 19 patients with localized Ewing's sarcoma

The initial diagnostic work-up included chest x-ray, skeletal survey, bone scan, liver and renal function tests and electrocardiogram (EKG). Pedal lymphangiography was carried out in patients with tumor located either in the pelvis or in the lower limbs (total 9). Bone marrow aspiration was carried out in 4 of 19 patients.

The treatment protocol is summarized in Figure 2. Radiotherapy was delivered using ^{60}Co teletherapy. The entire bone involved and the sorrounding tissues received an initial dose of 4,000 rad (1,000 rad per week). Subsequently, smaller fields were irradiated to a total tumor dose of 4,500-6,500 rad in relation to the site of primary involvement. In one patient the primary tumor (rib) was surgically removed and radiotherapy was delivered to the tumor area with a total tissue dose of 5,500 rad. In another patient, 5 years old, with primary involvement of the mandible, radiotherapy was not included in the treatment program following radical surgical excision.

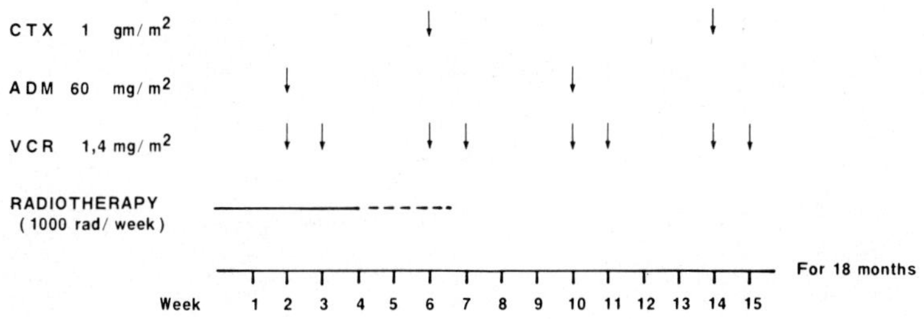

Fig. 2: Treatment schedule for localized Ewing's sarcoma

Chemotherapy was administered according to the dose schedule represented in Figure 2. All drugs were injected intravenously. The total dose of ADM was planned not to exceed 540 mg/m^2 (i.e. 9 cycles at the full dose of 60 mg/m^2). Chemotherapy was entirely administered in the out patient clinic of the Institute. All patients were carefully controlled with bimonthly roentgenograms of chest and skeleton. Chemistry and EKG were repeated every 4 months.

RESULTS

In all patients combined treatment induced a prompt complete remission of symptoms and physical signs of disease. A radiologically documented partial recalcification of the bone lesion was also observed in all patients. At the time of present analysis, 14 of 19 patients (74%) are free of disease with a follow up observation ranging from 6^+ to 35^+ months from the start of treatment. Figure 3 shows the actuarial disease-free survival.

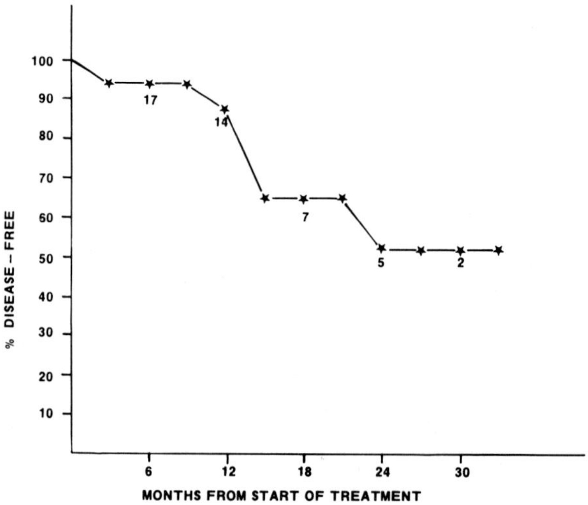

Fig. 3: Disease-free survival after combined radiotherapy-chemotherapy

In the 5 patients with relapse, new manifestations of disease were first detected in lungs (2), bones (1), lungs and bones (1) and brain (1). Four patients showed clinical evidence of metastases while on treatment after 2, 13, 14 and 14 months. The fifth patient relapsed 6 months after completion of all therapy, i.e. 2 years from the start of combined approach. This patient is currently free of disease 6 months after subsequent treatment with radiotherapy to bone lesions and chemotherapy with CTX, VCR, and CCNU. The other 4 patients who had relapse while on chemotherapy failed to respond to further chemotherapy with CCNU, procarbazine and actinomycin D (Act. D). Local tumor recurrence was clinically observed only in one patient and it became evident 4 months after the occurrence of pulmonary metastases. Two patients with primary involvement of metatarsus and humerus and who were considered to be in clinical complete remission, were surgically re-explored after 8 and 12 months, respectively from completion of radiotherapy and while on chemotherapy, because of bone fracture. In one patient the histologic specimen revealed residual malignant cells.

Side effects can be summarized as follows. Nausea and vomiting occurred almost always within few hours from each drug exposure. Combination chemotherapy produced alopecia in all patients. As far as bone marrow suppression is concerned, no patient developed severe leukopenia (leukocytes count less than 2,000 per cu.mm.) and/or severe thrombocytopenia (platelets count less than 75,000 per cu. mm.). No EKG abnormalities were documented. Two patients developed severe fibrosis in the soft tissues (upper arm and thigh) which were subjected to irradiation. While on chemotherapy one patient became pregnant. Therapeutic abortion was performed at the third month. The histologic examination of the uterine scraping showed the presence of hydatiform mole.

COMMENT

Our findings show that a definite improvement in the disease-free survival of patients with clinically localized Ewing's sarcoma can be achieved with combined treatment modality, when results are retrospectively compared with those achieved by radiotherapy alone[2]. In fact, a projected disease-free survival of 52% at two years from the start of treatment is significantly superior to that of 15-25% achieved with local modalities[4,10]. As shown in Table 1, our data are comparable to those obtained by other authors who have employed various schedules of combination chemotherapy as adjuvant treatment for Ewing's sarcoma.

TABLE 1

SUMMARY OF CURRENT RESULTS IN LOCALIZED EWING'S SARCOMA TREATED WITH ADJUVANT CHEMOTHERAPY

Author	Ref.	Combined treatment	Disease-free survivors/ treated	Time from start of treatment (months)
HUSTU et al. (1972)	5	Radiotherapy VCR+CTX	10/15	4^+ - 91^+ (median 19^+)
FERNANDEZ et al. (1974)	4	Radiotherapy VCR+CTX	6/19	12^+ - 46^+
JOHNSON et al. (1975)	6	Radiotherapy VCR+CTX+ADM CNS prophylaxis	12/15	median 24^+
JAFFE et al. (1976)	7	Radiotherapy VCR+CTX+Act. D	7/9	4^+ - 54^+
ROSEN et al. (1976)	8	Radiotherapy or surgery VCR+CTX+ADM+Act. D	15/19	15^+ - 66^+ (median 37^+)
Present series (1977)		Radiotherapy VCR+CTX+ADM	15/19	6^+ - 35^+ (median 16^+)

The chemotherapeutic agents employed for the combined treatment of Ewing's sarcoma included CTX, VCR, ADM and Act. D. The drugs were administered in a wide range of schedules. Our multiple drug regimen was selected on the basis of favourable results observed in the treatment of advanced disease. The reason for including ADM in the combination was based on the high response rate obtained when this drug was administered alone in patients resistant to conventional agents[11,12]. The cyclical regimen employed in our combined approach also proved to be well tolerated and devoid of significant marrow toxicity.

As observed in other studies utilizing adjuvant chemotherapy, a very low incidence of local recurrences was documented. This event represented one of the most important reasons for relapse in patients treated solely with radiotherapy or conservative surgery[4,10]. It is conceivable that the improved local control was due to the effects of combined treatment, along with the improved technique of irradiation.

Although present findings allow to state that adjuvant treatment has improved the outlook of Ewing's sarcoma with clinically undetectable metastases, two important points remain to be further clarified:

1. The actual cure rate of adjuvant treatment. In fact, follow up observation longer than two years for all patients is required, since new manifestations of disease usually occur during the first two years from diagnosis.
2. The optimal treatment program. It is necessary to establish the most effective therapeutic association in order to achieve the best results in term of disease-free survival at the expense of minimal disabling side-effects.

REFERENCES

1. Boyer, C.W. Jr. (1967) Cancer 20, 1602-1606.
2. Nesbit, M.E. (1976) CA, 26, 174-180.
3. Sutow, W.W. et al. (1971) Cancer Chemother. Rep. 55, 67-78.
4. Fernandez, C.H. et al. (1974) Cancer 34, 143-148.
5. Hustu, H.O. et al. (1972) Cancer 30, 1522-1527.
6. Johnson, R.E. and Pomeroy, T.C. (1975) Am. J. Roentgen. 123, 583-587.
7. Jaffe, N. et al. (1976) Cancer 38, 1925-1930.
8. Rosen, G. (1976) Ped. Clin. N. Amer. 23, 183-213.
9. Gasparini, M. et al. (1977) Tumori, in press.
10. Macintosh, M.J. et al. (1975) J. Bone Joint Surg. 57, 331-340.
11. Oldham, R.K. and Pomeroy, T.C. (1972) Cancer Chemother. Rep., Part 1, 56, 635-639.

12. Bonadonna, G. et al. (1975) Cancer Chemother. Rep., Part 3, 6, 231-245.

Adjuvant Therapy of Cancer, S.E. Salmon and S.E. Jones eds.

PRIMARY CHEMOTHERAPY IN THE MANAGEMENT OF PELVIC RHABDOMYOSARCOMA IN INFANCY AND EARLY CHILDHOOD

Daniel M. Hays, M.D., and Jorge Ortega, M.D.
Departments of Surgery and Pediatrics, University of Southern California
School of Medicine, Los Angeles, California

SUMMARY

Since 1968, 10 infants and pre-adolescent children with rhabdomyosarcoma; primary in the bladder, prostate or vagina, have been treated by a regimen of initial intensive chemotherapy and a limited use of radiotherapy and surgery. Therapy has consisted of between two and three years of chemotherapy; initially, vincristine, dactinomycin, and cyclophosphamide (Pulse VAC), at times supplemented with adriamycin. Four of the 10 patients have received radiotherapy, to the pelvis only (3) or the total abdomen (1). Surgery has consisted of limited endoscopic excisions or biopsies, in the case of tumors primary in the bladder or prostate; and partial vaginectomy and simple hysterectomy, in the case of vaginal-uterine tumors.

Two patients are more than seven years, and five additional patients between one and one-half and four years since diagnosis, without evidence of disease. One patient is less than one year from diagnosis on the chemotherapy regimen. Two patients have had urinary diversion, including one exenteration, for failure to respond to the chemotherapy regimen.

One patient died secondary to the effects of chemotherapy. The remaining nine are alive, seven of them without evidence of disease.

BACKGROUND

Chemotherapy is the prime modality of therapy in disseminated rhabdomyosarcoma. It has also been employed in children with "unresectable" primary tumors, as noted by Marshall, 1956[1], Pratt, 1969[2], Tefft and Jaffe, 1973[3], Ghavimi, Exelby, D'Angio, Whitmore, Lieberman, Lewis, Mike, and Murphy, 1973[4], and Holton, Chapman, Lackey, Hatch, Baum, and Favara, 1973[5]. In these patients, when initial surgery has been unsuccessful, the aim has been to reduce the volume of tumor with chemotherapy, with or without radiotherapy, and follow (when possible) by extirpative surgery. Such cases with pelvic rhabdomyosarcoma have been described by Wilbur, Sutow, Sullivan, Castro, Kaizer, and Taylor, 1971[6], Mackenzie, Sharma, Whitmore, and Melamed, 1971[7], Tank, Fellmann, Wheeler, Weaver, and Lapides, 1972[8], Kumar, Wrenn, Fleming, Hustu, Pratt, and Pinkel, 1975[9], and Jaffe, Weinstein, Cassady, and Traggis, 1976[10]. A number of these patients with "unresectable" rhabdomyosarcoma of the pelvis in which such a regimen has been employed, have had extended periods of tumor-free survival.

Our series of patients with pelvic rhabdomyosarcoma treated by a primary chemotherapy regimen, without initial laparotomy, was begun in 1968 and previously reviewed in 1975[11]. In scattered clinics throughout the world small groups of children with primary pelvic rhabdomyosarcomas, which could be regarded as "resectable" by modern standards, have subsequently been treated by regimens of primary chemotherapy. A total of 23 such patients are known to the authors, but only three are described in reports[12]. Approximately one half of these patients are alive more than two years following diagnosis. The results of such therapy in children with vaginal rhabdomyosarcomas have been superior to those with tumors primary in the prostate or bladder. In at least 75% of the tumors there has been a major reduction in tumor size. In many instances this has involved a complete elimination of gross tumor by chemotherapy alone, or chemotherapy with irradiation. In some cases all tumor tissue has been destroyed as demonstrated by repeated biopsies of the area. It is also apparent that some of these tumors have <u>not</u> responded to a significant degree to chemotherapy regimens, including Pulse VAC. Some series have employed no radiotherapy. All successful chemotherapy programs include multiple agents and a period of several years of chemotherapy.

In some patients in these series, although the bladder is physically present following the chemotherapy-radiotherapy regimens, its function is grossly disturbed and cystectomy and urinary diversions have been required after the child was apparently tumor free.

CLINICAL SERIES

Included in this series are only those patients who (a) had biopsied rhabdomyosarcoma apparently primary in the bladder, prostate, or vagina and adjacent uterus; (b) were infants or pre-adolescent children at the time therapy was initiated; (c) demonstrated no evidence of distant dissemination; and (d) in whom a vigorous chemotherapy regimen preceded radiotherapy or surgery (except biopsy). All qualified patients treated by this regimen at Childrens Hospital of Los Angeles (1969-1976) are included as well as one treated at another institution (#5).

The patient age range was .7 to 7.5 years at diagnosis. The series included two females with vaginal-uterine tumors, seven males with bladder or prostate primary sites, and one "female" with a form of testicular feminization and a tumor primary in the urogenital sinus. The actual site of origin is indefinite in some cases as noted in the next section. Conventional staging is of little significance in these patients and they cannot be compared with patients staged by exenteration or laparotomy.

Although there were many additions to and departures from the outlined chemotherapy program, the regimen below was standard as initial therapy and is referred to as Pulse VAC in Table 1.

Each Course of Therapy (q 3-5 weeks)

VCN	1.5 mg/m^2	IV push (Days 1 and 8)
CYX	300 mg/m^2	IV push (Days 1, 3 and 7)
ACD	600 mcg/m^2	IV push (Days 1, 2, 3, and 4)

The aim of the program, which developed during the course of this series, included an initial attempt to destroy the tumor by courses of Pulse VAC administered as rapidly as possible. If reduction in tumor size reached a plateau, either local irradiation or the addition of adriamycin to the chemotherapy regimen followed. Only four of these patients received radiotherapy at any time during the course (Table 1). Surgery in primary tumors of the bladder-prostate consisted of repeated cystoscopic examinations with excisions of tissue for biopsy purposes. Tumors primary in the vagina-uterus were treated by partial vaginectomy and simple hysterectomy, at a stage when the tumor was no longer palpable.

Among six patients who are at present (1977) more than 40 months since diagnosis, four have no evidence of disease (NED); one had been without evidence of disease for 19 months when lost to surveillance in 1975; and one succumbed to infection during the course of chemotherapy.

Table 1

PRIMARY CHEMOTHERAPY SERIES CHLA

#	Sex, Age at onset (years)	Primary Site	Stage	Chemo-therapy	Duration	Radiotherapy	Surgery	Observation Period Total	Observation Period w/o CEM	Comment
1	M 2.5	B-P	I-II	P-VAC VCN	22 mon. 13 mon. (35 mon.)*	2500r/abd. 4000r/pelv.	Cysto.** only	90 mon.	54 mon.	NED
2	F 1.5	V-U	I-III	P-VAC ACD-CYX	8 mon. 22 mon. (30 mon.)	0	Hyst. Vag.	76 mon.	46 mon.	NED
3	M 7.5	B-P	II-III	P-VAC	2 mon.	0	Cysto. only	2 mon. TOX.	0	DEAD (TOX.)
4	M 2.0	B-P	I-II	P-VAC ADM CYX	5 mon. 12.5 mon. 16.5 mon. (34 mon.)	3515r/pelv.	Cysto. only	54 mon.	20 mon.	NED
5	F 4.0	V-U	II-III	P-VAC	26 mon.	4000r/pelv.	Hyst. Vag.	40 mon.	14 mon.	NED
6	M 3.0	B-P	II-III	IRS-E	19 mon.+	3119r/pelv.	Cysto. only	19 mon.{}	0	NED
7	M 3.0	B-P	II-III	P-VAC + ADM	16 mon. 13 mon.+	0	Ileal "loop"	30 mon.	0	NED (Failure)
8	M 2.5	B-P	I-II	P-VAC	18 mon.+	0	Cysto. only	18 mon.	0	Alive with local tumor
9	F*** 3.0	V-V	I-II	P-VAC ADM	8 mon. 15 mon.+	0	Anterior Exenter.	23 mon.	0	NED (Failure)
10	M .7	B-P	I-II	P-VAC ADM	5 mon. 2 mon.+	0	Cysto. only	7 mon.	0	Alive with local tumor

* Total Period of Chemotherapy ( )
** Cystoscopy with Biopsy
*** Testicular Feminization Syndrome

B-P Bladder or Prostate
V-U Vagina or Cervix Uteri
V-V Vulva or Vagina

{} Lost to Follow-Up
\+ Still on Therapy

The four patients seen since that time have had periods of observation ranging from seven to 30 months. Two of these are NED, and two alive with palpable local tumor. Two of these are regarded as "failures", in that urinary diversion has been required, and in one case an anterior exenteration performed. Although these patients have not been successful from the point of view of avoiding diversion (or exenteration) they are without evidence of disease on chemotherapy regimens at the present time.

COMMENT

Once a regimen of simple biopsy and primary chemotherapy for these tumors is adopted; both traditional staging (except for Stage IV, i.e., known distant disseminated disease) and even identification of primary site may be uncertain. They cannot be directly compared with patients in which staging has been based on exenteration prior to chemotherapy, or even a laparotomy. After successful chemotherapy all patients become, in effect, Stage I. What stage these lesions were originally, as opposed to what stage they were after most of their volume has been destroyed by chemotherapy, is unknown. The distinction between a bladder trigone versus a prostatic primary may be uncertain. Even determination of the site of origin between the vagina and the cervix uteri may be unclear in a specimen removed after a successful chemotherapy regimen. Although it is probable that when a massive tumor is reduced to a small nodule the site of the latter may be assumed to be the site of the primary tumor, this is unproven.

The decision as to the major modality of therapy in the initial two cases in this series was influenced by a parental objection to an exenterative procedure. The regimen described was then adapted for this form of childhood rhabdomyosarcoma, a type in which the mortality has been relatively low[13] but the morbidity and post-surgical disability, high.

The results in this series must be compared with the results of the more conventional therapeutic regimen, i.e., exenteration, followed by local irradiation and then adjuvant chemotherapy (usually VAC) for two years. The results of such regimens in localized disease (as staged by exenteration specimens) may be excellent[14], when evaluated only on the basis of survival. The advantages of the elimination of exenteration and of intensive pelvic irradiation from the scheme of therapy, however, are of major significance and this will only be possible employing a primary chemotherapy regimen.

Patients who require urinary diversions to the skin were regarded as "failures" for the purposes of this study, although both patients in which this was required are alive. One of them is without known tumor. Thus it would appear that a primary chemotherapy regimen does not necessarily produce a detrimental effect on survival, even when it must be abandoned and urinary diversion or exenteration employed. The most devastating adverse effects on the urinary bladder are produced by combinations of chemotherapy and irradiation. If the latter can be eliminated from routine management of these patients, the possibility of retaining a normally functioning bladder, will be enhanced.

REFERENCES

1. Marshall, V.F.: Pelvic exenteration for polypoid myosarcoma (sarcoma botryoides) of the urinary bladder of an infant. Cancer 9:620, 1956.

2. Pratt, C.B.: Response of childhood rhabdomyosarcoma to combination chemotherapy. J. Ped. 74:791, 1969.

3. Tefft, M., Jaffe, N.: Sarcoma of the bladder and prostate in children. Rationale for the role of radiation therapy based on a review of the literature and a report of 14 additional patients. Cancer 32:1161, 1973.

4. Ghavimi, F., Exelby, P.R., et. al.: Combination therapy of urogenital embryonal rhabdomyosarcoma in children. Cancer 32:1178, 1973.

5. Holton, C.P., Chapman, K.E., et. al.: Extended combination therapy of childhood rhabdomyosarcoma. Cancer 32:1310, 1973.

6. Wilbur, J.R., Sutow, W.W., et. al.: Successful treatment of inoperable embryonal rhabdomyosarcoma. Ped. Res. 5:408, 1971.

7. Mackenzie, A.R., Sharma, T.C., et. al.: Non-extirpative treatment of myosarcomas of the bladder and prostate. Cancer 28:329, 1971.

8. Tank, E.S., Fellmann, S.H., et. al.: Treatment of urogenital tract rhabdomyosarcoma in infants and children. J. Urol. 107:324, 1972.

9. Kumar, A.P.M., Wrenn, E.L., et. al.: Preoperative therapy for unresectable malignant tumors in children. J. Ped. Surg. 10:657, 1975.

10. Jaffe, N., Weinstein, H., et. al.: Primary treatment with vincristine, actinomycin D and cyclophosphamide (VAC) and radiation therapy for unresectable rhabdomyosarcoma in children. ASCO Abstracts, pg. 284, 1976.

11. Rivard, G., Ortega, J., et. al.: Intensive chemotherapy as primary treatment for rhabdomyosarcoma of the pelvis. Cancer 36:1593, 1975.

12. Kumar, A.P.M., Wrenn, E.L., Jr., et. al.: Combined therapy to prevent complete pelvic exenteration for rhabdomyosarcoma of the vagina or uterus. Cancer 37:118, 1976.

13. Sutow, W.W., Sullivan, M.P., et. al.: Prognosis in childhood rhabdomyosarcoma. Cancer 25:1384, 1970.

14. Grosfeld, J.L., Smith, J.P., et. al.: Pelvic rhabdomyosarcoma in infants and children. J. Urol. 107:673, 1972.

Section VII

SARCOMA AND MELANOMA

Adjuvant Therapy of Cancer, S.E. Salmon and S.E. Jones eds.

ADJUVANT THERAPY IN MELANOMA AND SARCOMAS

Donald L. Morton, Frederick R. Eilber, E. Carmack Holmes,
Courtney M. Townsend, Jr., Joseph Mirra, and Thomas H. Weisenburger
Division of Oncology, Department of Surgery
University of California, Los Angeles, California 90024
United States

INTRODUCTION

Surgical procedures have been first order treatment for patients with melanoma or sarcoma. Although this method had considerable success for early Stage I melanoma (disease confined to primary site), there was a high rate of treatment failure in the later stages of melanoma[1,2] and undifferentiated skeletal or soft tissue sarcomas.[3-7] Even when local control could be achieved, these patients usually developed and succumbed to distant metastases of their disease. Thus, it has been obvious for some time that certain patients with both diseases have certain clinico-pathological features which can lead to a high incidence of treatment failure due to systemic metastases and/or local recurrence. This paper will briefly summarize our attempts to develop effective pre- and postoperative adjuvant therapy for patients with Stage II melanoma and for patients with skeletal and soft tissue sarcomas.

<u>Immunotherapy for Stage II melanoma</u>: Patients with Stage II melanoma (disease metastatic to regional lymph nodes) have a high rate of treatment failure despite lymphadenectomy. Such failures usually are not the result of uncontrolled primary or even regional disease, but, instead, are caused by clinically undetectable distant metastases. Because the rate of disease recurrence in these patients is approximately 70% at two years following operation for their primary tumor, it must be assumed that these occult metastases were present at the time of initial evaluation. In order to improve treatment results for patients with Stage II malignant melanoma, a clinical trial was started to assess the effects of adjuvant immunotherapy.

A prospective randomized trial of postoperative adjuvant immunotherapy was initiated to compare no additional therapy following operation with postoperative BCG alone or BCG plus an allogeneic melanoma cell vaccine. To date, 90 patients have been admitted to the trial since August 1974 after extensive examination that included history, chest x-ray, CBC, selected blood tests, liver, brain and bone scans to assess stage and extent of disease.

All patients underwent excision of their primary melanoma site with at least a 5 cm margin in all locations except the face, along with simultaneous regional lymphadenectomy. All patients in this study had histologically proven evidence of metastasis to regional nodes and, therefore, were categorized as Stage II malignant melanoma. Patients were stratified on the basis of age, sex, site of primary melanoma, and whether the nodes were thought to be involved with metastatic melanoma on clinical examination. The results of the randomization according to these stratification factors are given in Table I.

TABLE 1

MELANOMA: PATIENT INFORMATION AND TYPE OF TREATMENT

Factor	Group 1 BCG No. Pts.	Group 2 Tumor Cell + BCG No. Pts.	Group 3 Control No. Pts.
Number	32	29	28
Age (mean years)	44	40	42
Sex			
Male	23	23	21
Female	9	6	7
Site Distribution			
Head & Neck	5 (16%)	3 (10%)	6 (21%)
Extremity	7 (22%)	6 (20%)	7 (25%)
Trunk	16 (50%)	16 (53%)	12 (43%)
Unknown	4 (12%)	4 (17%)	3 (11%)
Lymph Node Status			
Clinicall positive	21	22	22
Clinically negative	11	7	6

Systemic immunotherapy was begun two to six weeks following the operation. Group 1 received BCG alone (Tice strain, Chicago Research Laboratories), given at a dosage of $1\text{-}2 \times 10^8$ organisms by the tine technique to each axilla and groin, and circumferentially around the primary site, at weekly intervals for twelve weeks and then biweekly thereafter. Group 2 received BCG plus allogeneic melanoma cells. In this procedure, BCG was given as described above followed by intradermal injection of 1×10^8 allogeneic tissue-cultured melanoma cells into the same areas at each time interval. The tumor cell vaccine was admixed with 1×10^6 organisms of Glaxo BCG during the first 2 inoculations, but not thereafter. Control patients, Group 3, received no additional therapy following their initial operative procedure. All patients were followed at monthly intervals with physical examination, CBC, SMA and chest x-rays. None were lost to follow-up. Patients who developed recurrence continued their particular adjuvant therapy in addition to chemotherapy with dimethyl-triazeno-imidazole-carboxamide (DTIC) combined with 1-3-bis(2-Chloroethyl)-1-nitrosourea (BCNU), or 1-(2-Chloroethyl)-3-cyclohexyl-1-nitrosourea (CCNU).

When the control patients were compared to patients who received adjuvant immunotherapy, the proportion of patients who had recurrent disease was higher (50%) than in either of the immunotherapy groups (41% and 34%, respectively). If the groups were compared by the proportion of patients who died, the control group had 36% deaths versus 19% in the BCG alone group, or 24% in the BCG plus tumor cell vaccine group. No patient developed systemic BCG infection and/or granulomatous hepatitis secondary to BCG administration which required discontinuation of therapy. For the most part, side effects consisted of transient malaise and low grade fever occurring on the day of immunization, and local reactions at the site of BCG administration. Such complications have responded to decreased dosages of BCG.

Patients receiving BCG and melanoma cell vaccine did develop additional complications related to the vaccine itself. Seven patients contracted hepatitis B infection, presumably from the human serum in which the melanoma cells were grown. All of these patients subsequently recovered completely from the hepatitis as evidenced by normal liver function tests and the disappearance of hepatitis B antigen from their sera.

Multimodality therapy for skeletal and soft tissue sarcoma: Surgical therapy has been the accepted method for management of most skeletal and soft tissue sarcomas of the extremity, although it has been associated with frequent treatment failure. Even when local control was achieved, over 50% of the patients with soft tissue sarcomas and 80% of the patients with skeletal sarcomas eventually developed and succumbed to distant metastases of their disease. Thus, single modality therapy for skeletal and soft tissue sarcomas with operation alone is followed by unacceptably high rates of treatment failure. Fortunately, new adjuvant treatment techniques have been developed that seem to have activity against these neoplasms.

Postoperative radiation therapy has dramatically reduced the incidence of local recurrence of soft tissue sarcomas, and preoperative continuous intra-arterial Adriamycin has been found to be effective for both soft tissue and skeletal sarcomas.[4] Postoperative adjuvant therapy with high dose Methotrexate and Citrovorum rescue and/or Adriamycin has reduced the incidence of pulmonary metastases from osteosarcomas and adjuvant immunotherapy with BCG and allogeneic sarcoma cell vaccine has lowered the incidence of distant metastases from soft tissue sarcomas.

Encouraged by the early results from these new treatment modalities for skeletal and soft tissue sarcomas, we began a clinical trial in November 1975 to evaluate the toxicity and therapeutic effectiveness of intra-arterial infusion of Adriamycin followed by moderate-dose radiation therapy before operation as a part of a program of multimodality therapy for patients with skeletal and soft tissue sarcomas of the extremities. Our purpose was to determine if it was possible to achieve preoperative in situ tumor destruction before adequate tumor resection, in order to preserve a functional extremity and to determine if postoperative adjuvant chemotherapy would improve disease-free survival.

Thirty-one consecutive patients with skeletal (14) and Stage III or IV soft tissue sarcomas (17) were entered into this study. Fifty-two patients served as controls -- 37 had amputation only (18 osteosarcoma and 19 soft tissue sarcoma), and 15 had amputation followed by chemotherapy (9 osteosarcoma and 6 soft tissue sarcoma). These control patients either were seen before effective chemotherapy was available or preferred standard surgical therapy (amputation) to experimental therapy. The histologic classification and type of therapy are listed in Table II.

TABLE II

HISTOLOGY AND TREATMENT OF SARCOMA PATIENTS

HISTOLOGY	TREATMENT CATEGORY Surgery	 Surgery + Adjuvant Chemo.	 IA Chemo. + XRT., Surgery + Adjuvant Chemo.
SOFT TISSUE SARCOMAS:			
Rhabdomyosarcoma	4	2	4
Undifferentiated sarcoma	4	1	5
Synovial cell sarcoma	3	2	1
Liposarcoma	3	1	5
Fibrosarcoma	3	-	1
Malignant fibrous histiosarcoma	1	-	-
Giant cell sarcoma	1	-	-
Neurofibrosarcoma	-	-	1
TOTAL	19	6	17
SKELETAL SARCOMAS:			
Osteosarcoma	16	6	12
Fibrosarcoma	1	1	-
Giant cell	1	-	1
Fibrous histiocytoma	1	2	-
Ewing's	1	-	1
TOTAL	20	9	14

Prior to treatment all patients had the following studies performed: CBC, SMA-12, electrocardiogram, chest radiographs, whole lung tomography, bone scans, and arteriography of the primary tumor. The stage of the soft tissue sarcomas was determined from incisional biopsy tissue using the staging method of the American Joint Commission for Cancer Staging.[4] The number of patients in each stage, the site of the tumor, and type of treatment are presented in Table II.

The group of patients who received radical amputation and postoperative adjuvant chemotherapy were given Adriamycin, 45 mg/M^2 I.V. on each of two consecutive days. Fourteen days later, high dose Methotrexate, 200 mg/kg as a four hour infusion was administered, followed four hours later by calcium leukovorin rescue.

The 31 patients who were treated with preoperative Adriamycin chemotherapy and radiation therapy had percutaneous arteriography performed by the Seldinger technique. The catheter was left in place in the major vessel supplying the extremity for the Adriamycin infusion. All patients received a total dose of 90 mg of Adriamycin over three days (30 mg/24 hours), suspended in 30 ml of normal saline, by continuous infusion with a Harvard pump.

Radiation therapy was begun the day following the intra-arterial infusion of Adriamycin. A 6-MEV linear accelerator was used to deliver 3500 rads to the mid-tumor plane in ten equal fractions over 12-15 calendar days. Each day the complete anatomic region of the tumor (e.g. the entire thigh) was treated by PA and AP parallel opposed fields. One week after the completion of radiation therapy, radical *en bloc* resection was performed as previously described[3] with at least one muscle or fascial plane between the tumor and the surgical margin. If the tumor originated in or invaded a muscle, the entire muscle group was removed from origin to insertion. Major vessels and nerves were resected if invaded by tumor, or preserved by dissection in a subadventitial plane where adequate margins could be obtained in this manner. In osteosarcoma patients, the diseased bones were replaced by cadaver allografts obtained from the tissue bank of the National Naval Medical Center, Bethesda, Maryland. Limb salvage was accomplished in 94% of patients with either skeletal or soft tissue sarcomas. All patients received postoperative adjuvant chemotherapy of Adriamycin - high dose Methotrexate for 4-28 months (median 14.5 months) alone or combined with immunotherapy of BCG and allogeneic sarcoma cell vaccine (no differences in response have been seen between these two groups so they are combined for the purposes of this paper).

To assess the effects of the Adriamycin/radiation therapy regimen on the histological characteristics and viability of the treated tumors, multiple representative sections of pretreatment and post-treatment specimens were examined. The pathologist had no prior knowledge of the type of treatment, if any. As a further control, slides from operative specimens treated by operation alone and representative of the types of tumors treated by the present approach were also examined for evidence of cellular necrosis. For all specimens, visual estimates of the amount of tumor cell necrosis present on each slide area were determined and averaged for the total number of slides reviewed and the percent necrosis calculated for each specimen.

Histologic examination of pretreatment biopsy specimens showed average necrosis of 4.3% compared to an average of 75%-90% necrosis in specimens after the combination of Adriamycin and radiation. In nine patients, no viable tumor cells were present. While this result is impressive, it must be emphasized that viable tumor cells were present in the majority of patients treated. Therefore, the radical surgical resection must be performed with meticulous technique.

DISCUSSION

Thus, to date, preliminary results of two clinical trials of adjuvant therapy for patients with Stage II melanoma and for patients with skeletal or soft tissue sarcomas appear to indicate some success in dealing with clinically undetectable metastases. In melanoma, even though the data suggest that immunization with the combination of BCG and tumor cell vaccine might be slightly better than BCG alone, the improvement is minimal at best. Therefore, even though adjuvant immunotherapy may be a first step in improved treatment, it is clear that more effective adjuvant programs must be developed.

On the other hand, results from the multimodality trials for skeletal and soft tissue sarcomas have been much more dramatic despite the fact that most of these patients have been under treatment for less than two years.

The multidisciplinary management for primary skeletal and soft tissue sarcomas described in this series has produced exciting results. Limb salvage without local recurrence is certainly gratifying for the patient and most satisfying for the surgeon. Obviously, there are many unresolved questions regarding this type of treatment, but these can only be answered by a longer period of follow-up.

The importance of continued adjuvant postoperative chemotherapy or chemo-immunotherapy cannot be overemphasized. It is obvious that few patients succumb to an uncontrolled extremity sarcoma. Death is usually due to disseminated disease in the lungs. Since most of the metastases appear within 24 months following resection of the primary tumor, it is likely that subclinical microscopic metastases were probably present at the time of initial treatment. Since these metastases govern the ultimate survival of the patient, it should be apparent that systemically active adjuvant therapy must become the determining factor for effective treatment. The dramatic results obtained from adjuvant chemotherapy for skeletal sarcomas appear to be possible for soft tissue sarcomas as well. At this point, it is too early to evaluate the additive value of immunotherapy over the results obtained by chemotherapy alone.

REFERENCES

1. Eilber, F.R., Morton, D.L., Holmes, E.C., Sparks, F.C., and Ramming, K.P.: Adjuvant immunotherapy with BCG in treatment of regional-lymph node metastases from malignant melanoma. New Eng. J. Med. 294:237-240, 1976.

2. Morton, D.L., Holmes, E.C., Eilber, F.R., Sparks, F.C., and Ramming K.P.: Adjuvant immunotherapy of malignant melanoma: Preliminary results of a randomized trial in patients with lymph node metastases. Raven Press, New York (1977), in press.
3. Morton, D.L.: Soft tissue sarcomas. In Cancer Medicine, J. F. Holland and E. Frei III (eds), Lea & Febinger, Philadelphia, 1974, pp. 1845-1861.
4. Morton, D.L., Eilber, F.R., Townsend, C.M., Jr., Grant, T.T., Mirra, J., and Weisenburger, T.H.: Limb salvage from a multidisciplinary treatment approach for skeletal and soft tissue sarcomas of the extremity. Ann. Surg. 184:268-278, 1976.
5. Townsend, C.M., Jr., Eilber, F.R. and Morton, D.L.: Skeletal and soft tissue sarcomas: Treatment with adjuvant immunotherapy. J. Am. Med. Assoc. 236: 2187-2189, 1976.
6. Eilber, F.R., Townsend, C.M., Jr., Weisenburger, T.H., Mirra, J.M. and Morton, D.L.: Preoperative intra-arterial adriamycin and radiation therapy for extremity soft tissue sarcomas: A clinico-pathologic study. World Book Medical Publishers (1977), in press.
7. Grant, T.T., Eilber, F.R., Mirra, J., Weisenburger, T.H. and Morton, D.L.: Limb salvage in malignant skeletal sarcomas of the extremities. J. Bone and Joint Surg. (1977), in press.

ACKNOWLEDGEMENT

This investigation was supported by grants CA12582, CA05262, NIH contracts CB-53941, CB-64076-TQ, awarded by the National Cancer Institute, DHEW, and Medical Research Services, Sepulveda Veterans Administration Hospital.

Adjuvant Therapy of Cancer, S.E. Salmon and S.E. Jones eds.

ADJUVANT CHEMOTHERAPY IN OSTEOSARCOMA OF ADULTS

A SOUTHWEST ONCOLOGY GROUP STUDY

William K. Murphy, M.D.,* Robert S. Benjamin, M.D.,** Harmon J. Eyre, M.D.+
Tate Thigpen, M.D.,∝ John P. Whitecar, Jr., M.D.,∿
Gonzalo Uribe-Botero, M.D.,§ Lawrence H. Baker, D.O.,†
Edmund A. Gehan, Ph.D.,∞ and Jeffrey A. Gottlieb, M.D.Φ

SUMMARY

A combination chemotherapy adjuvant regimen utilizing four drugs (CYVADIC) has been used in the treatment of 24 patients with osteosarcoma without metastatic disease following primary surgery. The treatment included cyclophosphamide, vincristine, doxorubicin (Adriamycin) and dacarbazine (DIC) repeated every three weeks and was considered completed when a total dose of 450 mg/M^2 had been reached. Treatment was initiated as soon as possible after definitive surgery. Eight of these patients were treated in a pilot study and of these, 5 remain free of recurrent disease at 29 to 40 months from diagnosis. An additional 16 patients have now been treated in a similar manner on a formal Southwest Oncology Group (SWOG) protocol. Of these, 3 have developed pulmonary metastases and 13 remain free of recurrent disease at 2 to 23 months from diagnosis.

INTRODUCTION

Until recent years treatment of primary osteosarcoma consisted almost exclusively of surgical removal. Results of this therapy were uniformly poor with the

---

Presented at the International Conference on the Adjuvant Therapy of Cancer, March 2-5, 1977, Tucson, Arizona.
From the University of Texas System Cancer Center, M.D. Anderson Hospital and Tumor Institute at Houston, Texas.
This investigation was supported in part by the following DHEW grants: SWOG No. CA10379, CA13238, CA16385, CA12014, and CA11430 from the National Cancer Institute
*Assistant Internist, Assistant Professor of Medicine.
**Assistant Internist, Assistant Professor of Clinical Pharmacology.
+Assistant Professor of Medicine, University of Utah, School of Medicine, Salt Lake City, Utah.
∝Assistant Professor of Medicine, Chief, Section of Oncology, University of Mississippi, School of Medicine, Jackson, Mississippi.
∿Clinical Associate Professor of Medicine, University of Texas School of Medicine, San Antonio, Texas.
§Assistant Professor of Pathology, V.A.Hospital and Baylor College of Medicine, Houston, Texas
†Associate Professor of Oncology, Wayne State University, School of Medicine, Detroit, Michigan.
∞Biometrician, SWOG, Professor of Biometrics, M.D.Anderson Hospital and Tumor Institute, School of Medicine, Houston, Texas
ΦDeceased
Address reprints. Wm. K. Murphy, M.D., M.D. Anderson Hospital and Tumor Institute Houston, Texas 77030

majority of patients suffering relapse, usually in the form of pulmonary metastases in less than 18-24 months.[1] Five year survival was 20% or less. The addition of preoperative irradiation did not affect the outlook.[2] Beginning in the 1960's but more prominently in the early 1970's chemotherapy was tried in metastatic osteosarcoma. Initially results were not particularly encouraging although some responses were seen primarily with alkylating agents. Sutow, et al, initiated adjuvant treatment as early as 1963 utilizing phenylalanine mustard but without notable success.[3] A later study by the same group in 1968, utilizing vincristine, actinomycin D and cyclophosphamide resulted in long-term survival of 3 of 11 patients (27%).[4] Subsequent studies in metastatic osteosarcoma demonstrated the activity of Adriamycin, DIC and combination chemotherapy with response rates of 10-40%.[5,6] The combination of Adriamycin and DIC seemed to affect response rate and survival favorably, more than doubling survival in responders.[6] In a parallel development high dose methotrexate with citrovorum factor rescue was found to achieve a similar response rate in advanced disease.[7]

More recently in a study by the Southwest Oncology Group utilizing cyclophosphamide, vincristine, Adriamycin and DIC in advanced sarcoma a response rate of 50% + was obtained in a small group of patients with soft tissue and boney sarcoma[8] With the availability of reasonably effective chemotherapy in advanced osteosarcoma the current adjuvant study was proposed and initiated.

PATIENTS AND PROCEDURES

An initial interinstitutional pilot study was started in 1973 and later, in 1975, was expanded into an official Southwest Oncology group study. Patient eligibility was essentially the same for both groups and required a pathologically confirmed diagnosis of osteosarcoma, the performance of definitive surgical therapy and the absence of any demonstrable metastatic disease. Patients with prior chemotherapy were excluded, as were patients with metastatic disease who had been rendered surgically free of disease by additional surgery. Informed consent was required of all patients. Although age restrictions were not imposed, it was intended that patients under the age of 15 be entered on the Southwest Oncology Group pediatric adjuvant osteosarcoma protocol. An abnormal electrocardiogram and/or a history of significant cardiac disease was not considered an absolute contraindication to treatment. In the presence of such findings each patient was considered individually. Additional requirements were, normal bone marrow, hepatic and renal function. Prior to treatment all patients had a complete history and physical, complete blood count with differential and platelet counts, SMA-12, urinalysis, bone scan, skeletal survey, PA and lateral chest x-ray, full lung tomograms and an electrocardiogram.

Treatment as outlined in Table 1 was initiated as soon as possible after surgery and it was intended that the maximum time lapse be no more than 30 days unless complications of surgery prevented earlier initiation of therapy. Treatment was repeated every 22 days if myelosuppression would permit (absolute granulocyte count of > 2000/cu mm and platelet count > 100,000/cu mm and rising).

TABLE 1.
CYVADIC DOSE SCHEDULE

Drug	Dose	Schedule
Vincristine	1.5 mg/M^2 (Max. 2 mg) IV	Weekly x6, then d-1 of each course
Adriamycin	40 mg/M^2 IV x4 then 60 mg/M^2 IV	d-2 of courses 1 through 4 d-2 q 3 weeks of a total of 450 mg/M^2*
Cyclophosphamide	400 mg/M^2 IV	d-2 of each course, q 3 weeks
DIC	200 mg/M^2 IV	d 1-5 of each course of the first 4 courses only, q 3 weeks

*When the total of 450 mg/M^2 of Adriamycin was reached, all chemotherapy was discontinued.

Because of the adjuvant and experimental nature of the chemotherapy, dosage escalation was not permitted except for the increase in Adriamycin dosage upon completeion of the 4 cycles of DIC. Reduction of dosage, however, was allowed depending on myelotoxicity (for Adriamycin, cyclophosphamide and DIC) or neurotoxicity (for vincristine). Significant evidence of cardiac toxicity was considered an indication for discontinuation of Adriamycin, as was hemorrhagic cystitis for cyclophosphamide.

All patients were followed at regular intervals with examinations, chest x-rays, blood counts and chemistries, urinalyses and electrocardiograms. Other studies were repeated on indication except for comprehensive reevaluation upon completion of the scheduled chemotherapy. Evidence of metastatic disease was considered an indication of treatment failure and, when confirmed, resulted in change of therapy.

Concurrent controls were not employed because of the relatively small number of patients available for study, and because of the high liklihood that therapy would be beneficial. A group of 106 patients treated with surgery only (to first metastases) at M.D. Anderson Hospital were utilized as controls for statistical purposes. These patients were between the ages of 14 and 68 and were seen between 1950 and 1973 (Fig. 1).

Between June, 1973, and October, 1974, nine patients were entered on the pilot

CYVADIC study from 4 Southwest Oncology Group member institutions. The official SWOG protocol was opened in March, 1975, and currently remains open. A total of 18 patients have been entered on study in this group. In the combined group there were 13 males and 12 females with a median age of 19 years (range 12 to 68 years). All of the patients in the pilot study were eligible and had osteosarcoma of the extremity. Included in the group study are 1 patient with pelvic osteosarcoma (extensive), 1 patient with osteosarcoma arising in Paget's disease, 1 patient with extraosseous sarcoma (biceps) 1 patient with Down's Syndrome and 1 patient who had preoperative radiation therapy. All patients had pathologically confirmed osteosarcoma but the variant pathologic types are not presently identifiable. Distribution of primary site is indicated in Table 2.

TABLE 2.

PRIMARY SITE

Femur	11
Tibia	6
Humerus	4
Biceps	1
Calcaneous	1
Pelvis	1
Ulna	1

RESULTS

Results for the pilot study, the Southwest Oncology Group study and combined results are tabulated in Table 3. The patient labelled a major protocol violation did not complete 4 courses with DIC, took therapy at widely varying intervals and took less than 300 mg/M^2 of Adriamycin. He relapsed at 12 months but is still alive at 27 months following additional chemotherapy and staged bilateral thoracotomies. The patient indentified as refusing chemotherapy refused further chemotherapy after 1 full course. His current status is unknown.

Relapse in the 6 patients indicated occurred at 3,3,12,17,18 and 28 months. The interval to initiation of chemotherapy is of some interest. The median interval was 18 days with a range of 10 to 136 days. Only one patient in the SWOG study had an interval over 30 days (57 days) and the relapses are apparently unrelated to the interval. In the pilot study, including the patient classified "MPV", there are 6 patients with an interval to chemotherapy over 30 days. Three of the four relapses are in this group.

TABLE 3.

RESULTS OF CYVADIC ADJUVANT OSTEOSARCOMA STUDY

Status	Pilot	SWOG 74-40	Combined
On-study	9	18**	27**
Inevaluable	1(MPV)*	1(Refused R_x)	2
Too early	0	1(N.E.D.)	1
Evaluable	8	16	24
Relapsed	3	3	6
Disease Free	5(62%)	13(81%)	18(75%)

* Major protocol violation.

** Includes patient with pelvic primary who relapsed at 2-3 months.

The disease free intervals for patients who have not relapsed are outlined in Table 4. If only patients on-study for 4 months or over were considered, the median duration of disease-free interval would be 22 months and there has been only one relapse beyond this time.

TABLE 4.

DISEASE FREE INTERVAL

Median (Pilot)	34 mo. (29-40 mo.)
Median (SWOG)	12 mo. (2-23 mo.)
Median (Combined)	19 mo. (2-40 mo.)
All Patients (mo.)	2,2,3,3,4,4,12,15, 19,19,21,23,23,29, 30,34,35,40

The toxicity encountered with this chemotherapy is what might be expected: nausea and vomiting, alopecia, peripheral neuropathy and myelosuppression. There have been no cases of cardiotoxicity and none suspected so far. Patient acceptance has been remarkably good with 1 patient stopping after 1 course and 1 patient taking therapy erratically and incompletely. Hemorrhagic cystitis has not been encountered. One patient had vincristine discontinued because of neuropathy. Myelosuppression has been moderate. The median lowest white count has been 2300/cu mm (range 1300-4500/cu mm), median lowest absolute neutrophil count 1200/cu mm (range 100-2100/cu mm) and median lowest platelet count 215,000/cu mm (range 154,000-487,000/cu mm). There have been no cases of sepsis and no reported cases of hospitalization for fever with neutropenia.

Compared with the historical data at M.D. Anderson Hospital the disease free interval for patients onthe CYVADIC study (pilot + SWOG) is significantly better with a P-value of 0.002 (see Figure 1). Included in the data for the study group are the patient classified as "MPV" and the patient with the pelvic primary, both of whom have relapsed. None of the patients in the control group had pelvic primary osteosarcoma (all are extremity primaries).

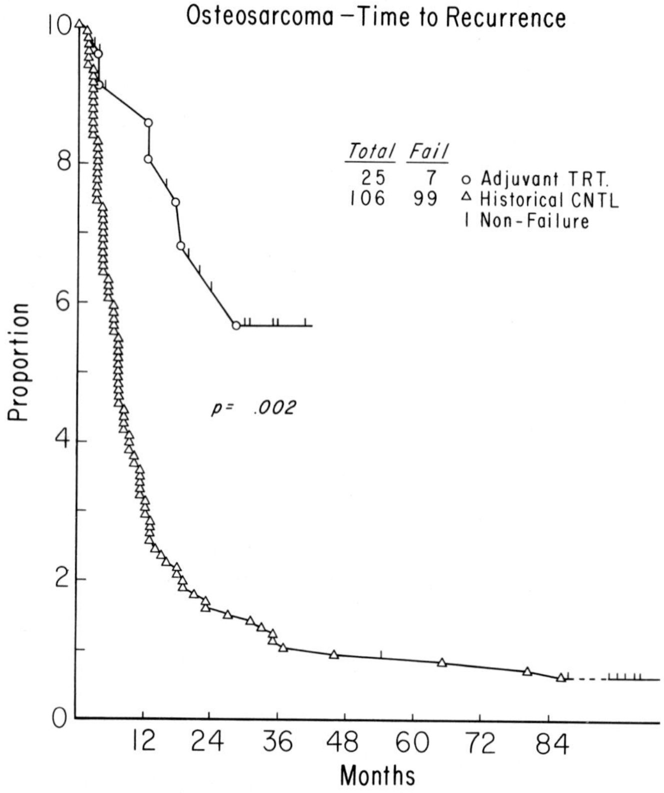

Fig. 1 Comparison of disease free survival in historical control and study group.

DISCUSSION

In evaluating the impact of adjuvant therapy on patients with primary, non-metastatic osteosarcoma, many things must be taken into account. Survival, as such, can no longer be compared with that of historical controls. Therapy of metastatic disease now is much more effective than in the past, having been altered by newer modalities of treatment: alternate effective chemotherapy, surgical intervention in metastatic disease, immunotherapy and combined treatment with chemotherapy and radiation therapy. Disease free interval or interval to first metastasis seems to be the more relaible measure of the efficacy of adjuvant therapy. The prognostic factors involved here make analysis complex. Age, site, pathologic type, surgical procedure and technique, interval from diagnosis to adjuvant therapy, symptomatic interval, sex, immunologic status and many other variables, including the intensity and variations of adjuvant therapy may play an important role in the outcome of adjuvant therapy. In a recent review by Uribe-Botero, et al, age was found not to be a significant variable.[9] In the study presented pathologic variant and surgical approach are certainly not adequately considered among the prognostic factors. Immunotherapy may be of value in the adjuvant therapy of primary osteosarcoma[10] but is not included in the majority of the on-going chemotherapy studies.

It seems evident that adjuvant chemotherapy has significantly prolonged the disease-free interval in primary osteosarcoma.[11 12 13 14] In so doing it has undoubtedly prolonged survival, although other factors may also have contributed to a significant extent. Late relapses have apparently become more frequent, perhaps even the pattern of relapse may have been altered.[15] Despite the promise of current adjuvant studies there certainly is no room for complacency or retrogressive studies at this point. Newer surgical approaches are being utilized, as are pre-surgical chemotherapy and combination chemotherapy-radiation therapy. On-going studies must be followed up and newer combined approaches must be utilized in the attempt to achieve a higher rate of cure in this devastating malignant disease.

BIBLIOGRAPHY

1. Lockshin, M.D., and Higgins, I.T.T., (1968): Prognosis in osteogenic sarcoma. Clin. Orthop. 58:85-101.
2. Friedman, M.A., and Carter, S.K., (1972): The therapy of osteogenic sarcoma-Current status and thoughts for the future. J. Surg. Oncol. 4:482-510.
3. Sutow, W.W., et al, (1971): L-phenylalanine mustard (NSC-8806) administration in osteogenic sarcoma--An evaluation of dosage schedules. Cancer Chemotherapy Rep. 55:151-157.
4. Sutow, W.W., et al.,(1975): Study of adjuvant chemotherapy in osteogenic sarcoma. J. Clin. Pharmacol. 15:530.
5. O'Bryan, R.M., et al., (1973): Phase II evaluation of adriamycin in human neoplasia. Cancer 32:1-8.
6. Gottlieb, J.A., et al., (1972): Chemotherapy of sarcomas with a combination of adriamycin and dimethyltriazino imidazole carboxamide. Cancer 30:1632-1638.
7. Jaffe, N., (1972): Recent advances in the chemotherapy of metastatic osteogenic sarcoma. Cancer 30:1627-1631.
8. Gottlieb, J.A., et al., (1974): An effective new 4-drug combination regimen (CY-VA-DIC) for metastatic sarcomas. Proc. of the Amer. Soc. of Clinc. Onc. 15:162.
9. Uribe-Botero, G., et al: Primary osteosarcoma of bone: A clinicopathologic investigation of 243 cases with necropsy studies in 54. Am. J. Clin. Path., (in press).
10. Kinney, T.R., and Chung, S.M.K., (1974): Advances in the treatment of tumors arising in bone. Seminars in Onc. 1:47-55.
11. Sutow, W.W., et al., (1975): Adjuvant chemotherapy in primary treatment of osteogenic sarcoma. Cancer 36:1598-1602.
12. Jaffe, N., et al, (1974): Adjuvant methotrexate and citrovorum-factor treatment of osteogenic sarcoma. N. Engl. J. Med. 291:994-997.
13. Cortes, E.P., et al, (1974): Amputation and adriamycin in primary osteosarcoma. N. Engl. J. Med.291:998-1000.
14. Rosen, G., et al, (1974): Vincristine (VCR), high dose methotrexate (HDMTX) with citrovorum factor (CF) rescue, cyclophosphamide (CY), and adriamycin (ADR) cyclic therapy following surgery in childhood osteogenic sarcoma. Proc Am. Assoc. Cancer Res. 15:1972.
15. Data presented at the Osteosarcoma Study Group meeting, N.C.I., Bethesda, Maryland, January 19, 1977.

Adjuvant Therapy of Cancer, S.E. Salmon and S.E. Jones eds.

SURGERY AND ADRIAMYCIN FOR PRIMARY OSTEOGENIC SARCOMA: A 5 YEAR ASSESSMENT

Engracio P. Cortes, M.D., James F. Holland, M.D., and Oliver Glidewell
for
Cancer and Leukemia Group B
Scarsdale, New York, 10583

INTRODUCTION

Although surgical therapy has been the accepted method for the management of primary osteogenic sarcoma, it has been associated with a dismal 20% 5-year survival rate (1). At the time of potentially curative surgery, it has been shown that osteosarcoma cells are already in the blood circulation (2). This may explain why 80% of the patients eventually develop and succumb to distant metastases.

Prior to 1970 the role of chemotherapy in metastatic osteogenic sarcoma was minimal. Although gratifying objective responses were occasionally seen with mitomycin C, L-phenylalanine mustard, cyclophosphamide or actinomycin D, these results were exceptional and usually brief (1).

Adriamycin, a cytotoxic antibiotic derived from streptomyces peucetius var. caesius, was introduced for clinical trials in the United States by Farmitalia, Milan, Italy in 1968. In 1972, we initially reported the activity of adriamycin in a small series of patients with osteosarcoma that had metastasized to the lungs (3,4). Encouraged by this therapeutic result in metastatic osteosarcoma, the Cancer and Leukemia Group B (CALGB) reported the preliminary results of a study initiated in 1971 using intermittent adriamycin treatment shortly after radical surgical amputation of primary osteosarcoma in an effort to apply chemotherapy when the body burden of tumor cells was lowest (5,6).

The present paper reports the 5-year follow-up of amputation and adriamycin in primary osteogenic sarcoma undertaken by CALGB.

METHODS AND MATERIALS

The criteria for entry to the study included: a) histologically proven osteosarcoma, characterized by osteoid or bone apposed to tumor cells (none of the patients had parosteal osteosarcoma, chondrosarcoma, fibrosarcoma, radiation induced osteosarcoma, or osteosarcoma after Paget's disease, all of which have different clinical courses (7)); b) surgically resectable primary tumor without roentgenologic evidence of metastases; c) a minimum leukocyte count of $4000/mm^3$ and platelet count of $100,000/mm^3$ and; d) blood urea nitrogen and creatinine less than 25 and 1.5 mg per 100 ml, respectively.

Hematologic, biochemical, and electrocardiographic examinations, chest x-ray and tomography, and bone survey were conducted before, during, and after therapy to monitor possible tumor recurrence and drug toxicity.

Drug Dosage and Schedule

Adriamycin is supplied in a 10 mg vial. Each vial was diluted with 5ml of sterile saline and the calculated dose was injected as an intravenous bolus.

Four to 14 days after amputation of the primary lesion, or as soon as wound healing was complete, adriamycin was given at a dose schedule of 30 mg per square meter of body surface daily for three successive days repeated every four to six weeks for six courses. The total cumulative dose of adriamycin was 540 mg. per square meter over a period of five to seven months. Thereafter, patients remained untreated.

The response to therapy was measured by the disease-free interval after the first course of adriamycin. Treatment failure was defined as unequivocal roentgenologic evidence of disease recurrence.

A leukocyte count of less than $1000/mm^3$ resulting from adriamycin administration required the reduction of succeeding doses of adriamycin to 25 mg per square meter daily for three days. No dose adjustment was to be made if the leukocyte nadir was over $1000/mm^3$ unless an accompanying complication such as septicemia occurred. Any reduction of adriamycin dose at this leukocyte nadir of over 1000 cells/mm^3 was considered a dose violation.

Radical amputation, i.e. complete removal of the involved bone was required. Cross-bone amputation of the involved long bone may be an inadequate procedure and was considered a surgery violation.

From November 1971 to December 1975, 102 patients from twenty-one institutions were entered into the study. Fourteen patients were disqualified: six had overt metastases; four were never started on adriamycin; one each had parosteal osteosarcoma, osteosarcoma arising from Paget's disease, inadequate records, and seqential adriamycin and high dose methotrexate treatment. The remaining 88 patients form the basis of this réport.

RESULTS

Of the 88 patients, 52 were male and 36 female. Their ages ranged from 4 to 66, with a mean and median age of 14 and 15 years, respectively.

The primary sites of osteosarcoma in these 88 patients are shown in Table 1. The lesion in 65 cases (73%) was localized around the knee joint.

TABLE I

FREQUENCY OF PRIMARY SITE

Femur		47
Distal	44	
Middle	3	
Tibia		26
Proximal	21	
Distal	5	
Fibula, Proximal		4
Humerus		6
Rib		3
Mandible		1
Iliac Spine		1
		88

The CALGB has no historical control of its own in primary osteosarcoma treated with surgery alone. We use the data reported by Marcove et al (8), Jaffe et al (9), and Sutow et al (10) as historical comparison groups. In these 3 series, approximately 20% of patients were free of metastases at 60 months. The median onset of pulmonary metastases occurred at 6 to 8.5 months (Figure 1).

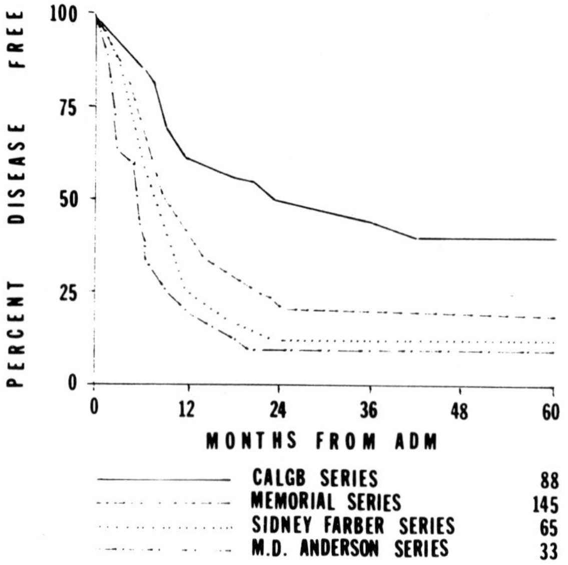

Fig. 1. Percentage of patients with osteosarcoma remaining disease free after adriamycin (CALGB series) and after operation alone.

In the adriamycin treated group, 43 of 88 (48.8%) had relapsed (38 pulmonary metastases, 3 local recurrences, and 2 bone metastases). At 60 months, 39% of the treated patients were expected to be free of disease as determined by the life table method. The median onset of recurrence was 20 months.

For reasons unrelated to a nadir of leukocytes below 1000 cells/mm^3, 16 of the 88 patients (Table 2) had their adriamycin dose reduced. Ten of these 16 (62.5%) have relapsed. Of 17 patients whose involved bones were not completely removed and of 8 who had both inappropriate dose reduction of adriamycin together with a subradical surgical procedure, 11 (64.7%) and 6 (75%) have relapsed, respectively. No protocol violation in terms of dose or extent of amputation occurred in 47 patients in the present series; among these 47, 16 (34%) have relapsed.

TABLE 2

CHARACTERISTICS OF 88 OSTEOSARCOMA PATIENTS ACCORDING TO PROTOCOL VIOLATION

CATEGORY	NO PROTOCOL VIOLATION	PROTOCOL VIOLATION
Total Number	47	41
Mean Days from Diagnosis to Surgery	12	10
Mean Days from Surgery to ADM	23 (20% > 21 days)	21 (15% > 21 days)
Mean Age	18 (42% < 16 yrs.)	21 (66% < 16 yrs.)
Male (Percent)	62	56
Tumor Site	Number (Percent)	Number (Percent)
Femur	18 (38)	29 (70)
Tibia	18 (38)	8 (20)
Fibula	4 (9)	0 (0)
Humerus	4 (9)	2 (5)
Other	3 (3)	2 (5)
Tumor Size	Number (Percent)	Number (Percent)
< 5 cm	10 (28)	6 (24)
5-10cm	16 (46)	11 (44)
>10 cm	9 (26)	8 (32)
Size not recorded	12	16

The following characteristics influenced disease-free status as projected by life table method at 4 years: a) adriamycin dose violation, 22 % b) surgery violation, 28%,c) adriamycin dose and surgery violation, 18% and; d) no violation (full adriamycin dose and complete removal of involved bone) 51% (Figure 2). The probability that the total groups with protocol adherence and protocol violation would have this disparate relapse rate based on chance alone is remote ($P < .003$).

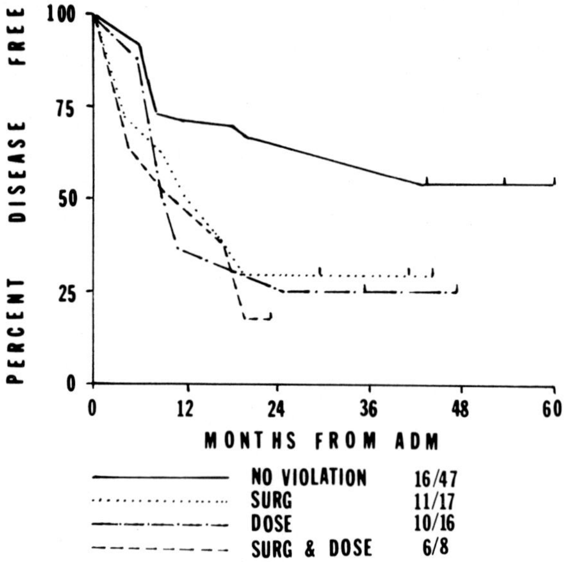

Fig.2. Percentage of patients disease free according to protocol violation (vertical lines indicate individual patients free of disease from last relapse).

Pulmonary metastases appeared in 17 of 88 patients before the completion of six courses of adriamycin therapy. Of 46 patients who have been observed for a year or more, 9 (19.5%) have relapsed. After two or more years, only one of 22 (4.5%) has developed pulmonary metastases, and this occurred at 42 months after the start of adriamycin therapy.

The higher recurrence rates of patients violating the protocol compared to those who were properly treated was also true for various primary sites, both sexes, and irrespective of age. While such factors as femur versus tibia-fibula and male versus female did not show significant difference in disease-free interval, the group of patients less than 16 years of age treated according to the protocol had a longer projected disease-free interval than patients over 16 years of age. At 48 months, 62.5% of patients less than 16 years old were expected to be disease-free compared to 37% in those over 16 years of age (Figure 3). The better prognosis of patients under 16 years compared to older patients was also seen in the protocol violation group.

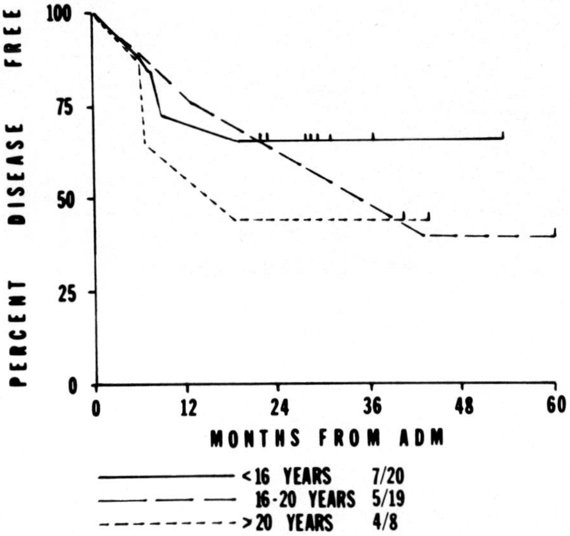

Fig.3. Percentage of patients with no protocol violation disease free according to age at time of diagnosis.

The disease-free interval for patients with a primary tumor of various sizes treated according to the protocol is shown in Figure 4. At 48 months, 87% of patients with lesions ranging from 5 to 10 cm in maximum diameter were expected to be free of disease. In contrast, tumor lesions less than 5 cm or more than 10 cm in diameter had projected disease-free status in substantially fewer patients.

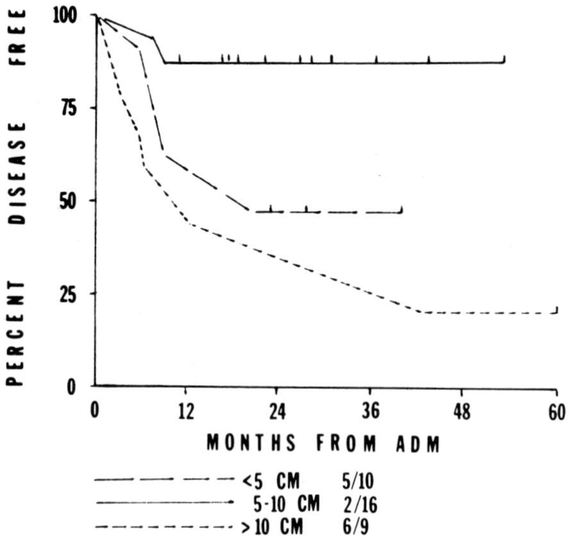

Fig. 4. Percentage of patients with no protocol violation disease free according to tumor size.

The characteristics of the primary tumors arising from the femur in 47 patients with or without protocol violation are shown in Table 3. A greater number of cases and a higher percentage of patients less than 16 years of age and tumors less than 5 cm in diameter were found in the protocol violation group compared to the protocol adherent group. All the rest of the listed characteristics seemed to be comparable between the two groups including mean days from diagnosis to surgery, mean days from surgery to adriamycin, male:female ratio and the percentage of tumor lesions ranging from 5 to 10 cm in diameter.

TABLE 3

CHARACTERISTICS OF 47 OSTEOSARCOMAS ARISING FROM THE FEMUR ACCORDING TO PROTOCOL VIOLATION

	NO PROTOCOL VIOLATION		PROTOCOL VIOLATION	
CATEGORY	NO. CASES	%	NO. CASES	%
Total Cases	18		29	
Sex				
Male	12	66	18	62
Female	6	33	11	38
Age				
< 16 years	9	50	19	65.5
16-20	6	33	8	27.5
> 20	3	16.6	2	6.8
Mean	20		14	
Median	15		14	
Tumor Size				
< 5 cm	2	14	5	26
5-10 cm	7	50	9	47
>10 cm	5	30	5	26
Size not recorded	4		10	

At 48 months, the disease-free interval in the protocol violation group was predicted to be 31% versus 48% in the protocol adherent group (Figure 5).

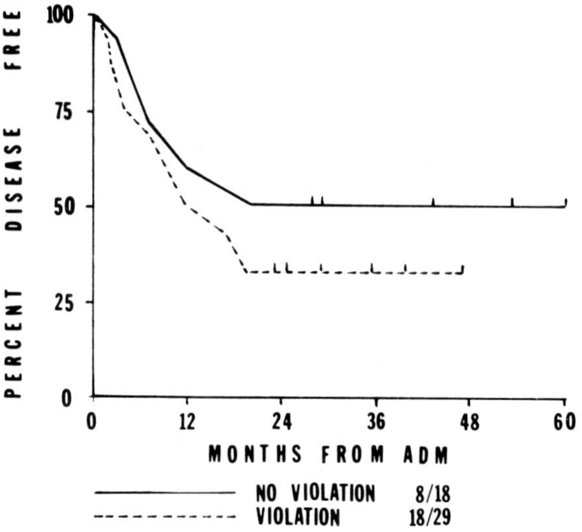

Fig. 5. Percentage of patients with femoral lesions remaining free of disease with or without protocol violation.

Pulmonary metastases are usually the first evidence of recurrent osteosarcoma. The published data of Marcove et al (8) on 145 patients less than 21 years of age with operable osteosarcoma of the extremities were used as a historical comparison group. Only 19% were free of pulmonary metastases at 60 months after operation. In the present series of 39 patients less than 21 years of age treated with full adriamycin dose and complete removal of the involved long bone 52% were projected to be free of pulmonary metastases at that time.(Figure 6).

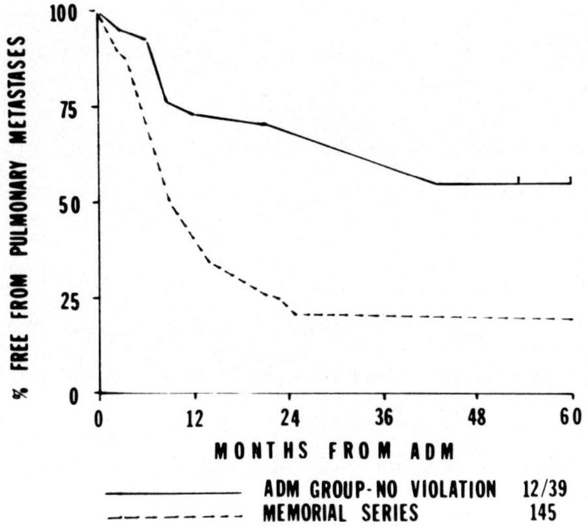

Fig. 6. Percentage of patients less than 21 years of age with operable long bone lesions remaining free from pulmonary metastases after adriamycin or surgery alone.

The toxicity from adriamycin was tolerable. Transient capital alopecia occurred in 100%, leukopenia <3000 cell/mm^3 in 60%, nausea and vomiting in 50%, stomatitis in 45%. Pneumonia occurred in one patient. In another patient, delayed wound healing complicated by a local wound infection was noted during adriamycin administration. Transient electrocardiographic changes in the form of premature atrial and ventricular beats occurred in 10%. Twenty patients of the 88 did not finish six courses of adriamycin because of relapse (18) or refused (2). Of the 68 patients who did finish the six courses of adriamycin. two developed congestive heart failure. One patient had a simultaneous onset of fatal pulmonary metastases and congestive heart failure two months after the completion of 540 mg/m^2 of adriamycin. At autopsy, a mural thrombus in the ventricle and interstitial fibrosis of the myocardium were noted. The other patient developed irreversible congestive heart failure 3 months after 540 mg/m^2 of adriamycin was completed. She died one month after the onset of heart failure. At autopsy, a metastatic lesion to the heart and metastases in the lungs were demonstrated which had not been previously noted by roentgenographic studies.

A 16 year old girl who completed the six courses of adriamycin, delivered a normal child at age 21 years.

DISCUSSION

The concept that chemotherapeutic agents are most effective when the body burden of tumor cells is lowest was summarized recently by Schabel (11). Chemotherapeutic agents, when they are effective, work by first-order reaction kinetics; that is, they kill a fixed fraction of exposed tumor cells. Studies of tumor cell growth kinetics indicate that the growth fraction (viable cells undergoing active cell replication divided by total number of cells) is inversely related to population size. The theoretical implication of this observation is that cure by chemotherapeutic drugs is more likely in an adjuvant setting than when the tumor has clinically recurred. That this concept is also true for human cancer is evident in Wilms' tumor (12), in which a combination of operation and chemotherapy prolonged the disease-free interval and increased the cure rate. The same phenomena may be true for breast cancer (13, 14, 15).

In osteogenic sarcoma, surgery alone or in combination with radiotherapy had repeatedly achieved a 5-year survival rate of approximately 20%. Although there is unanimous agreement that cross-bone amputation of the femur is the proper surgery for osteosarcoma arising from the proximal tibia, there are arguments regarding the level of amputation for lesions arising from the distal femur. Nevertheless, regardless of the type of surgical procedure, the 5-year survival rate of lesions arising from the femur remains the same (16). Local recurrence in the femoral stump, however, occurred in 7 of 38 (16%) patients treated by amputation through the femur as reported by Sweetnam (17), whereas disarticulation of the hip for femoral tumor in 30 patients was accomplished without local recurrence. This finding supports the "skip" metastases reported by Enneking and Kagan (18). They demonstrated that simultaneous, secondary, smaller foci of osteosarcoma, anatomically separate from the primary lesion, occurred in 10 of 40 osteosarcoma patients. These "skip' lesions were found either in same bone or on the opposing side of the adjacent joint, rather than in distant portions of the skeleton. In our present series, no local recurrence occurred in 63 patients whose involved long bones were completely removed. One patient, however, had contralateral tibial metastases at 9 months and another with dose violation had tumor extension to the homolateral acetabulum at 8 months from a primary osteosarcoma arising during pregnancy in the distal femur. One of 23 patients who had subradical surgery for osteosarcoma of the long bones had local recurrence at 19 months. Of five patients with osteosarcoma of the trunk (ribs (3) and iliac spine and mandible), the latter two have relapsed locally, presumptively because of limitation on radical extent of surgery.

In our previous reports (4, 6), although 7 of 17 patients with pulmonary metastases from osteosarcoma previously untreated with an anthracycline antibiotic responded to adriamycin therapy, none of four patients with measurable bony lesions showed any objective tumor shrinkage. In the present series, despite full doses of adriamycin in 17 patients who had subradical surgery , 11 have relapsed (10 with pulmonary metastases and one locally). It is possible that the remaining unresected involved bone contains "skip" or micrometastases not completely eradicated by adriamycin which were responsible for the pulmonary metastases and local recurrence upon termination of therapy. Whether this observation is also true in other adjuvant chemotherapeutic programs is not known.

Lowering the dose of adriamycin to avoid leukopenia was also associated with higher recurrence of disease than in patients who received full adriamycin dose. This extremely dose-dependent antitumor activity of adriamycin is consistent with our earlier reports in metastatic osteosarcoma (3, 4, 6,). Further evidence that this adriamycin dose-dependent antitumor activity exists in osteosarcoma was confirmed by Gottlieb (19). He reported that all 5 patients with primary osteosarcoma treated by amputation and adriamycin at $50 mg/m^2$ per course every three weeks, developed pulmonary metastases.

The series reported by Scranton et al (20) showing a better prognosis in females with osteosarcoma treated with surgery alone than in males is not seen in our adriamycin treated patients. McKenna et al (7) reported that tumor size correlated well with survival. In their series, osteosarcomas less than 5 cm diameter had a 40% 5-year survival rate compared to 17, 4 and 0% survival in lesions ranging from 5 to 10, 10 to 15, and over 15 cm, respectively. In our present report, it is uncertain why patients with a tumor of less than 5 cm in diameter had a shorter disease-free interval than those with lesions ranging from 5 to 10 cm. As might be expected from McKenna's data, however, over 10 cm in diameter had the worst prognosis, despite the full adriamycin dose and complete removal of the involved bone, with only 19% projected to survive 5 years.

The conclusion that full doses of adriamycin and complete removal of the involved bone in osteosarcoma are the most effective ways to assure successful adjuvant therapy is supported by a longer disease-free interval in patients without protocol violation compared to those with protocol violations in every prognostic category. This conclusion is reinforced by the effect of therapy in lesions of a single site, the femur. Despite less favorable balance of prognostic factors, of age and tumor size, the disease-free interval in the protocol adherent group is still significantly longer than in patients who violated the protocol.

The toxicity from adriamycin has been well tolerated. The high risk of serious cardiomyopathy in patients receiving a total cumulative dose of adriamycin over 550 mg/m^2 (21) made us limit the cumulative dose to 540 mg/m^2 in this study. Nevertheless, at this dose level, two of 68 patients developed congestive heart failure. Both of these patients, however, were found to have pulmonary metastases which may have contributed to their cardiac dysfunction. None of 20 patients with less than 540mg/m^2 developed cardiac failure.

The effect of adriamycin on reproductive function is not well studied. The delivery of a normal child by one of our patients indicates that ovarian damage is not absolute. Whether the delayed recurrence observed for up to 5 years in this report will result in cure remains to be proved in a year or two of further follow-up. The test that only a single relapse had occurred so far after two years of observation lends credence to this proposition. There is no doubt, however, that the increase in disease-free interval resulting from this treatment compensates for the toxicity, inconvenience, and expense of adriamycin therapy. By the same token, the failure to adhere to the protocol and the appearance of metastases in 50% clearly indicate this is only a step along the way, and we are now investigating other programs.

REFERENCES

1. Friedman, M.A., and Carter, S.K.: The Therapy of Osteogenic Sarcoma: Current Status and Thoughts for the Future. J. Surg. Oncol. 4:482-510, 1972.
2. Brenhovd, I.O., Roger, V., and Hoeg K.: Circulating Tumor Cells in Osteosarcoma. Colston Paper No. 24: Bone Certain Aspects of Neoplasia Price, C.H.G., and Rose, F.G.M., eds). London, Buttersworth and Co., 1972, pp 245-249
3. Cortes, E.P., Holland, J.F., Wang, J.J. and Sinks, L.F.: Doxorubicin in Disseminated Osteosarcoma. JAMA 221: 1132-1138, 1972.
4. Cortes, E.P., Holland, J.F., Wang, J.J. and Sinks, L.F.: Chemotherapy of Advanced Osteosarcoma. Colston Paper No. 24: Bone Certain Aspects of Neoplasia (Price, C.H.G., and Rose, F.G.M., eds). London, Buttersworth and Co,1972, pp 265-280.
5. Cortes, E.P., Holland, J.F., Wang, J.J., et al: Amputation and Adriamycin in Primary Osteosarcoma. N. Engl. J. Med. 291: 998-1000, 1974.
6. Cortes, E.P., Holland, J.F., Wang, J.J. and Glidewell, O.: Adriamycin (NSC123127) in 87 Patients with Osteosarcoma. Cancer Chemother. Rep. Part 3. 6:305-313, 1975.
7. McKenna, R.J., Schwinn, C.P., Soong, K.Y., et al: Sarcoma of the Osteogenic Series (Osteosarcoma, Fibrosarcoma, Chondrosarcoma, Parosteal, Osteogenic Sarcoma, and Sarcomata Arising in Abnormal Bone): An Analysis of 552 Cases. J. Bone Joint Surg.48: 126, 1966.

8. Marcove R. C., Mive V., Hajek J. V., et al: Osteogenic Sarcoma in Childhood. N.Y. State J. Med. 71:855-859, 1971.

9. Jaffe,N., Frei, E. III, Traggis,D., et al: Adjuvant Methotrexate and Citrovorum Factor Treatment of Osteogenic Sarcoma. N. Engl. J. Med. 291:994-997, 1974.

10. Sutow, W. W., Sullivan, M.P., Fernbach D. J., et al: Adjuvant Chemotherapy in Primary Treatment of Osteogenic Sarcoma. Cancer 36: 1598-1602, 1975.

11. Schabel F. M. Jr.: Concepts for Systemic Treatment of Micrometases. Cancer 35: 1524, 1975.

12. Fernbach, D.J., and Martyn, D.T.: Role of Dactinomycin in the Improved Survival of Children with Wilms' Tumor. JAMA 195: 1005-1009, 1966.

13. Fisher, B., Carbone, P., Economou, S.G. et al: L-phenylalanine Mustard (L-PAM) in The Management of Primary Breast Cancer: A Report of Early Findings. N. Engl. J. Med. 292: 117-122, 1975.

14. Bonadonna G., Brusamolino E., Valagussa P., et al : Combination Chemotherapy As An Adjuvant Treatment in Operable Breast Cancer. N. Engl. J. Med. 294: 405-410, 1976.

15. Cooper, R. G., Holland, J. F. and Glidewell, O. Breast Cancer: Surgery and Chemotherapy in Primary Treatment. (submitted).

16. Lewis, R.J. and Lotz,M.J.: Medullary Extension of Osteosarcoma: Implications for Rational Therapy. Cancer 33: 371-375, 1974.

17. Sweetnam,R.: Amputation in Osteosarcoma. J Bone Joint Surg (Br.) 55: 189-192, 1973.

18. Enneking W. F. and Kagan A. : "Skip" Metastases in Osteosarcoma. Cancer 36: 2192-2205, 1975.

19. Gottlieb J.: Personal Communication.

20. Scranton, P.E., DeCicco,F.A., Totten R.S., et al: Prognostic Factors in Osteosarcoma. Cancer 36: 2179-2191, 1975.

21. Cortes, E.P., Lutman, G., Wanka, J., et al: Adriamycin (NSC-123127) Cardiotoxicity: A Clinicopathologic Correlation. Cancer Chemother. Rep. (Part 3), 6: 215-225, 1975.

22. Rosen, G., Murphy, M.L., Huvos, A.G., et al: Chemotherapy, En Bloc Resection, and Prostetic Bone Replacement in The Treatment of Osteogenic Sarcoma. Cancer 37: 1-11, 1976.

23. Pratt C., Shanks E., Hustu O., et al: Adjuvant Multiple Drug Chemotherapy for Osteosarcoma of the Extremity Cancer 39: 51-57, 1977.

Adjuvant Therapy of Cancer, S.E. Salmon and S.E. Jones eds.

EFFECTS OF ADRIAMYCIN IN THE ADJUVANT TREATMENT OF OSTEOSARCOMA

Marco Gasparini, Franca Fossati-Bellani,
Leandro Gennari, Gianni Bonadonna
Istituto Nazionale Tumori, Milano
Italy

INTRODUCTION

The cure rate achieved with local treatment modality (amputation, radiotherapy, or both) in clinically localized osteogenic sarcoma does not usually exceed 20%[1]. In fact, most patients show a progressive clinical evidence of lung metastases during the first 12 months following surgery with a median disease-free survival ranging from 6 to 10 months[1,2,3]. This high incidence of early clinical dissemination prompted many investigators to administer as adjuvant treatment those chemotherapeutic agents which were proven to be effective in inducing objective response in patients with radiological evidence of distant metastases[1]. The intent of combined treatment approach is to eradicate the subclinical foci of disease which are present in the large majority of patients at the time of initial diagnosis[2,3,4].

Adriamycin (ADM) is known to be one of the most effective drugs in the treatment of advanced osteosarcoma[5,6]. For this reason, from 1974 we have combined ADM with radical surgery as an adjuvant treatment for clinically localized osteosarcoma.

PATIENTS AND METHODS

From March 1974 to September 1976, 12 consecutive patients with histologically proven diagnosis of "classic" osteogenic sarcoma were treated in our Institute with amputation followed by ADM. Other two patients with the histologic diagnosis of parosteal osteosarcoma were also treated with this combined approach. The main clinical features are described in Table 1. In 9 of 12 patients the age ranged between 10 and 15 years.

TABLE 1

MAIN CLINICAL FEATURES OF 12 PATIENTS WITH OSTEOGENIC SARCOMA

Age (years)	7.5 - 40		
Male/female ratio	7/5		
Primary involvement	Tibia 4 Humerus 1	Femur 4 Radius 1	Fibula 1 Pelvis 1
Initial symptoms ⟶ amputation	20 - 270 days (median 60)		

In Table 2 are summarized the most important data concerning treatment. After amputation, ADM was injected at the single intravenous dose of 75 mg/m^2. In absence of treatment failure chemotherapy was continued in the out patient clinic every 4 weeks for a total of 6 to 8 months. The total dose of ADM was planned not to exceed 600 mg/m^2. At the present moment, all patients have completed their adjuvant chemotherapy.

TABLE 2

MAIN TREATMENT FEATURES OF 12 PATIENTS WITH OSTEOGENIC SARCOMA

Amputation	transmedullary	4 (femur)
	disarticulation	2 (pelvis, humerus)
	above the joint proximal	6 (tibia, radius, fibula)
Amputation ⟶ chemotherapy	1-12 days (median 5)	
Cycles of ADM per patients	4-9 (median 8)	
Total dose of ADM per patient	285-600 mg/m^2 (median 525 mg/m^2)	

RESULTS

Figure 1 shows the actuarial disease-free survival of patients with osteogenic sarcoma. As of January 31, 1977, four patients showed relapse at 1, 4, 8 and 21 months following amputation. Eight patients (66%) remain continuously free of disease from 6^+ to 31^+ months. In contrast, 3 of 4 patients with relapse have already died of progressive disease after 5, 6 and 8 months, respectively from the diagnosis of primary treatment failure. None of the 4 patients treated with transmedullary amputation showed local recurrence in the stump, while 1 patient had lung metastases after 1 month from surgery. New manifestations of disease were documented in 3 patients in the lungs and in 1 patient in the skeleton (humerus). The fourth patient subsequently developed multiple bilateral lung metastases. Two patients showed relapse while on chemotherapy. The other two patients did so once ADM was discontinued. They had received only 6 of the 8 planned courses of adjuvant treatment. The disease-free survival could not be correlated to duration of symptoms before surgery, site of initial involvement, type of surgery and interval between amputation and start of chemotherapy.

Neither of the two patients with parosteal sarcoma showed recurrence after 8^+ and 31^+ months from amputation.

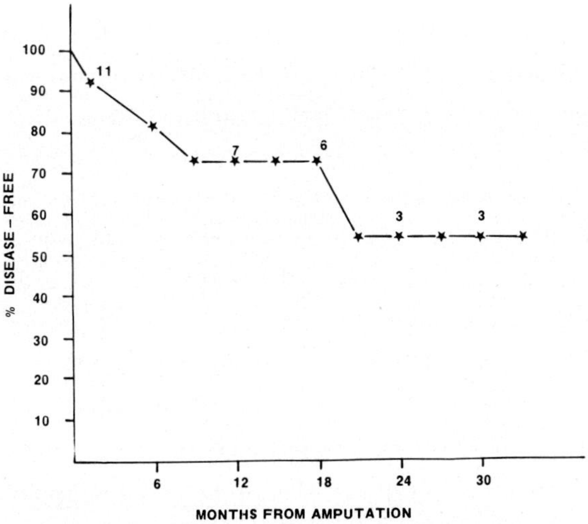

Fig. 1: Disease-free survival after amputation plus adriamycin

Treatment with ADM was, in general, well tolerated and dose reductions were seldom required. No patient showed a leukocyte count below 1,000 per cu.mm. In only one patient platelet count fell below 100,000 per cu.mm. No problem related to wound healing was recorded. All patients showed complete alopecia and in no instance were episodes of infection or stomatitis observed. No drug-induced amenorrhea was documented in 4 menstruating females. Aspecific and transient electrocardiographic changes occurred in 2 patients. At the present time, no episode of cardiomyopathy was observed.

DISCUSSION

In recent years, various adjuvant treatments were attempted in osteosarcoma following amputation or segmental resection in selected patients. None of the published reports have indicated the treatment of choice. However, available data showed that encouraging results are being obtained with single agent and combination chemotherapy[2,3,4,7]. For the time being, adjuvant immunotherapy alone seems not to be effective in preventing the development of clinical metastases[8]. The studies utilizing either ADM[4] or high-dose methotrexate (HD-MTX)[3] were those providing the first sound evidence of the real effectiveness of the combined treatment approach. The updated results of Cortes et al.[4] showed a 50% projected disease-free survival at 20 months from surgery in 21 patients treated with ADM alone (30 mg/m^2 for 3 consecutive days every 4 weeks). In their series, 13 of 21 patients were continuously free of disease for a period ranging from 5^+ to 33^+ months. Jaffe et al. employing HD-MTX preceeded by 2 mg/m^2 of Vincristine (VCR) reported that 60% of 12 patients with classic osteogenic sarcoma with local control were free of disease from 2^+ to 4.5^+ years[9]. Sutow et al.[2] utilized two polidrug regimens. The first combination (CTX, VCR, PAM and ADM or COMPADRI I) resulted in a 56% (24 of 43 patients) disease-free survival with a follow up observation ranging from 12 to 61 months. The second treatment (CTX, VCR, PAM, ADM and HD-MTX, or COMPADRI II) obtained a 67% (20 of 30 patients) disease-free survival with a follow up observation ranging from 12 to 26 months.

In spite of the small number of patients suitable for analysis, our present series supports the evidence that adjuvant treatment with ADM is effective in prolonging the disease-free status in patients with "classic" osteogenic sarcoma. Published results fail to indicate that in osteosarcoma adjuvant combination chemotherapy is definitely superior to single agent treatment. Furthermore, the improvement in the free interval is probably not sufficient to establish, at the present moment, the actual cure rate of combined modality approach. In fact, there is a possibility that adjuvant treatment can only delay the appearance of new disease manifestations, as exemplified by the occurrence of some late metastases after the second year[10]. Only a long-term analysis will clarify this crucial point. On the basis of the above mentioned considerations, we think that treatment with ADM is justified in the combined approach for osteogenic sarcoma. The drug is undoubtly effective in this tumor, it can be administered on an out patient basis, and its toxicity is predictable and reversible provided the cumulative dose does not exceed 550-600 mg/m^2.

REFERENCES

1. Friedman, M.A. and Carter, S.K. (1972) J. Surg. Oncol. 4, 482-510.
2. Sutow, W.W. et al. (1976) I. Bone Joint Surg. 58-A, 629-633.
3. Jaffe, N. et al. (1974) New Engl. J. Med. 291, 994-997.
4. Wang, J.J. and Cortes, E.P. (1975) Conflicts in Childhood Cancer, L.F. Sinks and J.O. Godden (eds) Alan R. Liss, Inc. pub. New York, 303-313.
5. Cortes, E.P. et al. (1972) Colston Paper No. 24, Bone-Certain Aspects of Neoplasia, C.H.G. Price and F.G.M. Ross (eds) London, Buttersworth and Co., 265-280.
6. Gottlieb, J.A. et al. (1975) Cancer Chemother. Rep. (part 3) 6, 271-282.
7. Rosen, G. et al. (1976) Cancer 37, 1-11.
8. Eilber, F.R. et al. (1975) Clin. Orth. 3, 94-100.

9. Jaffe, N. (1977) International Symposium on Recent Advances in Cancer Treatment, European Organisation for Research on Treatment of Cancer (EORTC), Bruxelles, Sept. 1976, Raven Press, New York (in press).
10. Sutow, W.W. (1976) Lancet I, 856.

Adjuvant Therapy of Cancer, S.E. Salmon and S.E. Jones eds.

THE TRANSFER FACTOR THERAPY OF STAGE II MALIGNANT MELANOMA

R.M. Bukowski, J. S. Hewlett, and S. Deodhar
Cleveland Clinic Foundation
9500 Euclid Avenue
Cleveland, Ohio 44106

Malignant melanoma is a disease where intense study of immunologic mechanisms and the role of immunotherapy has taken place during the past 10 years. Two observations have provided the basis for these investigations, namely, the spontaneous regression of primary malignant melanomas[1], and of metastatic lesions[2]. Multiple immunotherapeutic agents have been used in the treatment of disseminated malignant melanoma, and subsequently as adjuvants following surgical resection of stage II disease. One of these, transfer factor, was first described by Lawrence 20 years ago. This agent appears to transfer delayed hypersensitivity to non-immune recipients from immune donors. Its exact molecular structure and mechanism of action remain undetermined. Use of transfer factor in patients with disseminated malignant melanoma[3] and reports of responses to it form the basis for its use as adjuvant therapy. This report describes our experience with transfer factor as an adjuvant following surgical resection of stage II malignant melanoma.

Materials and Methods: Patient population: 29 patients with Stage II malignant melanoma have been entered in the study. Sixteen patients were randomized to no treatment and 13 patients to transfer factor. Stage II malignant melanoma was defined as metastatic disease in lymph node areas regional to the primary lesion and/or cutaneous or subcutaneous metastases greater than 3 cm from the original primary lesion on the same extremity. One patient withdrew from the study and the resulting 28 patients form the basis for this report. The characteristics of transfer factor treated and control patient groups are given in the following table (Table I).

Table I: Patient Characteristics

		Age	Lymph Node Status			Time of Stage II Diagnosis	
	M/F	(mean)	1 - 4	5	Other[1]	Presentation	Recurrence
TF Group	7/6	49.6	6	5	2	2	11
Control Group	11/4	53.2	10	2	3	4	11

[1]Cutaneous disease and/or nodal status unknown.

Clinical Studies: Following surgical resection of recurrent disease and radical lymphadenectomy, if indicated, all patients were studied to exclude residual disease. Staging procedures involved a chest x-ray, liver, bone, and EMI scans, and bone marrow biopsy. Lymphangiograms were performed when indicated.

If all initial studies were negative, the patient was considered eligible for the study. The patients were seen at intervals of 28 days for the first three months and at intervals of three months thereafter. A physical examination was performed each time, and evidence of recurrent disease recorded. The duration of the disease-free interval and survival for each patient was noted. Recurrent disease was proved by biopsy when possible.

Immunologic Studies: All studies were obtained prior to beginning any immunotherapy, and at least seven days following any surgical procedure. Immmunologic parameters measured included the following: 1) delayed hypersensitivity to five recall antigens (monilia, intermediate PPD, dermatophytin O, varidase and mumps); 2) percentage and absolute number of T-lymphocytes (E rosettes), activated T-lymphocytes (E' -rosettes) by the method of Wybran, et al[4], and B-lymphocytes (lymphocytes with complement receptors or EAC-rosettes, and bearing surface immunoglobulin or SIg); 3) lymphocyte blast transformation to plant mitogens, namely, phytohemagglutinin (PHA), pokeweed mitogen (PWM), and Concanavalin A (Con-A); 4) Quantitative serum immunoglobulins (IgG, IgA and IgM); and 5) lymphocyte cytotoxicity to cultured melanoma cells by the method of Hellstrom, et al[5]. The methods used in all these assays have all been described in previous publications[6]. These studies were obtained prior to entrance into the study, on day 28, 58, 84 and subsequently every three months.

Transfer Factor Preparation: Transfer factor donors were either cohabitants or unrelated subjects demonstrating greater than 75% cytotoxicity against cultured melanoma cells employing the microcytotoxicity assay. White cells were obtained by leukophoresis employing an Aminco continuous-flow blood cell separator. Dialyzable transfer factor was then prepared by the method of Lawrence[7]. The dialysate was lyophilized and reconstituted with sterile saline. The transfer factor was stored in individual vials containing one unit (equivalent to the amount prepared from 1×10^9 leukocytes) at 4° C. All transfer factor donors were skin tested to five recall antigens (following initial leukophoresis).

Transfer Factor Treatment Schedule: Thirteen patients have been randomized to receive transfer factor. The schedule employed involved the administration of one unit of transfer factor by the intramuscular route on days 1, 8, 15, 22, 36,50, and every 28 days thereafter. The transfer factor was continued until recurrent disease was documented.

Results: The study is ongoing and the results reported are a preliminary analysis of the immunologic data, disease free intervals, and survival of the first 28 patients on the study.

Immunologic Data All immunologic data in the transfer factor and control groups is summarized in Tables II, III, IV and V. In Table II, the various lymphocyte subpopulations are listed. Both the absoulute and relative values for total lymphocytes and several lymphocyte subpopulations for the first 56 days of the study are outlined. No significant differences between the absolute and relative values for total lymphocytes and T-lymphocytes were noted between the immunotherapy and the control groups (EAC- and SIg-lymphocytes not listed in Table II, also demonstrated no changes). Also, no significant changes in any lymphocyte subpopulation occurred in the group receiving transfer factor following its administration. One interesting observation, however, was that of the 13 patients who received transfer factor, eight demonstrated a 10% or greater rise in the absolute number of activated T-lymphocyte rosettes (E'-rosettes) whereas only three of 15 patients not receiving transfer factor demonstrated this ($p < .05$). When the absolute value for E'-rosettes was compared in the two groups, it can be seen that a progressive decrease occurred in the control group whereas in the transfer factor treated group it appeared to remain stable.

TABLE II: Immunologic Data - Lymphocyte Subpopulations

	TF Group			Control Group		
	Day Number					
Lymphocyte Type	0	28	56	0	28	56
Total Lymphocytes (20-45)[1]	1828[2]± 499	1654± 499	1658± 740	1717± 376	1412± 436	1564± 523
	(27.0)[3]	(24.8)	(28.5)	(26.4)	(24.2)	(23.4)
E-rosettes (75±5.3)	1245± 198	1197± 399	1060± 550	1149± 265	969± 385	1082± 406
	(69.0)	(72.5)	(63.7)	(67.0)	(67.0)	(76.1)
E'-rosettes (43.3 ± 6.9)	787± 380	745± 260	760± 430	809± 245	702± 227	737± 329
	(42.5)	(44.7)	(44.3)	(45.8)	(49.9)	(47.6)

[1]Normal values, 24 control subjects.

[2]Absolute value -- ± mean standard deviation.

[3]Relative value -- mean %.

Table III outlines the mitogen responses found in the transfer factor and control groups. The responses were expressed as percent transformation. A progressive increase in the mitogen responses in the transfer factor group occurred during the first 56 days, and at that point the values for PHA and PWM were significantly greater than the control group ($p < .05$). The Con A reponses also demonstrated a progressive increase, however, because of the large standard deviation, the results were not significantly different at day 56.

TABLE III: Immunologic Data - Mitogen Studies

Mitogen Type	TF Group			Control Group		
	Day Number					
	0	28	56	0	28	56
PHA	70.6[1]± 11.0	72.1± 7.6	74.2[2]± 6.7	64± 12.6	64± 11.2	62.1[2]± 14.7
CON A	62.8± 7.9	64.2± 12.2	66'.0± 33.0	61.5± 13.3	56 ± 10.6	55.3± 7.60
PWM	27.2± 6.20	28.4± 9.9	27.9[3]± 4.1	26.7± 8.3	24.6± 8.6	20.8[3]± 11.7

[1]Percent blast transformation ± standard deviation.

[2]Significant difference, $p < .01$. [3]Significant difference, $p < .05$.

Table IV outlines the lymphocyte cytotoxicity results and serum immunoglobulin levels in both groups. Levels for lymphocyte cytotoxicity against a melanoma cell line (M.B. cell line) were greater in the transfer factor group than the control group, however, these differences were not significant. No differences in serum immunoglobulin levels were found following transfer factor treatment, and no differences between the transfer factor group and the control group were noted.

TABLE IV: Immunologic Data: Lymphocyte Cytotoxicity and Serum Immunoglobulins.

	TF Group			Control Group		
	Day Number					
	0	28	56	0	28	56
Lymphocyte Cytotoxicity	64.0[1]± 24.4	69.1± 25.6	57.6± 27.1	60.8± 26.1	58.9± 22.8	49.8± 14.9
IgG (1380± 255)[2]	1130[3]± 447	1138± 385	1059± 161	975± 315	1034± 156	1109± 180
IgA (156± 92)	267± 83	254± 82	275± 87	338± 198	330± 165	384± 250
IgM (145 ± 105)	151± 79	163± 84	153± 49	104± 70	102± 49	118± 75

[1]Percent melanoma cell destruction vs M.B. cell line ± standard deviation.

[2]Normal range: Mg% ± standard deviation. [3]Mg% ± standard deviation.

Finally, delayed hypersensitivity skin testing was performed in all patients before and during treatment. It was not always possible to determine whether transfer of delayed hypersensitivity occurred since criteria for choosing a donor were not related to his pretreatment skin test reactivity, however, this was seen in three instances. Pretreatment skin tests in the transfer factor, control group and 45 normal subjects are outlined in Table V. The group of patients with malignant melanoma demonstrated reactivity equivalent to that in the normal subjects.

Following transfer factor administration the number of positive skin tests appeared to increase when compared to the control group.

Table V: Immunologic Data: Delayed Hypersensitivity

Patient Group		Antigen Type				
		PPD	Mumps	Varidase	Monilia	Dermatophytin
TF:	Day 0[1]	1/10[2]	2/6	9/10	8/10	2/10
	Day 28	4/10	3/6	9/10	10/10	1/10
Control:	Day 0	1/14	4/10	11/14	14/14	3/14
	Day 28	1/14	3/9	8/14	13/14	1/14
Normal		4/40	24/36	35/40	38/40	5/40

[1] Day of Study. [2] No. positive/no tested; positive equivalent to 5 x 5 mm induration at 24 to 48 hrs.

Response and Survival Data: Figures 1 through 4 illustrate the disease-free intervals and survival for the transfer factor and control groups. The curves were calculated using the Kaplan-Meier Life Table method and differences between curves were determined using the generalized Wilcoxon test performed by computer analysis. Figure 1 illustrates the disease-free intervals. Three subgroups were studied: those treated with transfer factor, the control group, and those treated with transfer factor who demonstrated absolute increases of activated T-lymphocytes (E'). No significant difference between the disease free intervals in the groups treated with transfer factor and the control group were noted ($p < .3$). When patients demonstrating increased levels of activated T-lymphocytes were compared to the control group, an increase in the median disease-free interval was noted but this was not significant ($p < .2$).

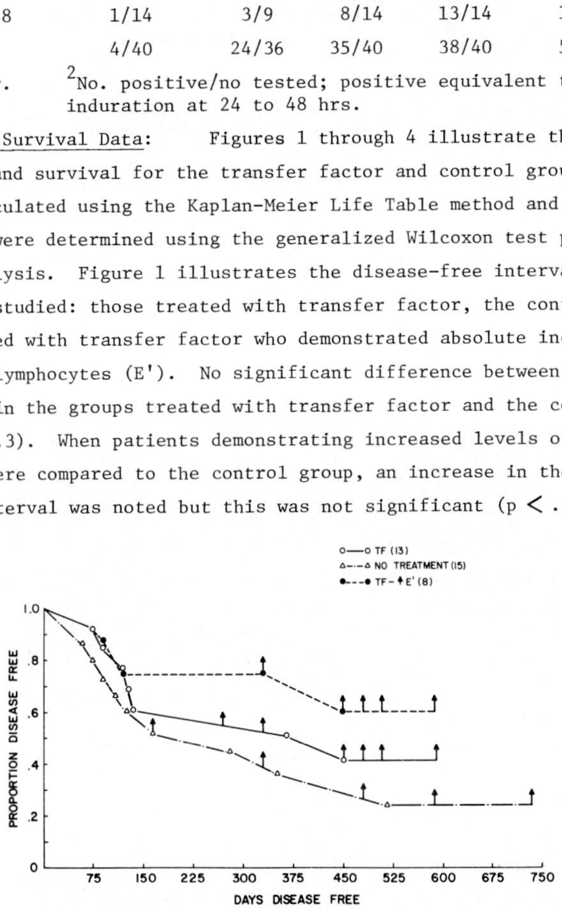

Figure 1: Disease-free interval in patients with stage II malignant melanoma.

Survival in patients with stage II melanoma is depicted in Figure 2. Again the group treated with transfer factor, the control group and the transfer factor group demonstrating increased levels of activated T-lymphocytes (E') are outlined. No significant differences between the survival in the transfer factor group and control group are apparent. When the transfer factor group demonstrating increased levels of activated T-lymphocytes is compared to the control group, an increase in the survival is noted, which is not quite statistically significant ($p < .1$).

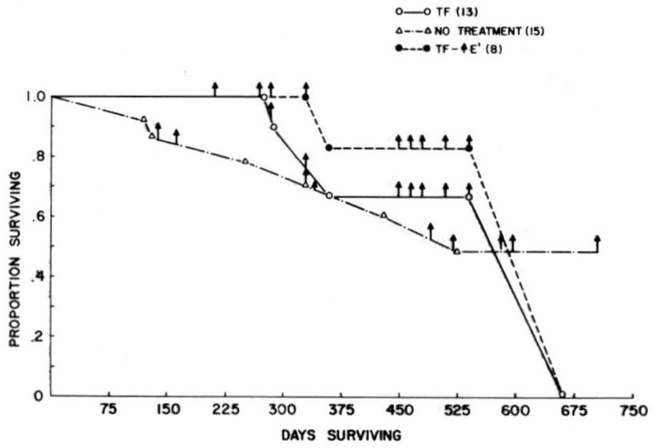

Figure 2: Survival in patients with stage II malignant melanoma.

When prognostic factors were examined for the 28 patients it was apparent that the control group contained a greater number of patients with one to four positive lymph nodes (10) compared to the immunotherapy group (6). For this reason disease-free and survival data was examined for the patients in both groups who demonstrated one to four positive lymph nodes. This data is outlined in Figures 3 and 4. Figure 3 shows the median disease-free interval has not been reached for the transfer factor group, and in the control group it is 320 days. The two disease-free interval curves are not yet statistically different ($p < .1$).

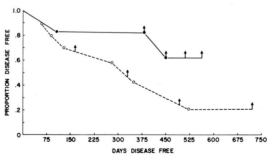

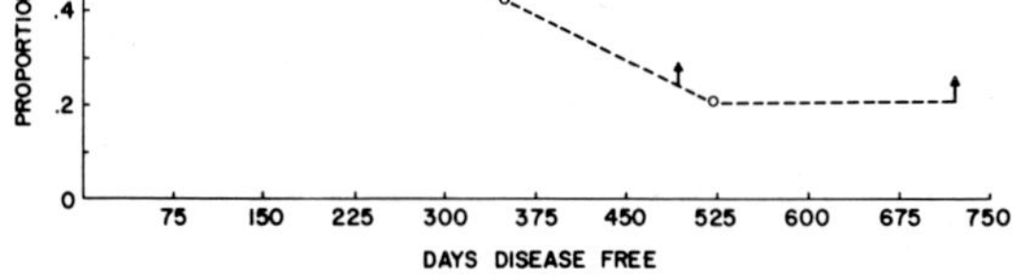

Figure 3: Disease-free intervals in patients with one to four lymph nodes involved.

Figure 4 shows the survival data in this same group of patients. Those treated with transfer factor demonstrated a significantly better survival than did the control group ($p < .05$). The median survival in the control group is 440 days and has not been reached in the transfer factor group.

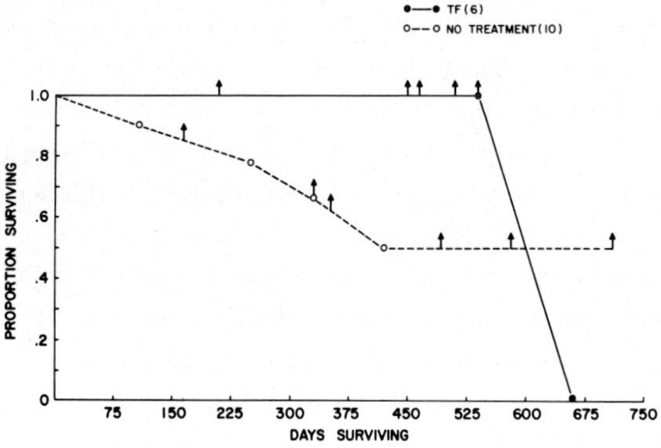

Figure 4: Survival in patients with one to four lymph nodes involved.

In view of the difference observed in patients demonstrating increased levels of activated T-lymphocytes (E'), the disease free and survival data for the transfer factor group were examined. Patients were divided by whether an increase ($\geq 10\%$) in absolute number of activated T-lymphocytes occured by day 56. Table VI lists the median disease free and survival data for these groups.

TABLE VI: Median Disease Free Intervals and Survival In Transfer Factor Treated Patients.

	Number Patients	Disease Free (days)	Survival (days)
Increased E'	8	>450	>450
Decreased E'	5	120	340

The disease free interval and survival curves are significantly different for both groups ($p < .05$) and demonstrate definite improvement in the patients with increased levels of activated T-lymphocytes.

Discussion: The nature and composition of transfer factor remains unsettled. Evidence has been presented demonstrating various nonspecific effects of transfer factor in a treated group when compared to a control group. Increases in the number of activated T-lymphocytes and plant mitogen responses have been found. Examination of the delayed hypersensitivity data also demonstrates a trend towards an increase in the number of positive skin tests in the group receiving transfer factor. These data appear to support the hypothesis of nonspecific effect of transfer factor when used as an immune adjuvant in this setting.

The study was originally designed to detect any adjuvant effects of transfer factor in patients with stage II malignant melanoma. The overall results (Figures 1 and 2) show no benefit for the group receiving transfer factor. However, if one of the biologic effects of transfer factor is to increase the number of activated T-lymphocytes, then the group of patients with this phenomenon showed an increase in the disease-free interval and survival approaching statistical significance. When prognostic factors are considered, those patients with the lowest tumor burden, namely those with one to four lymph nodes positive at the time of surgical resection of their disease showed an increase in the disease-free interval for the transfer factor group which as yet is not statistically significant because of the small number of patients. A definite increase in survival in transfer factor treated patients with one to four lymph nodes positive was seen. Finally, a statistically significant difference between the disease-free interval and survival was found in transfer factor patients who demonstrated increased activated T-rosettes compared to those that did not.

This study is early, and the number of patients in each arm is small. However, certain trends and differences are apparent and the study is being continued. At present, results would appear to demonstrate a nonspecific immunologic effect of transfer factor, and an apparent improvement in survival and disease-free intervals in those patients with minimal tumor burdens and those demonstrating a biologic effect of transfer factor. Larger numbers of patients will be needed to confirm these findings and demonstrate any potential usefulness of transfer factor preparations in patients with malignant melanoma.

Acknowledgement: Supported by PHS Grant CA-13916.

BIBLIOGRAPHY

1. Smith, J.L., Stehlin, J.S.: Spontaneous regression of primary malignant melanoma with regional metastases. Cancer, 18:1399-1415, 165.

2. Everson, T.C., Cole, W.H.: Spontaneous Regression in Cancer. Philadelphia, Saunders, 1966, pp. 1-560.

3. Spitler, L.E., et al: Transfer factor therapy of malignant melanoma. Clin. Res. 21:221, 1973.

4. Wybran, J., et al: Rosette-forming cells, immunologic deficiency diseases, and transfer factor. NEJM, 288:710-713, 1973.

5. Hellstrom, I., Hellstrom, K.E.: In Vitro Methods in Cell-Mediated Immunity. New York, Academic Press, p 408, 1971.

6. Bukowski, R.M., et al: Lymphocyte subpopulations in Hodgkin's disease. Am. J. Clin. Path., 65:31-39, 1976.

7. Lawrence, H.S.: Transfer factor in cellular immunity. New York, Academic Press, Harvey Lectures, series 68, pp 239-350, 1973.

Adjuvant Therapy of Cancer, S.E. Salmon and S.E. Jones eds.

MALIGNANT MELANOMA (STAGE IIIB): A PILOT STUDY OF ADJUVANT CHEMO-IMMUNOTHERAPY

T. A. McPherson, A. H. G. Paterson, D. Willans and M. Watson
Departments of Medicine and Pathology
W. W. Cross Institute and University of Alberta
Edmonton, Alberta, Canada

INTRODUCTION

Patients with regional lymph node involvement (Stage IIIB) from malignant melanoma have a 5-year survival of 15-25% after surgical removal of all apparent disease, and about a 6% recurrence-free 5-year survival. Those with clinically palpable, histologically positive nodes, undergoing "therapeutic dissection," have a 5-year survival of about 19%, whereas those with clinically nonpalpable, histologically positive nodes, undergoing "elective dissection," have a 5-year survival of about 55%[1]. Thus, systemic adjuvant therapy is clearly warranted in Stage IIIB melanoma--especially in those with clinically positive nodes.

The treatment of metastatic melanoma with chemotherapy is disappointing, with short-term objective remissions being observed in from 16 to 31% with DTIC[2], and from 16[3] to 21%[4,5] with the nitrosoureas. Metastatic melanoma may, in a few cases, be responsive to chemo-immunotherapy with DTIC and BCG[6], and the disease-free interval and survival of Stage IIIB disease may be improved with BCG immunotherapy[7,8]. DTIC in usual doses is only moderately immunosuppressive[9], but it is possible that the use of BCG immunotherapy might overcome nonspecific immunosuppression caused by chemotherapy, as well as stimulate "specific" immunity to melanoma because of cross-antigenicity between BCG and melanoma antigens[10]. Thus, there is some evidence to suggest that the use of DTIC and BCG, as well as, perhaps, the combination of DTIC and a nitrosourea plus BCG, might be beneficial in the adjuvant treatment of Stage IIIB melanoma following "therapeutic dissection."

We report here the results of an uncontrolled "pilot trial" to study the effect of DTIC plus BCG given by Heaf gun, or DTIC/BCNU/hydroxyurea plus BCG given orally, on the disease-free interval and survival of 30 Stage IIIB melanoma patients with no evident disease after treatment by therapeutic node dissection.

CLINICAL STUDY AND RESULTS

<u>Patients:</u> The clinical characteristics of the patients entering the study, in comparison with 33 Stage IIIB "historical controls" treated in Edmonton by therapeutic dissection of affected nodes alone between 1968 and 1972, are shown in Table 1.

TABLE 1. Clinical features of the treatment groups (D/BCG and DBH/BCG) and of a local historical control (HC)

WE = wide excision

WE + G = wide excision and graft

■ = 2 patients treated by amputation of finger, 1 by mid-tarsal amputation of the foot, 1 by node dissection, and 1 by wide excision, graft and radical node dissection

○ = 1 patient died melanoma-free of possible chemotherapy complication

△ = 1 patient died melanoma-free with pre-senile dementia

	W.W.Cross		
	D/BCG	DBH/BCG	HC
CLINICAL FEATURE	11	19	33
MEDIAN RANGE AGE (Yrs)	45 29-77	47 27-78	46 22-86
MALE (Nº)	8	10	17
FEMALE (Nº)	3	9	16
Site of Primary (Nº) Trunk	4	4	13
Head & Neck		2	10
Extremities	7	12	10
Unknown		1	
Clark's Level of Primary (Nº) III	1	4	
IV or V	5	7	
Unknown	5	8	
Treatment of Primary (Nº): WE	3	5	19
WE + G	8	9	13
Other		5■	
Time from Primary to Node Recurrence (months): Mean	17.6	23.9	11.9
Median	15	15	5
Range	1-48	0-90	0-84
Nº of Patients	11	19	33
Disease-Free Interv. Median	20	9	—
Range in months	4-29+	3+-31	
Nº Surviving	○4	△12	7
Survival Duration Median	20.8+	12+	11.5
Range in months	8-29+	6+-31+	2-60+

TABLE 2. Histological features of the primary lesion

	Good		Bad	
	D/BCG	DBH/BCG	D/BCG	DBH/BCG
Depth	0	2	9	13
Lymphocyt.	2	4	7	11
Mel.Type	7	7	2	8
Invasion	9	13	0	2
Ulceration	5	11	4	4
Cytology	4	6	5	9
TOTAL	27	43	27	47

Melanoma Type	Clark's Level III		Clark's Level IV	
	D/BCG	DBH/BCG	D/BCG	DBH/BCG
Nodular	0	3	2	5
Sup.Spread.	1	2	5	3
Other	1*	0	0	2**

*Invasive Intraepidermal Component.

**Acral Lentiginous Melanoma.

Growth Phase	Group	
	D/BCG	DBH/BCG
Radial	0	1
Intermed.	2	2
Vertical	6	9

Total Primary Melanomas Reviewed : D/BCH=9/11 ; DBH/BCG= 15/19.

Drugs: No patient had received prior chemotherapy for melanoma. The dose and schedule of DTIC/BCG (D/BCG) and DTIC/BCNU/hydroxyurea/BCG (DBH/BCG) is shown in Table 3.

TABLE 3

Week	1		4	5
Day	1 2 3 4 5 6 7 8 9 10	12 17	22 23 24 25 26	29 30 31 32 33
DTIC/ BCG	D D D D D #	# #	D D D D D	
DBH/ BCG	D D D D D O O O O O B H H H H H			D D D D D B H H H H H

DTIC/BCG : DTIC 250 mg/m^2 i.v. daily ; BCG (#) 40 mg by Heaf gun days 7, 12, 17 – X 12 courses
DBH/BCG : DTIC 150 mg/m^2 i.v. daily ; BCNU 150 mg/m^2 i.v. once ; Hydroxyurea 1500 mg/m^2 po daily ; BCG (O) 120 mg po daily – X6, then q3moX4.

In the D/BCG group, DTIC was given, as indicated, at a dosage of 250 mg/m^2 intravenously, with decremental doses given on subsequent courses if indicated by hematologic values, and BCG (Connaught, 40 mg in 1 ml of diluent) was applied in two strips from upper-scapular to iliac crest level in outwardly extending, paraspinal strips. The moist surface containing BCG was then perforated with multiple punctures (at least 20 sites) with a 20-needle Heaf gun. In the DBH/BCG group, DTIC and BCNU were given at a dosage of 150 mg/m^2 intravenously, and hydroxyurea at a dosage of 1,500 mg/m^2 orally, as indicated, also with appropriate decremental doses according to hematological values, and BCG was given orally in 5 ml of orange juice as indicated.

Side-effects--Chemotherapy: All patients suffered from nausea, and most from vomiting, during the course of chemotherapy. This was worse in the DBH/BCG group, and was most pronounced on the first day of the schedule when the patient received both DTIC and BCNU. The use of oral Largactil spansules (75 mg) well before the drugs, in addition to Stemetil, intramuscularly before, and as needed, was helpful in controlling these symptoms in some patients.

The white cell count (WBC), and platelet count (PC) were reduced in most patients. There was not, however, a significant difference in the values obtained prior to, and regularly after, treatment in those patients who did well on treatment as compared to those who did not (Table 4).

TABLE 4

	WBC (X10^3)			Platelets (X10^3)		
	Mean	Median	Range	Mean	Median	Range
Pre – Rx	6.6	6.2	3.7–9.4	287	275	152–520
Non-Progressor	4.4	4.4	2.9–6.0	239	230	133–338
Progressor	3.9	3.9	3.0–5.0	242	242	160–354

Three patients developed abnormal neurological symptoms and signs, unaccountable for by other known medical diagnoses. These consisted of amaurosis fugax in a 47-year old woman, transient hemiparesis and confusion in a 49-year old woman, and pre-senile dementia (with which he died) in a 45-year old man[11]. These were thought possibly to be related to DTIC, although all episodes occurred after several courses of DTIC, with no acute neurological abnormalities occurring in these, or other patients, during, or shortly after, DTIC administration.

Two patients died with no gross or microscopic melanoma at autopsy; one with pre-senile dementia, and the other of unknown cause after admission to her local hospital for "flu-like" symptoms. This latter patient was afebrile during her 24-hour admission, but hematologic values were nót obtained. Both patients were considered chemotherapy-related deaths. One patient dropped out of the trial of his own accord because of chemotherapy toxicity.

Side-effects--BCG: Heaf gun administered BCG was tolerated for the first six to twelve administrations in most patients (2-4 full protocol courses), but after this most patients found the reactions unacceptable, both aesthetically and because of pruritus and discomfort. However, no patients dropped out of the trial of their own accord because of BCG side-effects.

Oral BCG was well tolerated by all patients. Several noted mild epigastric distress, nausea, and a "flu-like" syndrome, with, in some, loose bowel motions, while on BCG. In addition, one patient developed mild ascites while on protocol. We have also noted the development of ascites shortly after commencing oral BCG in one other patient with Stage IVB melanoma[12], which may have been associated with enhancement of intra-abdominal tumor, or inflammatory responses in intra-abdominal tumor due to BCG. Gallium 67-citrate scanning has been a useful method for detecting progression of disease[13]. However, development of a peculiar homogeneous increase in uptake of Gallium 67-citrate in lungs, in the presence of normal lung X-rays and full lung tomography, has also been noted in several patients. In two patients, with this abnormality, tested for pulmonary function, single-breath diffusion studies have been clearly reduced, suggesting a diffuse abnormality of diffusion (Dr. N. Brown, University of Alberta, Edmonton, personal communication). One other patient, with an increased, homogeneous uptake of Gallium 67-citrate in the lungs, and a decreased single-breath diffusion test, but with a reticular-nodular abnormality on chest X-ray, was found to have cells suggestive of a granulomatous infiltrate, without evidence of melanoma, when cytology was done on a fine-needle aspirate of the lung[14]. The abnormality showed definite clearing with isoniazid treatment. Thus, the diffusion studies and Gallium 67-citrate scans might be indicative of the development of BCG-granulomatous infiltrates in the lungs in some patients on oral BCG. The question of whether the granulomatous infiltrates are surrounding microscopic foci of melanoma, or not, is not known, but might be answered by further studies on similarly treated patients with Stage I disease, treated with oral BCG, who are less likely to have microscopic foci of melanoma at the time of study.

Investigations: All patients were investigated by conventional hematological, biochemical and radiological examinations, as well as by liver and gallium scans, for the possibility of residual disease prior to entering the study, and at regular intervals while on study. In the early days of the study, immune status was monitored with skin tests to a standard battery of recall antigens, by a dose response study of lymphocyte transformation to PHA and PPD, and by CEA plasma levels. However, it soon became apparent that the absolute lymphocyte count in these patients, even on blood taken before chemotherapy, was closely correlated with the *in vitro* PHA response, and the *in vitro* PPD response was not helpful in separating patients who showed progressive disease from those who did not. In addition, CEA levels were not helpful. Thus PHA and PPD *in vitro* testing as well as CEA tests were abandoned. Dilutional skin tests to PPD were done regularly, but these results also failed, in general, to correlate with disease course. Several patients who have done well on therapy failed to convert to positive PPD, even when tested at a strength of 250 tuberculin units. We thought this might represent "immune deviation" of available immunocompetent cells such that an attack on melanoma antigens, cross-reactive with BCG, was occurring in some patients, but not in others. This possibility is supported by a similar finding in some of our regressor Stage IVB patients on BCG. On the other hand, some patients receiving oral BCG definitely showed an increase in PPD lymphocyte transformation and skin sensitivity to PPD, indicating that oral BCG could clearly cause increasing sensitivity to PPD.

Disease-free interval and survival: The censored disease-free interval, and survival, of the D/BCG, DBH/BCG, and combination of the two groups, as compared to our local historical control (HC) are shown in Figure 1. Figure 2 shows the cumulative survival rate as a proportion of patients on study for the combination of our two groups as compared to our historical control group. Statistical comparison of the censored disease-free interval and survival curves was made using the modified Wilcoxon test[15]. A significant difference at the 0.05 level was observed when the survival of the DBH/BCG group was compared to the historical control (Z = 2.249), but was not observed for the D/BCG vs. HC (Z = 1.733), DBH/BCG vs. D/BCG (Z = 0.157), or for the disease-free intervals of DBH/BCG vs. HC (Z = 1.93), D/BCG vs. HC (Z = 1.465), or DBH/BCG vs. D/BCG (0.025). The comparison of the survival curves between the combination of the D/BCG and DBH/BCG groups with the historical control was significant at the 0.01 level (Z = 2.597), and a similar comparison of the disease-free interval curves closely approached significance (Z = 2.175).

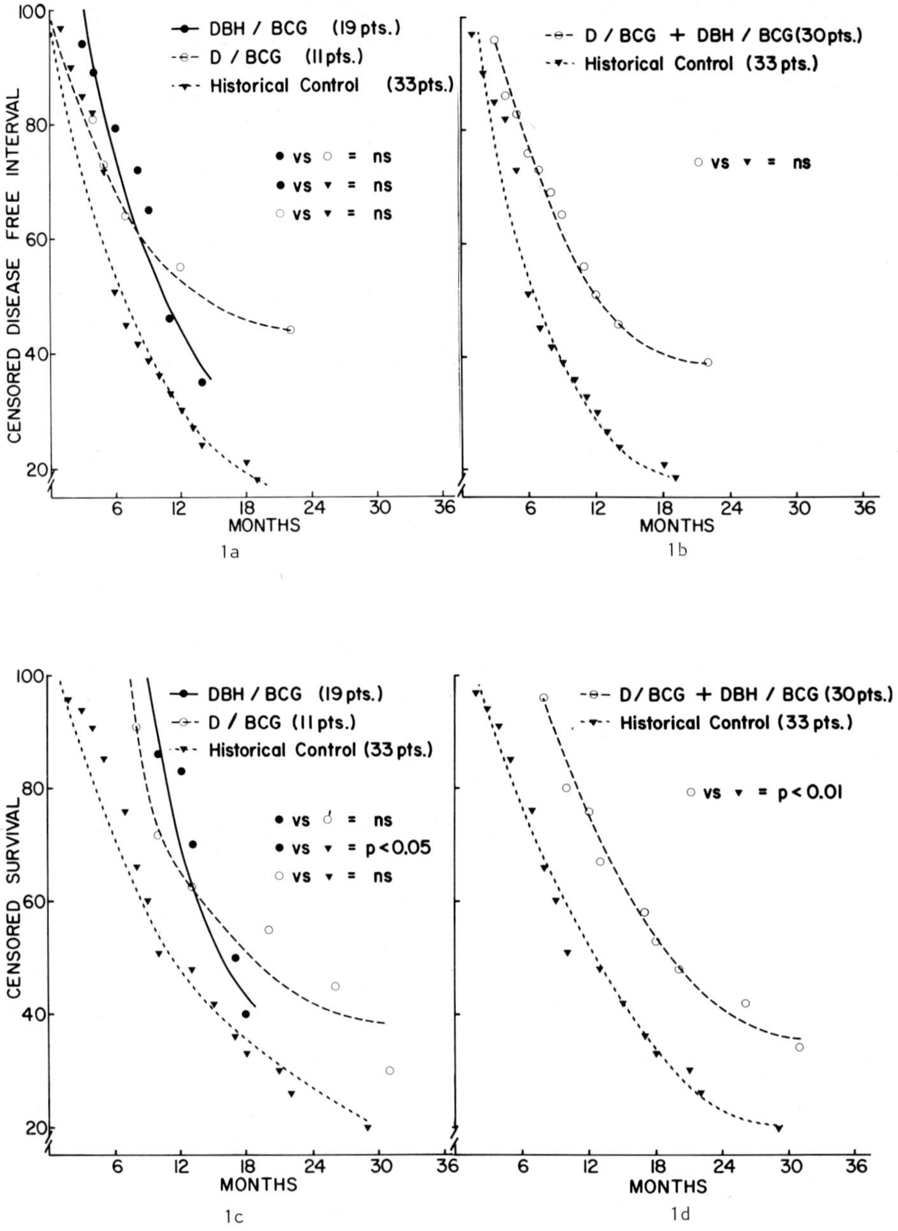

FIG. 1. Censored disease-free interval and survival of the treatment groups compared to each other and to a local historical control

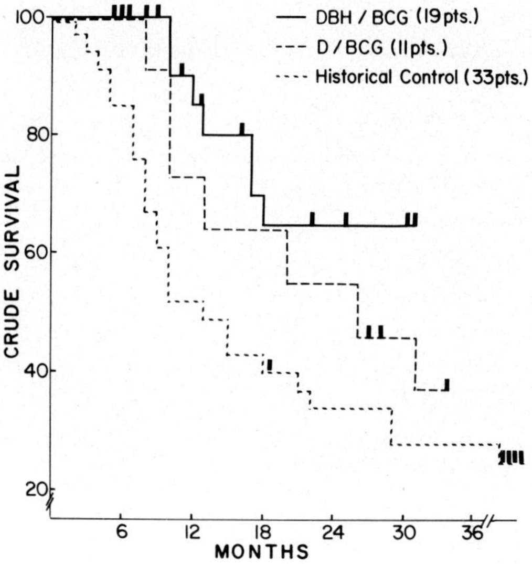

FIG. 2. Crude survival of the treatment groups compared to each other and to a local historical control

▌ = surviving patient

A comparison of the censored disease-free interval and survival curves for a historical control from an M. D. Anderson Hospital study[16] with those for the combination of our two treatment groups and with those for our historical control was performed. The disease-free interval curve of our treatment group was significantly different at the 0.001 level ($Z = 3.294$) from the M. D. Anderson group, but the survival curve comparisons were not significantly different ($Z = 1.385$). Our historical control was not significantly different from the M. D. Anderson group for either disease-free interval ($Z = 0.945$) or survival ($Z = 0.0941$).

DISCUSSION

It is not our impression that the use of adjuvant chemo-immunotherapy treatment of Stage IIIB malignant melanoma, as described in this report, was of sufficient therapeutic benefit to our patients to warrant a further, more definitive, study.

ACKNOWLEDGEMENTS

We thank the physicians and surgeons of Alberta, and particularly those participating in the Melanoma Clinic, for their help and for referring patients to this study. We also thank Drs. Shaw, Koch and Katakkar, and Ms. Melnychuk, for help in different aspects of the study, and Mr. Karl Liesner for preparing the illustrations. This study was supported, in part, by the Research Committee of the Provincial Cancer Hospitals Board, and by the Police Benevolent Society of Edmonton.

REFERENCES

1. DeVita, Jr., V. T. and Fisher, R. I. (1976) Cancer Treatment Rep. 60, 153-157.
2. Costanza, M. E., Nathanson, L., Costello, W. G., Wolter, J., Brunk, S. F., Colsky, J., Hall, T., Oberfield, R. A. and Regelson, W. (1976) Cancer 37, 1654-1659.
3. Cruz, Jr., A. B., Metter, G., Armstrong, D. M., Aust, J. B., Fletcher, W. S., Wilson, W. L. and Richardson, J. D. (1976) Cancer 38, 1069-106.
4. Ahmann, D. L., Hahn, R. G. and Bisel, H. F. (1974) Cancer 33, 615-618.
5. Young, R. C., Canellos, G. P., Chabner, B. A., Schein, P. S., Brereton, H. D. and DeVita, V. T. (1974) Clin. Pharmacol. Ther. 15, 617-622.
6. Gutterman, J. U., Mavligit, G., Gottlieb, J. A., Burgess, M. A., McBride, C. E., Einhorn, L., Freireich, E. J. and Hersh, E. M. (1974) New England J. Med. 291, 592-597.
7. Eilber, F. R., Morton, D. L., Holmes, E. C., Sparks, F. C. and Ramming, K. P. (1976) New England J. Med. 294, 237-240.
8. Eilber, F. R., Townsend, Jr., C. M. and Morton, D. L. (1976) Amer. J. Surgery 132, 476-479.
9. Bruckner, H. W., Mokyr, M. B. and Mitchell, M. S. (1974) Cancer Res. 34, 181-183.
10. Minden, P., Sharpton, T. R. and McClatchy, J. K. (1976) J. Immunol. 116, 1407-1414.
11. Paterson, A. H. G. and McPherson, T. A. (1977) Cancer Treatment Rep. 61, in press.
12. Nutting, M. G. and McPherson, T. A. (1976) New England J. Med. 295, 395.
13. Jackson, F. I., McPherson, T. A. and Lentle, B. C. (1977) Radiology 122, 163-167.
14. Schapira, D. V. and McPherson, T. A. (1977) New England J. Med. (in press).
15. Gehan, E. A. (1965) Biometrika (London) 52, 203-223.
16. Gutterman, J. U., McBride, C., Freireich, E. J., Mavligit, G., Frei, III, E. and Hersh, E. M. (1973) Lancet 1973, 1208-1212.

Adjuvant Therapy of Cancer, S.E. Salmon and S.E. Jones eds.
© 1977 Elsevier/North-Holland Biomedical Press, Amsterdam

IMMUNOTHERAPY OF MELANOMA WITH 2-4 DINITROCHLOROBENZENE (DNCB).

by S. MALEK-MANSOUR.
Hospital of Baviere (dermatology)
Liege - Belgium

Tumor specific antigens, capable of inducing a host immune response, have been demonstrated in various animal models. Moreover, there is increasing evidence that human cancers contain specific antigens which are immunogenic in the autologus host. Host immunologic response against these antigens may be important in the development of malignancy. As immune deficiency is a favorable condition for the development of neoplasia, cell mediated skin reactivity to various antigens was employed as screening technique in the follow-up of cancer. Moreover, skin tests for delayed sensitivity were used for evaluation of prognosis. On theoretical ground, it was thus reasonable to consider that stimulation of cell-mediated immunity should be beneficial in the treatment of malignancies. We report here on our seven year experience of the so-called "active non specific immunotherapy" in the therapy of metastatic or primary melanoma with DNCB.

MATERIALS AND METHODS.

DNCB was the artificial hapten chosen as immunotherapeutic agent as it was known to induce rapid sensitization of 95 % of normal recipients. Patients were, first, sensitized towards DNCB by applying in the scapulary region and for 48 hours a patch moistened with 20λ of a 3 per cent solution of the drug in acetone. A caustic reaction was observed.15 days later, sensitivity was estimated with a 48 hours application of a patch moistened with 20 λ of a 0.66 per cent of DNCB in acetone on the forearm. Unresponsive patients were submitted to additional sensitization. A patient was considered as been anergic, when no reaction was observed after four sensitizing patches had been applyied at 15 days intervals. All patients suffering from metastatic melanoma and studied so far, exhibited a reaction after the regular sensitization towards DNCB. For therapeutic use, DNCB was incorporated in an ointment containing 2 per cent (w/w) concentration and applied for 48 hours on skin sites of melanoma. The treatment was repeated at weekly intervals until complete disappearance of the tumor.

Patient ranged in age from 20 to 85 years. They had primary or metastatic melanoma with or without lymph node or visceral involvement.

Of the total of 47 cases studied, 7 did not have histological confirmation but were based on clinical diagnosis.

RESULTS

Locoregional intradermal metastases.

Ten patients who had locoregional intradermal metastases without visceral involvement were treated by local application of DNCB.

Two of them had been treated four years and 15 days before by a limited but complete excision of their primary melanoma. Four had been treated by wide excision with skin graft, followed by a lymph node dissection. One patient in this group had histological positive nodes while the remaining three cases were negative. These patients had recurrences after 1 year, 6 months, 1 year and 1 year respectively. Two patients were treated with a limited but complete excision of the primary tumor followed by a lymph node dissection. Both had positive nodes. Locoregional metastases appeared after 1 month and 4 years. One patient had the primary tumor coagulated 6 months before the apparition of locoregional metastases. One had received an immunotherapy of her primary melanoma by 3 applications of DNCB followed by a large excision and a skin graft.

All these patients had one to thirty intradermal locoregional metastases of melanoma (fig. 1). DNCB was applied for a range of 2 months to 3 years. For patients who had repetitive applications for a long period, therapy was stopped when clinical remission appeared. Of this group, 6 patients remain in complete remission (fig. 2) for a range of 1 to 6 years.

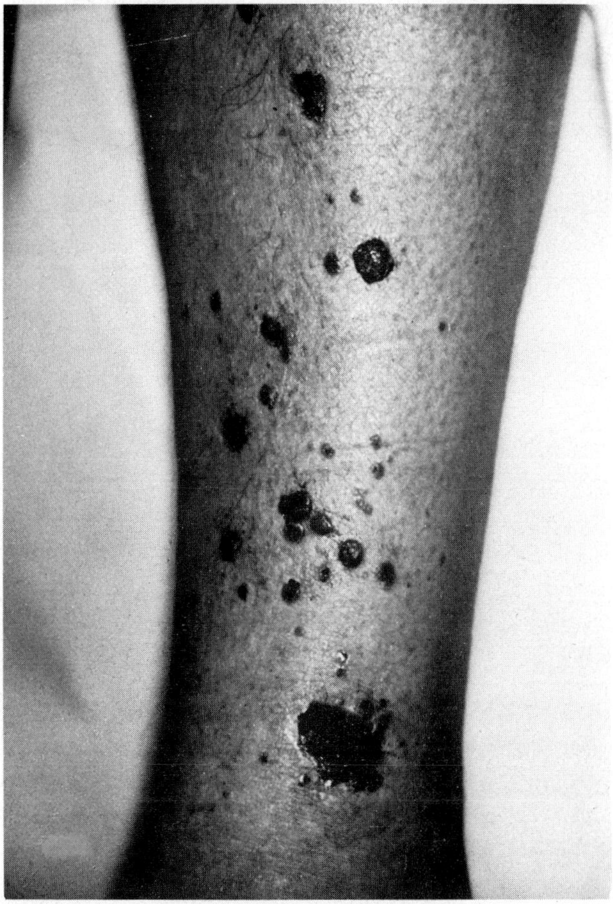

fig. 1 the leg before treatment

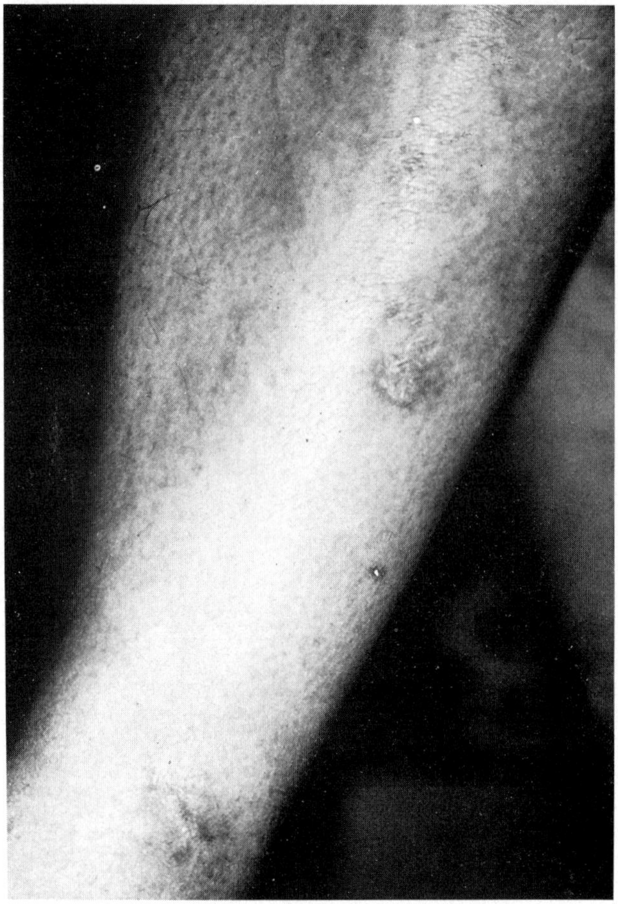

fig. 2   the leg after treatment

The remaining 4 cases had episodic local recurrences which are treated with DNCB. They have not presented signs of dissemination in from 2 - 3 years.

The median time of treatment of this group is 13.9 months and the median time of follow-ups is 39.2 months.

Primary melanoma (immunotherapy followed by surgery)

18 patients suffering from primary melanoma received 10 applications of DNCB followed by surgery, consisting of wide excision and a skin graft. The lymph node were not excised because there was no clinical evidence of involvement at the first consultation. Of this group, 15 are alive without recurrence with follow-up of more than three years. The remaining 3 patients died of metastases.

Primary melanoma (immunotherapy without surgery).

4 patients with primary melanoma were treated with DNCB alone without surgery. All four remain in complete remission for 45, 40, 33 and 31 months. Within this group, 1 had level 4 lesions, 1 had level 5 lesions and 2 had level 1 lesion by the Clark's classification.

Immunotherapy on widespread metastatic melanoma.

15 patients had generalized intradermal or hypodermal metastases and lymph node involvement : most of them had extensive visceral involvement. Some of these patients had received prior radiotherapy, chemotherapy or surgery.

All patients got intensive immunotherapy consisting of :

- local application of DNCB for the intradermal lesions ;
- injection of DNCB at 2 % in tween 80 for hypodermal lesions ;
- intradermal injection of 10^4 autologus cells of melanoma bound with DNCB ;
- surgery for the largest tumors.

Despite regression of treated cutaneous lesions, 13 of the cases have died of the melanoma with metastases : their survival ranges in a period between 2 months and 3 years. In this group, 3 patients had periods of regression of the tumor and clinical remission for several months.

One patient, with a primary melanoma on his leg, lymph node and liver involvement was treated with local applications of DNCB, without surgery and is still alive with a three year follow-up.

One other patient, seen for the first time with multiple cutaneous tumors, lymph node invasion, liver and lung metastases, was treated with DNCB. The tumors of this patient were randomized : those which had been treated with local application of DNCB regressed as well as the voluminous lymph node invasion. The tumors which were not treated and were chosen at distance from the treated ones also dissapeared. A year later, this patient, 75 years old, died of heart failure. The anatomo-pathological examination showed a destruction of all cutaneous and visceral tumors.

The histological examination of regressing tumors shows in all cases an extensive inflammatory reaction with enlarged blood vessels surrounded by a cellular reaction wherein monocytes predominated. Tumor tissue was invaded with a monocytic reaction disrupting contact between neoplastic cells. Numerous eosinophiles were also present. Sometimes, monocytes penetrate into the neoplastic cells. Melanophages were numerous. In sites of complete regression, only melanophages and a few lymphocytes remained without evidence of malignant cells. Generally, we did not observe this infiltrate in the patched subdermal or untreated lesions. Nevertheless, in our last case, the histological examination shows the same picture in all regressing tumors : the patched, the untreated and the visceral ones.

In view of our observation, we whish to evaluate the therapeutic efficiency of DNCB.

In the cases of intradermal metastases with poor prognosis, we observed a complete remission in 60 % of the cases and a very good result in 40 % of the cases. Four cases of primary melanoma have regressed completely with DNCB only. Of eighteen cases of primary melanoma treated by DNCB and surgery, 15 are in remission and 3 died with metastases. All these cases with visceral metastases died of melanoma except two cases. Nevertheless, some patients had a survival from 1-3 years ; the anatomic examination of one of the latter two cases showed destruction of visceral metastases : in the other cases, therapy was a failure, despite long survivals of some instances.

The mechanism of the apparent local effect of DNCB on intradermal lesions is not mediated through a caustic effect as the skin surrounding the neoplasma does not necrose. The therapeutic effect was confirmed by histological examination and suggested a delayed hypersensitivity mechanism. Furthermore, the involution of malignant tumors was encountered when direct contact was achieved between the drug and the neoplasma. DNCB, a potent immunogenic chemical, could well modify the surface of malignant or normal melanocytes and induce a delayed hypersensitivity reaction at the sites of binding with tissue materials. As DNCB is capable of reacting with any polypeptide containing free amino groups, it remains to the explained why a possible immune reaction of this type should preferentially involve melanocytes. In addition to the efficiency of DNCB by an immune reaction enhanced locally, the drug could also operate by increasing the overall immunologic defense mechanism of the patients. Such a possible immunological mechanism is certainly not sufficient to control generalized form of the malignancies. Much clinical and experimental work is still required to validate such a theory.

Nevertheless, the therapeutic efficiency of DNCB in the treatment of intradermal superficial metastatic melanoma appears sufficiently promising to warrant consideration in the management of such poor risk patients.

References

1. Helm, F. and Klein, E. : Effects of allergic contact dermatitis on basal cell epitheliomas. Arch.Derm., Chicago 91 : 142-144(1965)
2. Malek-Mansour S., Castermans-Elias S., et Lapière Ch.M. : Régression de métastases de mélanomes après thérapeutique immunologique. Dermatologica (Basel) 146-156 (1973).
3. Malek-Mansour S., Remission of Melanoma with DNCB treatment. The Lancet, September 1, 1973.
4. Malek-Mansour S., Castermans-Elias S., and Van Wyck R. : Immunotherapy of melanoma metastases by 2,4 dinitrichlorobenzene. Revue Institut Pasteur, Lyon, tome 6 n° 3, 185-194, 1973.
5. Van Wyck R., Rustin P., Malek-Mansour S., Castermans-Elias S., et Castermans A. : Résultats préliminaires du traitement immunochirurgical du mélanome primitif. Acta Chir. Belg. 1975, 74, 430-440.
6. Malek-Mansour S. et Lapière Ch.M. : La place de l'immunothérapie dans le traitement du mélanome. Méd. et Hyg. 32 : 1296-1298, 1974.

Section VIII

CANCERS OF THE HEAD AND NECK, THYROID AND BRAIN

Adjuvant Therapy of Cancer, S.E. Salmon and S.E. Jones eds.
© 1977 Elsevier/North-Holland Biomedical Press, Amsterdam

METHOTREXATE-LEUCOVORIN WITH IMMUNOTHERAPY AS ADJUVANT TO SURGERY AND RADIOTHERAPY IN STAGE III-IV HEAD AND NECK SQUAMOUS CANCER PATIENTS*

Samuel G. Taylor, IV,** David E. Bytell, George A. Sisson
Sharon Nisius, William D. DeWys
Northwestern University
Chicago, Illinois 60611

INTRODUCTION

A previous pilot study of adjuvant chemotherapy with methotrexate and leucovorin has achieved a 71% two year disease-free (NED) survival in stage III and IV head and neck cancer.[1] These results, along with reports of synergistic effects from immunotherapy in this disease,[2,3] led to a collaborative effort to evaluate adjuvant chemoimmunotherapy in a prospective fashion.

METHODS

Patients were accepted for study if they had a diagnosis of squamous cell carcinoma of the head and neck region with stage III or IV disease based on the 1975 classification of the American Joint Commission for Staging and End Results Reporting (AJC).[4] To be eligible, all patients required a curative approach to

TABLE 1

STRATIFICATION VARIABLES: ADJUVANT CHEMOIMMUNOTHERAPY IN HEAD AND NECK CANCER

1. Skin test reactivity
   - A. ≥10 mm induration
   - B. <10 mm induration
2. Prognostic category
   - A. 31-50% estimated 3 year NED
   - B. 11-30% estimated 3 year NED
   - C. 0-10% estimated 3 year NED
3. Histologic differentiation
   - A. Well or moderately well
   - B. Poorly differentiated or anaplastic
4. Standard therapy
   - A. Surgery
   - B. Radiation therapy
   - C. Both

* Supported in part by grants from the American Cancer Society, Illinois division, 75-41 and 77-21, and from the National Cancer Institute 2-R10-CA-17145 and 1-P02-CA-15145.

** Recipient of an American Cancer Society Junior Faculty Clinical Fellowship.

treatment with radiation therapy and/or surgery. Stratification variables (Table 1) included: 1) skin test reactivity to a battery of four common recall antigens, 2) prognostic category based on disease site of origin and stage, 3) histologic differentiation of the cancer and 4) the planned approach with surgery and radiation therapy.

Skin tests consisted of Mumps, Candida 1:100, intermediate PPD and Veridase 25 units and were measured at 48 hours. The sum of the mean diameter of all tests was utilized to classify the patient as reactive ($\geq$10mm) or non-reactive (<10mm).

Estimation of the prognostic category was based on 3 year NED survival statistics of the AJC (1965, 1972, 1976) and the reported experience with peristomal recurrences.[5] Table 2 details the division of patients based on site of disease and stage.

The technique of randomization was to use a log book with a page for each possible combination of variables. The initial treatment entry on each page was randomized using a table of random numbers. Subsequent treatment entries alternated between the two therapy options. The name and stratification variables of each patient accepting the protocol were telephoned to a protocol secretary who entered the name in the next consecutive treatment space for that stratification group. This technique assured even distribution of patients into each treatment

TABLE 2

PROGNOSTIC CATEGORIES FOR ADJUVANT CHEMOIMMUNOTHERAPY STUDY

Patients were divided into risk groups based on AJC (1965, 1972, 1976) and[5].

Site	Stage	Estimated 3 Year NED Survival		
		0-10%	11-30%	31-50%
Buccal Mucosa, Floor Mouth, Alveolar Ridge, Ant. Tongue	III			X
	IV	X		
Palate, Naso-, Oro-, hypo-pharynx	III		X	
	IV	X		
Sinus	III		X	
	IV	X		
Supraglottic Larynx	III			X
Glottic Larynx	III			X
Subglottic Larynx	III		X	
All Larynx	IV	X		
Peristomal Recurrence	Above		X	
	Lat. or below	X		

option despite a large number of stratification variables, while keeping the treatment section blinded to the investigators.

Patients were randomized to receive chemotherapy or chemoimmunotherapy. The chemotherapy consisted of methotrexate 60 mg/M^2 q 6h x 4 doses given on Day 1. Six hours after the last dose, leucovorin 39 mg was given orally every 6 hours for 2 doses and then 9 mg every 6 hours for 6 doses. The methotrexate-leucovorin cycle was repeated on Days 5 and 9 provided no oral ulcerations were present, the white count was above 2,500/mm^3 and platelets were greater than 75,000/mm^3. If no mucositis was present and the white count was greater than 4,000/mm^3 and platelets were greater than 125,000/mm^3 the dosage of methotrexate was escalated on Day 5 to 90 mg/M^2 for 4 doses and on Day 9 to 120 mg/M^2 for 4 doses. The leucovorin dosage remained constant. Two week courses were repeated every 3 months for one year, except that, after completion of radiation therapy or surgery, an interval of at least 6 weeks was required prior to starting the next course of treatment. Dosage of methotrexate at the beginning of each course was 60 mg/M^2 q 6h x 4 independent of prior dose escalation to allow for reduced tolerance following surgery or radiation therapy.

Immunotherapy consisted of an autochthonous tumor cell vaccine and BCG. Tumor tissue was minced, passed through a 100 micron wire sieve and titurated in RPMI 1640 with 20% heat-inactivated, fetal calf serum to obtain a single cell suspension. Cells were washed and incubated in RPMI 1640 at 37°C with vibrio cholera neuraminidase (Behring Diagnostics, New Jersey), 25 units per 10^6 cells, for one hour and irradiated with 10,000 rads (4 Mev Linac linear accelerator). They were washed twice in phosphate buffered saline, concentrated to 1 x 10^7 cells per cc and stored frozen at -70°C in 0.1 cc amounts in tuberculin syringes. No proteolytic enzymes or antibiotics were used during preparation of the vaccine.

Tumor cells when available and BCG were given following radiation therapy and surgery, initially every two weeks for 6 treatments and then monthly for a total of one year. The tumor cells were given intradermally and the BCG was applied over this site using one vial of Tice strain BCG administered by multiple prong technique. Alternating sides of the neck and supraclavicular or shoulder areas were used.

Surgery was performed by one group of surgeons and conformed to the recommendations of "The Network for the Control and Rehabilitation in Patients with Head and Neck Cancer."

Radiotherapy was given by the therapists at Northwestern University and utilized a minimum of 6,500 rads tumor dosage in 7 weeks to be considered curative as a single modality. If used post-operatively a dosage of at least 6,000 rads was delivered to involved regions and 5,000 rads to high risk areas. All radiotherapy utilized megavoltage equipment, usually a Linac 4 Mev linear accelerator.

Usual supportive measures to ensure adequate nutrition were used during the study. Parental hyperalimentation was not included in this routine but was utilized for one patient with a T_4N_0 lesion of the hypopharynx-cervical esophagus who presented with obstruction and severe cachexia.

RESULTS

Thirty patients with stage III or IV head and neck squamous cancer accepted protocol treatment and were entered from December, 1974 to December, 1976. There were 10 stage III and 20 stage IV patients. Patient characteristics are summarized in Table 3. There was no difference between the treatment groups in any of the characteristics examined. Sixteen patients were randomized to receive chemotherapy and 14 chemoimmunotherapy. Five patients (all stage IV) failed to achieve a disease-free status and one has not completed treatment. They are not considered in the disease-free survival results but are included in the actuarial survival. The median duration of followup is 10 months.

Eight (67%) of 12 patients rendered disease-free in the chemotherapy only group continue NED. Ten (83%) of the 12 patients rendered disease-free in the chemoimmunotherapy group continue NED. One of the two patients who recurred in the immunotherapy group was the only patient considered to have inadequate radiotherapy. This patient had a T_3N_1 hypopharynx primary and was treated with radiotherapy after chemotherapy with a complete regression of disease. He refused to return for the remaining radiation therapy after receiving 5,000 rads and developed a recurrence 2 months later. There is as yet no difference between the two treatment groups in disease-free survival (Figure 1).

Four of 10 stage III patients have failed treatment because of recurrent disease (2 in each treatment group). Two of 14 stage IV patients have developed tumor recurrence after having achieved NED status (both in the chemotherapy only group). Tumor cell vaccine was available for 8 of the 14 immunotherapy treated patients. One patient who received vaccine and one who did not have recurred.

TABLE 3

PATIENT CHARACTERISTICS: ADJUVANT TRIAL OF CHEMOIMMUNOTHERAPY

Characteristic	Chemotherapy	Chemoimmunotherapy
Number	16	14
Age: mean (range)	55.4 (38-66)	59.6 (46-70)
Sex M/F	12/4	11/3
Oral Cavity & Oropharynx	6	5
Nasopharynx	1	0
Hypopharynx	5	4
Larynx	4	5
Stage III	5	5
Stage IV	11	9
Path: Well/Poor	13/3	12/2
Number not NED	4	2

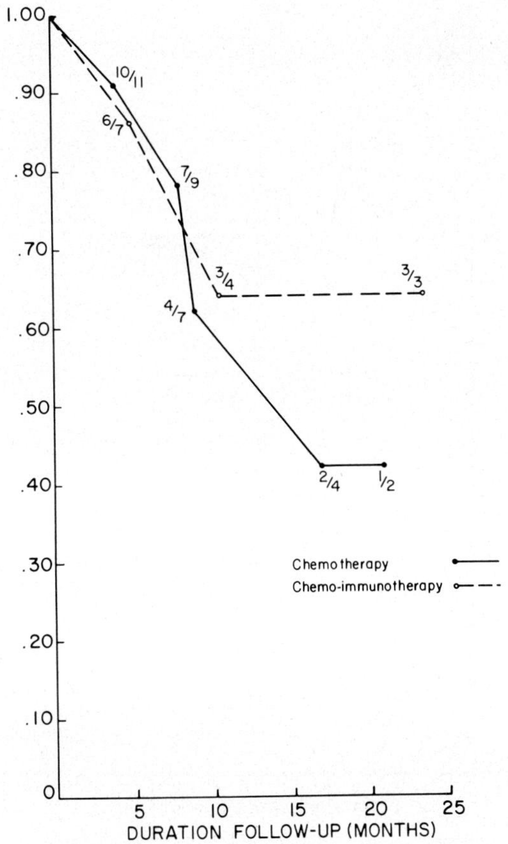

Fig. 1. Disease-free survival curves (Kaplan, Meier) for adjuvant chemotherapy and chemoimmunotherapy treated patients as a randomized study. All study patients with stage III or IV head and neck cancer rendered disease-free are included with results expressed as the proportion remaining NED.

Tumor response to chemotherapy was measured in 23 patients. Thirteen (57%) had greater than 25% tumor shrinkage during the 2 week course. This rapid tumor shrinkage was not related to NED survival with 9 of 15 patients (60%) who remained NED having rapid tumor shrinkage versus 4 of 8 patients who failed therapy having measurable shrinkage.

The 5 patients who failed to achieve NED status (17% of the 29 patients who have completed surgery and radiation therapy) failed because they were found to be inoperable at surgery and could not be salvaged with radiotherapy (3 patients)

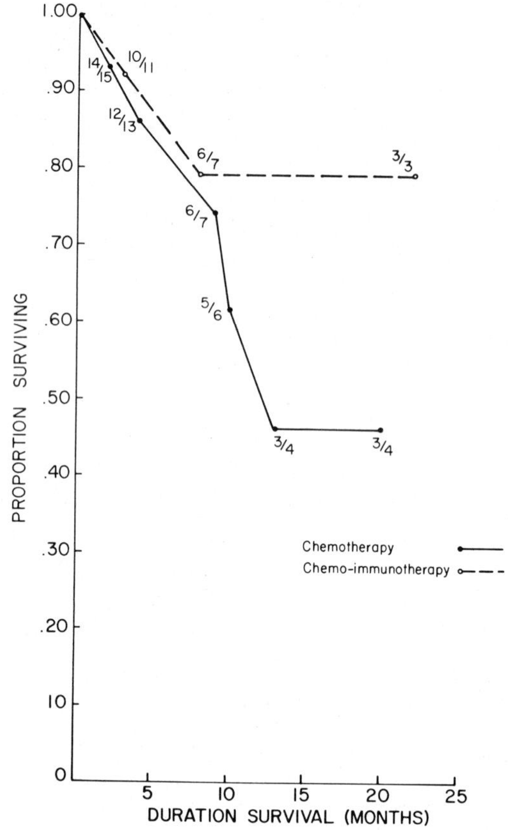

Fig. 2. Actuarial survival curves (Kaplan, Meier) for adjuvant chemotherapy and chemoimmunotherapy treated patients as a randomized study. All patients with stage III or IV head and neck cancer entered on study are included with results expressed as the proportion surviving.

---

or they failed radiotherapy and had tumor not encompassable by surgery (2 patients). Actuarial survival including these 5 patients who failed treatment and the 6 who recurred is shown in Figure 2. Although the results favor immunotherapy at this time, the short followup and small number of patients prevent any statistical conclusions.

TOXICITY

Twenty-seven patients with a history of no prior radiation therapy were assessed for toxicity to the initial course of methotrexate-leucovorin. Twenty-six (96%) received all three courses and 21 (78%) had some dose escalation (12 tolerated two escalations and 9, one). Skin toxicity was usually dose-limiting whereas hematologic toxicity was mild. Ten (37%) had moderately severe mucositis with mucosal ulcerations lasting usually less than 5 days and 13 (48%) had mild mucositis. Four patients (15%) had white counts less than 3,000, and 3 (11%) had platelet counts below 75,000/mm^3. Only one of these had a white count less than 1,000 and none had a platelet count less than 20,000. The usually mild hematologic toxicity made this regimen practical for pre-operative therapy.

One patient had a flap infection during chemotherapy requiring a delay of surgery. One patient with a history of gout experienced temporary azotemia with a BUN of 40mg% following the second cycle of methotrexate (the only patient who did not receive 3 cycles during the first course). Surgery could be performed one week following the methotrexate in all except 3 cases, and no surgical complications could be causally related to the chemotherapy. Radiotherapy could also be started immediately following chemotherapy. Chemotherapy given immediately prior to radiation therapy resulted in radiation dermatitis occurring earlier than expected and may have attributed to prolongation of the course of radiation in a few patients.

A second methotrexate course has been delivered to 15 patients following surgery or radiation therapy. Five patients were not yet due, 5 not NED, 3 refused a second course after surgery, and 2 recurred prior to the time for the next course. As shown in Table 4, tolerance to the second course of chemotherapy

TABLE 4

DOSE ADJUSTMENT DUE TO MUCOSAL TOXICITY FROM METHOTREXATE-LEUCOVORIN

A comparison of the first course with the initial post-operative and post-radiotherapy course

	Course 1	Course 2: No Radiotherapy	Course 2: S/P Radiotherapy
No. Cycles:			
2	1[a]	3	6
3	26 (96%)	3 (50%)	3 (33%)
Dose Escalation:			
None	6	1	7
Once	9 (78%, Once + Twice)	2 (83%, Once + Twice)	2 (22%, Once + Twice)
Twice	12	3	0
Mucositis:			
0	4	0	0
1	13	4	4
2-3	10 (37%)	2 (33%)	5 (56%)

a) Third cycle held because of BUN elevation to 40mg% in a patient with gout.

was reduced, especially in the radiation therapy-treated patients, due to increased mucous membrane toxicity. After surgery the percentage of patients able to tolerate 3 cycles of chemotherapy was reduced from 96% to 50%, although the percentage of dose escalations and of patients getting severe mucositis was similar to that during the first course of chemotherapy. However, after radiation therapy, only 3 of 9 patients (33%) tolerated 3 cycles with 2 (22%) having some dose escalation. Despite this marked dosage reduction mucosal ulcerations occurred in 5 patients (56%) after radiotherapy. Subsequent courses after the second course were better tolerated but still required substantial dosage reduction over the pre-radiotherapy or surgery course. Hematologic toxicity was usually mild, comparable to that during the first course.

DISCUSSION

The study design of this randomized trial using estimated prognostic categories allowed stratification of patients into a manageable number of subsets while accounting for the multiplicity of sites and stages possible in head and neck cancer, each with its own risk of treatment failure. Stratification by each site and stage would have resulted in an impractical number of stratification variables. If several different sites with different prognoses were combined into a small number of "regions," patients having a high risk of recurrence would have been intermixed with those having a lower risk. Either alternative would have caused an imbalance in each treatment group requiring several hundred patients to obtain an equal distribution of risk factors. Division of patients into risk categories was further justified by a recent cooperative study of methotrexate in a large series of patients that demonstrated no difference in response to methotrexate based on disease site when tumor burden determined by stage and ambulatory status was considered (in our adjuvant study all patients were ambulatory).[6]

The survival results have been encouraging in the short period of followup. Other adjuvant methotrexate studies have demonstrated improved NED survival in the first 6 to 8 months but by 12 to 18 months this gain was no longer apparent.[7,8] We have not encountered such frequent recurrences after one year in our pilot study which now has a median followup of 26 months. That study revealed a 71% NED survival in stage III and IV head and neck cancer patients at two years.[1] A possible explanation for the difference in results from other studies is the use of dosage escalation to toxicity prior to surgery or radiation therapy. Only one of our patients has received parental hyperalimentation, a patient with a T_4 obstructing hypopharyngeal-cervical esophogus lesion who has been followed 5 months, so this therapeutic adjunct cannot explain the improved survival in our series. We are beginning a randomized trial at another institution to establish the effectiveness of this chemotherapy program.

Repeated two week courses of methotrexate-leucovorin after radiation therapy or surgery were given in this study. Because head and neck squamous cancer is often initially sensitive to chemotherapy but rapidly develops resistance, repeated intensive courses were thought to possibly be more advantageous than a prolonged maintenance schedule. No conclusions about the value of this approach can yet be made. We have found markedly reduced tolerance to the same chemotherapy given after radiation therapy, resulting in reduced dosage and increased toxicity. It is doubtful that an effective dosage of methotrexate can be given in the period of time immediately following radiation therapy. Any adjuvant chemotherapy trial utilizing methotrexate and radiation therapy should thus strongly consider giving an intensive chemotherapy course prior to radiation therapy as a part of the protocol design.

The immunotherapy resulted in no local complications other than pain from the injection with local erythema and pruritus as described with BCG alone. The cell vaccine usually resulted in a localized area of more intense erythema, pustule formation and occasionally ulceration. Neuraminidase-treated and subsequently frozen cells have been found to be as effective as viable, non-frozen cells in an animal model system[9] and the addition of BCG is synergistic.[10] Although the current results favor chemoimmunotherapy using BCG and the neuraminidase-treated autochthonous tumor cells, the study is still too early to reach definite conclusions about the value of this approach.

REFERENCES

1. Taylor, S.G., IV, Bytell, D.E., et al: Methotrexate with leucovorin as an adjuvant to surgery and radiotherapy in local advanced squamous carcinoma of the head and neck. Submitted to Amer. Soc. Clin. Oncol. for the XIII Annual Meeting, 1977.
2. Donaldson, R.C.: Methotrexate plus bacillus Calmette-Guerin (BCG) and isoniazid in the treatment of cancer of the head and neck. Amer. J. Surg. 124:527-534, 1972.
3. Richman, S.P., Livingston, R.B., et al: Chemotherapy versus chemoimmunotherapy of head and neck cancer: Report of a randomized study. Cancer Treat. Rep. 60:535-539, 1976.
4. Chandler, J.R., Guillamondegui, O.M., et al: Clinical staging of cancer of the head and neck: A new "new" system. Amer. J. Surg. 132:525-528, 1976.
5. Sisson, G.A., Bytell, D.E., et al: Mediastinal dissection - 1976: Indications and new techniques. Laryngoscope (In press).
6. DeConti, R.C.: Phase III comparison of methotrexate with leucovorin vs. methotrexate alone vs. a combination of methotrexate plus leucovorin, cyclophosphamide and cytosine arabinoside in head and neck cancer. Proc. Amer. Soc. Clin. Oncol. XII Annual Meeting, C-46:248, Toronto, 1976.

7. Sancho, H., Richard, J.M.: Une politique suivie d'essais therapeutiques dans le probleme de la chimiotherapie intra-arterielle des tumeurs de la sphere O.R.L. Bulletin du Cancer 61:257-264, 1974.
8. Tarpley, J.L., et al: High dose methotrexate as a pre-operative adjuvant in the treatment of epidermoid carcinoma of the head and neck. A feasibility study and clinical trial. Amer. J. Surg. 130:481-486, 1975.
9. Rios, A., Simmons, R.L.: Experimental cancer immunotherapy using a neuraminidase-treated non-viable frozen tumor vaccine. Surgery 75:503-507, 1974.
10. Simmons, R.L., et al: Immunospecific regression of methylcholanthrene fibrosarcoma using neuraminidase. III Synergistic effect of BCG and neuraminidase-treated tumor cells. Ann. Surg. 176:188-194, 1972.

Adjuvant Therapy of Cancer, S.E. Salmon and S.E. Jones eds.

WEEKLY HIGH DOSE METHOTREXATE WITH LEUKOVORIN RESCUE AS INITIAL ADJUVANT THERAPY IN ADVANCED SQUAMOUS CELL CARCINOMA OF THE HEAD AND NECK: A PILOT STUDY

Susan W. Pitman, Daniel Miller, Ralph Weichselbaum, Emil Frei, III,
Sidney Farber Cancer Institute and Joint Center for Radiation Therapy,
Harvard Medical School, Boston, Massachusetts

SUMMARY

Initial experience with weekly high dose Methotrexate with Leukovorin rescue (MTX-LCV) in advanced recurrent or metastatic squamous cell carcinoma of the head and neck is presented. The 75% tumor response rate and high therapeutic index prompted a trial of MTX-LCV as initial adjuvant therapy in high risk non-metastatic patients. Results in 10 patients confirm the high response rate to MTX-LCV, and the low incidence of myelotoxicity and mucositis, when concurrent urinary alkalinization is employed. Optimum aggressive combinations of surgery and radiation therapy have not been compromised by initial MTX-LCV administration. Cytoreduction with MTX-LCV may be used initially in combined therapy for high risk squamous cell carcinoma of the head and neck.

INTRODUCTION

Despite aggressive surgical therapy, local irradiation, or a combination of both modalities, advanced squamous cell lesions of the head and neck continue to have notoriously poor three-year NED rates because of local recurrence and distant metastatic disease. There is some evidence that the addition of chemotherapy might improve local control and cure (7). The most effective single agent in squamous cell carcinoma of the head and neck is methotrexate (MTX). Responses to intermittent MTX therapy are comparable both with weekly injections of 30-40 mg/M^2 and with higher doses (250 mg - 1 g/M^2) with leukovorin rescue administered either weekly or at more frequent intervals (1,6). We, therefore, decided to test the therapeutic efficacy of an even higher dose rate of methotrexate with leukovorin rescue (MTX-LCV), by administering the drug weekly, at higher doses than previously used, and with concurrent urinary alkalinization (9) to patients with recurrent or metastatic squamous cell carcinoma of the head and neck, and, if shown to be more effective or to have an improved therapeutic index, to administer adjuvant MTX-LCV to advanced but localized lesions prior to treatment with radiation and/or surgery. We report here the results of these trials.

PATIENTS AND METHODS

Twenty-nine patients, listed in Table 1, with biopsy-proven squamous cell carcinoma of the head and neck were treated with MTX-LCV administered weekly as an out-patient regimen.

TABLE 1

WEEKLY MTX-LCV: PATIENT PROFILE

	GROUP A*	GROUP B**
# Patients	19	10
Age Range/Median (yrs)	(36-77)58	(35-69)56
Prior Radiation	17(89%)	0
Prior Chemotherapy	2(10%)	0
MTX-LCV # Courses	176	42
1 g/M^2	52	6
3 g/M^2	65	20
7.5 g/M^2	59	16
Range/Patient	1-23	1-8
Median/Patient	9	4
Mean/Patient	9	4

* Recurrent or metastatic disease
** Initial adjuvant patients

All patients were required to have a creatinine clearance greater than 60 ml per minute and a normal IVP. Nineteen (Group A) had advanced disease, either locally recurrent in the primary or regional nodes, or metastatic, beyond the scope of surgery or radiotherapy. All but two of these patients had received prior radiotherapy.

Ten others (Group B) who were seen in a multidisciplinary Head and Neck Clinic and who were staged as any T primary with N_3 nodes, or a T_3, T_4 primary with any nodal stage, were treated with MTX-LCV as outlined in Figure 1, prior to definitive surgery or radiotherapy. Pathology was reviewed in all cases. All tumors in Group B were graded as well to moderately well differentiated squamous cell carcinoma.

Figure 1

Schema of Therapeutic Approach to Advanced Non-Metastatic Patients

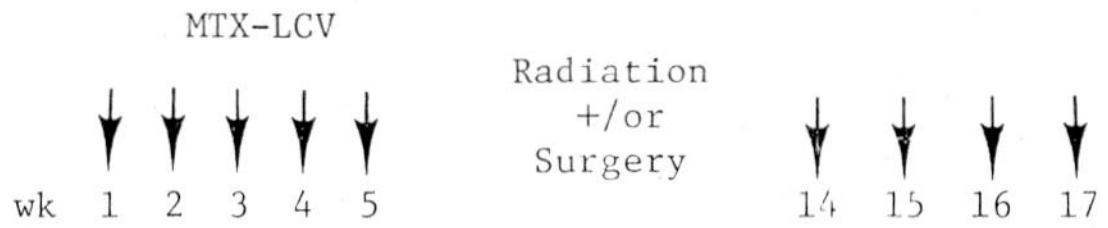

The treatment schema for MTX-LCV is outlined in Figure 2. MTX was given as an intravenous push in doses ranging from 1 to 7.5 g/M^2. The earliest eight patients began at 1 g/M^2, subsequent patients at 3 g/M^2 and 7.5 g/M^2. Starting dose was continued for all subsequent weekly treatments, unless there was evidence of stable or progressive disease, when MTX dose was escalated. Calcium leukovorin was administered 24 hours later, 10 mg/M^2 IV, followed by 10 mg/M^2 orally every 6 hours for 12 doses. Stat creatinine and MTX levels were obtained at 24 hours. The stat 24 hour serum creatinine determination was always compared to the baseline serum creatinine (prior to the first course) to assess change in renal function, if any, after each course. Evidence of nephrotoxicity prompted an increase in dose rate of leukovorin, from the usual dose, outlined above, to 100 mg p.o. or intravenously q. 3 h. until serum MTX concentration fell below 1×10^{-7}Molar, a procedure shown to be effective in aborting toxicity (5). Serum MTX determinations were used only if the 24 hr. serum creatinine had risen more than 50%: a 24 hour MTX level above the median for a given dose prompted an increase in the LCV dose rate, while a level below the median allowed rescue to proceed normally.

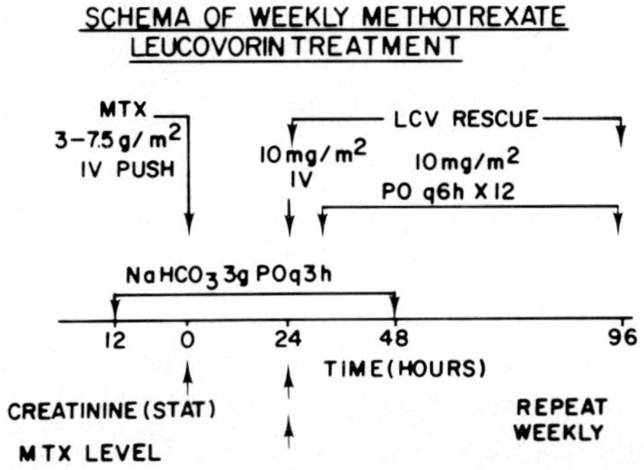

Figure 2: MTX-LCV Schema

Urinary alkalinization was begun the night before MTX administration. Patients were instructed to keep their urine pH greater than or equal to 7, using out-patient Combistix monitoring. They were instructed to maintain adequate hydration at home, and immediately prior to MTX administration were given one liter of D5W while waiting for the results of a stat creatinine, which was obtained by finger-stick on the morning of each weekly drug administration. Group B patients in the pilot adjuvant study were seen in a multidisciplinary Head and Neck Clinic immediately after initial diagnosis, and subsequently thereafter during chemotherapy, during irradiation, and before any decisions regarding surgery.

Radiation was delivered on a 4-MEV linear accelerator at 180-200 rad fractions 5 times per week.

Nephrotoxicity was defined as a greater than 50 percent rise in serum creatinine above the baseline prior to MTX administration. Myelosuppression was defined as a white count less than or equal to 2×10^3 cells/mm^3 and/or platelet count less than or equal to 1 x 10^5 platelets/mm^3. The criteria for tumor evaluability for response were as follows: (1) the presence of objectively measurable disease; (2) the administration of at least two weekly courses of MTX; and (3) no other concurrent therapy, as with irradiation. Complete response was defined as complete disappearance of all measurable disease. Partial response was defined as a greater than 50 percent reduction in the product of perpendicular tumor diameters, as compared with initial measurements.

RESULTS

The tumor response and toxicity to MTX-LCV are summarized in Table 2. Four patients were inevaluable because of absence of measurable disease, inadequate follow-up, or termination after one course because of myelosuppression.

Table 2

WEEKLY MTX-LCV: TUMOR RESPONSE AND TOXICITY

Tumor Response	Group A	Group B	Toxicity	Group A	Group B
# Eval.	16	9	Total # Courses	176	42
# Responders	12(75%)	7(78%)	Myelotoxicity*	7(4%)	3(7%)
Complete	1	0	Mucositis	3(2%)	1(2%)
> 50%	11	7	Nephrotoxicity	1**	0
< 50%	1	2	Nausea/Vomiting	13(7%)	5(12%)
Duration Range (wks)	(7-25+)	--			
Median	13	--			

* WBC ≤ 2000/mm^3 +/or plt ct ≤10^5
**Toxicity aborted with ↑↑ LCV dose rate

In the Group A recurrent and metastatic disease patients, the overall response rate of 75 percent included responses of primary disease, lymph node disease, lung parenchymal involvement, and skin subcutaneous nodules. Two patients with recurrence initially judged as inoperable, had tumor regression such that subsequent local excision was possible. The regimen was well tolerated. The seven myelotoxic courses occurred in six Group A patients, four of whom had pretreatment hematocrits less than or equal to 30%, raising the possibility of folate deficiency in this subpopulation of patients as a predisposing factor to myelosuppression. Four patients experienced headache following MTX administration, and both had had prior radiation to the nasopharynx.

Tumor response in the Group B adjuvant patients was prompt and dramatic, occurring often within a week of therapy, usually within three weeks of MTX initiation. Of the seven responders, five achieved greater than 75 percent reduction in tumor mass prior to initiation of radiation and surgery. The two patients who achieved less than 50 percent tumor regression received 1 g/M^2 MTX. All others received 3 or 7.5 g/M^2. Early experience with one debilitated patient who was given 8 initial courses and in whom initial partial response after 5 courses was followed by stabilization and possibly progression, led us to limit the number of courses per patient to 3-5. After three courses, patients were re-evaluated and a joint decision made to continue for another 1-2 courses. The low incidence of patient morbidity during MTX-LCV treatment is evident from Table 2. Two of the 10 patients had a pretreatment hematocrit less than or equal to 30%; the three myelotoxic episodes occurred in these two patients. Nausea and vomiting, experienced by two patients, was mild.

Table 3

RADIATION AND SURGERY FOLLOWING MTX-LCV IN 10 PATIENTS

PT	STAGE(UICC)	SITE	PRIMARY	NECK/SUPRACLAV	SURGERY
	OROPHARYNX				
RH	T_3N_0	Posterior tongue	7020/58d	4140r/36d	None
MM	T_3N_0	Posterior tongue	4400r/41d	4000r/36d	Composite resect.
JK	T_3N_0	Posterior tongue	5140r/67d	4140r/47d	Composite resect.
DW	T_2N_3	Posterior tongue	7000r/in prog.	4140r/35d	
LK	T_2N_3	Uvula, soft palate	7000r/in prog.	4000r/27d	Composite resect.
	HYPOPHARYNX				
WZ	T_3N_1	Post Pharyng wall	6980r/58d	1980/20d	Rad. Neck Dissect. (bilateral)
JB	T_3N_0	Post Pharyng wall	5600r/52d 7000r/in prog.	4000/29d	
	ORAL CAVITY				
GA	T_3N_0	Alveolar ridge	540r	360r	Composite resect.
FB	T_3N_2	Anterior tongue	6800r/80d	4000r/41d	None
	LARYNX				
ME	T_1N_3	Supraglottis	4400r/in prog.	4400r/29d	

Table 3 demonstrates the subsequent irradiation and surgery by site and stage of disease. The degree of radiation mucositis was comparable to that seen with radiotherapeutic regimens without MTX. Radiation was begun within 5-10 days following the last course of MTX-LCV in most cases. No delay in initiation of planned irradiation because of toxicity was necessary. Radiation was limited to 500 rads in one instance following composite resection of an alveolar ridge tumor because of edema of tissues within and adjacent to the radiation portal occurring within 20 minutes following three separate fractions given at weekly intervals, associated with erythema in the area. Neither antihistamine nor steroid treatment ameliorated this response, which was felt to be an idiosyncratic synergy possibly post surgical lymphatic obstruction, although MTX irradiation synergy cannot be excluded. The two patients who experienced a less than 50 percent response to MTX-LCV, failed also to respond to irradiation, requiring surgery sooner than originally planned.

Surgery was performed within 5-10 days following drug treatment. No compromise of a surgical procedure was seen by one of us (DM), nor was delay in surgical wound healing seen. Tumor necrosis, including marked reduction in tumor formerly invading bone, was seen in two surgical specimens following MTX-LCV treatment.

DISCUSSION

Weekly MTX-LCV was studied in patients with both advanced recurrent or metastatic squamous cell carcinoma of the head and neck, most of whom had had prior irradiation, and in a smaller group of de novo patients who had had no prior therapy. The high response rate of 75 percent in both groups indicates that MTX, given on a weekly schedule and in doses ranging from 1 to 7.5 g/M^2 with leukovorin rescue is the single most active agent in this disease to date.

The rationale for the use of MTX-LCV is that in poorly perfused or transport resistant tumors, cytotoxic intracellular drug concentrations can be obtained without intolerable host toxicity. Free intracellular MTX is a critical factor in MTX inhibition of tetrahydrofolate (THF) synthesis and THF-dependent processes. Only with high dose MTX regimens can critical levels of free intracellular MTX be generated, levels which are necessary in Ehrlich ascites and in L-1210 to inhibit nucleic acid and protein synthesis (4).

The high therapeutic index is superior to other MTX regimens, either orally (8), intravenously (6), or intravenously with lower doses of MTX-LCV (1). This low incidence of myelotoxicity and mucositis is related to concurrent urinary alkalinization, which has decreased the incidence of MTX-induced nephrotoxicity (10). Its safety makes it an ideal choice for adjuvant treatment of locally advanced but non-metastatic disease.

In contrast to other attempts to use MTX prior to irradiation, the use of MTX in this trial did not appear to (1) delay initiation of irradiation or (2) increase the severity of radiation mucositis. Surgical procedures were not compromised by drug given as little as a week before nor was surgical wound healing delayed. These results indicate that preoperative chemotherapy with MTX-LCV is feasible and may render surgery and radiotherapy more effective by reducing tumor size. The importance of tumor size as a determinant of therapeutic response has long been recognized clinically (2). Experimentally, in the Lewis lung and EMT-6 tumor systems, small tumors have been considerably more radiosensitive than large ones, with a correspondingly lower hypoxic fraction (3,11). Initial cytoreduction with MTX-LCV may likewise render squamous cell carcinoma more radiosensitive.

The relatively short median duration of response (13 weeks) in the group with recurrent or metastatic disease suggests the development of drug resistance. Theoretically, administration of MTX prior to surgery or radiation may allow for the development of resistant clones which may then make adjuvant therapy of microscopic disease more difficult. While the results are too preliminary to know whether survival will be changed, failure to affect survival in the advanced non-metastatic group of patients, when sufficient numbers of patients are accrued, might be due to the development of such drug resistance. The results are too preliminary to know whether long-term side effects may be encountered.

REFERENCES

1. Capizzi, R. L., DeConti, R. C., Marsh, J. C. and Bertino, J. R.: Methotrexate therapy of head and neck cancer: Improvement in therapeutic index by the use of leucovorin "rescue". Cancer Res. 30:1782-1788, 1970.
2. Fletcher, G. H.: Elective irradiation of subclinical disease in cancers of the head and neck. Cancer 29:1450-1454, 1972.
3. Fu, K. K., Phillips, T. L., Wharam, M. D.: Radiation response of artificial pulmonary metastases of the EMT 6 tumor. Int. J. Radiation Oncology, Biology, Physics 1, 257-260, 1976.
4. Goldman, I. D.: Analysis of the cytotoxic determinants for methotrexate: A role for "free" intracellular drug. Cancer Cehmother. Rep. 6:51-61, 1975.
5. Howell, S., Pitman, S. W., Blair, H., Frei, E., III: Clinical-pharmacologic approaches to MTX-toxicity. In preparation.
6. Leone, L. A., Albala, M. M., and Rege, V. B.: Treatment of carcinoma of the head and neck with intravenous methotrexate. Cancer 21:828-837, 1968.
7. Lustig, R. A., DeMare, P. A., and Kramer, S.: Adjuvant methotrexate in the radiotherapeutic management of advanced tumors of the head and neck. Cancer 37:2703-2708, 1976.
8. Papac, R. J., Jacobs, E. M., Foye, L. V., Jr., and Donohue, D. M.: Systemic therapy with amethopterin in squamous cell carcinoma of the head and neck. Cancer Chemother. Rep. 32:47-54, 1963.
9. Pitman, S. W., Landwehr, D., Jaffe, N., and Frei, E., III: Methotrexate-Citrovorum: effect of alkalinization on nephrotoxicity and of weekly schedule on response. Proc. Amer. Assoc. Cancer Res. 17:129, 1976.
10. Pitman, S. W., Parker, L. M., Tattersall, M. H. N., Jaffe, N., and Frei, E., III: Clinical trial of high dose methotrexate (NSC-740) with citrovorum factor (NSC-3590) -- toxicologic and therapeutic observations. Cancer Chemother. Rep. 6:43-49, 1975.
11. Shipley, W. U., Stanley, J. A., and Steel, G. G.: Tumor size dependency in the radiation response of the Lewis lung carcinoma. Cancer Res. 35:2488-2493, 1975.

Adjuvant Therapy of Cancer, S.E. Salmon and S.E. Jones eds.
© 1977 Elsevier/North-Holland Biomedical Press, Amsterdam

MULTIMODALITY TREATMENT FOR HIGH RISK THYROID CARCINOMA

Brian G. M. Durie, M.D.[*†], Dorothea Hellman, M.D.,
Robert E. O'Mara, M.D.[††], James Woolfenden, M.D.[**]
Mark Kartchner, M.D. and Sydney E. Salmon, M.D.[†]

From the Health Sciences Center
University of Arizona
Tucson, Arizona 85724

INTRODUCTION

Thyroid neoplasms contribute only 1% to overall cancer incidence. However, about 4% of people in the United States have nodular thyroid glands (1). Since there is always the question of malignancy in a thyroid nodule, the approach to thyroid neoplasms takes on a significance beyond its natural incidence. This significance has recently been enhanced by increased awareness of thyroid carcinoma associated with prior head and neck irradiation (2). The fact that papillary carcinoma, which accounts for the majority of cases in most series, has a generally good prognosis, has inhibited the development of definitive approaches to therapy (3). Nonetheless, from the comprehensive clinicopathologic studies of Woolner et al (4), Beaugie et al (3), Fransilla (5,6), Staunton and Greening (7), Stratton Hill (8), and Chong et al (9), it has become clear that, depending primarily upon histology, stage of disease and the age of the patient, there is a notable incidence of recurrent and metastatic disease with death from cancer related causes.

A higher risk of recurrence is associated with anaplastic histology, follicular cell type with moderate to marked vascular invasion, papillary with extra-nodal spread, and medullary with extracapsular spread (3-9). Although each individual treatment modality has contributed to improved prognosis (7,10-13), patients with high risk features have continued to have recurrent disease and die of thyroid carcinoma. In an effort to eliminate residual disease after initial definitive surgery and produce long term disease-free survival, our team at the University of Arizona has developed a combined modality approach including thyroid hormone suppression, radio-iodine, chemotherapy and immunotherapy. We report results of treatment in our first fifteen high risk patients to establish the feasibility and initial areas of success in this approach.

---

* Scholar Leukemia Society of America
† Section of Hematology and Oncology, University of Arizona, Tucson, Arizona
** Section of Nuclear Medicine, University of Arizona, Tucson, Arizona
†† Chief, Division of Nuclear Medicine, University of Rochester Medical Center, Rochester, New York 14642

MATERIALS AND METHODS

A total of sixty-five patients were seen and evaluated by members of the multimodality team in Tucson which included an endocrinologist (D.E.H.), surgeon (M.K.), nuclear medicine specialists (R.E.O'M. and/or J.W.) and oncologists (B.G.M.D. and S.E.S.). Fifty patients did not satisfy the high risk criteria and were therefore not eligible for the multimodality protocol. The high risk criteria used are outlined in Table 1.

Table 1
HIGH RISK CRITERIA

HISTOLOGY
- Anaplastic
- Papillary: Extra Nodal Spread
- Follicular: Moderate - Marked Vascular Invasion
- Medullary: Nodal or Extra Nodal Spread

Other Factors
- Age
- Resectability of primary
- Extent of metastases
- Disease activity

The primary criteria were the histologic features. However, no patient under age 40 yrs was included unless additional high risk features were present including such factors as: primary unresectable, progressive disease with convential therapy and extra nodal, extra capsular spread. Patients over age 40 yrs were treated essentially in adjuvant fashion. Fifteen patients satisfied the high risk criteria and the details are listed in Table 2.

Treatment

Surgery was the primary treatment modality. If at all possible, total or subtotal thyroidectomy with local positive node dissection was carried out. However, in cases 2 and 3, biopsy only was possible because the tumors were large, vascular and invasive. In cases 1, 5 and 13, only limited thyroid resection could be accomplished. The extent of residual disease postoperatively was established on clinical examination, soft tissue x-rays of the neck, ^{131}I scans (14), ^{111}Indium-bleomycin scans (15), plasma calcitonin levels before, during and after calcium infusion (16) and plasma and urine polyamine levels (17).

Table 2

DETAILS OF 15 CASES

	Age (yrs)	Sex	Surgery	^{131}I mCi	Response to Therapy	Months on Protocol
Anaplastic (A)						
1	76	F	ST* PND†	300	CR	24
2	28	F	B**	750	PR***	41
3	64	F	B	0	CR	12
4	72	M	ST PND	150	PR	2
Papillary (P)						
5	73	F	ST PND	0	PR	6
6	23	F	T††	750	NR	42
7	34	M	T	700	PR	14
8	44	F	ST	450	PR	12
Follicular (F)						
9	20	M	ST PND	300	CR	33
10	40	M	ST PND	450	CR	22
11	65	F	ST	150	PR	6
12	55	F	ST	150	CR	6
Medullary (M)						
13	55	M	ST PND	0	PR	17
14	48	M	ST	0	PR	22
15	28	F	ST	0	NR	10

* ST = subtotal thyroidectomy
† PND = positive node dissection
** B = biopsy only
†† T = total thyroidectomy
*** See text for discussion and figure 2

Radioiodine Searches and Therapy

Within two to four weeks postoperatively or at the time of referral, radioiodine searches were performed after oral doses of 5 millicuries of ^{131}I. If significant abnormal uptake were detected, a treatment dose of 100-150 millicuries was administered on an inpatient basis following current Atomic Energy Commission license and National Council on Radiation Protection and Measurement guidelines (18). All patients, either after the treatment dose or negative search scan, were given oral L-thyroxine in a dose range 0.2-0.4 mg daily.

Following the general treatment plan outlined in Figure 1, repeat diagnostic searches were carried out at three month intervals following withdrawal from exogenous thyroid hormone replacement and documentation of a rise in endogenous T.S.H. to >50 μI.U./ml. Again, if significant residual uptake was detected, a further treatment dose of 100-150 millicuries was administered. The maximum cumulative dose administered to any patient was 750 millicuries (patients 2 and 6). When search scans became negative, they were repeated at six monthly intervals.

Chemotherapy

All the fifteen patients with high risk pathologic features received the combination chemotherapy schedule (Figure 1). Baseline studies included pulmonary function studies and cardiac evaluation which comprised clinical examination, chest x-ray, 12 lead EKG, echocardiography, phonocardiography and determination of systolic time interval.

The chemotherapy was initiated immediately after the ^{131}I search (if negative) or ^{131}I treatment dose. The adriamycin 40 mg/M^2 was given intravenously on day 1. Melphalan (as 2 mg tablets) was given orally in a dosage of 6 mg/M^2/day on days 3-6. The vincristine 1 mg and bleomycin 15 mg were given intravenously on day 14. The bleomycin was given 30 minutes after the vincristine. As already indicated, a 1 mg I.V. test dose of bleomycin was given initially. For fever >100°F benadryl 50 mg plus Tylenol were used as necessary. Ten courses of the combination therapy were given resulting in total doses of 400 mg/M^2 adriamycin and 150 mg (total) of bleomycin.

Maintenance Therapy

After initial induction, maintenance using melphalan plus bacillus Calmette Guerin (B.C.G.) immunotherapy was begun provided there had been satisfactory initial response. A satisfactory response was defined as complete (CR: no evidence of residual disease) or partial (PR: <50% decrease in measurable disease). Melphalan given in a dosage of 10 mg/M^2/day for 4 days every 28 days was continued for 6 months. B.C.G. immunotherapy using Pasteur high viability vaccine by scarification using 1 ampule ($6 \pm 4 \times 10^8$ organisms) per scarification was given on days 7 and 14 of each cycle being reduced to once/month after the first 2-3 months depending upon the severity of reactions and patient tolerance. Baseline and follow-up skin testing was performed as previously reported (19). The B.C.G. immunotherapy was given for a total of 1 year. Thereafter, patients have been followed off all therapy.

Figure 1

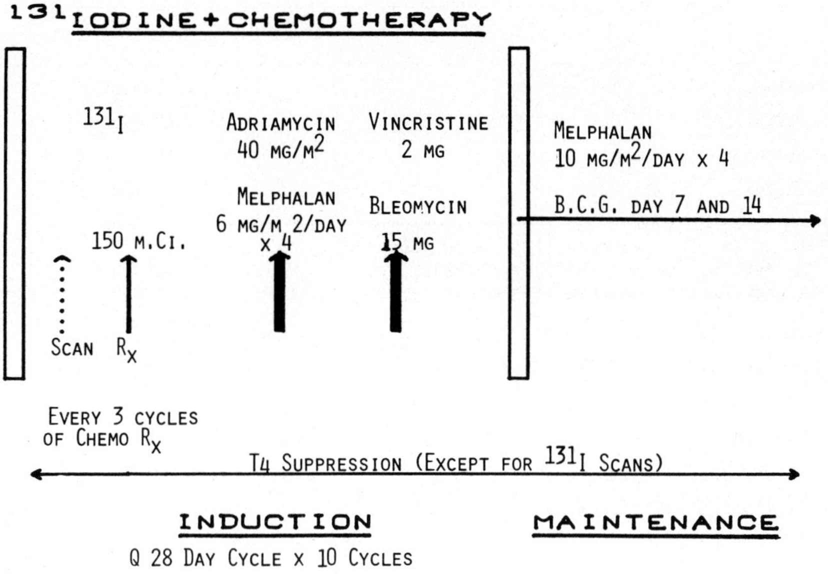

The details of the multimodality program are outlined in diagrammatic form. The "every 3 cycles" refers to the ^{131}I scans and treatment doses (Rx) if necessary. Chemotherapy is given on a 28 day cycle with adriamycin on day 1, melphalan days 3-6 and vincristine and bleomycin day 14. T_4 suppression is oral L-thyroxine 0.2-0.4 mg per day.

RESULTS

Response to Therapy

Good responses to therapy were seen in all histologic categories. However, as summarized in Table 3, responses in the anaplastic and follicular categories were more striking with two out of four and three out of four complete responses respectively. In the papillary and medullary categories, responses tended to be slower and less complete, there being definite residual disease in all patients treated so far.

Table 3

SUMMARY OF RESULTS

	CR	PR	NR	Mean survival to date
Anaplastic	3	1	0	20 months
Papillary	0	3	1	19 months
Follicular	3	1	0	17 months
Medullary	0	2	1	16 months

*CR No current evidence of disease; complete response
PR Partial response; 50% regression; definite residual disease
NR No evident response to therapy

The pattern of response was interesting and probably clinically relevant. Figure 2 illustrates the serial radioiodine search scans in patient 2 with anaplastic carcinoma. Initially, only a few follicular elements were seen histologically and ^{131}I uptake was limited. However, after several courses of combination chemotherapy, the more differentiated follicular elements became more evident as manifested by intense ^{131}I uptake on scans two and three. With further ^{131}I therapy plus ongoing chemotherapy, these more differentiated elements were largely eliminated.

Evaluation of Residual Disease

Serially, during therapy, every effort was made to establish the presence or absence of residual disease. In patients 5, 6, 7, 8, 11, 13, 14 and 15, residual disease was clearly evident on clinical examination, routine x-rays, ^{131}I scan or plasma calcitonin assay. In patient 2 the only evidence of disease was a tiny focus of uptake in the left thyroid bed area with a 5 millicurie ^{131}I thyroid search preceded by T.S.H. stimulation. Patients 1, 3, 9, 10 and 12 had no demonstrable disease. In patients 1, 9 and 10, greater than two fold increases in urinary spermidine levels with chemotherapy had given early evidence of excellent response to therapy (17), all five patients with complete response and return of urinary and plasma polyamine levels to well within the normal range. Other routine parameters including clinical examination, soft tissue x-ray, ^{131}I scan, and ^{III}Indium bleomycin scan were also normal in these complete responders.

Figure 2 Serial ^{131}I Scans in a Patient with Anaplastic Carcinoma with Follicular Elements

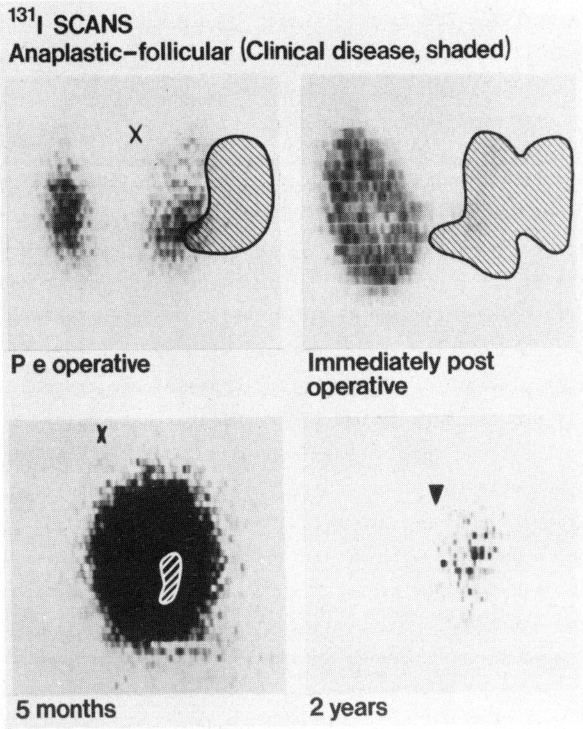

These are serial scans on patient number 2. Scan 1 is pre-operative. X is the thyroid cartilage. The shaded area is the "cold" lesion palpable clinically. Scan 2 is post-operative by which time the tumor mass (shaded) is much larger. Scan 3 is 5 months later when the palpable mass has shrunk to the size of the white shaded area, but there is dramatic ^{131}I uptake. Scan 4 is 2 years post-operatively during maintenance therapy when no palpable mass remained and there was only minimal ^{131}I uptake.

Side Effects of Treatment

The treatment program was remarkably well tolerated. Alopecia was mild-moderate and entirely reversible. Myelosuppression was mild with no associated bleeding nor significant infections. Occasional fever with bleomycin was easily controlled. One patient (number 6) had mild vincristine neuropathy. After one dose of ^{131}I (150 millicuries), patient number 2 had transient enlargement and tenderness of the salivary glands. Adriamycin cardiotoxicity was monitored by means of serial 12 lead electrocardiograms, echocardiography and phonocardiography as well as determination of systolic time intervals. No persistent abnormalities developed as a result of adriamycin therapy even in the patient with pre-existant aortic stenosis. Of interest and as recently reported (20), reversible impairment in systolic time intervals were noted with thyroid hormone withdrawal as preparation for thyroid scans. The next doses of adriamycin were withheld until cardiac function had been documented to have returned to normal.

DISCUSSION

This is the first report of attempted comprehensive multimodality therapy for high risk thyroid carcinoma. Although controversy persists with regard to the elements of optimal initial treatment including surgery, high radioiodine and external irradiation (7, 10-13), there is no doubt that even with maximal prior efforts, patients in the high risk categories have continued to have relapsing disease and die from thyroid carcinoma (21, 22). We have combined what is generally accepted as maximal convential therapy with our own formulation of combination chemotherapy plus B.C.G. immunotherapy. Based upon the potential high morbidity of very radical surgery and the knowledge that postoperative therapy would be used to treat residual disease, subtotal thyroidectomy with limited node dissection was selected as the surgical procedure of choice. Since postoperative ^{131}I therapy has been shown to improve survival in patients over 40 years of age and in patients with metastatic or extra thyroid cervical disease, ^{131}I was incorporated into the protocol for patients with functional metastases or residual disease (23-26). All patients received replacement, suppressive doses of L-thyroxine in an effort to inhibit recurrent tumor growth.

The selection of drugs for the adjuvant chemotherapy was based upon prior published experience with single agents in patients with advanced disease (27). Drugs with evident activity included adriamycin, melphalan, vincristine and bleomycin (27, 28, 29). Melphalan was selected as an alkylating agent with known additive effects to those of adriamycin and structural similarity to thyroid hormones (30). Vincristine and bleomycin were used on day 14 of the treatment schedule in an effort to take advantage of any tumor recruitment or synchronization following initial cell kill with the adriamycin-melphalan. B.C.G. immunotherapy was added as a potentially helpful adjunct with reported benefit in terms of prolongation of disease free interval in a variety of solid tumors (31).

In the current pilot study, patients with high risk carcinoma of all histologic types were treated. The patients with anaplastic carcinoma clearly benefited from our program. All patients showed evidence of response and the median survival was 20 months. This result is particularly encouraging in view of rather disappointing prior experience in similar patients using a variety of approaches (7, 28). Because such tumors are frequently highly invasive and vascular definitive surgery is rarely possible as in Cases 2 and 3 in the present series. Postoperative external irradiation has found limited success largely because of the high tumor growth fraction and the conventional low fractionation radiation schedules. Perhaps with higher fractionation schedules, better cell kill could be accomplished as recently reported for melanoma (32). There have, however, been reports of successful irradiation-chemotherapy combinations. Wallgren and Norin (33) reported a 9 month remission using a combination of external irradiation, 5-fluorouracil and cyclophosphamide in a 70 year old woman with anaplastic carcinoma. Rogers _et al_ (34) obtained remissions in 3 of 6 patients using external irradiation plus actinomycin D. Our combination chemo-immunotherapy approach would seem to have been at least as successful as this latter report. The absence of any detectable residual disease in 2 of 4 patients at 12 and 24 months would seem to indicate the possibility of prolonged remission. The finding of delayed intense radioiodine uptake (Figure 2) justifies the inclusion of ^{131}I in the regimen and makes follow-up ^{131}I scanning an absolute requirement.

The elimination of all residual disease in three of four patients with vascular invasive (moderate-marked) follicular carcinoma was also very encouraging. Since 50% of patients with this type of histology can be expected to die from thyroid carcinoma within 5 years, our results would seem to indicate a potentially important advance in therapy. As discussed by Halnan (35), early adjuvant therapy with this degree of effectiveness could well produce cure where similar therapy in the presence of a much higher tumor burden would be inadequate. Only time will tell if this type of schedule can, in fact, be curative; however, promising results in other tumor types treated in adjuvant fashion, would seem to justify a larger study in patients with invasive follicular carcinoma.

Results in patients with papillary and medullary carcinoma were less promising. Although 3 patients with extrathyroidal papillary carcinoma showed evidence of response, none came close to complete response. This certainly calls into questions the early aggressive treatment of such patients who, depending upon age, have at least a 50-60% 10 year survival (4, 6). However, patients 6 and 7 had extensive prior ^{131}I therapy over several years which could have precluded subsequent response to chemotherapy. The long, rather indolent course, also suggests a low growth fraction which might have made any response less obvious. In patients 5 and 7, progressive disease led to the instigation of combined therapy. In patients 6 and 8, therapy could conceivably have been withheld until complications of advancing disease, when and if such developed, necessitated treatment. Further follow-up will be necessary to evaluate the possible benefits of early treatment.

The medullary carcinoma cases proved to be the least responsive of all to therapy despite a published report of excellent regressions with adriamycin as a single agent (28). Since medullary carcinoma with node involvement is associated with significant morbidity and mortality (8, 9), it would be beneficial to have active adjuvant type therapy available. However, unless more promising results are found in a few more patients just starting off on protocol, more effective combined modality treatment will have to be sought. Fortunately, in familial cases, detected at an early stage, using screening calcitonin assay (16), in the absence of nodal metastases, early aggressive surgery can produce an 86% 10 year survival (9).

In summary, effective combined modality therapy has been developed for both anaplastic and follicular carcinomas. The regimen is sufficiently well tolerated to justify early adjuvant type treatment with reasonable hope of extended disease free survival or cure. In patients with papillary and medullary carcinomas, results were less promising, but may serve as a basis for more effective multimodality treatment. Perhaps the most significant finding was the successful integration of multiple specialities in the treatment of thyroid carcinoma. This early aggressive approach can hopefully serve as a model for combined modality approaches in other institutions.

REFERENCES

1. DeGroot, L.J. Thyroid carcinoma. Symposium on Current Concepts of Thyroid Disease. Med Clin North Am 59:1233-1261, 1975.
2. Favus, M.J., Schneider, A.B., et al. Thyroid cancer occurring as late consequence of head-and-neck irradiation. N Engl J Med 294:1019-1025, 1976.
3. Beaugie, J.M., Brown, C.L., et al. Primary malignant tumours of the thyroid: the relationship between histological classification and clinical behaviour. Br J Surg 63:173-181, 1976.
4. Woolner, L.B. Thyroid carcinoma: pathologic classification with data on prognosis. Semin Nucl Med 1:481-502, 1971.
5. Fransilla, K. Value of histologic classification of thyroid cancer. Acta Pathol Microbiol Scand 225:1-76, 1971.
6. Franssila, K.O. Is the differentiation between papillary and follicular thyroid carcinoma valid? Cancer 32:853-864, 1973.
7. Staunton, M.D. Greening, W.P. Treatment of thyroid cancer in 293 patients. Br J Surg 63:253-258, 1976.
8. Hill, C.S., Jr., Ibanez, M.L., et al. Medullary (solid) carcinoma of the thyroid gland: an analysis of the M.D. Anderson Hospital experience with patients with the tumor, its special features, and its histogenesis. Medicine 52:141-171, 1973.
9. Chong, G.C., Beahrs, O.H., et al. Medullary carcinoma of the thyroid gland. Cancer 35:695-704, 1975.

10. Johnston, I.D.A. The surgery of thyroid cancer. Br J Surg 62:765-768, 1975.
11. Editorial. Thyroid cancer. Br Med J 1:113-114, 1976.
12. McCowen, K.D., Adler, R.A., et al. Low dose radioiodide thyroid ablation in postsurgical patients with thyroid cancer. Am J Med 61:52-58, 1976.
13. Kagan, A.R., Nussbaum, H., et al. Thyroid carcinoma: Is postoperative external irradiation indicated? Oncology 29:40-45, 1974.
14. Pochin, E.E. Radioiodine therapy of thyroid cancer. Semin Nucl Med 1: 503-515, 1971.
15. Lilien, D.L., Jones, S.E., et al. A clinical evaluation of indium-111 bleomycin as a tumor-imaging agent. Cancer 35:1036-1049, 1975.
16. Jackson, C.E., Tashjian, A.H., Jr., et al. Detection of medullary thyroid cancer by calcitonin assay in families. Ann Int Med 78:845-852, 1973.
17. Durie, B.G.M., Salmon, S.E., et al. Polyamines as markers of response and disease activity in cancer chemotherapy. Cancer Res 37:214-221, 1977.
18. U.S. Atomic Energy Commission Byproduct Material License No. 05-00046-13, Amend. 34, Condition No. 7, and National Council on Radiation Protection and Measurement, Report No. 37, Chapter 4, "Release from the hospital of patients containing radioactive material," 1970.
19. Jones, S.E. and Salmon, S.E. Chemotherapy versus chemoimmunotherapy in non-Hodgkin's lymphomas. Int Conf Adj Chemoth 61, March 5, 1977.
20. Crowley, W.F., Ridgway, E.C., et al. Noninvasive evaluation of cardiac function in hypothyroidism. N Eng J Med 296:1-6, 1977.
21. Silverberg, S.G., Hutter, R.V.P., et al. Fatal carcinoma of the thyroid: histology, metastases, and causes of death. Cancer 25:792-802, 1970.
22. Heitz, P., Moser, H., et al. Thyroid cancer: a study of 573 tumors and 161 autopsy cases observed over a thirty-year period. Cancer 37:2329-2337, 1976.
23. Varma, V.M., Berierwaltes, W.H., et al. Treatment of thyroid cancer. Death rates after surgery and after surgery followed by sodium 1-131. JAMA 214: 1437, 1970.
24. Jackson, G.L., Blosser, N.M. Surgical and radioiodide therapy in thyroid carcinoma. Pa Med 74:77, 1971.
25. Leeper, R.D. The effect of 1-131 on survival of patients with metastatic, papillary or follicular thyroid carcinoma. J Clin Endocrinol Metab 36:1143, 1973.
26. Bricout, P., Kilber, R.S. Experience in the management of thyroid carcinoma by 1-131. J Can Assoc Radiol 24:323, 1973.
27. Gottlieb, J.A., Hill, C.S., et al. Chemotherapy of thyroid cancer. An evaluation of experience with 37 patients. Cancer 30:848-853, 1972.

28. Gottlieb, J.A., and Hill, C.S., Jr. Chemotherapy of thyroid cancer with adriamycin. Experience with 30 patients. N Eng J Med 290:193-197, 1974.

29. Harda, T., Nishikawa, Y., et al. Bleomycin treatment for cancer of the thyroid. Am J Surg 122:53-57, 1971.

30. Tobias, J.S., Parker, L.M., et al. Adriamycin/cyclophosphamide and adriamycin/melphalan in advanced L1210 leukemia. Br J Cancer 32:199-207, 1975.

31. Gutterman, J.U., Mavligit, G.M., et al. Immunotherapy of breast cancer, malignant melanoma, and acute leukemia with BCG: prolongation of disease free interval and survival. Cancer Immunol Immunother 1:99-107, 1976.

32. Habermalz, H.J. and Fisher, J.J. Radiation therapy of malignant melanoma. Experience with high individual treatment doses. Cancer 38:2258-2262, 1976.

33. Wallgren, A. and Norin, T. Combined chemotherapy and radiation therapy in spindle and giant cell carcinoma of the thyroid gland. Acta Radiologica Therapy Physics Biology 12:17-20, 1973.

34. Rogers, J.D., Lindberg, R.D., et al. Spindle and giant cell carcinoma of the thyroid: a different therapeutic approach. Cancer 34: 1328-1332, 1974.

35. Halnan, K.E. The non-surgical treatment of thyroid cancer. Br J Surg 62: 769-771, 1975.

Adjuvant Therapy of Cancer, S.E. Salmon and S.E. Jones eds.

COMBINATION CHEMOTHERAPY AND DELAYED SPLIT COURSE RADIATION THERAPY IN MALIGNANT GLIOMAS: A PRELIMINARY REPORT

*Harvey Alan Gilbert, MD, **Leonard Sadoff, MD, ***David Eder, MD, ****Karen Cove, MD, *****John Wagner, MD, *A. Robert Kagan, MD, *Herman Nussbaum, MD, *Paul Chan, MD, *Aroor Rao, MD

*From the Department of Radiotherapy, **the Department of Internal Medicine, ***the Department of Neurosurgery, ****the Department of Pathology, and *****the Department of Neurology, Kaiser Permanente Medical Center, Los Angeles, California 90027.

INTRODUCTION

This is a preliminary report of a non-randomized combination multi-agent chemotherapy and split course radiation regime in the treatment of Grade III and IV gliomas. The survival results are preliminary. Postsurgical Karnofsky level and anatomic site will be shown to be prognostic factors which significantly describe patients with gliomas. A "control" group of patients seen consecutively with the protocol patients but not referred for treatment will also be evaluated in order to demonstrate that a serious selection problem must be dealt with if we are to gain insight into what type of patients constitute a given protocol population as well as those excluded from protocol.

I. METHODS

Forty-nine consecutive adult patients were seen at the Southern California Permanente Medical Group/Kaiser Hospitals within an 18 month period, with a diagnosis of glioma Grade III and IV of the supratentorial region.

Of these, 29 were treated by an institutional protocol and received at least one course of chemotherapy and radiation therapy.

Twenty patients were not treated by protocol and were treated by the following methods: Three of these patients received 1 course of chemotherapy only, 1 received full course radiation only and 16 were treated with varying doses of Decadron. Exclusions were for: 1) Deterioration after Decadron and surgical decmompression; 2) coma or hemiplegia postsurgery; 3) meningitis.

Primary Diagnosis:

All patients had a preoperative diagnostic work-up using either computerized axial tomography and/or an extensive neuroradiologic approach. All tumors were classified as to radiologic presence of tumor neovascularity. Approximately 50% of the tumors in this study were considered "hypovascular" on arteriography.

Tissue was obtained on all patients but two and subtotal resection if possible was always performed.

TREATMENT

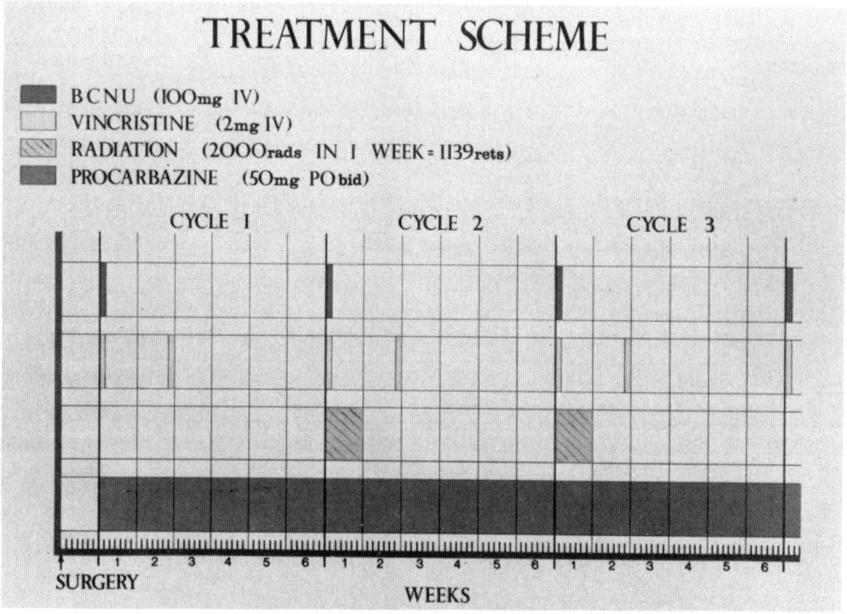

1. Chemotherapy (Figure 1)

Prior to starting radiation therapy with its resultant vasculitis, the initial treatment of patients was 3-drug chemotherapy for 6 weeks. The first cycle was started by the end of the 7th postoperative day. BCNU was given at 100 mg IV on day 1 of each 6 week cycle. Two mg of Vincristine IV was given on day 1 and day 14 of each cycle. Procarbazine was given at doses of 100 mg a day by mouth on a continuous daily basis. This multiagent chemotherapy was continued at 6 weekly intervals until death or tumor relapse. Previous use of these drugs was reported by Gutin[1] and Avellanosa.[2]

2. Decadron

Most patients were on Decadron at least through their first course of radiation therapy.[3] Some few patients who did not respond to usual doses of Decadron, 16 mgms/day or less, were placed on higher doses with a maximum of 64 mgms/day. There were 3 patients who failed to respond at 16 mgms and had excellent responses at higher dose levels.[4] These dose dependent responses were usually short lived.

3. Radiation therapy

Besides having some theoretical biologic advantages rapid split course irradiation requires fewer patient trips (10) than conventional irradiation (more than 30). This treatment was delivered as whole brain radiation therapy on our 4 mev Clinac linear accelerator from day 42 to day 47 (2000 rads) and day 84 to day 89 (2000 rads). The dose was calculated at the midplane and 400 rads were given daily for 5 consecutive treatment days. Two fields per day were treated. Patients treated in this fashion (2000 rads in 5 fractions = 1139 rets) can develop self-limited but severe headaches if not on Decadron. Previous use of delayed radiation has been described by Avellanosa.[2]

4. Measurement Parameters

We feel that survival is only one parameter that should be determined in the life of a patient with a malignant glioma.

a. Functional Level

The most critical factor in the functional capability of a brain tumor patient was the ability to get out of bed and initiate self care. This would correspond with a Karnofsky index of 60 or greater. If one takes all the months of a patient's life that are spent in a Karnofsky level above 60 (ambulatory) and divides this by the total number of months of survival, a ratio will be obtained which shows the percent of life spent in an ambulatory status.

b. Survival

Both individual survival as well as the alive/dead ratio (number of patients alive/number dead) illustrates this parameter.

c. Prognostic Factors

Factors evaluated for prognostic significance are patient age (more or less than 60 years of age), motor impairment such as paresis on initial examinatiion, anatomic site in the brain (parietal and basal ganglia versus other sites), Karnofsky functional scale at the end of the first postoperative week (ambulatory and functional versus predominantly bedridden) and histologic grade (Grade III vs. IV). We did not use extent of resection as a prognostic factor because our surgeons always attempted subtotal resection unless in their opinion this would produce detrimental neurologic deficit. Size of lesions in centimeters was not reliable.

RESULTS

The only selection criteria stated in the protocol was an adult (> 18 years old) with a malignant supratentorial brain tumor who accepted and by the judgement of the physician could tolerate the protocol regimen. Not one patient refused the protocol.

TABLE I

PATIENT CHARACTERISTICS

		29 Protocol		20 Nonprotocol	
		Alive	Dead	Alive	Dead
Anatomic Site	Parietal or basal ganglia	5	7	3	12
	Other	11	6	3	2
Histologic Grade	Grade III	7	5	4	6
	Grade IV present	9	8	2	8
Patient Age	Greater than 60	4	8	2	6
	Less than 60	12	5	4	8
Presence of Paresis on Diagnosis	Presented with paresis	9	5	2	10
	No paresis	7	8	4	4
Post-surgical Karnofsky	Ambulatory (Karnofsky 50)	14	10	3	0
	Non-ambulatory (Karnofsky 50 or less)	2	3	3	14
Total		16	13	6	14

Out of a total of 49 patients seen during this period, 20 (40%) failed decompression and Decadron and were considered too ill to be included in the protocol. The composition of the protocol and nonprotocol groups is very different (Table I). Patients that were not entered on protocol had an inferior postsurgical Karnofsky status and the location of tumor was usually in the parietal or basal ganglia areas.

Survival

Figure 2

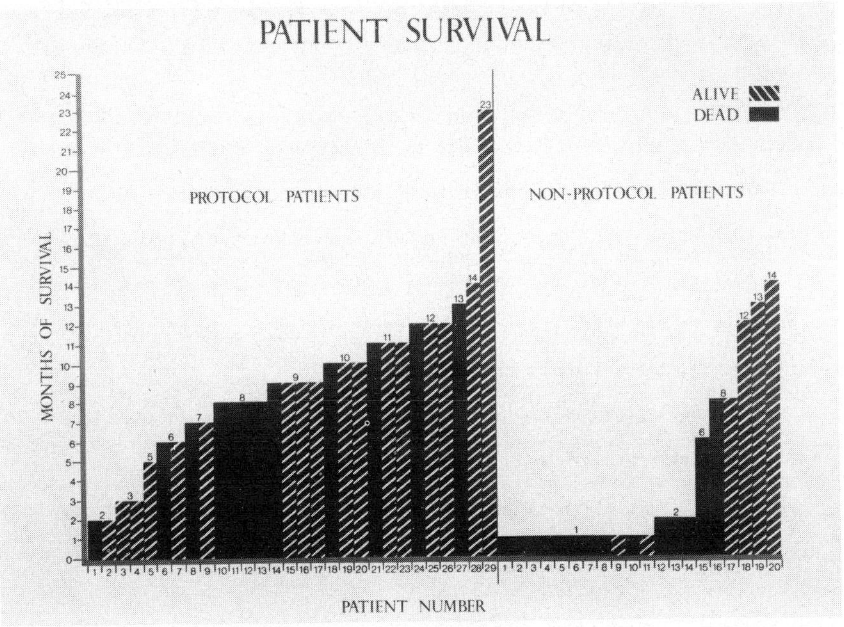

Figure 2 demonstrates the trend towards earlier death in the nonprotocol population. Median survival in the protocol population has not been reached. The alive/dead ratios are 1.23 (16/13) for the protocol group and .42 (6/14) for the nonprotocol group. We feel that for our entire glioma population the presence of initial paresis, the presence of a non-ambulatory status (low Karnofsky) postoperatively and the location of the lesion in the parietal area are factors adversely affecting the alive/dead status as well as exclusion from the protocol. For patients, though, who make it on to the protocol, the most critical factors influencing survival appear to be age and site. We are hopeful that as more patients are accrued, we will be able to predict in advance the good treatment responders in the protocol group using these parameters.

Grade of tumor,[5,6] initial presence of cranial nerve deficit and seizures,[7] age,[7] and radiation dose[6] have been quoted as having prognostic value. Walker[7] found that grade and site in the brain exhibited no effect on survival. The difference in survival between the protocol and nonprotocol patient groups we feel may be due more to selection than treatment.

Median survival for the entire group of patients is now in excess of 9.5 months.

Quality of Life

We calculated the percent of life spent in a functional ambulatory status - defined as Karnofsky 60-100 - for the protocol and nonprotocol populations. The protocol population spent approximately 80% in an ambulatory status (Karnofsky 60 or better), whereas the nonprotocol group spent 42% above that level. When one attempts to see which prognostic factors most adversely affect a Karnofsky 60-100 level, the following trends are seen:

1. In the protocol group an age above 60 years old and a low postsurgical Karnofsky status below 60.
2. In the nonprotocol group the presence of initial paresis, age over 60, Grade IV, postsurgical Karnofsky 60 status and parietal lobe lesions.

Treatment Toxicity

The toxicity from chemotherapy was minimal. Table II demonstrates the toxicities requiring dosage alteration or temporary omission of drugs. There was no serious morbidity or mortality. Fifteen out of 29 protocol patients required alteration of therapy. One unusual toxicity was found. This was a serious but reversible cardiac arrhythmia apparently induced by IV BCNU induction in a debilitated patient during his first injection.

TABLE II

TOXICITY SECONDARY TO CHEMOTHERAPY

(29 patients)

	Patients
Leucopenia	11
Skin Rash	5
Severe Paresthesias	1
Severe Vomiting	4
Phlebitis	1
Severe Fatigue	2
Herpes Zoster	2

Total number of patients requiring alteration of therapy = 15

Unusual complications: 1 ventricular cardiac arrhythmia with BCNU injection. 1 severe steroid myopathy.

CONCLUSIONS

1. Patient selection accounted for approximately 40% of all glioblastoma multiforme patients being consciously or unconsciously excluded from our protocol treatment.
2. The common characteristic shared by those patients not entered on protocol is a nonimproving non-ambulatory postsurgical status at the end of the first week postop, not responding to Decadron or surgical decompression and commonly associated with a parietal lobe lesion.
3. The multi-agent chemotherapy given produced no major complications. Fifteen out of 29 protocol patients required alteration in the drug schedule planned. Preliminary survival results are favorable.
4. The quality of survival measured by the percent of total life spent in a functional ambulatory status is distinctly superior in the protocol patients (80%) versus the nonprotocol (42%). This may be due primarily to patient selection.
5. In order to permit comparison of results from different institutions

future reports should describe patients with respect to postcraniotomy status, site of lesion, presence or absence of paresis, above or below 60 years of age, grade and most important, patients diagnosed as glioma Grades III and IV but excluded from complete treatment.

ACKNOWLEDGMENT:

We wish to acknowledge the following doctors: K. Fuchs, K. Ro, S. Hoshek, S. Stavropoulos, F. Latino, F. Cassidy, N. W. Davidson, I. Ali, E. Oktay, F. Gabriel, A. Bredt, N. Helman, A. Radcliffe.

REFERENCES

1. Gutin, P. et al (1975) Phase II Study of Procarbazine, CCNU, and Vincristine Combination Chemotherapy in the Treatment of Malignant Brain Tumors. Cancer 35:1398-1404.

2. Avellanosa, A. et al (1976) Chemotherapy before Radiotherapy in the Treatment of Malignant Gliomas of the Central Nervous System. Proceedings of Twelfth Annual Meeting of American Society of Clinical Oncology May 4-8, Toronto, Ontario, Canada.

3. Gutin, P. (1975) Corticosteroid Therapy in Patients with Cerebral Tumors: Benefits, Mechanisms, Problems, Practicalities. Seminars in Oncology 2: 49-56.

4. Renaudin, J. et al (1973) Dose dependency of Decadron in patients with partially excised brain tumors. J. Neurosurg. 39:302-305.

5. Sheline, G. (1976) The Importance of Distinguishing Tumor Grade in Malignant Gliomas: Treatment and Prognosis. Intl. J. Radiation-Oncology-Biology-Physics 1:781-786.

6. Salazar, O. et al (1976) High Dose Radiation Therapy in Treatment of Glioblastoma Multiforme: A Preliminary Report. Intl. J. Radiation-Oncology-Biology-Physics 1:717-727.

7. Walker, M. and Gehan, E. (1976) Brain Tumor Study Group. Presented at the Modern Concepts in Brain Tumor Therapy, Laboratory and Clinical Investigations, Atlanta, Georgia, Feb. 26-28.

Adjuvant Therapy of Cancer, S.E. Salmon and S.E. Jones eds.
© *1977 Elsevier/North-Holland Biomedical Press, Amsterdam*

ADJUVANT CHEMOIMMUNOTHERAPY IN CENTRAL NERVOUS SYSTEM TUMORS

A Preliminary Report With An In Depth View Into Tumor-Host Immunobiologic Interactions

S. DeCarvalho, M.D., Ph.D., A. Kaufman, M.D. and A. Pineda, M.D.
Belmont Medical Clinic and Bellwood General Hospital
Bellflower, California 90706

INTRODUCTION

The immunobiology of the neural tissues and their neoplasms has to be viewed in the context of the nature of these tissues when compared to others. Elements of their specific nature include: a) their origin in the neuroectoderm and the local mesenchyme under its organizing influences[1]; b) their biochemical and biophysical differentiation which lead to the requirement for insulation from local migration or homing of surveilling T lymphocytes (immunologically privileged site) and even shielding against many molecular species (hemato-encephalic barrier). A unique morphogenetic interrelation is also continuously operative whereby neural cells influence the proliferation of endothelial cells, a property which is reflected in the apparent malignant induction by the tumor on cells or species of cells other than their own strict histologic kind[2]. Even tumors metastatic to the brain may undergo these influences; for instance, lymphocytes from a patient with intracerebral metastatic melanoma became cytotoxic to other glioblastoma cells[3]. Yet, despite these specific features, the general immunologic behavior of neural tumors is similar to that of other tumors, in regard to antigenicity, response to cytotoxic antibody or antibody-dependent cytotoxicity and to cell-mediated immunity. However, being a privileged site precludes access to specifically primed T cells from other sources and to other antigens; also, being beyond the blood-brain fence isolates it from access to specific immunoglobulins (passive immunotherapy). The mesenchymal origin of the glia gives its cells macrophagic properties. Non-specific immunotherapeutic stimulation of these cells has a better chance of making them aggressive killers of neoplastic cells. During chemoimmunotherapy an important correlation has been described between bone marrow macrophage precursors and antitumor macrophage cytotoxicity[4].

Antigenicity of brain tumors (astrocytin), loss of antigenicity and cross-reaction with non-neural tumors are well established[5,6,7,8]. Depressed or even abolished cell-mediated immunity is a frequent clinical feature of growing brain tumors[9,10,11]. This important aspect of neural tumor immunobiology is reviewed in detail by Harris and Synkovics[2] and will not be discussed much further here. Worth emphasizing is the reported existence in the sera of brain tumor patients of an IgG that strongly inhibits PHA lymphocyte blastogenesis and skin sensitization to brain tumor extracts[9,10] but this inhibition may extend to cytotoxicity to non-neural tissues. Complement-activating cytotoxic antibodies to gliomas and astrocytomas have been described in the serum of these patients[12].

Attempts at specific passive and active immunotherapy of human brain tumors have yielded results ranging from partially effective[8] to totally ineffective[13,14,15], respectively. Increased effectiveness was seen when the antibody was armed by coupling it with a chemotherapeutic agent[16]. These difficulties may be more inherent to the general immunobiology of tumors than to the specific immunobiologic characteristics of brain tumors since specific immunotherapeutic attempts with other tumors have only met with equally unsatisfactory or inconclusive results.

Non-specific therapeutic immunopotentiation (NSTI) has, thus, become the subject of wider efforts because it is less prone to abrogation by serum factors such as specific immunoblockers, immunoregulatory effects of certain α-globulins[17] and to antigenic modulation, simplification, loss or drift and to enhancement and tolerogenesis (Fig. 1). Above all, it has provided most of the promising therapeutic effects, not only in the now classical studies of Gutterman and Klein in skin neoplasms[19] but also in many other solid tumors including colo-rectal, lung, breast and brain[2,20].

The rationale for non-specific immunostimulation by BCG has been extensively analyzed[19] and it will be only expanded in synoptic form here (Fig. 1). Experimentally, Albright et al.[21] demonstrated that, in the intracerebral murine glioma model, CCNU and early immunization following tumor challenge were additive in producing significant increase in survival time. Our own work with nitrosoureas and BCG, still not widely utilized[22], is a clinical pilot study based on this concept.

MATERIALS AND METHODS

CCNU was always given at 130 mg/m^2/6 weeks starting 2 weeks after surgery and about the same time or 1 week preceding radiotherapy. Base line studies, beyond the initial diagnostic work up, included computerized axial cranial tomography, isotopic brain scan, skull X-rays, electroencephalography and neurologic examination. These were repeated every 6 to 12 weeks.

Immunologic profiling consisted of absolute lymphocyte count, PHA lymphocyte transformation testing, quantitation of serum immunoglobulins and intradermal test doses of BCG (Glaxo Danish substrain, liophylized preparation from E. Lilly Co.); 0.1 ml of the reconstitute was given intracutaneously 1 week post-operatively. Lack of progression to inflammatory stage was taken as indication of depressed hypersensitivity and macrophage suppression.

In this series CCNU was given a maximum of 5 times in 2 patients and a maximum of 3 times in all the others with most receiving only a second dose. BCG was given at 0.5 ml intradermal in the forearms at weekly intervals but withheld for as long as previous sites were still frankly inflammatory with exudation. Thus,

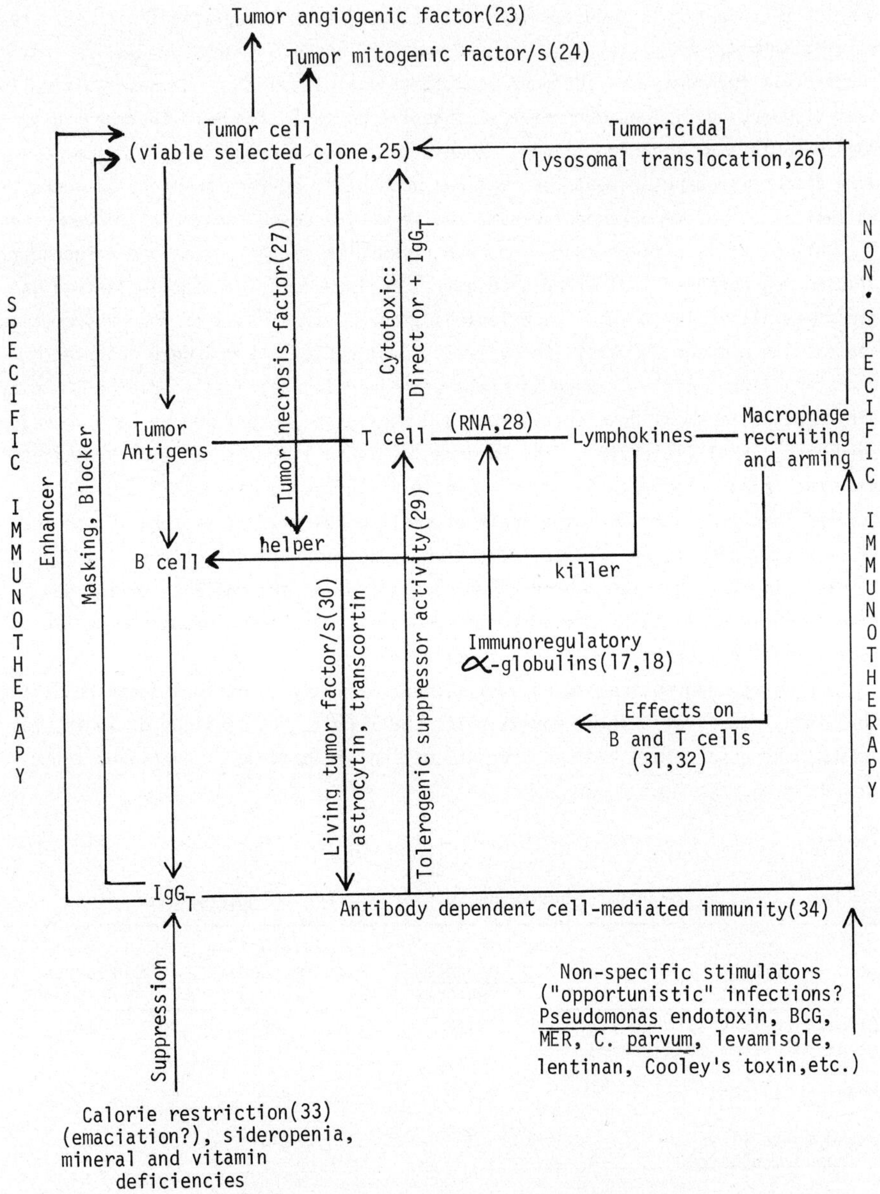

Fig. 1. Complex homeostatic immunobiologic reactions of the host in response to clonal selection and growth of tumor cells.

none of these patients received more than a total of 8 inoculations with most receiving 3 to 4.

Criteria for remission included asymptomatic status with no demonstrable malignant disease, conditions much more stringent than those for mere therapeutic response (50% tumor size reduction). When a remission was attained CCNU and BCG were discontinued but repeat observations were still carried on every 12 weeks. At indications of recurrence the same regime was resumed. Only 2 astrocytoma and 1 medulloblastoma patients have required resumption of the regime and a second remission was obtained indicating no acquired resistance. The medulloblastoma patient was also reirradiated. BCG lesions after several weeks of cold suppuration healed with pigmented scars. No systemic complications of BCG were observed.

Patients who initially were severely depressed in their cell-mediated immunity (no response to small dose intradermal BCG challenge) were found to have increased serum and spinal fluid IgG. This observation is in line with that of Brooks _et al._[9] and Young[10] referred to above. Previous studies by Mitsuoka[35] and ourselves[36] had indicated the usefulness of small doses of cyclophosphamide to reverse B cell inhibition of T cell function. One week after a course of 5 days of 200 mg daily by mouth they would become better responders while serum IgG declined. Some patients became better responders as the chemoimmunotherapeutic regime went on without the cyclophosphamide push.

Late marrow depression, never very severe, was only seen in patients requiring more than 2 doses of CCNU. Prophylactic, small (10^9) transfusions of leukocytes in subleukopenic stages avoided discontinuation of the drug or even drug reduction[37].

RESULTS

TABLE 1

ADJUVANT CHEMOIMMUNOTHERAPEUTIC REGIME OUTCOMES

Tumor	# Responses / # Patients	Survival time of responders (Years)	# Recurrences / # Responses
Gliomas (grades III and IV, 2 glioblastoma multiforme)	4/8	>5	2/4
Medulloblastomas	2/2	>4	1/2
Ependymomas (1 is an ependymoblastoma)	3/3	>3	0/3
Sarcomatous meningioma	1/1	>2	0/1
Pituitary adenomas, extrasellar	4/4	>4	0/4
	Total=14/18	Mean>3.9 (Weighted,#38)	Total=3/14

DISCUSSION

Brain tumor chemotherapy before the nitrosoureas was greatly disappointing[39]. With the introduction of these liposoluble agents, able to transpose the blood-brain barrier, the era of neurochemotherapy was started[40]. Their therapeutic effectiveness in recurrent neural tumors is now well established.

Adjuvant therapy of brain tumors may be directed to macrodeposits as well as to microdeposits of malignant cells rather than primarily against micrometastatic disease as in other malignancies. In this sense (like BCG) it is more strictly adjuvant (potentiator) of other therapies directed towards the primary tumor than a prophylactic measure against early recurrence.

Early attempts at adjuvant (starting on the 3rd post-operative week) CCNU therapy following surgery and radiation in brain tumors by the European Organization for Research and Treatment of Cancer (EORTC) Brain Tumor Group[41] did not appear to deter recurrence and did not differ from the benefits of surgery and radiation

TABLE 2*

COMPARATIVE INFLUENCE OF COMBINATION THERAPIES (SURGERY, RADIATION, NITROSOUREAS AND BCG) ON MEDIAN SURVIVAL TIME ON ALL NEURAL TUMORS

Therapeutic Modality	# Responses / # Patients	Median Survival Time (Weeks)	Reference
S		6	39
R		12	39
S + R		18	45 (Holland and Frei, 1973)
S + R		30	39
S + R + T_3		60	39 (Griem _et al_., 1976)
S + R + C_{Rec}	4/16	30	41 (EORTC, 1976)
S + R + C_{Rec}		41	40 (Walker _et al_., 1972)
S + R + C_{Adj}	16/22	48	46 (Carter _et al_., 1974)
" " "		-	44 (Goldsmith _et al_., 1974)
" " "		47	43 (Weir _et al_., 1976)
S + R + C_{Adj}		50	41 (EORTC, 1976)
S + R + I_{Rec}		-	Takakura (as quoted in #2, p. 526)
S + R + I_{Adj}		-	
S + R + C_{Adj} + I_{Adj}	14/18	170 (p<.001,#38)	

*Abbreviations:

S - Surgery R - Radiation T_3 - Triiodothyronine

C - Chemotherapy by CCNU at 130 mg/m^2/6 weeks

C_{Rec} - Same for recurrence C_{Adj} - Same as adjuvant

I - Immunotherapy with intradermal BCG 0.5 ml/weekly or less

(S + R). When administered after recurrence only 4 of 16 patients achieved remission lasting an average of 30 weeks. Second responses in recurring medulloblastomas treated with procarbazine-vincristine-CCNU were obtained in 10 of 12 patients but lasted only 2 to 18 months[42]. Other results[43], however, point more definitely to the benefit of concurrent radiation and CCNU.

Control of primary brain tumors has been one of the most frustrating areas of cancer treatment, affecting about 12,000 people annually in the United States[44]. Hence the continuous search for improved methods. Griem _et al._[39] in a controlled study introduced triiodothyronine in large doses as a radiosensitizing agent. Compared to S + R alone, with a median survival time of 30 weeks, the 18 study subjects on S + R + T_3 had double median survival time on less radiation. An important, recent experiment in specific _curative_ immunotherapy with a murine neuroblastoma was carried out by Byfield _et al._ in which antibody-dependent cellular cytotoxicity (ADCC) was utilized. All tumor cells that can recognize the Fc portion of a xenogeneic specific IgG antibody to tumor cells can be "armed" with it and become specifically cytotoxic to that tumor. Such cells included lymphocytes, monocytes, macrophages and neutrophils. This significant result may provide means to manipulate non-specific immunocytes into becoming specific tumoricidal agents[34].

Initial depression of cellular immunity may be the overriding factor in the final outcome of any form of therapy. Adjuvant non-specific immunostimulation appears to have been the key element in the increased survival of responders in this, yet to be enlarged, series.

SUMMARY

18 patients of both sexes and in the biphasic age incidence of 4 to 60 years were treated with CCNU-BCG concurrently with radiation therapy following surgery for excision and/or biopsy. Comparison is made with results from the literature of patients treated with surgery and radiation only. Thus, in 2099 malignant gliomas the median survival time was 4.5 months with only 10% alive at 18 months[45]. In our small series 4 out of 8 high grade malignant gliomas are alive after 5 years with 3 asymptomatic. The median survival time for medulloblastomas is given as about 5 years. 2 of 2 of our medulloblastoma patients are alive after 4 years. For malignant ependymomas the median survival time is 2 to 3 years. 3 out of 3 in our series are alive and asymptomatic after 3 years; 4 out of 4 invasive pituitary adenomas are alive and well after 4 years. The remainder is a sarcomatous meningioma going into the 3rd year. 2 of the gliomas and 1 of the medulloblastomas required repetition of the chemoimmunotherapy. In none was there maintenance therapy. Considering the inherent difficulties in evaluating therapies for neural tumors and the smallness of our sample, it is felt that these observations, though of interest, require continuation with increasing numbers. The key to these results appears to be the reversion of the initial depression of cellular immunity

which seems to determine the outcome of all other forms of therapy. The complex homeostatic immunobiologic reactions of the host to the antigenic modulation of the tumor pertinent to immunotherapy are summarized in synoptic form.

REFERENCES

1. Darlington, C. D. (1959) In: Genetics and Cancer (13th Symposium on Fundamental Cancer Research). Univ. Texas Press, Austin, Texas.
2. Harris, J. E. and Synkovics, J. C. (1976) The Immunology of Malignant Disease. The C. V. Mosby Co., St. Louis, Mo., p. 469.
3. Levy, N. L., Mahaley, M. S., Jr., and Day, E. D. Cancer Res. (1972) 32, 477.
4. Fisher, B. and Wolmak, N. Cancer Res. (1976) 36, 2241.
5. Catalano, L. W., Jr., Harter, D. H. and Hsu, K. C. Science (1972) 175, 180-182.
6. Trouillas, P. Lancet (1971) ii, 552.
7. Wickremesinghe, H. R. and Yates, P. O. Br. J. Cancer (1971) 25, 711.
8. DeCarvalho, S. Cancer (1963) 16, 306-330.
9. Brooks, W. H., Netsky, M. G., Normansell, D. E., et al. J. Exp. Med. (1972) 136, 1631.
10. Young, H. F. Surg. Neurol. (1976) 5, 19.
11. DeCarvalho, S. Z. f. Allergie u. Immunitätsfschg. (1969) 137, 276.
12. Quindlen, E. A., Dohan, F. C., Jr. and Kornblith, P. L. Surg. Forum (1974) 25, 464.
13. Mahaley, M. S., Jr. J. Neurosurg. (1971) 34, 458.
14. Bloom, H. J. G., Peckham, M. J., Richardson, A. E., et al. Br. J. Cancer (1973) 27, 253.
15. Bloom, H. J. G. Cancer (1975) 35, 111.
16. DeCarvalho, S. Nature (Lond.)(1964) 202, 255-258.
17. Menzoian, J. O., Glasgow, A. H., Nirnberg, R. D., et al. J. Immunol. (1974) 113, 266.
18. Glaser, M., Ofek, I. and Nalken, D. Immunol. (1972) 23, 205.
19. Bast, R. C., Jr., Zbar, B., Borsas, T. and Rapp, H. J. N. Engl. J. Med. (1974) 290, 1413-1420 and 1458-1469.
20. Internat. Conf. on Immunotherapy of Cancer. Ann. N. Y. Acad. Sci. (1976) 277, Part III.
21. Albright, L., Madigan, J. C., Gaston, M. R. and Houchens, D. P. Cancer Res. (1975) 35, 658.
22. International Registry of Tumor Immunotherapy. Compendium of tumor immunotherapy protocols, No. 4 (1976). Intern. Cancer Res. Data Bank, Informatics, Inc., Washington, D. C.
23. DeCarvalho, S. In vitro angiogenic activity of RNA from leukemic lymphocytes. Angiology: Journal of Vascular Diseases (In the press).

24. Stockdale, F. and Hsuch, H. W. The Cancer Letter (1976) 2, 7.
25. Nowell, P. Science (1976) 194, 23-28.
26. Bucana, C., Hoyer, L., Hobbs, B., Breisman, S., McDaniel, M. and Hanna, M. G., Jr. Cancer Res. (1976) 36, 4444.
27. Hoffmann, M. K., Green, S., Old, L. J. and Oettgen, H. Nature (Lond.)(1976) 263, 416-417.
28. Paque, R. E. Cancer Res. (1976) 36, 4530.
29. Andersson, L. C., Binz, H. and Wigzell, H. Nature (Lond.)(1976) 264, 778-780.
30. Price, M. R. and Baldwin, R. W. (1975) In: Cancer, A Comprehensive Treatise, 4. F. Becker (Ed.). Plenum Press, New York, p. 224.
31. Schrader, J. W. J. Exp. Med. (1973) 138, 466.
32. Watson, J., Trenkner, E. and Cohn, M. J. Exp. Med. (1973) 138, 699.
33. Fernandes, G., Yunis, E. J. and Good, R. A. Nature (Lond.)(1976) 263, 504-507.
34. Byfield, J., Zerubavel, R. and Fonkalsrud, E. Nature (Lond.)(1976) 264, 783-785.
35. Mitsuoka, A., Baba, M. and Morikawa, S. Nature (Lond.)(1976) 262, 77-78.
36. DeCarvalho, S. Pulsating, low dose, cyclophosphamide reversal of lack of reaction to intradermal BCG in anergic cancer patients (Abstract). 18th Ann. Meet. Soc. Hematol. (In the press).
37. DeCarvalho, S. Small leukocyte-transfusions during subleukopenic stages of patients under chemotherapy. Prevention of severe leukopenia and extension of the therapeutic index of myelotoxic agents (Abstract). 19th Ann. Meet. Am. Soc. Hematol. (In the press).
38. Alder, H. L. and Roessler, E. B. (1972) Probability and Statistics, 5th ed. W. H. Freeman and Co., San Francisco, Ca.
39. Yung, W-K., Steward, W., Marks, J. E., Griem, M. L. and Mullan, J. F. Intern. J. Radiation Oncol. Biol. Biophys. (1976) 1, 645.
40. Walker, M. D. and Gehan, G. A. Proc. Am. Assoc. Cancer Res. (1973) 13, 67.
41. Hildebrand, J., Brochi, J., Calliauw, L., Le Mevel, B., Resche, F., et al. Eur. J. Cancer (1976) 12, 41.
42. Wilson, C. B. and Levin, V. A. CCNU with procarbazine and vincristine in the treatment of malignant brain tumors. Audiotape: Vol. 1, Side 2 (1976) Bristol Laboratories, Syracuse, N. Y.
43. Weir, B., Band, P., Urtasun, R., Blain, G., McLean, D., Wilson, F., Mielke, B. and Grace, M. J. Neurosurg. (1976) 45, 129.
44. Goldsmith, M. A. and Carter, S. K. Cancer Treatment Revs. (1974) 1, 153.
45. Holland, J. and Frei, E., III. (1973) Cancer Medicine. Lee & Feabiger, Philadelphia, Pa., p. 1396 and references.
46. Wasserman, T. H., Slavik, M. and Carter, S. K. Cancer Treatment Revs. (1974) 1, 131.

Section IX

LYMPHOMA

Adjuvant Therapy of Cancer, S.E. Salmon and S.E. Jones. eds.

THE ROLE OF ADJUVANT MOPP IN THE RADIATION THERAPY OF HODGKIN'S DISEASE: A PROGRESS REPORT AFTER EIGHT YEARS ON THE STANFORD TRIALS

by

Saul A. Rosenberg, M.D.
Henry S. Kaplan, M.D.
Eli Glatstein, M.D.
Carol S. Portlock, M.D.

Division of Oncology, Department of Medicine
and the Division of Radiation Therapy, Department of Radiology,
Stanford University School of Medicine, Stanford, California 94305

INTRODUCTION

In August, 1968, controlled clinical trials were initiated at Stanford University to test the value and establish the role of adjuvant MOPP chemotherapy following radiation therapy for Hodgkin's disease. These studies were expanded in 1970 to include the most favorable settings of the disease. Detailed descriptions of the trials and preliminary results have been published in 1972[1,2] and 1975[3]. These trials were extensively modified in May, 1974. The present report provides a 2.5 to 8.5 year follow up for the 241 patients on these studies as of February 1, 1977.

PATIENTS AND METHODS

The details of the study[1,2,3], histopathologic criteria[4], diagnostic methods[5] and staging designations[5,6] have appeared in previous reports.

Two hundred forty three previously untreated patients, all pathologically staged (PS) with exploratory laparotomy and splenectomy, stages IA through III_SB have been randomized within each stage to receive irradiation, either alone or followed by six cycles of combination chemotherapy utilizing nitrogen mustard, vincristine, procarbazine and prednisone (MOPP).

Acknowledgements: These studies would not have been possible without the involvement of many of the authors' colleagues in the Departments of Diagnostic Radiology, Nuclear Medicine, Surgery and Surgical Pathology and their Fellows and Nurses in Medical Oncology and Radiotherapy. Statistical and computer assistance was provided by Messrs. Robert Bassett and Loarn Thoelecke.

This work was supported, in part, by Grants CA-05838, CA-08122, and CA-05008 from the National Cancer Institute, National Institutes of Health, Bethesda, Md. The reporting of this investigation has been supported, in part, by Grant CA-19892, National Cancer Institute, Department of Health, Education and Welfare.

Details of the radiation fields, dose and fractionation employing a 6-MeV linear accelerator are described in earlier reports. A dose of 4400 rads delivered in a minimum of 4 weeks was given to all sites of known disease in all of the four different treatment plans. The fields and dose planned to apparently uninvolved sites were different for the various subgroups as previously described[3].

Patients randomized to receive adjuvant MOPP chemotherapy were given the first cycle after an interval of 30 to 60 days following completion of their radiotherapy, with a planned course of six cycles. Details of drug dosage and criteria for dose modification can be found in previous reports. Since 1973, prednisone has been eliminated from the combination chemotherapy for patients who had received mediastinal irradiation. This policy was adopted because of the observation that occasional patients appeared to have aggravation or the initial appearance of clinically severe radiation pneumonitis and/or pericarditis associated with abrupt corticosteroid withdrawal[7]. A recent retrospective analysis has shown no loss of chemotherapy efficacy when nitrogen mustard, vincristine and procarbazine (MOP) is used instead of MOPP[8].

Curves for the probability of freedom from relapse (FFR) and survival have been calculated by the method of Kaplan and Meier[9]. Tests for significance between FFR and survival curves are reported using the method of Gehan[10].

Survival data have been calculated from the date of the patients' first visit to Stanford Medical Center. FFR duration has been calculated both from the completion of radiotherapy and the completion of all therapy, but for simplicity is shown only from the patient's first visit.

RESULTS

Of the total group of 243 patients, 125 patients were randomized to receive irradiation alone and 118 to receive adjuvant chemotherapy MOP(P) following completion of the radiation therapy. Two patients in the adjuvant group refused to continue with the planned chemotherapy program and are not included in the analysis of results. Both patients are alive and one is known to be free of evident disease. Two patients, both randomized to receive adjuvant chemotherapy, have died, and were shown at autopsy to have diffuse histiocytic lymphoma. In retrospect the pathologists felt the initial diagnoses of Hodgkin's disease were incorrect. However, both patients are included in the analysis. Ten of the 28 patients who have died did not have clinical or postmortem evidence of Hodgkin's disease. None of these deaths has been excluded in the survival results reported.

Table I shows the eight year actuarial probability of freedom from relapse (FFR) and survival for each pathologic stage of the disease. The figures are for six years for those with stage IA and IIA disease. Actuarial curves for survival and FFR are shown in Figures 1-4. Patients with limited extranodal extension of the disease, the E-lesion of the Ann Arbor system, or involvement of the spleen, are included with the lymph node extent of disease. Survival and FFR analyses have been calculated separately for patients with E-lesions and are the same as those without E-lesions in each treatment group.

As has been reported from earlier analyses there is a highly significant improvement in FFR in all stages and studies as a result of adjuvant MOP(P) chemotherapy, except for patients with PS IB and IIB disease. However, there are no differences in the curves of survival in any stage or trial group as measured by the Gehan test at the 5 per cent level.

The survival curves, however, appear to be diverging after the third year for those with PSIIIB disease, for the entire group with systemic symptoms(B) and for the total study group of 241 patients. The Gehan p-values for the differences in survival of these groups are of borderline significance when calculated after 4.0 years favoring the adjuvant MOP(P) groups. For those with PS IIIB disease, p (Gehan)=.10 after 4.0 years (Figure 2); for all B patients, p (Gehan)=.06 after 4.0 years (Figure 3); and for all patients, p (Gehan)=.11 after 4.0 years (Figure 4). The standard errors of the final observations for these pairs of survival curves of borderline significance are shown in the Figures and in Table I.

DISCUSSION

It is not surprising that a chemotherapy program capable of producing prolonged complete remissions of clinically evident Hodgkin's disease[11], should be successful as an adjuvant for presumed occult disease. The chemotherapy program, however, is prolonged, difficult and has known and potential dangers. The value of an adjuvant chemotherapy is only tentative, even when significant prolongation in freedom from relapse has been demonstrated. This advantage must be translated into clear survival benefits for the various initial disease settings.

This is especially true for Hodgkin's disease in which radiation therapy can cure a majority of patients with PS IA, IIA, IB, IIB and IIIA disease, including those with limited extranodal disease (the E-lesion of the Ann Arbor system) and/or involvement of the spleen. Between 70 and 90 per cent of these patients do not require adjuvant chemotherapy to effect a clinical cure and therefore will have received chemotherapy unnecessarily to improve the initial cure rate by the 10 to 25 per cent projected by these studies. Only in the group of patients with pathologic stage IIIB is the FFR rate following radiotherapy alone so poor (seven per cent after four years) that chemotherapy is clearly indicated. The question for patients with PS IIIB disease is not if chemotherapy should be used as an adjuvant, but how radiotherapy might best be integrated into a plan in which chemotherapy is the major treatment.

For patients with PS IA, IIA and IIIA disease the improvement in FFR is highly significant (70 versus 90 per cent at eight years, p=.002) but a significant survival benefit is not yet definitive [88 ± 5.7 versus 92 ± 5.2 per cent at eight years, p (Gehan)=.34]. In these groups the question remains whether or not combination chemotherapy should be reserved for the approximately 30 per cent who will relapse after subtotal or total nodal radiotherapy.

The results of the trial for patients with PS IB and IIB disease are of special interest. All patients received total nodal irradiation including pelvic fields despite a negative staging laparotomy. Radiotherapy has resulted in an 81.5 ± 8.5 per cent FFR rate at eight years in this subgroup. It is difficult to demonstrate an improvement on this result with adjuvant chemotherapy (87.3 ± 6.9 per cent) because the radiotherapy has proved so successful and the size of the groups too small to demonstrate small significant differences.

The major argument against the routine adoption of adjuvant MOP(P) chemotherapy in the radiation management of Hodgkin's disease has been the prolonged, difficult, expensive treatment program with considerable acute morbidity, not yet justified by a clear survival benefit. A serious concern has been the sterility produced in virtually all male patients treated with six cycles of MOP(P) chemotherapy.

There has also been the suggestion that non-lymphomatous malignancies, especially acute myelogenous leukemia will be increased in patients who have received combined chemotherapy and radiotherapy for Hodgkin's disease[12]. In this series of 241 patients, four have developed second malignancies in the 2.5 to 8.5 year period of follow-up. One patient developed progressive renal transitional cell carcinoma, five years after radiation therapy for PS III_SB disease, one year after MOP therapy for relapse in the bone marrow. He had no Hodgkin's disease at autopsy. Another developed carcinoma of the colon two years after radiotherapy for PS III_SA disease. She did not receive chemotherapy and had no Hodgkin's disease at autopsy. One patient, still alive, developed acute myelogenous leukemia, without clinical recurrence of Hodgkin's disease, five years after radiotherapy and adjuvant MOPP for PS IIA disease. A fourth patient developed a fatal myeloproliferative disorder five years after radiotherapy for PS IIA disease, one year after MOP therapy for relapse of disease in lymph nodes.

In a larger series of 1005 patients with Hodgkin's disease treated at Stanford, there were 25 examples of second malignancies occurring after treatment[13]. The incidence was 2.2 per cent in patients receiving radiotherapy alone and 3.1 per cent in the 341 receiving both radiotherapy and chemotherapy during a follow-up period of 2 to 15 years. There have been six examples of acute myelogenous leukemia seen to date, all in the group receiving combined modality therapy, an incidence of 1.8 per cent, but only one in a patient who received chemotherapy as an adjuvant.

TABLE I

HODGKIN'S DISEASE CLINICAL TRIAL

The Value of Adjuvant MOPP (CT) in the Radiation Therapy (RT) of Pathologic Stages I, II, and III Disease

(actuarial percentages at eight years, as of February 1977)

Pathologic Stage*	Number of Patients	Freedom from Relapse			Survival		
		RT	RT + CT	p (Gehan)	RT	RT + CT	p (Gehan)
**IA, IIA,	87	70	86	.02	87	97	.46
IB & IIB	50	81	87	.57	87	92	.92
IIIA	60	71	96	.03	85	88	.30
IIIB	44	7	50	.04	40 ± 12.8	67 ± 10.3	.62 (.10)***
All A's	147	70	90	.002	88	92	.34
All B's	94	45	70	.05	63 ± 8.9	80 ± 5.9	.62 (.06)
All I, II & III	241	61.6	81.5	.0009	77.7 ± 5.3	87.5 ± 3.7	.46 (.11)

* includes E and S subgroups of Ann Arbor system

** actuarial percentages at 6 years

*** p (Gehan) in ( ) calculated after 4.0 years

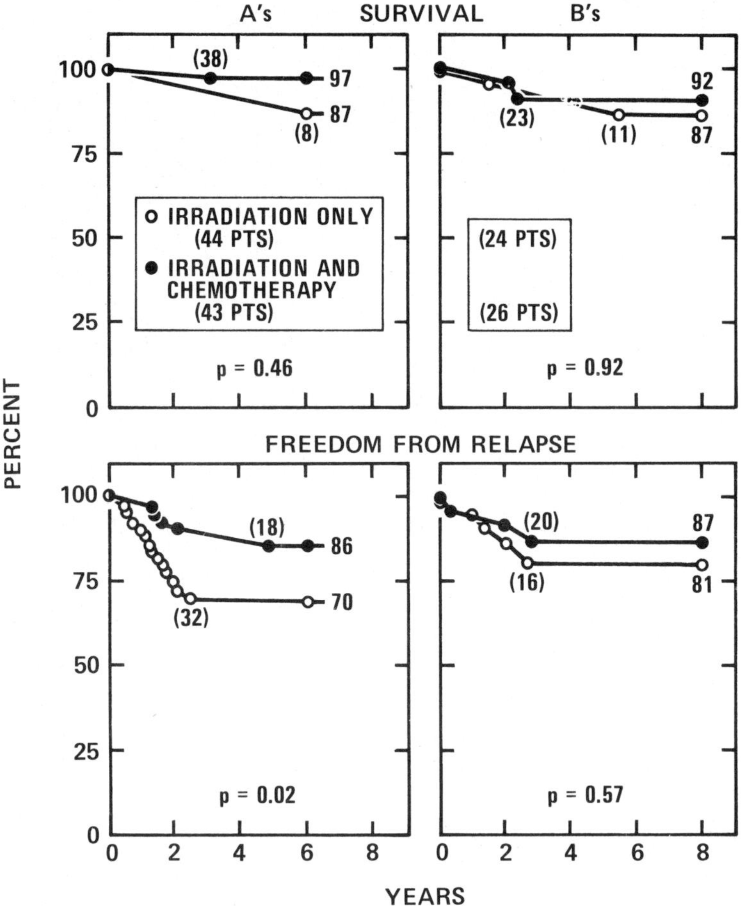

Fig. 1. Actuarial survival and freedom from relapse curves of randomized clinical trials of adjuvant MOP(P) in the radiation management of pathologic stages I and II Hodgkin's disease with (B) and without (A) systemic symptoms as of February, 1977. ( ) indicate numbers of patients at risk at the final calculations, no events occurring thereafter. p-values are by the method of Gehan[10]

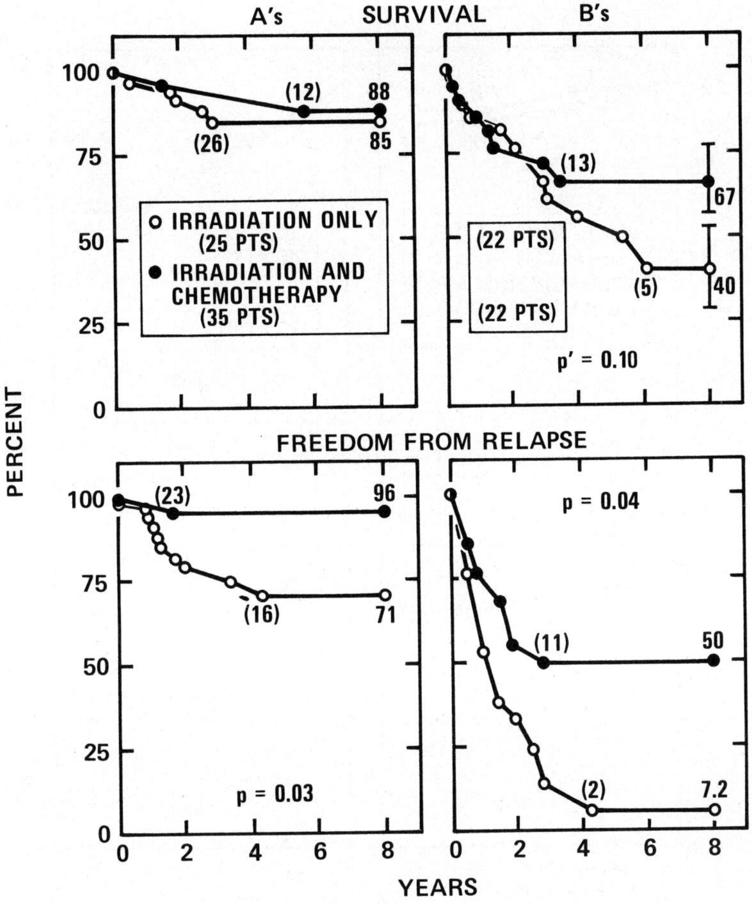

Fig. 2. Actuarial survival and freedom from relapse curves of randomized clinical trials of adjuvant MOP (P) in the radiation management of pathologic stage III Hodgkin's disease with (B) and without (A) systemic symptons as of February, 1977. ( ) indicate number of patients at risk at the final calculations, no events occurring thereafter. Standard errors shown for the final calculation at that point. p' is Gehan value after 4.0 years.

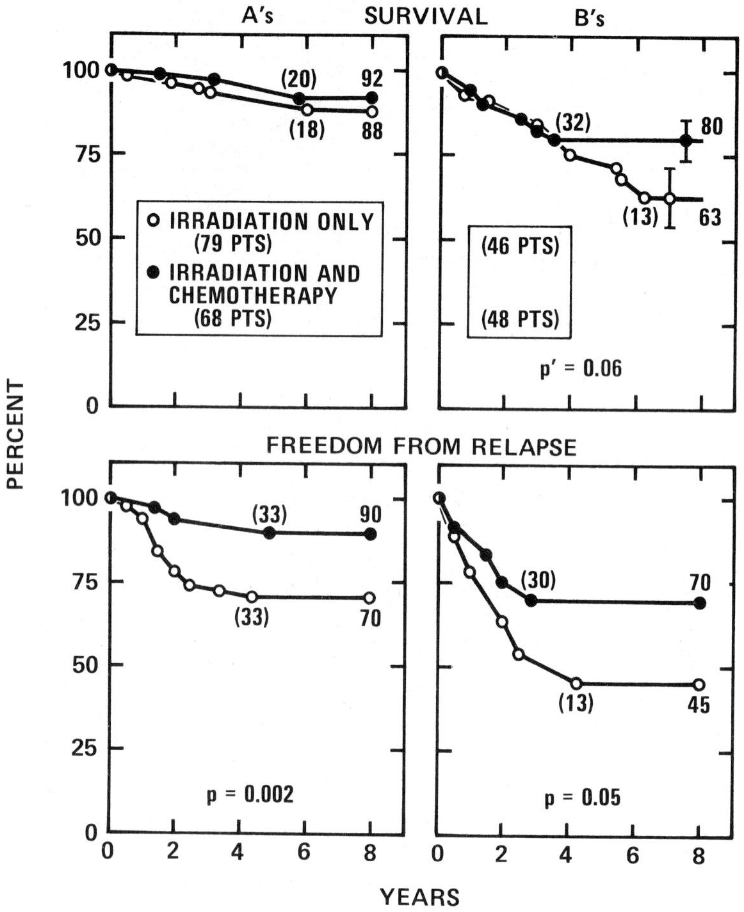

Fig. 3. Actuarial survival and freedom from relapse curves of randomized clinical trials of adjuvant MOP (P) in the radiation management of pathologic stages I, II and III Hodgkin's disease with (B) and without (A) systemic symptoms as of February, 1977. ( ) indicate number of patients at risk at the final calculations, no events occurring thereafter. Standard errors shown for the final calculation at that point. p' is Gehan value after 4.0 years.

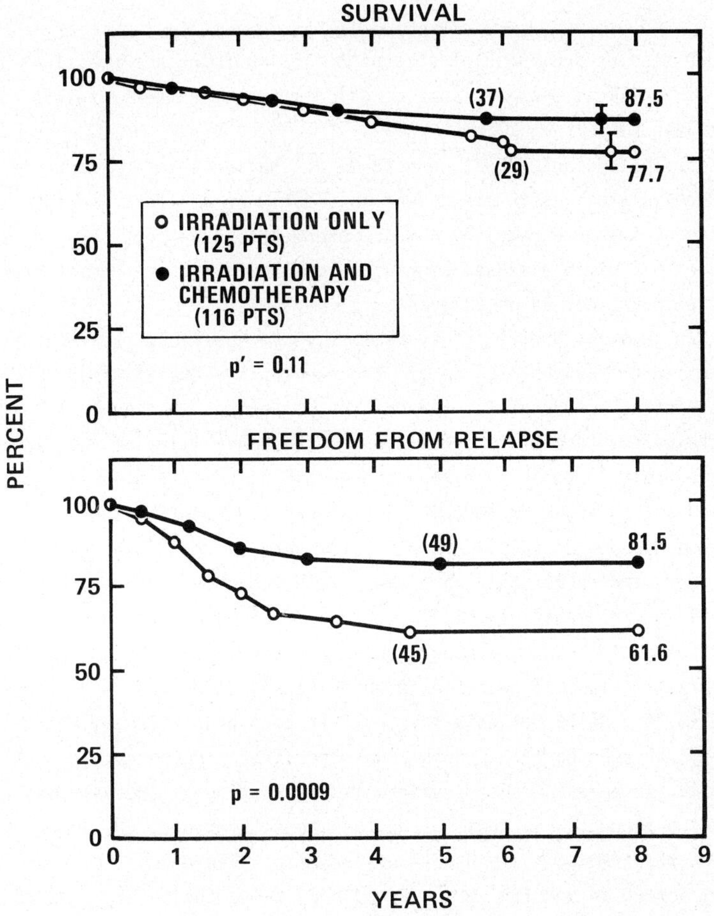

Fig. 4. Actuarial survival and freedom from relapse curves of randomized clinical trials of adjuvant MOP (P) in the radiation management of pathologic stages I, II and III Hodgkin's disease as of February, 1977. ( ) indicate number of patients at risk at the final calculations, no events occurring thereafter. Standard errors shown for the final calculation at that point. p' is Gehan value after 4.0 years.

CONCLUSIONS

These studies and those of others[14,15] raise important questions in the management of Hodgkin's disease, some of which must be tested by future careful clinical trials.

1) Should adjuvant MOP(P) be used in all patients following radiation therapy for Hodgkin's disease? The answer is clearly no at the present time. The survival benefits have required six or more years to project and are primarily for those with PS IIIB disease, a group which should receive chemotherapy as the major treatment, not as an adjuvant.

2) Can adjuvant MOP(P) safely replace very wide field radiotherapy programs for patients with favorable disease? The answer is a qualified yes. There has been no loss of effectiveness of the primary management when evaluated at six years. But the certainty of male sterility and the possibility of late acute myelogenous leukemia in those receiving the combined modality program should be considered in comparing the morbidities of the treatment options.

3) Can the use of adjuvant MOP(P) eliminate or reduce the need for diagnostic laparotomy and splenectomy in patients with Hodgkin's disease? The answer is probably no, at least at this time. The studies reported herein were all performed on patients who have undergone splenectomy and the conclusions may not be appropriately applied to patients who have not. For patients with systemic symptoms, PS IB and IIB patients have not yet been benefitted by adjuvant chemotherapy, whereas PS IIIB should always receive chemotherapy in their management program. In some instances, diagnostic laparotomy is the only way to distinguish these two groups. For those without systemic symptoms, the adjuvant program has not yet resulted in a clear survival benefit. Radiation fields are usually different for PS IA and IIA versus PS IIIA disease, the former treated with subtotal nodal fields (sparing the pelvis), and the latter with total nodal fields.

4) Can chemotherapy programs other than MOP(P) be used as an adjuvant for the radiation management of Hodgkin's disease? The answer is maybe. Certainly it would be desirable to reduce the acute morbidity and duration of the adjuvant program. It might also be safer to employ regimens without one or the other of the drugs in MOP(P) which might be most mutagenic (i.e. - procarbazine) or most responsible for the male sterility (i.e. - alkylating agent). However, such modifications of the adjuvant program will require careful randomized trials using MOP(P) as a control to demonstrate the new adjuvants' greater safety and tolerance without the loss of therapeutic benefit.

REFERENCES

1. Moore, M. R., Bull, J. M., Jones, S. E., Rosenberg, S. A. and Kaplan, H. S. (1972) Sequential radiotherapy and chemotherapy in the treatment of Hodgkin's

disease - A progress report. Ann. Intern. Med. 77:1-9.
2. Rosenberg, S. A., Moore, M. R., Bull, J. M., Jones, S. E., and Kaplan, H. S. (1972) Combination chemotherapy and radiotherapy for Hodgkin's disease. Cancer 30:1505-1510.
3. Rosenberg, S. A. and Kaplan, H. S. (1975) The management of stages I, II, and III Hodgkin's disease with combined radiotherapy and chemotherapy.
4. Lukes, R. J. (1971) Criteria for involvement of lymph node, bone marrow, spleen and liver in Hodgkin's disease. Cancer Res. 31:1755-1767.
5. Rosenberg, S. A. and Kaplan, H. S. (1970) Hodgkin's disease and other malignant lymphomas. Calif. Med. 113:23-28.
6. Carbone, P. P., Kaplan, H. S., Musshoff, K., Smithers, D. W., and Tubiana, M. (1971) Report of the Committee on Hodgkin's Disease Staging Classification. Cancer Res. 31:1860-1861.
7. Castellino, R. A., Glatstein, E., Turbow, M. M., Rosenberg, S. A., and Kaplan, H. S. (1974) Latent radiation injury of lungs or heart activated by steroid withdrawal. Ann. Intern. Med. 80:593-599.
8. Jacobs, C., Portlock, C. S. and Rosenberg, S. A. (1976) Prednisone in MOPP chemotherapy for Hodgkin's disease. Br. Med. Journal 2:1469-1471.
9. Kaplan, E. S., and Meier, P. (1958) Non-parametric estimation from incomplete observation. Am. Stat. Assoc. J. 53:457-480.
10. Gehan, E. A. (1965) A generalized Wilcoxon test for comparing arbitrarily singly-censored samples. Biometrika 52:203-233.
11. DeVita, V. T., Jr., Serpick, A. A., and Carbone, P. P. (1970) Combination chemotherapy in the treatment of advanced Hodgkin's disease. Ann. Intern. Med. 73:881-895.
12. Arseneau, J. C., Sponzo, R. W., Levin, D. L., Schnipper, L. E., Bonner, H., Young, R. C., Canellos, G. P., Johnson, R. E., and DeVita, V. T. (1972) Non-lymphomatous malignant tumors complicating Hodgkin's disease. N. Engl. J. Med. 287:1119-1122.
13. Kaplan, H. S., Glatstein, E. and Thoelecke, L. (1977) Unpublished observations
14. Tubiana, M. (1974) The place of radiotherapy in the treatment of malignant lymphoma. Clinics in Haematology 3:161-193.
15. O'Connell, J. J., Wiernik, P. H., Brace, K. C., Byhardt, R. W., and Greene, W. H. (1975) A combined modality approach to the treatment of Hodgkin's disease. Preliminary results of a prospective randomized clinical trial. Cancer 35:1055.

Adjuvant Therapy of Cancer, S.E. Salmon and S.E. Jones eds.
© 1977 Elsevier/North-Holland Biomedical Press, Amsterdam

ADJUVANT CHEMOTHERAPY AFTER RADIOTHERAPY IN STAGE I AND II HODGKIN'S DISEASE. E.O.R.T.C. Radiochemotherapy Cooperative Group.

Presented by G. Mathé, M. Tubiana and M. Hayat.
Institut de Cancérologie et d'Immunogénétique and
Institut Gustave Roussy, 94800-Villejuif, France.

As early as 1963, when the possibility of permanently curing patients suffering from Hodgkin's Disease was demonstrated, the problem arose of whether one could improve the quality of the results by combining the two major therapeutic weapons of the epoch, sequentially: radiotherapy and chemotherapy. Thus, in 1964, we suggested to the European Organisation of Research on the Treatment of Cancer (EORTC) the creation of a radiotherapy-chemotherapy group[+] to undertake such a study. At that time, data in the literature on the combination of radiotherapy and chemotherapy in stages I and II of Hodgkin's disease were few and fragmentary. In addition, in certain studies the radiotherapy had been too weak to be effective and, in others, the chemotherapy had been limited to a few injections of nitrogen mustard (1,2). This is why it seemed useful to carry out a randomised trial in which all stage I and II patients would have received an efficient radiotherapy, and one of the two groups of patients a long-term adjuvant chemotherapy.

[+]The chairmen of this cooperative group have been: M. TUBIANA (1964-1967), K. BREUR (1967-1969), B. van der WERF-MESSING (1969-1972), A. LAUGIER (General Secretary); M. HAYAT (Statistician).

Cooperative Centres have been, in France : C.A.C. Bordeaux (C. LAGARDE), C.A.C. Caen (S. ABBATUCCI), Lyon (J. Papillon, L. Revol), Paris : Hôtel-Dieu (J. BOUSSER), C.A.C. Rouen (H. PIGUET), Villejuif (G. MATHE, M. TUBIANA, J.L. AMIEL). In Belgium : Brussels Institut Jules Bordet (J. HENRY), Liège (R. LEMAIRE), Louvain (A. WAMBERSIE). In Holland : Amsterdam (K. BREUR, M. BURGERS), Leiden (P. THOMAS), Nijmegen (C. HAANEN), Rotterdam (B. van der WERF-MESSING, W.G. STENFERT KROESE).

The members of the histology review committee : R. GERARD-MARCHANT, J. van UNNIK, and of the lymphography review committee : R.W. KROPHOLLER, J.D. PICARD, P. PARKOVITS, J.L. CHASSARD.

MATERIALS AND METHODS

The principle of this trial ("H1 Trial") has already been reported and here we will summarize it only briefly. All the patients included in the trial presented with clinical stage I or II of Hodgkin's disease. They had been classified after a clinical and radiological examination, which included, in particular, an ilio-lumbar lymphangiogram, x-ray of the mediastinum and, if necessary, tomographic examination, liver function tests and, in a few cases, liver biopsy. A laparotomy was not specific and this was never done before treatment. On the other hand, many patients underwent hepatic and splenic scanning.

The involved areas and the intermediate adjacent areas of the same side of the diaphragm were irradiated at a dose of 4000 rads delivered in four weeks, at 1000 rads per week (3). In the cases where the clinical or radiological lesions were large, the dose to these areas was increased to 4500 rads by superimposition.

Four to six weeks after the end of irradiation, the patients in complete remission were randomly assigned to one of the two following groups: a) no complementary treatment or b) long-term chemotherapy of weekly intravenous injections of vinblastine for two years.

All the patients were examined regularly every six months. At the time of each consultation the patients were examined clinically and x-rays of the thorax and abdomen, and measurement of the erythrocyte sedimentation rate were performed. The date taken as that of the first relapse was either that on which the first clinical symptoms were noticed by the patient or were revealed by the various examinations, or that of the appearance of the first biological signs when the clinical symptoms appeared after the increase in the sedimentation rate.

The trial was started in 1964 and ended in 1970. Fourteen hospitals participated in it: six in France, five in Holland, and three in Belgium. There were 296 patients included in the study, and the preliminary results have already appeared in two publications (4,5,6) The group of patients followed, in particular at Villejuif, has been the object of a recent study.

Results

1. Effect of the treatment on the proportion of patients in first remission.

Figure 1 shows that the proportion of patients in first remission

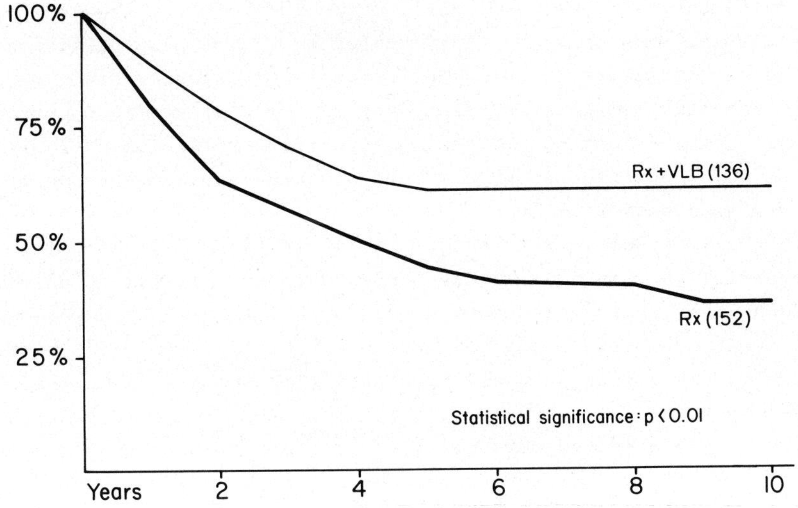

Fig. 1 Actuarial curve of first complete remission.
Rx = radiotherapy
VLB = vinblastine

TABLE I

TRIAL H_1 E.O.R.T.C.

LOCALISATION OF THE FIRST RELAPSE : (5 years follow-up)

	RADIO-THERAPY	RADIO-THERAPY + VELBE	TOTAL	STATISTICAL SIGNIFICANCE
PATIENTS AT RISK	154	138	292	
RECURRENCE IN AN IRRADIATED AREA	17 11%	8 6%	25	N.S.
RECURRENCE IN A NON IRRADIATED AREA	42 27%	20 15%	62	$p < 0.02$
EXTRA NODAL RECURRENCE	29 19%	22 16%	51	N.S.

N.S. NOT SIGNIFICANT

at the tenth year is significantly lower in the group treated by radiotherapy alone than in that treated by radiotherapy followed by long-term administration of vinblastine. For example, five years after the start of the treatment, 43% of the patients in the group treated with radiotherapy alone were in first remission as against 63% in the group treated by combined radiotherapy and chemotherapy administered sequentially.

This difference is not due to a delay in the appearance of relapses. Contrary to what has happened in certain trials in which the chemotherapy had been carried out only during a brief period (7), the difference between the proportions of patients in first remission in the two groups did not diminish with time and seems, on the contrary, to have a tendancy to increase. This suggests that the chemo-therapy used had permanently sterilised a considerable number of occult lesions. Moreover, one notices that relapses continue to arise until the ninth year in the group treated by radiotherapy alone, whereas they no longer arise after the fifth year in the group treated by the combined therapy.

2. Analysis of the different types of relapse.

Table I shows that the incidence of relapse in the non-irradiated lymphatic areas of the group treated by the combined therapy is about half that of the group treated by radiotherapy alone, and this difference is statistically significant.

The frequency of relapse in the irradiated lymphatic areas of the group treated by the combined therapy is also half that of the group treated by radiotherapy alone, but this difference is not significant on account of the small size of the sample. On the other hand, there is no significant difference in the frequency of the extra-lymphatic relapses, especially hepatic and splenic.

This contrast between the good effects of chemotherapy on the lymphatic lesions and the poor results, or lack of them, on the visceral lesions is, at first, surprising. Nevertheless, the majority of lymphatic relapses in the non-irradiated areas arise at the level of the lumbo-aortic lymph nodes as the great majority of patients presented with supra-diaphragmatic lesions and had a lymphography which was considered to be normal; the occult intra-lymphatic lesions were, therefore, small.

The methods of hepatic and splenic exploration (essentially scanning) are much less sensitive than those of the exploration of the lymph nodes. It is, therefore, possible that the size of the occult lesions was greater.

This would suggest that vinblastine chemotherapy had a favourable effect on small lesions and was less effective on more voluminous lesions.

The absence of late relapses in the group treated by the combined therapy is in favour of this hypothesis.

3. Interval between the start of treatment and relapse.

Ninety percent of relapses arise less than four years after the initial treatment. In the patients treated at Villejuif, a study of the interval between the beginning of the treatment and the time of relapse has been carried out. This interval is, on average, nine months longer in the patients treated by combined radio-chemotherapy than in those treated by radiotherapy alone. This difference is relatively short-lived. The doubling time of Hodgkin node lesions is of the order of a month in radiotherapy patients. A delay of nine months in the appearance of clinically detectable relapses shows that the effect of the chemotherapy on the number of tumoral cells is weak since the number of surviving cells would be of the order of 2‰ (a delay of 10 months, being 10 doubling times, would correspond to 1‰ of cells surviving). This confirms the inefficiency of this type of chemotherapy on voluminous lesions.

4. Percentage of patients surviving.

The proportion of patients surviving is the same in the two groups and is close to 70% (Fig. 2) after 10 years. It then seems to be stabilized, but one cannot, however, exclude the possibility of some later deaths.

The fact that the proportion of survivors is the same in the two groups, whereas the number of relapses is greater in the group of patients treated by radiotherapy alone, shows that, after relapse, one can cure (or keep alive) a greater number of patients in the group initially treated by the radiotherapy only. It must be noted, in this connection, that the interval between the first and second relapses is similar in the two groups (about 15.7 months in patients treated by radiotherapy + vinblastine, as against 18.5 months in those treated by radiotherapy alone).

Moreover, the same proportion of patients in the two groups presented with a second relapse after the first. These similarities are not surprising as the treatment of relapses was similar for the two groups.

The absence of difference in long-term survival, therefore, seems due to the difference in survival rate after the second relapse. As a hypothesis, one can ask oneself if the differences in rescue

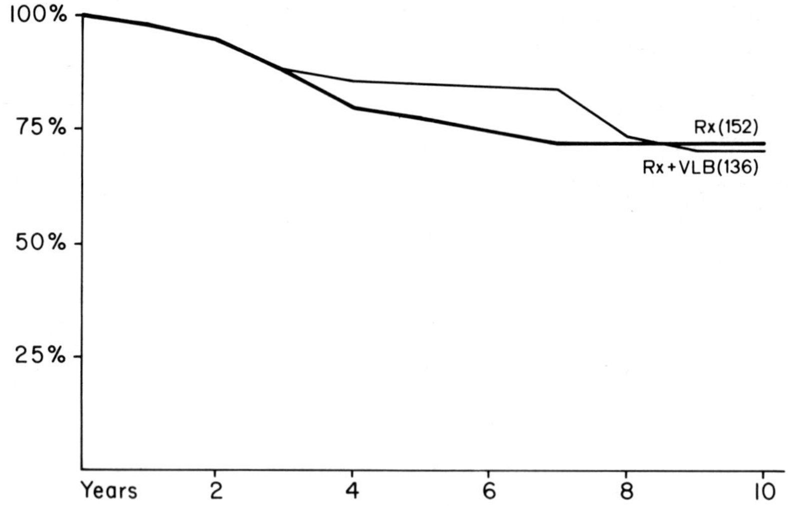

Fig. 2 Actuarial curve of survival.
Rx = radiotherapy
VLB = vinblastine

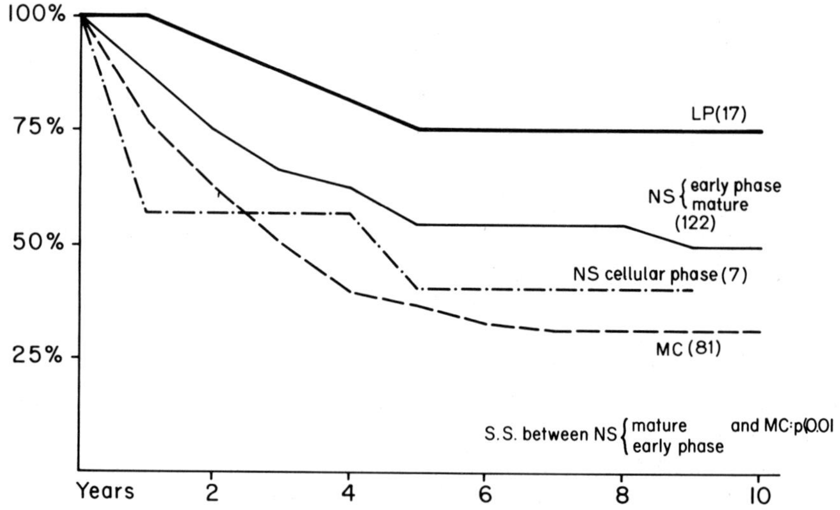

Fig. 3 Actuarial curve of first complete remission according to histology.
LP = lymphoid predominance
NS = nodular sclerosis
MC = mixed cellularity

capacity of the radiotherapy group are not particularly noticeable after the second relapse. They could be connected with differences in tolerance to the treatment. It is possible that the patients who received a two-year course of vinblastine after radiotherapy, followed by chemotherapy at the time of the first relapse, tolerate subsequent treatment less well than those who were initially treated by radiotherapy and received chemotherapy only at the time of first relapse.

5. Prognostic factors.

The question was whether the influence of prognostic factors could still be found in this sample of patients and whether the usefulness of chemotherapy was the same for the various prognostic groups.

a) Histologic type. The patients were classified according to the four histologic types of the Rye classification (8), and a significant correlation between the prognosis and the histologic type was regarded as much from the point of view of the percentage of patients in first remission (Fig. 3) as the percentage of patients surviving (Fig. 4). At 10 years, for example, more than 80% of the survivors are patients of 'good' prognostic histologic type, whereas, among the patients of mixed cellular histologic type, the percentage of survivors is only about 60%.

Chemotherapy appears more useful for the poor-risk histologic type (mixed cellularity) than for those histologic types indicating a good prognosis (nodular sclerosis and lymphocytic predominance) (Fig. 5). Moreover, the percentage of patients surviving is no different in the two therapeutic groups.

The percentage of relapses is also lower in the group of nodular sclerosis type patients treated by the combined therapy than in those treated by radiotherapy alone (Fig. 5). However, the difference is not statistically significant and, once again, there is no difference from the point of view of survival.

b) Influence of age and sex. The results are significantly less good in patients of more than 40 years of age. For men one observes both poor therapeutic results and greater effectiveness of adjuvant chemotherapy than for women.

c) Presence or absence of systemic symptoms have no significant influence on prognosis. On the other hand, the erythrocyte sedimentation rate for stage 1 is significantly correlated with prognosis, this being worse for patients with ESR of more than 70 mins. during the first hour.

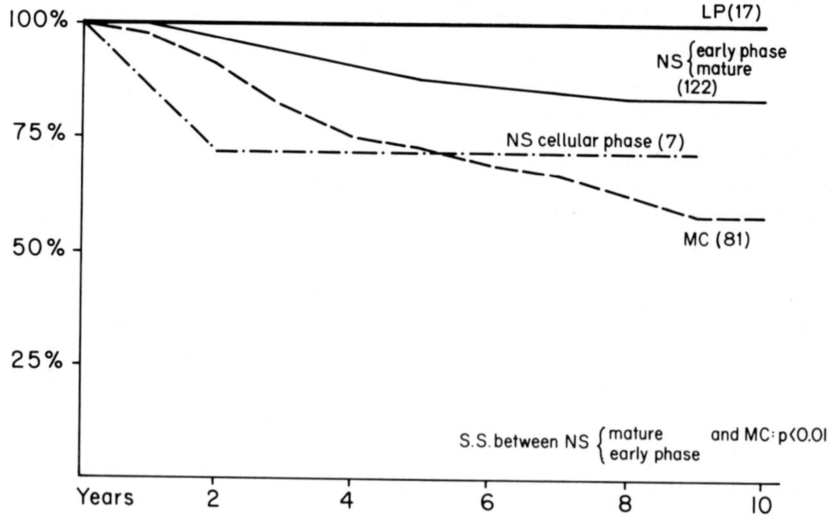

Fig. 4 Actuarial curve of survival according to histology.
LP = lymphoid predominance
NS = nodular sclerosis
MC = mixed cellularity

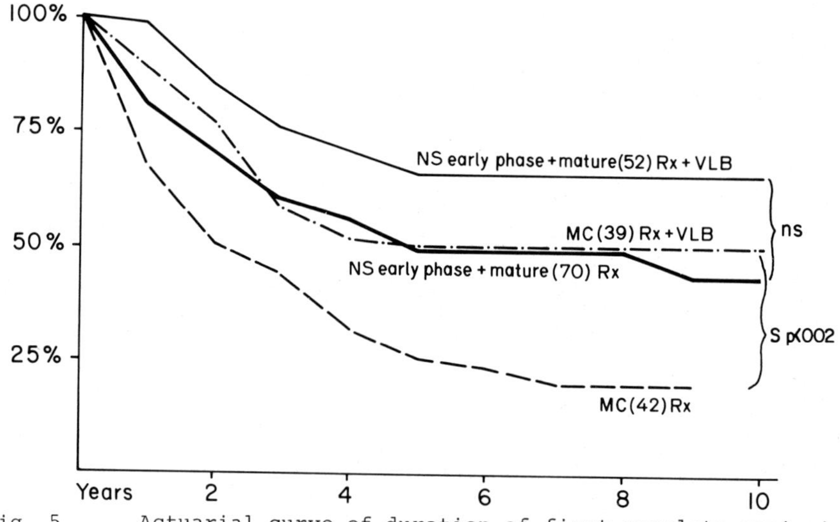

Fig. 5 Actuarial curve of duration of first complete remission according to histology and treatment.
NS = nodular sclerosis
MC = mixed cellularity
Rx = radiotherapy
VLB = vinblastine

d) Mediastinal involvement. The long-term results confirm our previous observations, according to which, for clinical stage II, the proportion of patients in first remission, like the proportion of patients surviving, is lower in patients with an uninvolved mediastinum than in those with an involved mediastinum.

In taking into account these different prognostic factors, which are also partially linked to each other, one can define two groups of patients: a) the so-called 'good' prognosis group, which is composed of subjects of less than 40 years of age, in whom the lesion is of the nodular sclerosis or lymphocytic predominance type, who have an involved mediastinum, are without general symptoms, and who have a sedimentation rate lower than 50 mm in the first hour; and b) the poor-risk group into which fall all the other patients.

For the good prognosis group, who represent about 40% of the patients, the proportion of relapses is low, about 30%, whereas for the so-called poor-risk group it is about 60% (Fig. 6). Chemotherapy is as efficacious in the good as in the poor-risk cases and reduces the frequency of relapses by half in both groups of patients. Survival is of the order of 85% at year 10 for the good cases and of about 65% for the poor-risk ones (Fig. 6).

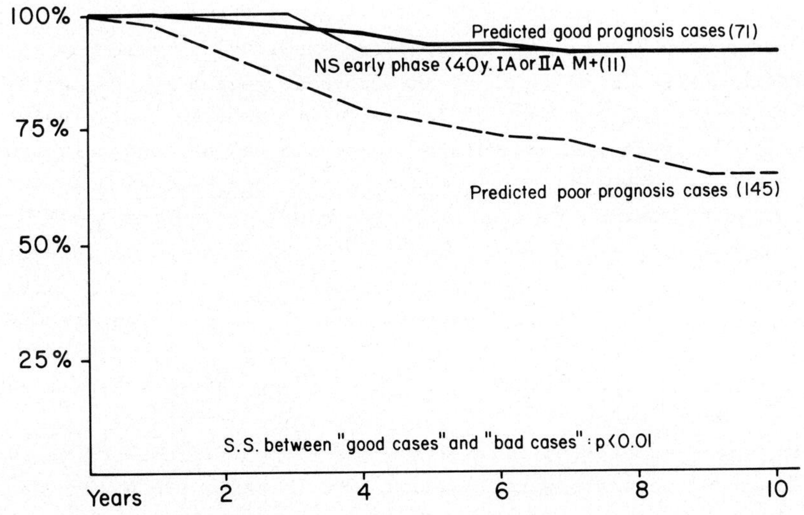

Fig. 6 Actuarial curve of survival according to prognosis factors.
M = mediastinal involvement

DISCUSSION

Two conclusions arise from this trial. The first is the effectiveness of long-term chemotherapy, even when given at moderate doses. Vinblastine applied during two years is capable of sterilizing the small lesions and of significantly reducing the frequency of relapses. Thanks to this therapeutic treatment combined with radiotherapy, about 80% of Hodgkin's disease patients of good prognosis are in first remission at the 10th year. The second fact which emerges from this study is the great frequency of relapses in the lumbo-aortic and extra-nodal regions. When interpreting this result one must take into account the fact that these patients have not undergone an exploratory laparotomy, and one can, therefore, assume that about 30% of them had a spleen involvement at the time of treatment.

In addition, this study demonstrates the inadequacy of the lymphography, which is not capable of revealing the numerous occult lesions and this explains the frequency of relapses in lumbo-aortic regions in patients who have not had long-term chemotherapy.

In view of the results of this first trial, a second trial was undertaken by the EORTC. The patients were randomly divided into two groups. In the first group of patients, a systematic laparotomy was performed with a splenectomy and biopsy of the lumbo-aortic and iliac nodes. In the second group, these examinations were not performed. After irradiation of the thoracic region by the mantle field technique, both groups of patients were treated: a splenic and lumbo-aortic radiotherapy in patients who had not had a laparotomy, and only a lumbo-aortic irradiation in those who had had one.

A long-term chemotherapy (vinblastine alone or vinblastine + procarbazine) was carried out only on patients of mixed cellularity or lymphocytic depletion histologic types.

The aim of this trial was two-fold: (1) to compare the effectiveness of splenic radiotherapy with splenectomy for the treatment of lesions of the spleen; (2) to analyse the prognostic significance of splenic involvement.

This trial was started in 1972 and was stopped at the end of 1976, when about 300 patients were included. It is still too early to present the results of this trial. However, the preliminary data show that the proportion of patients surviving and the proportion of relapses are not significantly different in the two groups. The efficacy of splenic radiotherapy, therefore, seems comparable to that of splenectomy. As for the sequelae of this radiotherapy, they are seen above all at the level of the upper part of the left kidney, but they seem slight and have no functional repercussions (9).

Furthermore, in the group of patients having undergone splenectomy one can study the prognostic significance of splenic invasion. The preliminary data on 260 patients indicate that the frequent nodal relapses in the non-irradiated areas, that is essentially at the level of the iliac or inguinal nodes, are seen only in cases with an invaded spleen (6 cases of iliac or inguinal extension among 36 patients), whereas they were not found in 88 patients whose spleen had not been involved. On the other hand, there is no significant difference between the two groups as far as extra-nodal extension is concerned (3 cases out of 88 patients in the group with negative splenectomy as against 1 case out of 36 patients in the group with positive splenectomy).

These data serve as the basis for the elaboration of a new protocol, which would include two groups: a group of cases with good prognosis, as defined above, and who would nevertheless undergo a laparatomy with splenectomy. They would not be definitively considered as of good prognosis unless no Hodgkin's tissue was found by the splenectomy. It seems, then, that for these patients one could be satisfied with a mantle irradiation eventually combined with an irradiation of the lumbo-aortic nodes. According to the data of the first trial, about 28% of relapses have been observed in such cases, but the experience acquired from the systematic splenectomies shows that the spleen must be invaded in about 20% of cases. The probability of relapse in patients not having an involved spleen must, therefore, not exceed 5% to 10% of cases. The data from the splenectomy - splenic radiotherapy trial give similar indications: a single extra-nodal relapse among 29 patients with negative splenectomy falls into this category. If one admits that at least one patient in two can eventually be permanently cured by an intensive chemotherapy, one could end up with a rate of cure superior to 95%, and with the treatment limited to a regional radiotherapy and not including any chemotherapy in 90% of patients. This is particularly important for young subjects as one then avoids all irradiation or lesion of the gonads by drugs.

In the group of poor-risk patients, in which all the other patients would be grouped, experience shows that one needs, at the very least, to extend the radiotherapy until it is a total lymphoid radiotherapy, combined eventually with chemotherapy.

This protocol will, therefore, enable one to adapt the severity of the treatment to the severity of the illness.

SUMMARY

The patients were staged after clinical and radiological examination. No laparotomy was performed. Radiotherapy was carried out using the mantle field or the inverted Y technique. The patients were randomly assigned to two groups: a) no further treatment, and b) a weekly injection of vinblastine for two years. Fourteen hospital centers participated, six in France, five in Holland and three in Belgium.

From 1964 to 1970, 296 patients were included in the study. The proportion of recurrence-free patients is significantly higher amongst those who received a long-term adjuvant chemotherapy. The incidence of recurrences in liver, spleen and lung and in irradiated areas does not differ between the two groups, but the incidence of reçurrence in non-irradiated para-aortic or iliac areas is significantly higher in the group of patients who did not receive chemotherapy. This suggests that only small aggregates of neoplastic cells, which were not visible on pretreatment lymphangiogram, were sterilised.

In spite of the high incidence of relapses in the group treated by radiotherapy alone, no difference in survival between the two groups was observed.

These results, as well as the preliminary ones of two other trials established as the logical consequences of this conclusion, are discussed.

REFERENCES

1. Clarysse A., Kenis Y., Mathé G. Cancer chemotherapy. Its role in the treatment strategy of hematologic malignancies and solid tumors. Heidelberg-New York, 1976, Springer Verlag.
2. Mathé G., Tubiana M. (eds). Natural history diagnosis and treatment of Hodgkin's disease. 2 vol., Copenhagen, 1973, Munksgaard.
3. Kaplan H.S. Radiology 1962, 78, 553.
4. E.O.R.T.C. Radiotherapy-Chemotherapy Group. Europ. J. Cancer 1972, 8, 553.
5. Tubiana M, Mathé G. Series Haematologica 1973, 6, 199.
6. E.O.R.T.C. Communication to European Congress, Radiology. Amsterdam, 1971, Excerpta Medica.
7. Hancock P.E.T., Austin D.E., Smith P.G. Lancet 1973, 1, 832.
8. Lukes R.J., Craver L.F., Hall T.C., Rappaport H., Ruben P. Cancer Res. 1966, 26, 1311.
9. Le Bourgeois J.P. Unpublished data.

Adjuvant Therapy of Cancer, S.E. Salmon and S.E. Jones eds.
© 1977 Elsevier/North-Holland Biomedical Press, Amsterdam

CHEMOTHERAPY AND TOTAL NODAL RADIOTHERAPY IN PATHOLOGICAL STAGE IIB, IIIA, AND IIIB HODGKIN'S DISEASE

Charles A. Coltman, Jr.*, Eleanor Montague** and Thomas E. Moon**

For The Southwest Oncology Group

*Wilford Hall USAF Medical Center, Lackland AFB, Tx. 78236

**The University of Texas System Cancer Center, Houston, Tx. 77030

SUMMARY

One hundred forty-four patients with Pathological Stage IIB, IIIA and IIIB Hodgkin's disease were treated with MOPP* followed by total nodal radiotherapy with an 87% (125/144) complete and 7% (10/144) partial response. Disease free survival is 76% (95/125) and overall survival is 86% (124/144) with follow-up to 335 weeks. The complete response rate, disease free, and overall survival did not differ for 3 or >3 cycles of MOPP (P=0.50; P=0.12; P=0.87 respectively). The complete response rate for patients with Stage II and III_N was significantly lower than Stage III_S and III_{NS} (P=0.04). The disease free and overall survival did not differ with respect to extent of disease (all P values >0.16). Life threatening toxicity occurred in 10 patients (4 leukopenia, 5 thrombopenia and 1 CNS) with no difference for 3 or >3 cycles of MOPP (P>0.22). These data show that 3 cycles of MOPP, followed by total nodal radiotherapy can be safely delivered to patients with intermediate stages of Hodgkin's disease with excellent disease free and overall survival.

INTRODUCTION

Properly applied radiotherapy is curative in a substantial proportion of patients with localized (Stage I and II) Hodgkin's disease (1,2). High dose combination chemotherapy (MOPP) is curative in as high as 40% of previously untreated patients with advanced (Stage IV) Hodgkin's disease with follow-up to 7 and 10 years (3,4). In 1971, when this Southwest Oncology Group Study was initiated, the disease free survival of patients with IIB and IIIB Hodgkin's disease treated with total nodal irradiation was considerably less favorable (5).

*Mechlorethamine, Oncovin, Prednisone and Procarbazine

This study was designed to combine MOPP chemotherapy with total nodal radiotherapy in laparotomy Staged IIB, IIIA and IIIB Hodgkin's disease. The sequence of MOPP followed by radiotherapy was chosen to determine the safety and effectiveness with which total nodal radiotherapy could be delivered following MOPP chemotherapy. Further objectives were to promptly control B symptoms and to reduce bulk disease and thus minimize the size of the radiotherapy ports. This single arm Phase I Study allowed for the gradual escalation of the dose of MOPP from 3 to 6 cycles as tolerance to radiotherapy was demonstrated.

MATERIALS AND METHODS

Patients with biopsy proven Hodgkin's disease with Ann Arbor Pathological Stage IIB, IIA and IIIB Hodgkin's disease who had received no prior therapy, were eligible for this study. Each patient gave informed consent. Preoperative Clinical Staging included isotope scans, metastatic bone survey, and lymphogram. Pathological Staging included percutaneous bone marrow biopsy and liver biopsy, if liver involvement was suspected. All those with negative biopsies underwent a staging laparotomy, splenectomy, wedge and needle biopsies of the liver and appropriate lymph node biopsies. Only after complete pathological staging were patients eligible for entry into the study. The tissue from the diagnostic lymph node biopsy was submitted for review by the Pathology Panel and Repository Center for Lymphoma Clinical Studies. Those found to have other than Hodgkin's disease were considered not eligible for the study.

The initial treatment consisted of 3 cycles of MOPP as previously reported (6). A minimum of four weeks, or until marrow recovery (maximum of ten weeks), elapsed from the last course of MOPP to the start of radiotherapy. All patients received total nodal radiotherapy, except for those treated at the M.D.Anderson Hospital where total abdominal radiotherapy, rather than the inverted Y port, was employed (7/144 patients). The minimum requirements for radiotherapy included: (1) A supervoltage radiation source of at least 2 MEV. (2) A time dose relationship of at least 750 rads tumor dose per week in five fractions. (3) Essential axis tumor dose estimation at levels of clinical interest. (4) Beam verification films. (5) Radiation therapy to be discontinued with a white blood count of less than

2000 per μL or platelet count less than 60,000 per μL. (6) Each participating institution to have their radiotherapy dose measurements and calculation monitored by the Radiological Physics Center.

The area of major and symtomatic involvement prior to chemotherapy was the first area to be treated with radiotherapy. In the majority of patients, the disease above the diaphram was treated first with anterior and posterior extended (mantle) fields excluding normal lung. In the presence of residual large mediastinal masses the field was reshaped periodically to avoid unnecessary irradiation to the lung. 4000 rads tumor dose was delivered in all involved areas in four to five and one-half weeks (not below 750 rads tissue dose per week) and additional boost was delivered thru reduced fields to residual disease at the discretion of the therapist.

Radiation below the diaphram started from 6 to 8 weeks following completion of the mantle port. The abdominal field covered the inquinal, femoral and deep iliac nodes bilaterally together with the paraortic nodes and the splenic pedicle. Treatment to the abdominal nodes was done in one course, or, in patients with poor tolerance to radiation therapy (poor tolerance to chemotherapy, excessive weignt loss and continuing disability), abdominal treatment was given in two courses. In that case, the upper two thirds of the abdominal nodes were treated first and, following a 4 to 8 week break, the pelvic and fermoral nodes. With total abdominal radiotherapy a 3000 rad tissue dose was delivered in 4 to 5 weeks and an additional 1000 rad tumor dose delivered thru reduced fields to residual disease.

Following termination of treatment patients were followed in unmaintained remission at monthly intervals for six months, two month intervals for six months, four month intervals for two years and yearly thereafter or until relapse. After 11 months of case accural the number of courses of MOPP administered was increased to 4 cycles. Five months later an analysis indicated that there was no significant difference in the ability to deliver radiotherapy following 3 or 4 cycles of MOPP and the dose was escalated to 5 and subsequently 6 cycles.

RESULTS

A total of 179 eligible patients were entered on to this study between April

1971 and February 1975. Thirty-five were considered not evaluable, four, because of inadequate data and 31 because of a major protocol violation. The protocol violations were relative to the administration of radiotherapy. Nineteen patients who had splenic and/or splenic node involvement, identified at staging laparotomy, failed to have treatment adminstered to a splenic pedicle port. Twelve patients did not begin radiotherapy to the pelvic nodes in spite of good marrow reserve

One hundred forty-four patients are considered partially or fully evaluable. One hundred twenty-five (87%) of the 144 patients had a complete response and an additional ten patients (7%) had a partial response giving a complete + partial response rate of 94% (135/144). Table 1 shows the distribution of patients by the extent of disease as well as their response to therapy.

TABLE 1

RESPONSE BY EXTENT OF DISEASE

STAGE	NO. PTS. (%)	CR (%)	PR (%)	
II	21 (15)	17 (81)	2 (10)	
III_N	25 (17)	19 (76)	3 (12)	P = 0.04*
III_S	34 (24)	30 (88)	1 (03)	
III_{NS}	64 (44)	59 (92)	4 (06)	

* Difference in Complete Response Rate

Stage III_N are those patients with disease limited to lymph nodes. III_S are those with only splenic involvement below the diaphragm and III_{NS} those with nodal and splenic involvement below the diaphragm. The distribution of 19 selected pre-treatment characteristics in these four staging groups is comparable, except that all Stage II patients had B symptoms (in accordance with the protocol) and Stage III_N had more patients <20 years of age (P=0.09) and fewer caucasians (P=0.06). The complete response rate was lower in the two groups with disease limited to lymph nodes (II and III_N) than in those with splenic involvement (III_S and III_{NS} (P=0.04). The characteristics which may account for these differences are symptom status, and an absolute lymphocyte count >1000 (all P values <0.08).

Table 2 shows the response rate with respect to the number of cycles of MOPP.

TABLE 2

RESPONSE BY EXTENT OF MOPP

CYCLES OF MOPP	NO. PTS. (%)	CR (%)	PR (%)	
3	68 (47)	62 (91)	4 (06)	*P=0.50
> 3	70 (49)	63 (90)	2 (03)	
< 3	6 (04)	0 (00)	4 (67)	

* Difference in complete response rate

Only six patients received two cycles of MOPP prior to radiotherapy and none of them achieved a complete response. The distribution of patient characteristics is comparable in the two large treatment groups. There is no difference in response rates (P=0.50).

Table 3 shows the complete response rate by histological type and extent of disease. One hundred-ten patients have had histological review and in 98% of instances the Pathology Review Panel confirmed the diagnosis of Hodgkin's disease. There was, however, only 52% concurrence when the contributing institution pathologist's and the review hematopathologist's cell type interpretations were compared.

TABLE 3

RESPONSE BY CELL TYPE AND EXTENT OF DISEASE

CELL	TOTAL		II	III_N	III_S	III_{SN}
TYPE*	NO. (%)	CR (%)	CR (%)	CR (%)	CR (%)	CR (%)
LP	7(05)	7(100)	0(00)	4(100)	1(100)	2(100)
NS	74(55)	60(81)	13(81)	7(64)	15(83)	25(86)
MC	49(36)	44(90)	1(50)	5(71)	10(91)	28(97)
LD	5(04)	5(100)	1(100)	0(00)	1(100)	3(100)

*LP = Lymphocyte predominant; NS = Nodular sclerosis; MC = Mixed cellular: LD = Lymphocyte depleted.

The majority of patients had nodular sclerosis (55%) and mixed cellular disease

(26%). There is no difference in the total complete response rate with respect to histology. There is a suggestion that the complete response rate for mixed cellular disease is lower in patients with Stage II and III_N (P=0.066).

Table 4 shows the complete response rate by symptom status and extent of disease.

TABLE 4

RESPONSE BY SYMPTOM STATUS AND EXTENT OF DISEASE

SYMPTOM STATUS	TOTAL NO.(%)	CR(%)	II CR(%)	III_N CR(%)	III_S CR(%)	III_{NS} CR(%)
A	69(48)	62(90)	0(00)	12(92)	16(84)	33(86)
B*	74(52)	62(84)	17(81)	7(58)	13(93)	26(93)

* P = 0.004

There is no difference in total complete response rate with respect to symptom status. Again, there is a significantly lower complete response rate in the symptomatic patients with Stage III_N disease (P=0.04).

When the whole group is considered there is no difference in complete response rate with respect to sex, age, race, histological type (as determined by pathological review), symptom status, clinical stage, white blood count or performance status. There is, however, evidence that the complete response rate differs with respect to absolute lymphocyte count (P=0.02), and weight loss (P=0.02). Favorable patient characteristics are an absolute lymphocyte count of >1,800 and no weight loss.

The median time to complete response for all patients is 12 weeks. There is no significant difference in time to complete response when considered with respect to extent of disease (all P values > 0.45) or number of courses of MOPP (P=0.05). Seventy-six percent of those who achieved a complete response (95/125) remain free of disease while the Kaplan and Meyer response duration estimate curve plateaus at 70% with follow-up to 250 weeks. The last relapse occurred at 175 weeks. There is no significant difference in complete response duration with respect to extent of disease (all P values > 0.16) of number of cycles of MOPP (all P values > 0.12). There is no evidence of a difference in survival with respect to stage (all P values > 0.16) or number of cycles of MOPP (P=0.87).

There have been a total of 3 fatalities due to toxicity in this study. One patient developed a thrombotic thrombocytopenic purpura-like syndrome with a central nervous system death and two patients, who received 4 cycles of MOPP followed by radiotherapy, had fatal thrombopenia. Seven additional life threatening toxicities occurred; 4 granulocytopenia (< 500/μL) and 3 thrombocytopenia (<50,000/μL). Additional mild to moderate toxicity included neuropathy, nausea, vomiting and alopecia. Combining severe, life threatening and fatal toxicities there is no difference in toxicity rate by the number of cycles of MOPP or the extent of disease (both B values > 0.22).

Marginal recurrances were noted in 10 patients (6 neck, 1 axilla and 3 hilum of lung). Six of those were irradiated and are now without disease. Five localized recurrences occurred within the radiotherapy field (2 axilla and neck and 1 L-2 vertebral body). The remaining relapses were disseminated.

The abdominal radiotherapy was prolonged by more than a week longer than scheduled in 21 patients because of cytopenias, but was completed in all cases. The dose administered to the pelvic ports was lower than scheduled (when a split course was given) in 32 patients. The median dose delivered to the pelvis in those 32 was 2000 rads.

The Radiological Physics Center Dosimetry Review of the participating institutions showed that, of 133 patients reviewed, 97 (73%) were within ± 5% of the reported dose.

DISCUSSION

This Phase I study was the initial combined modality study of the Southwest Oncology Group in which medical, surgical and radiation oncologists worked together. As the study progressed, a true sense of collaboration developed which has made a sound foundation for subsequent combined modality efforts of the group. The dose ranging aspect of this study was related to the tolerance to total nodal radiotherapy following escalating doses of MOPP chemotherapy. Although abdominal radiotherapy was delayed in 21 patients and pelvic irradiation never completed in 21 patients, there was no correlation with the number of cycles of MOPP chemotherapy administered. The question of tolerance to total nodal radiotherapy alone was not tested in this study, but such delays and incomplete therapy are not as common as those noted in this study. Further follow-up will identify the need for full therapeutic doses of radiotherapy to the pelvis.

The symtomatic control was prompt following the administration of MOPP. Reduction in the size of mediastinal masses with chemotherapy allowed smaller than planed ports in many patients resulting in preservation of normal lung. This was particularly important in children.

These data show that MOPP chemotherapy, followed by total nodal radiotherapy can be given to patients with Stage IIB, IIIA and IIIB Hodgkin's disease with excellent survival. These data are at least as good as total nodal radiotherapy followed by MOPP chemotherapy and are clearly better than radiotherapy alone (1,2,5). Chemotherapy plus total nodal radiotherapy is now being compared to chemotherapy alone in these stages of Hodgkin's disease (SWOG 7518).

REFERENCES

1. Rosenberg, S.A. and Kaplan, H.S. (1975) The Management of Stages I,II,and III Hodgkin's Disease With Combined Radiotherapy and Chemotherapy. Cancer 35:55-63.
2. A Colaborative Study. (1976) Survival and Complications of Radiotherapy Following Involved and Extended Field Therapy of Hodgkin's Disease, Stages I and II. Cancer 38:288-305.
3. Devita, V.T. Jr., Canellos, G., et al. (1976) Chemotherapy of Hodgkin's Disease with MOPP: A 10 Year Progress Report. Proc ASCO. 17:269 (Abst).
4. Coltman, C.A.Jr., Frei, E. et al. (1976) MOPP Maintenance vs. Unmaintained Remission for MOPP Induced Complete Remission of Advanced Hodgkin's Disease: 7.2 Year Follow-up. Proc ASCO. 17:289 (Abst).
5. Johnson, R.E., Thomas, L.B., et al. (1970) Preliminary Experience With Total Nodal Irradiation in Hodgkin's Disease. Radiology 96:603-608.
6. Frei, E. III, Luce, J.K., et al. (1973)Combination Chemotherapy in Advanced Hodgkin's Disease - Induction and Maintenance of Remission. Ann. Intern. Med. 79:376.

Adjuvant Therapy of Cancer, S.E. Salmon and S.E. Jones, eds.

ADJUVANT CHEMOTHERAPY WITH CVP AFTER RADIOTHERAPY (RT) IN STAGE I-II NON-HODGKIN'S LYMPHOMAS

Angelo Lattuada, Gianni Bonadonna, Franco Milani, Alberto Banfi,
Pinuccia Valagussa, Mario De Lena, and Silvio Monfardini
Istituto Nazionale Tumori, Milano
Italy

INTRODUCTION

In spite of extensive use of new staging procedures and of improvement of radiotherapeutic techniques, the cure rate of localized (stage I-II) non-Hodgkin's lymphomas remains unsatisfactory. Considering the whole eterogeneous group of non-Hodgkin's lymphomas, the overall 5-year survival for stage I-II patients treated with primary radiotherapy (RT) does not exceed, in general, 50%. This figure varies according to clinical presentation (e.g. nodal or extranodal) and histopathologic subgroup. Most relapses occur within two years from completion of RT and the incidence of extranodal manifestations is very high[1]. Therefore, to eradicate the subclinical foci of lymphoma cells chemotherapy appears indicated in conjunction with radiotherapy which remains the best available tool to sterilize the clinically visible tumor.

In this paper we report the results of a prospective controlled study where RT was compared to sequential RT-chemotherapy modality.

PATIENTS AND METHODS

From October 1972, to December 1975, a total of 113 previously untreated adults with histologically proven diagnosis of non-Hodgkin's lymphoma and classified as stage I-II disease were started on RT. The histopathologic classification employed in this study was that of Rappaport. The staging procedures and the clinical classification utilized were those proposed at Ann Arbor for Hodgkin's disease. Ninety nine patients (88%) were considered suitable for this comparative study. In fact, ten patients (9%) showed new manifestations of disease while on RT. The remaining 4 patients had protocol violations. Table 1 summarizes the main clinical and histopathological features of 99 evaluable patients.

TABLE 1

MAIN CHARACTERISTICS OF EVALUABLE PATIENTS

	RT		RT+CVP	
	No.	%	No.	%
Total evaluable	51		48	
Sex M	28	55	30	62
F	23	45	18	38
Age (median, yrs.)	50	(19-73)	52.5	(19-73)
Histology				
Nodular pattern	12	23	15	31
Diffuse pattern	38	75	32	67
Lymphocytic group	13	25	14	29
Non-lymphocytic group	37	73	33	69
Unclassifiable	1	2	1	2
Stage				
Pathological	50	98	47	98
Clinical	1	2	1	2
I	23	45	23	48
II	28	55	25	52
Clinical presentation				
Nodal	24	47	26	54
Waldeyer's ring	15	29	11	23
GI tract	5	10	5	10
Other extranodal	7	14	6	13

Four weeks after completion of RT patients in clinical complete remission were randomized to receive either no further therapy or 6 cycles of CVP. RT was given using ^{60}Co teletherapy. In 26% of patients the RT fields encompassed with large margins the involved regions. In 74% (control group 37 patients, CVP group 36) RT was delivered to the involved areas as well as to the proximal adjacent lymph-node-bearing region (regional extended radiotherapy). Table 2 briefly describes the extent of prophylactic irradiation which was dependent upon the site of primary involvement. The involved areas received 4,000 rad at the schedule of 800-1,000 rad in 5 days per week. The non involved areas received 3,000-3,500 rad.

TABLE 2

EXTENT OF PROPHYLACTIC IRRADIATION

Primary involvement	Extent of irradiation
Waldeyer's ring	Cervical region, bilateral
Cervical, unilateral	Waldeyer's ring + cervical, contralateral
Axilla, unilateral	Supraclavicular, ipsilateral
Inguinal, unilateral	Iliac, ipsilateral + para-aortic
Extranodal (GI, testicle, etc.)	Regional lymph nodes

CVP was administered according to the original dose schedule of Bagley et al.[2]. Cyclophosphamide (CTX) was given po from day 1 to 5 at the dose of 400 mg/m^2, vincristine (VCR) iv on day 1 at 1.4 mg/m^2 and prednisone (PRD) from day 1 to 5 at 100 mg/m^2. Treatment was recycled on day 22. A dose attenuation schedule was utilized in the presence of marrow depression on day 22. Patients showing treatment failure after RT were started on CVP. In both groups, patients resistant to CVP were treated with ABP (adriamycin, bleomycin, prednisone).

COMPARATIVE TREATMENT FAILURE AND SURVIVAL

Primary treatment failure at 36 months from completion of RT is summarized for both groups in Table 3. There was a significant difference in the total failure in favor of combined modality compared to single modality (P = 0.02). The breakdown according to the main histologic subgroups showed a statistical advantage of CVP therapy only for patients with diffuse lymphoma.

The comparative treatment failure is graphycally illustrated in Figure 1. It is noteworthy that in the group given RT alone most patients showed relapse during the first six months from completion of the irradiation program.

TABLE 3

TREATMENT FAILURE AT 36 MONTHS FROM COMPLETION OF RADIOTHERAPY
(Actuarial analysis)

	RT		RT+CVP		P*
	%	±SE	%	±SE	
Total failure	50.9	7.5	27.6	7.2	0.02
Histology					
Nodular pattern	35.2	14.0	29.6	12.5	0.77
Diffuse pattern	56.4	8.8	27.4	9.1	0.01
Lymphocytic group	60.0	16.8	20.3	13.4	0.25
Non-lymphocytic group	46.3	8.1	31.3	8.7	0.15
Unclassifiable	-		-		
Stage					
I	38.4	11.0	9.9	6.7	0.10
II	62.9	10.0	44.8	11.5	0.13

*Calculated on time distribution SE: Standard Error

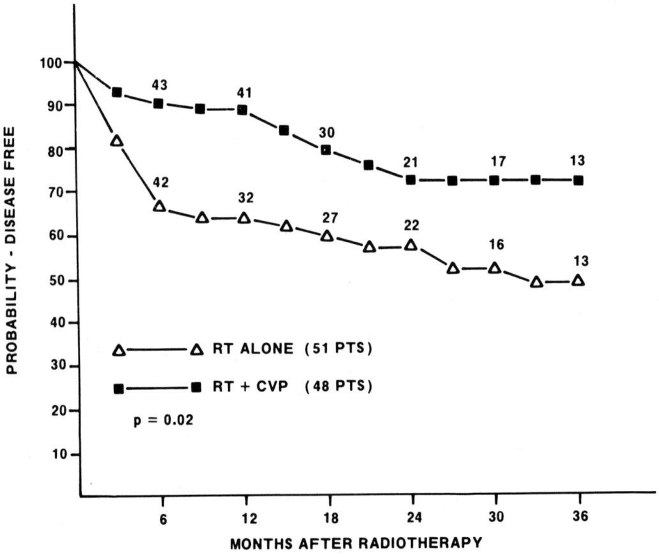

Fig. 1: Treatment failure time distribution in all patients

Table 4 presents the sites of first relapse. True and marginal recurrences were almost nihl. In both treatment groups the highest incidence of relapse occurred either in distant (transdiaphragmatic) nodal sites or in extranodal areas. Patients with nodular lymphoma showed a higher incidence of nodal relapse (4/6) compared to patients with diffuse lymphoma (11/27).

TABLE 4

SITE OF FIRST RELAPSE

	RT	RT+CVP
Marginal recurrence	0	1 (9%)
Nodal extention	13 (54%)	3 (27%)
Transdiaphragmatic	8	2
Extranodal extention	11 (46%)	7 (64%)
GI tract	4	1
Skin	3	2
Bone marrow	0	2
Other sites	4	2
TOTAL	24	11

Figure 2 presents the overall survival curves for both treatment groups. At 36 months from starting RT, 68.5% of patients treated with RT alone are still alive compared to 80.9% of those who were given the combined modality approach ($P = 0.11$). The reason for the lack of significant difference in the 3-year survival between the treatment groups could, in part, be attributed to vigorous and effective secondary therapy which was promptly instituted upon primary treatment failure.

TOXICITY

The irradiation program was, in general, carried out without acute complications. Late sequelae from RT were observed in two patients. They consisted of small intestinal occlusion due to radiation fibrosis.

During treatment with CVP bone marrow suppression represented

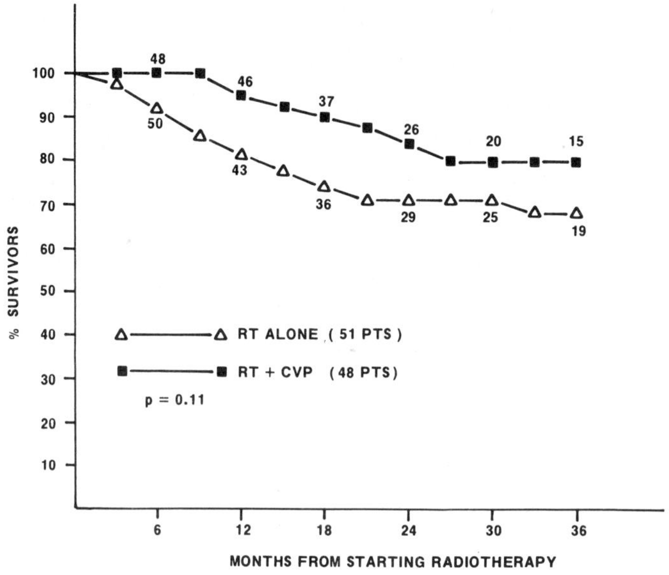

Fig. 2: Overall survival in stage I-II non-Hodgkin's lymphomas

the dose limiting factor in most patients. However, severe leukopenia and/or thrombocytopenia were minimal thus allowing the administration of a high percent of optimal dose (CTX 82%, VCR 87%, PRD 96%).

CONCLUSIONS

Although our series consisted of an eterogeneous group of diseases considering the various cytologic subgroups, the results of present study indicate that 6 cycles of adjuvant CVP significantly improved the overall 3-year relapse rate when sequentially combined to local or regional extended RT. The most consistent information is based on findings observed in the subgroup with diffuse histology which represented more than 70% of the entire series. The small number of patients evaluable in each subgroup prevents to draw practical conclusions for each histologic category.

Many questions remain to be answered. The first concerns the extent of RT. The analysis of the pattern of recurrence confirms once more that in diffuse non-Hodgkin's lymphomas extended RT is not routinely indicated because of the high incidence of recurrence in extranodal sites. For this reason, RT is best limited to involved and regional lymph node-bearing regions with the specific intent to sterilize the bulky (visible) disease with tissue doses ≥ 4,000 rad. Considering the incidence of new disease manifestations occurring during primary RT (9%) and the frequency of relapses within 6 months from completion of irradiation (33.3%), it is conceivable that chemotherapy could have been more effective if administered at an earlier phase than utilized in this study. Therefore, on the basis of present results, we suggest for diffuse lymphomas a combined modality approach employing split-course chemotherapy. As currently used in our Institute, treatment should initiate with three cycles of combination chemotherapy (CVP or BACOP) to produce a substantial control of occult disease before starting RT.

In contrast to diffuse lymphomas, nodular lymphomas usually run a slow course and show tendency to recur in nodal areas. Therefore, for this group of lymphomas we would suggest a more extensive use of prophylactic RT (total nodal irradiation) to be followed by prolonged adjuvant chemotherapy.

The type of chemotherapy to be employed in the combined modality approach also represents an unsolved problem. Several effective combinations are presently available for the treatment of advanced non-Hodgkin's lymphomas[1]. However, none of them can yet be regarded as the regimen of choice for all histopathologic subgroups of the Rappaport classification. CVP was employed in the present study since in a previous controlled trial[3] it was found to be effective in stage IV lymphocytic (CR 58%) and histiocytic lymphomas (CR 36%). However, recent results in diffuse histiocytic lymphomas have shown a higher incidence of complete remission with combinations including adriamycin (HOP, CHOP, BACOP), Methotrexate or Ara-C[1]. As in the treatment of advanced disease, it is conceivable that adjuvant therapy may include different forms of combination chemotherapy for patients with unfavourable histology and single agent chemotherapy (e.g. oral alkylating agents) for those with nodular and differentiated lymphomas[4]. A similar parallelism could be applied to the problem of the duration of adjuvant treatment. The natural history of diffuse histiocytic lymphomas would suggest that 6 to 8 cycles of an aggressive cyclic chemotherapy could be sufficient to achieve cure in a high percent of patients[5,6]. On the contrary, the group of lymphocytic and nodular lymphomas have tendency to show a pattern of relapse over time and therefore they would require a prolonged drug administration to assure either cure or a sustained disease-free status.

REFERENCES

1. Bonadonna, G. et al. (1976) Eur. J. Cancer 12, 661-673.
2. Bagley, C. et al. (1972) Ann. Int. Med. 76: 227-234.
3. Monfardini, S. et al. (1977) Med. Ped. Oncol. (in press).
4. Portlock, C. et al. (1976) Blood 47, 747-756.
5. De Vita, V.T. et al. (1975) Lancet 1, 248-250.
6. Schein, P.S. et al. (1976) Ann. Int. Med. 85, 417-422.

Adjuvant Therapy of Cancer, S.E. Salmon and S.E. Jones eds.

COMBINED MODALITY TREATMENT IN THE MALIGNANT LYMPHOMAS

Eli Glatstein, M.D.*
Carol Portlock, M.D.**
Saul A. Rosenberg, M.D.+
Henry S. Kaplan, M.D.***

From the Division of Radiation Therapy, Department of Radiology and the Division of Oncology, Department of Medicine, Stanford University School of Medicine, Stanford, California 94305

* Assistant Professor, Division of Radiation Therapy
** Assistant Professor, Division of Oncology Department of Medicine
\+ Professor and Chief, Division of Oncology, Department of Medicine Cancer Biology Research Laboratory
*** Professor of Radiology and Director, Cancer Biology Research Laboratory

This work was supported by Research Grants CA-05008, CA-08122 and CA-05838 from the National Cancer Institute, National Institutes of Health, Bethesda, Maryland.

INTRODUCTION

In the treatment of the non-Hodgkin's lymphomas, the diagnostic evaluation, optimal treatment, and prognosis remain controversial. The purpose of this communication is to present preliminary results of ongoing prospective randomized studies in patients with non-Hodgkin's lymphomas that test the value of combined modality treatment. The histopathologic classification system used is that of the Rappaport scheme[1]; the studies are concerned with adult patients, i.e., over fifteen years of age, and the staging classification is that of the Ann Arbor scheme proposed for Hodgkin's disease[2]. Biopsies with both nodular and diffuse elements in the same node have been considered as nodular[3].

Since the most likely sites of failure following radiotherapy appear to be unirradiated nodes or extranodal sites[4], and since the most likely sites of failure following chemotherapy alone appear to be the sites of known involvement[5], a series of randomized prospective clinical trials was initiated in July of 1971 at Stanford.

MATERIALS AND METHODS

Details of the rationale, clinical evaluation, and preliminary results of treatment have been published elsewhere [6,7]. Biopsy evidence of tumor classified according to the Rappaport classification system was required. All patients included in the studies were under 65, had no prior treatment, and had no concurrent medical condition which was thought to limit the patients' ability to withstand extensive diagnostic or therapeutic procedures. For all patients, the diagnostic evaluation included routine laboratory studies, bipedal lymphangiography, multiple additional radiographic procedures and an adequate marrow biopsy. In all patients who did not have overt evidence of stage IV disease following such work-up, exploratory laparotomy was used for staging, with multiple lymph node biopsies, liver biopsies and splenectomy, as well as an open bone marrow biopsy, unless the patient had been explored for diagnosis elsewhere prior to his referral to Stanford.

RESULTS

For patients with favorable histology (i.e., NLWD, NLPD, NM, AND DLWD) who had pathologic stage I or II disease following the extensive work-up including laparotomy, either involved field radiotherapy or total lymphoid radiotherapy (mid-plane dose in excess of 4,000 rads) was used. The survival at five years was excellent in both groups with only one death being seen and that from unrelated intercurrent disease. Only one relapse was detected following the involved field treatment and none following total lymphoid treatment. However, because of the small number of patients (only 15) who had pathologic stage I or II disease of favorable histologic type and because of the relatively short period of follow-up, no conclusion can yet be made concerning the relative merits of the two treatment regimens.

Patient with pathologic stage I or II non-Hodgkin's lymphoma of unfavorable histologies (NH, DLPD, DM, DH, AND DU) were randomized between total lymphoid irradiation alone and total lymphoid irradiation followed by six cycles of adjuvant chemotherapy. For those patients who had diffuse histiocytic lymphoma, the adjuvant chemotherapy was a combination of cytosine arabinoside, adriamycin, and 6-thioguanine (CAT), a regimen with a response rate of approximately 75% in patients with diffuse histiocytic lymphoma [6,7]. For all the other histologies on this particular study, the adjuvant chemotherapy consisted of cytoxan, vincristine and prednisone (CVP)[8]. After five years, the survival on both arms was approximately 70%, without any detectable benefit in those patients who received six cycles of adjuvant chemotherapy. Approximately 60% of patients on both arms remained free of any relapse. Thus, for local and regional lymphoma of unfavorable histologic types, six cycles of the adjuvant chemotherapies employed in these studies did not prove beneficial in either survival or freedom from relapse. Moreover, the results of total lymphoid irradiation appeared surprisingly good in this group of patients with unfavorable histology.

For patients with pathologic stage III non-Hodgkin's lymphomas of relatively favorable histologies, a similar study was devised whereby all patients received total lymphoid irradiation and half were randomized to receive adjuvant CVP chemotherapy for six cycles. No significant difference was seen in survival (approximately 75% at four years in both arms) or in the freedom from relapse (approximately 60% at four years in both arms); thus, no obvious improvement was detected with the addition of six cycles of adjuvant CVP chemotherapy in these patients with pathologic stage III disease.

For patients with stage IV non-Hodgkin's lymphomas of favorable histologies, a prospective three-armed study was initiated which compared the results of A) intensive CVP chemotherapy, B) combined modality treatment consisting of two or three cycles of CVP followed by high dose total lymphoid irradiation followed by additional CVP, and C) single agent chemotherapy consisting of oral cytoxan or chlorambucil. At five years, the survival was excellent in all three arms with approximately 80% of the patients surviving at five years. However, the probability of freedom from relapse was only about 35% in all three arms. No obvious superiority was seen in either intensive treatment arm over what was achieved by the conservative single agent approach; relapses appeared to occur at a relatively constant rate, regardless of the treatment employed. Not only did this study fail to show superiority for aggressive treatment over conservative management in patients with stage IV disease of favorable histologic types, but it also serves to emphasize the necessity for carefully controlled studies in patients with such disease in whom survival benefits are often ascribed to aggressive treatment programs.

For patients with non-Hodgkin's lymphomas of unfavorable histologies of stage III or IV extent, treatment was randomized between either combination chemotherapy alone or a combined modality approach consisting of intensive chemotherapy for two or three cycles followed by high dose total lymphoid irradiation followed by additional chemotherapy. For patients with DH or DU, the chemotherapy employed was CAT; for all other histologies on this study, the chemotherapy employed was CVP. The survival of patients receiving chemotherapy alone was 24% at four years compared to 47% of the patients at 5 years following combined modality treatment. The probability of freedom from relapse, however, was generally disappointing. Only 9% of patients randomized to chemotherapy alone continued in their first remission at four years. Of patients who had been randomized to the combined modality arm, 24% remained in their first remission at five years. These data suggest that the combined modality approach may have a role to play in advanced stages of non-Hodgkin's lymphomas of unfavorable histologies, although the optimal sequence of combining the two modalities remains to be established.

COMMENTS

Recently, for patients with advanced stages of unfavorable histologies, we have reduced the dose of irradiation to 3,000 rads instead of 4,000 rads and have begun a program[7] of alternating two cycles of combination chemotherapy with separate periods of radiation to the mantle (or mini-mantle, which is a supramediastinal field), upper abdominal[9], and pelvic fields. Such an alternating sequence of two modalities of treatment, which requires close cooperation between various specialists, appears to have potential for further improvement in the results of treatment for patients with non-Hodgkin's lymphomas.

REFERENCES

1. Rappaport, H., Winter, W.J., and Hicks, E.B.: Follicular lymphoma - a re-evaluation of its position in the scheme of malignant lymphomas, based on a survey of 253 cases. Cancer 9:792-821, 1956.
2. Carbone, P.P., Kaplan, H.S., Musshof, K., Smithers, D.W., and Tubiana, M.: Report of the committee on Hodgkin's disease staging classification. Cancer Res 31:1860-1861, 1971.
3. Warnke, R., Kim, H., Fuks, Z., and Dorfman, R.F.: The coexistence of nodular and diffuse patterns in nodular non-Hodgkin's lymphomas: Significance and clinico-pathologic correlation. Submitted for publication.
4. Fuks, A., Glatstein, E., and Kaplan, H.S.: Patterns of presentation and relapse in the non-Hodgkin's lymphomata. Brit. J. Cancer 31 (suppl. II): 286-297, 1975.
5. Schein, P.S., Chabner, B.A., Canellos, G.P., Young, R.C., and DeVita, V.T.: Non-Hodgkin's lymphoma-patterns of relapse from complete remission after combination chemotherapy. Cancer 35:354-357, 1975.
6. Rosenberg, S.A. and Kaplan, H.S.: Clinical trials in the non-Hodgkin's lymphomata at Stanford University. Experimental design and preliminary results, Brit J. Cancer 31 (suppl. II).
7. Glatstein, E., Donaldson, S.S., Rosenberg, S.A., and Kaplan, H.S.: The potential for combined modality therapy in malignant lymphomas. Cancer Treatment Reports, in press.
8. Bagley, C.M., Jr., DeVita, V.T., Jr., Berard, C.W., and Canellos, G.P.: Advanced lymphosarcoma: Intensive cyclical combination chemotherapy with cyclophosphamide, vincristine, and prednisone. Ann Int. Med 76:227-234, 1972.
9. Goffinet, D.R., Glatstein, E., Fuks, Z., and Kaplan, H.S.: Abdominal irradiation of non-Hodgkin's lymphomas. Cancer 37:297 - 2805, 1975.

Adjuvant Therapy of Cancer, S.E. Salmon and S.E. Jones eds.
© 1977 Elsevier/North-Holland Biomedical Press, Amsterdam

ADJUVANT IMMUNOTHERAPY WITH BCG IN LYMPHOMA

Stephen E. Jones, M. D.
Sydney E. Salmon, M. D.
Section of Hematology and Oncology
Department of Internal Medicine
University of Arizona College of Medicine
Tucson, Arizona 85724

INTRODUCTION

The concept of employing immunostimulating or immunomodulating agents as an adjuvant to chemotherapy or radiotherapy for patients with malignant lymphoma appears to be well founded. Lymphomas arise from the cells of the immune system, and clinical manifestations can be related to immunocompetence of the host[1-4]. Several reports of clinical studies involving immunotherapy are available[5]. Of the trials of immunotherapy reported to date, some are anecdotal and most of the others represent early attempts at immunotherapy which cannot be interpreted in terms of our present standards for the conduct of adequately controlled clinical studies[6-8]. Only three trials meet our minimal criteria for assessing the results of immunotherapy (e.g., adequate numbers of evaluable patients and properly selected control groups, matched for critically important prognostic factors like stage of disease, histology, age, and type of treatment other than immunotherapy)[9-11].

The first trial which appears to be evaluable was the one involving BCG by scarification for patients in remission after receiving cyclophosphamide for Burkitt's lymphoma[9]. African Burkitt's lymphoma was one of the first tumors which was judged to be curable with chemotherapy alone. Although cyclophosphamide produced initial complete remission rates of 95%, approximately two-thirds of the patients relapsed within one year[12]. This fact prompted a controlled trial of immunotherapy with BCG as a non-specific immunostimulant in an effort to prevent relapse. Eighty patients with African Burkitt's lymphoma were entered into this trial between 1971 and 1973. Only 40 of the 80 patients were judged evaluable for the effects of BCG. Twenty-one patients in remission received lyophilized Pasteur Institute BCG (3×10^8 organisms) by scarification on rotated limbs every 4 days for 7 doses and then weekly for 6 doses (a total of 10 weeks of immunotherapy); 11 patients in this group relapsed. Nineteen patients who received no further therapy served as controls and 11 of these patients relapsed. The authors noted that BCG caused in creased reactivity to skin test recall antigens 4 weeks after chemotherapy but concluded that BCG did not prolong remission duration or affect survival in Burkitt's lymphoma[9].

The second evaluable trial is being conducted by the Eastern Oncology Group (ECOG)[10]. In 1972, ECOG began a clinical trial to examine the benefit of BCG in prolonging remission duration in patients with advanced Hodgkin's disease who achieved a complete remission (CR) with one of 2 drug combinations. Several important controls were incorporated into this study such as routine pathology review and stratification randomization procedures designed to balance treatment groups with respect to major prognostic factors. The preliminary results of 264 evaluable patients entered on this trial were recently presented by Bakemeier et al[10]. One hundred and eighty-five patients (70%) achieved a complete remission with chemotherapy and the remission rates were similar for both remission induction programs. One hundred and twenty-four patients have entered the maintenance phase of this study and until the study is completed or until there is a significant difference, the results remain coded. The treatment plan is shown below:

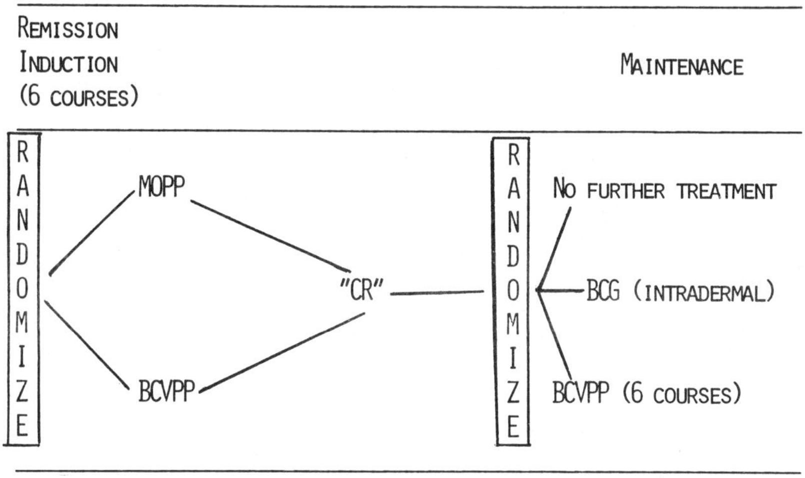

Fig. 1. Treatment schema for Eastern Oncology Group Study 2472 for patients with advanced Hodgkin's disease. MOPP = combination chemotherapy with nitrogen mustard, vincristine (Oncovin), procarbazine, and prednisone. BCVPP = chemotherapy consisting of BCNU, cyclophosphamide, vincristine, procarbazine and prednisone.

Patients who were assigned maintenance treatment with BCG received 0.1 ml of Tice strain BCG (2 x 10^6 viable units) intradermally at 1, 2, 4 and 6 months after chemotherapy was discontinued. The preliminary results of this study indicate that neither BCG by intradermal administration nor maintenance chemotherapy have prolonged remission duration compared to the patients who received no further treatment after induction.

In this study Bakemeier et al.[10] reported that BCG was generally well tolerated despite the intradermal route of administration. The investigators were concerned that the infrequency of administration of BCG was low compared to studies in other types of tumors[13] and that this fact alone may have been responsible for their inability to show benefit with BCG in patients in complete remission. Accordingly, ECOG has initiated a new study (ECOG 1476) which employs a more frequent and more prolonged schedule of immunotherapy with BCG administered by tine technique for patients with Hodgkin's disease who achieve a complete remission with either chemotherapy or chemotherapy and radiation therapy.

The third evaluable trial of immunotherapy is the one we are conducting with the Southwest Oncology Group (SWOG). Preliminary results have been recently presented[12] and although still preliminary, they are updated in this report.

PATIENTS AND METHODS

In this study we are assessing the effect of BCG both as part of a remission induction regimen and as a means to prolong remission duration for those patients who achieved a complete remission (CR) of non-Hodgkin's lymphomas.

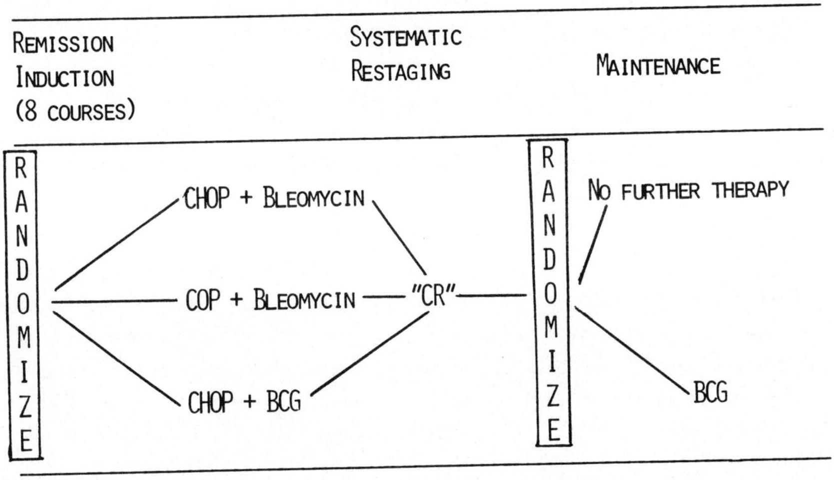

Fig. 2. Treatment schema for Southwest Oncology Group Study 7426/7427. See text for details.

Only patients with advanced disease (Stages III and IV) and no prior chemotherapy were eligible. It was required that pathologic material on all cases was to be reviewed by members of the Lymphoma Pathology Panel and Central Repository[14] and classified according to the Rappaport criteria[15]. Eligible patients were randomly assigned to treatment (stratified for nodular or diffuse histologies) as follows:

1. COP-Bleomycin (four drugs): cyclophosphamide (C), 125 mg/m^2 given orally daily for 14 days starting on Day 1; vincristine (Oncovin [O]), 1.4 mg/m^2 given intravenously (iv) on Days 1 and 8 (maximum of 2 mg per injection); prednisone (P), 100 mg/day given orally on Days 1-5; and bleomycin, 4 mg/m^2 given iv on

Days 1 and 8. Courses were repeated every 28 days if the peripheral blood counts were adequate.

2. CHOP-Bleomycin (five drugs): cyclophosphamide, 750 mg/m^2 given iv on Day 1; adriamycin (hydroxyldaunorubicin [H]), 50 mg/m^2 given iv on Dayl; vincristine, 1.4 mg/m^2 given iv on Day 1 (maximum of 2 mg per injection); prednisone, 100 mg/day given orally on Days 1-5; and bleomycin, 4 mg/m^2 given iv on day 1. Courses were repeated every 21 days if the blood counts were adequate[16].

3. CHOP-BCG (five drugs): same regimen as in CHOP-Bleomycin-therapy except for substitution of high viability Pasteur BCG (bacillus Calmette-Guerin) for bleomycin. BCG was given by scarification at a dose of 1 ampule ($6 \pm 4 \times 10^8$ viable units of Pasteur lyophilized BCG) on Days 8 and 15 of each 21-day treatment cycle. BCG scarifications were performed on extremities with a standard 5 x 5 cm grid of 10 scratches in each of 2 perpendicular directions. BCG sites were rotated with each dose so that all major lymphoid drainage pathways from upper and lower extremities were repetitively challenged. Doses of drugs and BCG were modified in accord with standard SWOG guidelines based on toxicity.

Remission induction consisted of 8 courses of treatment for responding patients. If they appeared to be in a complete remission after 8 courses, a careful "systematic restaging" examination was performed (which discovered occult persistent lymphoma in 18% of cases in apparent remission)[17]. Patients with confirmed remissions were then re-randomized to receive either no further treatment or BCG by scarification at monthly intervals for 18 months. Patients who relapse from the unmaintained remission group will likely provide some insights on the residual tumor stem cell burden after chemotherapy or chemoimmunotherapy induction. In addition to concomitant controls, an immediately prior historical control with CHOP alone also served for comparison with respect to remission induction[16].

RESULTS

Between October, 1974 and January, 1977, 589 patients with non-Hodgkin's lymphomas were entered on this trial. Three hundred patients registered on one of the 3 primary induction limbs of the study have had a final evaluation for response (i.e., have completed remission induction); the others are still receiving treatment. The results are given in Table 1.

TABLE 1

CHEMOIMMUNOTHERAPY OF NON-HODGKIN'S LYMPHOMA

SWOG 7426/7427

Preliminary Results (January, 1977): Remission Induction

Treatment	No. of Patients with final evaluations	No. with CR (%)	No. with PR (%)	PR + CR (%)
CHOP + BCG	91	54 (59%)	26 (29%)	(88%)*
CHOP + Bleomycin	91	52 (57%)	18 (20%)	(77%)*
COP + Bleomycin	118	70 (59%)	27 (23%)	(82%)*
Total	300	176 (59%)	71	

* The difference between overall response rates (CR + PR) is at the p = 0.09 level. CR = complete remission (with restaging); PR = partial remission.

There is no significant difference in the complete remission rates according to treatment. However, there is a difference in overall response rates (due to increased numbers of partial responses) in patients receiving chemoimmunotherapy with BCG ($p = 0.09$). For pathologically reviewed cases with nodular lymphomas, the complete response rate is 62% compared with a 55% complete response rate in diffuse lymphoma. Within major histologic types of lymphoma (pathology review completed) no significant difference in complete remission rates according to induction treatment is apparent.

All three induction treatment regimens have been generally well tolerated with the major toxicity being leukopenia. The COP + bleomycin regimen was associated with less toxicity ($p < 0.001$) than CHOP + bleomycin or CHOP + BCG. There was no difference in hematologic toxicity between CHOP + bleomycin or CHOP + BCG treatment. The administration of BCG was also well tolerated. Sixty-three percent of patients experienced no toxicity requiring modification of BCG frequency or dosage. No cases of systemic BCG infection or fatal BCG reactions have been encountered during remission induction.

To date, 46 relapses have been observed in patients achieving a complete remission (CHOP + BCG = 8; CHOP + bleomycin = 11; COP + bleomycin = 27). The duration of complete remission is longer for patients with nodular lymphoma compared to those with diffuse histologic types ($p = 0.08$). When the duration of remission is examined by major type of lymphoma and the type of initial treatment, no significant difference exists for patients with nodular lymphoma (although only 1 patient has relapsed after CHOP + BCG induction). However, the duration of complete remission induced with CHOP (CHOP + bleomycin or CHOP + BCG) is significantly longer for patients with diffuse lymphomas than that obtained with COP + bleomycin induction treatment ($p < 0.05$).

As of January, 1977, 175 patients who achieved a complete remission documented by restaging have been registered on the unmaintained or BCG immunotherapy limbs of this study. Of these, 129 are currently fully evaluable as detailed below:

TABLE 2

CHEMOIMMUNOTHERAPY OF NON-HODGKIN'S LYMPHOMA

SWOG 7426/7427

Preliminary Results (January, 1977): Remission Maintenance

	No. of Patients	No. of Relapses (%)
No further treatment	64	17 (28%)
BCG monthly	58	13 (23%)
Refused BCG (non-randomized)	7	1 (14%)

At this time there is no significant difference in relapse rates between BCG-maintained remission or unmaintained remission.

The overall survival of all partially and fully evaluable patients entered on this study (407 patients) is superior to that observed in the most recently completed study where 238 partially and fully evaluable patients received CHOP alone for remission induction ($p = 0.003$)[16]. In this study, there is no significant difference in survival in relation to the type of initial induction treatment. To date, 71 patients have died: 18 who received CHOP + BCG, 23 who received CHOP + bleomycin and 30 who received COP + bleomycin. The survival of patients with nodular lymphoma is superior to that observed with diffuse lymphoma ($p = 0.002$). For patients with diffuse lymphoma survival is independent of the initial induction treatment. However, for patients with nodular lymphoma, survival is somewhat better if they received CHOP + BCG compared to CHOP + bleomycin ($p = 0.10$) or COP + bleomycin ($p = 0.13$). Indeed, none of the patients who received CHOP + BCG have yet died.

DISCUSSION

Non-specific immune stimulation with BCG has received considerable attention in in recent years as a form of adjuvant cancer therapy. Chemoimmunotherapy with BCG has been evaluated in various types of cancers including melanoma, acute leukemia, breast cancer, and lymphoma. In most of these trials survival or duration of remission has been reported as improved by the addition of BCG to chemotherapy but rates of complete remission have not been increased[13]. Similar observations may eventually be confirmed in this carefully controlled study of chemoimmunotherapy for patients with non-Hodgkin's lymphoma, but the results are still too preliminary to be certain. With final evaluations of about one half of the cases entered on this study, we have demonstrated a significant improvement in overall survival compared to our most recently completed and otherwise comparable trial[16]. In addition, we have observed that the overall response rate (partial plus complete) is greater in patients receiving CHOP + BCG compared to treatment with either CHOP + bleomycin or COP + bleomycin, although there is no difference in complete remission rates. There is also a suggestion (not yet significant) that both remission duration and survival of patients with nodular lymphoma might be improved by the addition of BCG to CHOP chemotherapy compared to the regimens without BCG. This is interesting because nodular lymphoma patients appear to be more immunocompetent at the time of presentation[1] and may have better preservation of the T-dependent areas of lymphoid organs which could be relevant if the BCG immunotherapeutic effect is mediated through T lymphocytes.

After induction of complete remission we have not yet been able to demonstrate any advantage in terms of prolonging duration of complete remission by administering BCG at monthly intervals by scarification compared to no further treatment The majority of relapses observed to date have occurred early (average time from restaging to relapse is 4 months [range 1-12 months]) and many of the relapses appear to have occurred in patients whose restaging evaluations were not sufficiently thorough to detect persistent lymphoma[17]. Thus, a significant number of residual lymphoma stem cells may have persisted in these patients. Our choice of administering BCG at monthly intervals after restaging, in retrospect, may have been inadequate to enhance immunoreactivity in patients who did not receive the more intensive BCG stimulation during the remission induction phase. For instance, it might have been more appropriate to begin maintenance BCG at weekly intervals until strong reactions occurred, followed by reductions in the frequency of administration or dosage of BCG thereafter.

We must reiterate that the results of this study are still tentative as only half of the patients have been fully analyzed and the length of followup, even of these patients is still short. Much longer periods of observation and analysis of all cases in this ongoing trial will be of critical importance in assessing the role of adjuvant immunotherapy with BCG in the management of patients with non-Hodgkin's lymphoma.

REFERENCES

1. Jones, S., Griffith, K., Dombrowski, P., Gaines, J. (1977) Immunodeficiency in patients with non-Hodgkin's lymphomas, Blood (in press).
2. Hersh, E., Mavligit, G., Gutterman, J. (1976) Immunodeficiency in cancer and the importance of immune evaluation of the cancer patient, Med. Clin. N. Am. 60:623-639.
3. Jones, S., Durie, B., Salmon, S. (1973) Immunologic aspects of the hematologic neoplasms, Postgrad. Med. 54:209-216.
4. Young, R., Corder, M., Berard, C., DeVita, V. (1973) Immune alterations in Hodgkin's disease. Effect of delayed hypersensitivity and lymphocyte transformation on course and survival, Arch. Int. Med. 131:446-454.
5. Jones, S. The immunotherapy of human lymphoma. In Clinical Immunotherapy (A. F. LoBuglio, ed.). Marcel Dekker, Inc., New York (in press).

6. Hoerni, B., Chauvergne, G., Hoerni-Simon, M., et al. (1976) BCG in the immunotherapy of Hodgkin's disease and the non-Hodgkin's lymphomas, Cancer Immunol. Immunother. 1:109-112.
7. Mathe, G., Belpomme, D., Pouillart, P., et al. (1975) Preliminary results of an immunotherapy trial on terminal leukaemic lymphosarcoma, Biomedicine 23: 465-467.
8. Sokal, J., Aungst, C., Snyderman, M. (1974) Delay in progression of malignant lymphoma after BCG vaccination, N. Eng. J. Med. 291:1226-1230.
9. Magrath, I., Ziegler, J. (1976) Failure of BCG immunostimulation to affect the clinical course of Burkitt's lymphoma. Brit. Med. J. 1:615-618.
10. Bakemeier, R., Costello, W., Horton, J., DeVita, V. (1977) BCG immunotherapy following chemotherapy-induced remissions of stage III and IV Hodgkin's disease. In Immunotherapy of Cancer: Present Status of Trials in Man (W. D. Terry and D. Windhorst, eds.). Raven Press (in press).
11. Jones, S., Salmon, S., Moon, T., et al. (1977) Chemoimmunotherapy of non-Hodgkin's lymphoma with BCG. A preliminary report. In Immunotherapy of Cancer: Present Status of Trials in Man (W. D. Terry and D. Windhorst, eds.). Raven Press (in press).
12. Ziegler, J. (1972) Chemotherapy of Burkitt's lymphoma. Cancer 30:1534-1540.
13. Gutterman, J., Mavligit, G., Hersh, E. (1976) Chemoimmunotherapy of human solid tumors. Med. Clin. N. Am. 60:441-472.
14. Jones, S., Butler, J.,Byrne, G. et al. (1977) Histopathologic review of lymphoma cases from the Southwest Oncology Group. Cancer (in press).
15. Rappaport, H., Winter, W., Hicks, E. (1956) Follicular lymphoma: a re-evaluation of its position in the scheme of malignant lymphoma, based on a survey of 253 cases. Cancer 9:792-821.
16. McKelvey, E., Gottlieb, J., Wilson, H., et al. (1976) Hydroxyldaunomycin (adriamycin) combination chemotherapy in malignant lymphoma, Cancer 38:1484-1493.
17. Herman, T., Jones, S. (1977) Systematic restaging in the management of non-Hodgkin's lymphoma. Cancer Treat. Rep. (in press).

Adjuvant Therapy of Cancer, S.E. Salmon and S.E. Jones eds.

ADJUNCTIVE IMMUNOTHERAPY OF PATIENTS WITH MYCOSIS FUNGOIDES

Z. L. Olkowski, M.D., Sc. D., J. R. McLaren, M.D.,
P. McGinley, Ph.D., F. Bilek, M.D., and Marianne J. Skeen, M.S.
The Laboratory of Tumor Biology and Clinical Immunology
Winship Clinic for Neoplastic Disease
Emory University School of Medicine
Atlanta, Georgia 30322, U.S.A.

INTRODUCTION:

Mycosis fungoides, first described by Alibert (1), is a malignant lymphoproliferative disorder which often begins with non-specific scaly eruptions of the skin, progressing through multiple erythematous patches to plaques, ulcers and tumors. The time of progression varies from patient to patient and may last from a few months to several years. It eventually spreads to visceral organs and approximately 50% of these patients die within 3½ years after the biopsy diagnosis (2).

The therapy of this skin lymphoma has not altered the survival of these patients (2), although electron beam radiation therapy has been successfully used in patients with early stages of this disease to obtain long-term remissions (3,20). Availability of 18 MeV linear accelerators and dosimetry for rotational therapy (4) will hopefully increase disease free intervals in patients with mycosis fungoides.

Since most patients with a variety of malignant tumors present with impaired immunocompetence (5-13), considerable effort is being directed toward stimulating patients' immune systems following surgery or radiation therapy with the hope that it may result in an increased cure rate. Recently Levamisole, which has been shown to stimulate depressed immune systems, has been extensively evaluated as an immunomodulator (14).

Our earlier work as well as the work of Nordqvist and Kinney (15) and Lutzner et al (21) has shown that patients with mycosis fungoides have impaired cellular immunity. Since radiation therapy may further depress the immune systems of these individuals, we decided to test the efficacy and safety of Levamisole in stimulating cell mediated immunity of patients with mycosis fungoides who had had whole body electron beam radiation therapy and were clinically free of disease following this treatment.

MATERIAL AND METHODS

Patients: Twenty patients (10 males and 10 females) with biopsy proven mycosis fungoides (MF) Stages I, II, or III (staged according to Schein, 1974) were studied and 15 of these were placed on protocol. The time since diagnosis varied from 6 months to more than 10 years (see Graphs 1 and 2) prior to radiation therapy. These patients ranged in age from 38 to 72 years, had been treated in the past with topical nitrogen mustard, superficial radiation therapy, and several with total body electron beam therapy, and presented with recurrent disease at time of this study.

Treatment: Treatment consisted of whole body radiation with electrons, 400 rads per fraction once a week over a period of 6 weeks to a total dose of 2400 R with a boost to the axillary and perineal areas as well as to the soles of feet (7 patients); or daily, whole body treatments with electrons, 3000 R over a period of 4 to 5 weeks (13 patients). After remissions were obtained patients were placed on immunotherapy. Ten patients selected randomly received Levamisole 150 mg twice a week on 2 consecutive days and 5 patients received a placebo. Three patients in the control (placebo) group recurred after 8-16 weeks. At this point the code was broken for these individuals and following regression with re-treatment they were placed on Levamisole. The results of immunological evaluations of all patients and a control group, consisting of 82 healthy, age matched individuals are presented in Tables I, II, and III and clinical results in Graphs I and 2.

Immunological Evaluations: Lymphocytes were isolated from peripheral blood on a Ficoll-Hypaque gradient as described previously (6) giving a cell suspension consisting of 92-94% lymphocytes and 6-8% monocytes. The E-rosette assay for T-lymphocytes was performed using these isolated lymphocytes as previously described (6). Samples of patients' serum were assayed for IgE using commercially available radioimmunoassay kits, with results expressed in IU/ml. Transformation of lymphocytes in vitro was performed using a modification of the whole blood methods of Pauly et al. (16) and Pelegrino et al. (17). The results are expressed as a stimulation index (SI) which is the ratio of counts per minute in the PHA and pokeweed (PWM) mitogen-stimulated cultures to counts per minute for unstimulated lymphocytes. Cyclic AMP was evaluated using the method of Kuo et al. (18), using peripheral blood lymphocytes isolated by Ficoll-Hypaque gradients. Protein was determined according to Lowry. Results are expressed in pM of cAMP/mg cellular protein.

Statistical Analysis: To determine whether a healthy control group had significantly different average values for percentage and levels of T-lymphocytes, IgE, PHA, PWM, and cyclic AMP when compared with values obtained with various groups of patients with mycosis fungoides, preliminary one way analysis of variance was performed for each variable. Scheff's method of multiple comparison was then used to test hypotheses on mean differences (19). To determine whether there is a significant difference between patients with MF before radiation therapy, after radiation therapy, and on Levamisole or placebo, paired analyses were performed (19)

TABLE I

IMMUNE PARAMETERS + OF PATIENTS WITH MYCOSIS FUNGOIDES (M.F.)

		NO. OF CASES	T - CELLS % T	T - CELLS T LEVEL
HEALTHY CONTROLS		82	69.4 ± 6.8	1408 ± 434
MF BEFORE RADIATION THERAPY		14	49.9* ± 8.9	942* ± 314
MF AFTER RADIATION THERAPY		14	48.8* ± 9.4	665* ± 549
IMMUNOTHERAPY 8 - 12 WEEKS	PLACEBO	5	40.8* ± 4.4	1034* ± 399
IMMUNOTHERAPY 8 - 12 WEEKS	LEVAMISOLE	10	52.8* ± 8.1	839* ± 413

* Significantly different at the level $P < 0.001$

TABLE II

IMMUNE PARAMETERS + OF PATIENTS WITH MYCOSIS FUNGOIDES (M.F.)

		IgE I.U./ml	PHA S. I.	PWM S. I.
HEALTHY CONTROLS		< 100	150.5 ± 98.9 n = 31	40.1 ± 25.6 n = 30
MF BEFORE RADIATION THERAPY		95.9 ± 43 n = 8	2.1* ± 1.1 n = 6	1.1* ± 0.2 n = 6
MF AFTER RADIATION THERAPY		80.3 ± 34.0 n = 8	1.9* ± 1.0 n = 4	1.6* ± 0.8 n = 6
IMMUNOTHERAPY 8- 12 WEEKS	PLACEBO	62.7 ± 30.0 n = 3	Range 1.4 - 65 n = 5	Range 1.0 - 12 n = 5
IMMUNOTHERAPY 8- 12 WEEKS	LEVAMISOLE	73.8 ± 48.4 n = 5	Range 0.7 - 242 n = 10	Range 0.9 - 67 n = 9

* Significantly different at the level $P < 0.001$

\+ = mean ± 1 S.D.

n = No. of patients

RESULTS

Side Effects: In general, side effects reported by our patients were mild, consisting of increased temperature, nausea and metallic taste of water. The incidence and nature of these symptoms was similar to that described by us earlier (12). One patient, remaining free of disease, had to be removed from the protocol because of severe granulocytopenia, which improved after 4 days of hospitalization without specific treatment.

Immunological Evaluations: Prior to radiationtherapy all 20 patients with mycosis fungoides had percentages and levels of T-lymphocytes lower than control values. Fifteen of these patients matched after receiving a course of electron beam radiaton therapy had unchanged percentages and levels of T-lymphocytes from their pre-radiation values, but remained statistically different from the control group (Table I). The median time patients remained on Levamisole or on placebo before recurrence was approximately 13 weeks. In five individuals who received placebo provided by Jansen R&D the percentages of T-lymphocytes were significantly lower than in fifteen patients on Levamisole. However, there was no statistically significant difference in T-lymphocyte levels between these groups.

IgE levels in healthy controls was less than 100 IU/ml (Table II). In patients evaluated before radiation therapy, 3 patients had very high values of IgE: 1850 IU/ml, 4000 IU/ml, and 5000 IU/ml. These values were not used in calculating the mean and SD. The rest of the group had a mean IgE of 95.9 IU/ml which was not significantly different from control values. The same patients tested after radiation therapy had a mean of 80.3 IU/ml, which was not significantly different from pre-radiation or control levels. Radiation therapy did not reduce the very high levels of IgE observed in the 3 patients mentioned above. Mean IgE level in patients on placebo was a normal 62.7 IU/ml although one patient had 3600 IU/ml, which was not included in statistical analysis. The mean IgE level was 73.8 in patients undergoing Levamisole therapy.

Patients with MF tested before radiation therapy had a mean stimulation index by PHA of 2.1 (Table II), which is significantly different from the healthy control mean of 150.5. Mean stimulation index on the last day of radiaton therapy was 1.9, essentially that of pre-radiation values and significantly lower than controls. Two relatively high patients stimulation indices (51 and 65, but significantly lower than mean control values) were not included in the statistical analysis because the post radiation results were not available. The mean SI of 1.1 by pokeweed mitogen in patients before radiation therapy showed no change by radiation with a mean value of 1.6. Both values are significantly different from controls of 40.1. Again, one patient had a relatively high PWM stimulation index (38), but was excluded from statistical analysis because post radiation results were not available.

Seven individuals with mycosis fungoides tested before radiation therapy had 14.8 pM of cyclic AMP/mg protein in peripheral lymphocytes (Table III) which is significantly different from the mean control level of 47.4 pM/mg protein. Six patients tested after radiation therapy had a mean of 16.8 pM of cyclic AMP/mg protein, which was not significantly different from pre-treatment values, but remained lower than control values. The mean cyclic AMP level in the lymphocytes of 8 patients after 8-12 weeks of Levamisole therapy was 17.2 pM/mg of protein which is significantly lower than healthy controls but not statistically different from the values obtained before or after radiation therapy. Cyclic AMP level evaluated in one patient on placebo, was 12.76 pM/mg protein.

TABLE III

CYCLIC ADENOSINE MONOPHOSPHATE (cAMP) LEVELS IN LYMPHOCYTES OF PATIENTS WITH MYCOSIS FUNGOIDES (MF)

	NO. CASES	cAMP pM/mg.protein mean $\pm$ 1 S.D.
HEALTHY CONTROLS	15	47.5 $\pm$ 10.2
MF BEFORE RADIATION THERAPY	7	14.8* $\pm$ 7.6
MF AFTER RADIATION THERAPY	6	16.8* $\pm$ 11.1
MF AFTER RADIATION THERAPY ON LEVEMISOLE FOR 8 - 12 WEEKS	8	17.2* $\pm$ 5.4

* Statistically different from controls $P < 0.001$

Serial evaluations of immune profiles in individual patients may have predictive value which would aid in treatment management. In patients on the immune therapy protocol the percentages and the levels of T-cells and PHA-stimulated blastogenesis tended to increase in individuals during 4-8 weeks of Levamisole therapy. However, there was no evidence of a similar increase in placebo patients. Clinical recurrence of mycosis fungoides was usually preceded approximately 4-6 weeks by a decrease in percentage and levels of T-lymphocytes and PHA stimulated blastogenesis in vitro.

GRAPH I

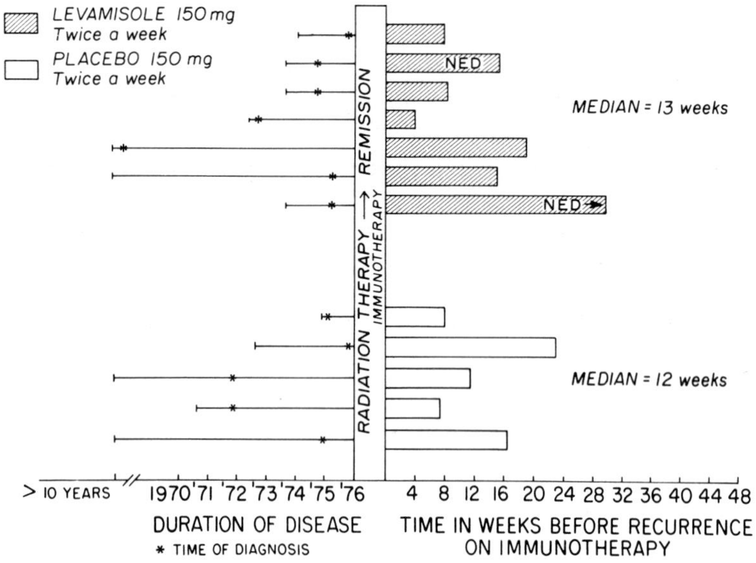

GRAPH 2

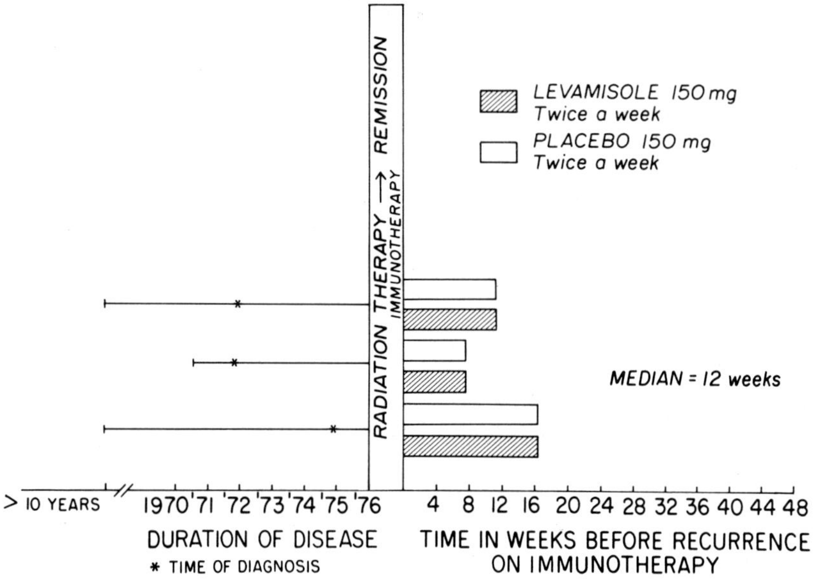

Clinical results are summarized in Graphs 1 and 2. No difference was observed between Levamisole and placebo patients with respect to disease free interval following radiation therapy (Graph 1). At time of recurrence the code was broken to determine whether or not patient was on active drug because of the possibility of an allergic skin reaction. Three such patients had been on placebo, and were treated a second time with radiation and then placed on routine Levamisole therapy. These data (Graph 2) revealed that the disease free intervals were equivalent for placebo and Levamisole treatment periods.

Two patients on Levamisole remained free of disease for 16 and 28 weeks, respectively. However, one of them had to be removed from the protocol because of granulocytopenia, which subsided without specific therapy after four days of hospitalization for reverse isolation.

DISCUSSION

The reason for poor stimulation of peripheral lymphocyte response to mitogens and mixed leukocyte reaction (15, 21), as well as the impairment of other functions of cell mediated immunity in patients with MF despite therapeutic approaches may lie within the lymphocyte itself. Our preliminary results, suggesting that decreased cAMP levels in lymphocytes from patients with MF remain at levels below control values after radiation therapy as well as after adjuvant immunotherapy with Levamisole support this hypothesis. In contrast, our earlier work (12, 13) indicated that patients with melanoma, squamous cell carcinoma and other solid tumors present with decreased cAMP levels and increased prostaglandin $F_2\alpha$-levels in peripheral lymphocytes. Surgical excision of the tumors resulted in a decrease of $PGF_2\alpha$-levels in patients with head and neck cancers and increase of cAMP levels in most patients. Levamisole, given for 8-18 weeks to patients who had impaired immunity but no clinical evidence of disease, resulted in further increase of cAMP to the control levels, which remained at this level in most of our patients in remission. Decrease of various immunological indices as well as sudden drop in lymphocyte cAMP levels usually preceded clinical recurrence of the tumor or metastasis by 6-8 weeks (13). Lack of positive clinical response of our patients with MF to adjuvant immunotherapy may be inherent in the lymphocytes inability to alter the adenyl cyclase-phosphodiesterase system, resulting in impaired translation of various cell membrane stimuli.

A series of elegant experiments, summarized by Ahmed (21), has shown that neoplastic T-cells from patients with Sezary syndrome were unable to respond to nonspecific mitogens, allogeneic cells, blastogenic factor and the mitogenic activity of anti-T serum. This lack of response was not secondary to the production of inhibitors. Our work, although preliminary, complements these results and suggests that the second messenger system of cyclic nucleotides in lymphocytes of patients with MF and Sezary syndrome may be responsible for immunotherapeutic failures in the cure of these skin lymphomas.

CONCLUSIONS:

1. Patients with mycosis fungoides Stage I, II, and III present with impaired immunity and decreased cyclic AMP levels in the peripheral lymphocytes.
2. The above values were unchanged by routine total body electron beam therapy with boosts to axilla and inner thigh and perineum.
3. Although Levamisole increased several parameters of cell mediated immunity in these patients increases of disease free intervals of Levamisole vs placebo treated patients were not observed.
4. Adjuvant Levamisole therapy did not produce an increase of cyclic AMP levels in these patients such as observed in patients with some solid tumors.

ACKNOWLEDGMENTS

This work was supported by a Grant from Winship Clinic. Our thanks are due to Miss Kris Wright, Mrs. Rainell Boswell, and Miss Wendy Hsiao for invaluable laboratory assistance, to Dr. M. Kutner for statistical analysis, to Ms. Peggy Firth for art work, and to Miss Nancy Fletcher for typing the manuscript.

Levamisole was supplied by Johnson and Johnson and help of Richard Berger, M.D. and Bob Edwards in this matter is gratefully acknowledged.

REFERENCES

1. Alibert, J.L.M. - Monographie des dermatoses, Ed. G. Bailiere, Paris, 1835, p. 413.
2. Epstein, E.H., et al. - Mycosis fungoides survival, prognostic features, response to therapy and autopsy findings. Medicine, 15, 61-72, 1972.
3. Bagshaw, M.A., et al. - Electron beam therapy of mycosis fungoides. California Med. 95, 292-297, 1961.
4. McGinley, P. Total body electron therapy utilizing a Linear Accelerator. Proc. of Varian Users Meeting, Callaway Gardens, Georgia, April 1976.
5. Dellon, A.L., et al. - Thymus dependent lymphocyte levels in bronchogeneic carcinoma; correlation with histology, clinical stage, and clinical course after surgical treatment. Cancer, 35, 687-698, 1975.
6. Olkowski, Z.L., and Wilkins, S. A. - T- lymphocyte levels in the peripheral blood of patients with cancer of the head and neck. The American Journal of Surgery, 130: 440-644, 1975.
7. Olkowski, Z. L., Powell, R. W., McLaren, J.R. - T-lymphocyte levels and immunoglobulins A,G, and M levels in patients with neoplastic breast diseases. Proc. 10th International Congress of Anatomists, Tokyo, Japan, August 25-30, 1975.

8. Olkowski, Z.L. and McLaren, J.R. - Immunocompetence of patients undergoing radiation therapy for breast cancer (abst.). Proc. of the 23rd Annual Meeting of the Radiation Research Society, Miami Beach, Fla., May 11-12, 1975.
9. Olkowski, Z.L., Murray, D.R., and McLaren, J.R. - Whither Immunocompetence? Journal of Medical Association of Georgia, June, 1975, p. 246-247.
10. Olkowski, Z.L., McLaren, J.R., and Mansour, K.A. - Immunocompetence of patients with bronchogenic carconoma. The Annals of Thoracic Surgery, 21: 546-551, 1976.
11. Olkowski, Z.L. and Nixon, D.W. - Immunological evaluation of breast cancer patients during chemotherapy. Proc of 3rd International Symposium on detection and Prevention of Cancer, New York, New York, April 26-May 1, 1976.
12. Wilkins, S.A. and Olkowski, Z.L. _ Immunocompetence of cancer patients treated with Levamisole. Cancer, Feb., 1977 (in press).
13. Olkowski, Z.L. - Cyclic Adenosine Monophosphate levels in lymphocytes from patients with melanoma and SCC of head and neck treated with Levamisole. Proc. Third International Conference of Modulation of Host Resistance in the Prevention or Treatment of Induced Neoplasia, Bethesda, Dec. 14-15, 1976.
14. Symoens, J. - An overview of Levamisole. ibid.
15. Nordqvist, B.C. and Kinney, J.P. - T and B cells and Cell Mediated Immunity in Mycosis Fungoides. Cancer, 37, 714-718, 1976.
16. Pauly, J.L., et al. - Whole blood culture technique for functional studies of lymphocyte reactivity to mitogens, antigens and homologous lymphocytes. J. Lab. Clinic. Med., 82, 500-512, 1973.
17. Pellegrino, M.A., Et al. - A rapid microtechnique for in vitro stimulation of human lymphocytes by PHA. Clin. Immunology and Immunopathology, 2, 67-73, 1973.
18. Kuo, J.F. and Greengard, P. - Cyclic Nucleotide Dependent Protein Kinases. VIII, An assay method for the measurement of adenosine 3'5' monophosphate in various tissues in the study of agents influencing its level in adipose cells. J. Biol. Chem., 245, 8067-8074, 1970.
19. Bahn, A.E. - Basic Medical Statistics. 5th Ed. Grune and Stratton, Inc. NY, 1972.
20. Fuks, Z., et al. - Prognostic signs and the management of the Mycosis Fungoides. Cancer, 32, 1385-1395, 1973.
21. Lutzner, M. (Moderator): Cutaneous T-cell lymphomas: The Sezary Syndrome, Mycosis Fungoides, and Related Disorders. NIH Conference. Ann.Int. Medicine, 83, 534-552, 1975.

Section X

PERSPECTIVES AND SUMMARY

Adjuvant Therapy of Cancer, S.E. Salmon and S.E. Jones eds.
© 1977 Elsevier/North-Holland Biomedical Press, Amsterdam

CURRENT TRENDS IN ADJUVANT THERAPY TRIALS FOR SOLID TUMORS

Arthur Louie, Stanislaw Mikulski, Daniel D. Von Hoff
Marcel Rozencweig, Franco M. Muggia
CTEP, DCT, National Cancer Institute
Bethesda, Maryland 20014

INTRODUCTION

Although adjuvant therapy has not been consistently encouraging, increasing knowledge of prognostic factors in early disease[1] and more effective systemic therapies in advanced disease have renewed interest in trials of this approach. This review analyzes current design concepts for adjuvant therapy trials in solid tumors. We define adjuvant therapy as systemic therapy designed to eradicate undectable tumor foci in patients apparently disease-free after surgery and radiotherapy.

MATERIALS AND METHODS

Protocols of 71 ongoing adjuvant clinical studies were reviewed in the Division of Cancer Treatment of the National Cancer Institute. The analysis is restricted to patient eligibility and stratification criteria and current trends in therapy.

RESULTS

The distribution of the 71 adjuvant trials by tumor type is summarized in Table I. Studies in 5 major tumor types (breast, GI, lung, bone sarcomas, and malignant melanoma) account for two-thirds of the studies, with most of them in breast and GI cancer. Chemotherapy which appears in 61 protocols, is the most widely used treatment modality. RT is given in 22 studies and is either randomly tested or allowed before randomization. Immunotherapy is tested in 15 studies, most of them in breast cancer and melanoma. An analysis by individual tumor type follows.

<u>Breast Cancer</u> (15 trials): Patient eligibility is quite uniform; all patients are treated with either a radical or modified radical mastectomy and all have positive lymph nodes. The only exception is the National Surgical Adjuvant Breast Project (NSABP #6) study of different types of surgery for breast cancer. Most studies have patient age limits of 70-75 years. Eligibility for radiotherapy (RT) is well specified; 8 studies exclude patients with prior RT, 4 studies allow and stratify for prior RT, and 2 studies include RT combined with chemotherapy. Generally, radioisotope scanning, mammography, and xerography for patient evaluation and follow-up are optional. Stratification is principally by nodal status, age, and menopausal status. Nodal status and age are used in the NSABP studies (#7-10); the other studies differ from each other by at least one stratification criterion.

Well studied treatments include L-PAM[2] and cyclophosphamide + methotrexate + 5-Fluorouracil (CMF) based combinations,[3,4] This is reflected in the drugs selected for these trials. Of note, all of the 5 "CMF" studies differ significantly in either dose, schedule, or duration of treatment. The only studies using hormonal therapy are found in the breast studies; both trials use tamoxifen + combination CT.

The most striking finding is the complete absence of untreated controls in these studies. Because preliminary reports suggested prolongation of disease-free interval with L-PAM or CMF new studies were designed without control arms; ongoing studies sometimes dropped existing control arms. It may be argued that this step was premature, since long term follow-up is incomplete.

Gastrointestinal Cancer (11 trials in gastric, large bowel, and rectal cancer) Most studies agree on the importance of microscopically negative margins at resection. Prior CT or RT is not allowed. There is disagreement on the need for en bloc resections which are required in only 4 of 11 studies; the rest allow discontinuous removal of tumor. There is little agreement concerning patients with ascites; 7 studies do not mention it, 3 specifically exclude such patients. Most studies set limits on the time between surgery and the start of adjuvant therapy. Stratification is by depth of tumor invasion, location of the primary, extent of surgery, and time between surgery and start of adjuvant therapy. Only depth of tumor invasion is used by more than half of the studies; the other criteria are used in only a minority of studies so there is substantial variability in stratification among these trials.

As in advanced disease, 5-FU[5] and MeCCNU[6], alone or combined[7], are the backbone of adjuvant therapy. Every CT study uses one or both drugs; 4 studies use the 2-drug combination exclusively. Seven studies have untreated control groups, 2 studies use immunostimulation, and all 3 rectal cancer studies use RT.

Lung Cancer (7 trials in non-small cell carcinoma): All studies select or stratify patients by cell type and disease stage; nearly all studies set minimal performance status standards. As in the GI studies, some minor stratification criteria, including type of surgery and histologic differentiation, introduce variability.

Treatment involves CT in 4 studies, RT in 2 studies, and immunotherapy in 1 study. All CT studies are randomized, with untreated control arms, and use CCNU alone or in combination with other agents. Duration of CT is 12 months for 1 study and 24 months for the other 3 studies. The 2 RT studies are randomized and 1 has an untreated control. Each study deals with a different stage or cell type and, thus, no study is directly comparable to another study in the group. The chemotherapeutic agents used are limited.

Bone Sarcomas (7 trials): The trials allow patient entry following bone biopsy confirmation of the diagnosis. Most studies clearly separate classical osteogenic sarcoma from other bone cancers. The main disagreement on patient entry concerns resected pulmonary metastases; 4 studies specifically exclude these patients while 3 studies allow entry if all metastases can be resected. Stratification criteria are highly variable and are not specified at all in 3 studies. In the other 4 studies a wide variety of minor criteria (location of the primary, histologic type, extent of disease, immune status, age, sex, tumor size, onset of adjuvant treatment, and prior treatment with RT) illustrate the non-uniform stratification. Notably, only 1 of the 3 studies allowing patients with resectable metastases stratifies separately for this group.

Study design is also quite variable. Four studies are randomized but only 1 has an untreated control group; 3 studies used historical controls. CT is used in all of the studies, usually in combination regimens. The most commonly used drugs are adriamycin, cyclophosphamide, and vincristine.

Melanoma (7 trials): Patient entry required histologically confirmed diagnoses with either no regional node metastases or metastases in only one regional node group. There was some controversy about entry of patients with recurrent but resectable disease; it was allowed in 4 studies, specifically excluded in 2 studies, and unspecified in the 1 study. Stratification is mainly by sex, presence or absence of node dissection, and time elapsed since surgery. Minor criteria include: tumor thickness, regional node status, skin test reactivity, and primary vs recurrent disease. Although not specifically listed as a criterion, histologic level was noted in 6 patients. Two studies did not specify stratification criteria.

Reports of successful therapy with BCG[8] have led to trials of immunostimulants; 5 trials employ BCG, C. parvum, or transfer factor. CT, most commonly DTIC alone or in combination, is used in 4 studies.

Genitourinary Tumors (6-4 bladder cancer and 2 testicular cancer). The bladder trials explore a variety of approaches: preoperative and postoperative RT, bladder instillation with thiotepa, and poly I: C. The testicular protocols explore RT and CT with vinblastine, bleomycin, and cis-platinum.

Ovarian Tumors (5 trials): The studies evaluate alkylating agent therapy, RT and combinations of the two. Only 2 of the 5 studies have untreated control groups. Four studies use melphalan as the alkylating agent.

Other Tumors (13 trials): These include studies for head and neck tumors, soft tissue sarcomas, pediatric solid tumors, and a few studies of "limited extent" brain tumors.

TABLE I
DISTRIBUTION OF ADJUVANT STUDIES IN THE MAJOR TUMOR TYPES

Tumor Type	# of Studies	Study Design: Randomized	Study Design: Untreated Control	Treatment Modalities Under Study[a]: CT	IT	RT	CT+IT	RT+CT
Breast	15	14	0	8[b]	0	0[d]	6[c]	1
Gastrointestinal	11	11	8	6	0	1	2	2
Lung	7	7	6	4	1	2	0	0
Bone Sarcomas	7	4	1	7	0	0	0	0
Melanoma	7	6	5	2	3	0[e]	2	0
Genitourinary	6	5	0	2	0	2	0	2
Ovarian	5	5	2	2	0	0	0	3
Other[f]	13	10	4	1	0	0	3	9
Total	71	62	26	32	4	5	13	17

a. CT = Chemotherapy; IT = immunotherapy; RT= radiotherapy
b. Includes one study of CT + hormonal therapy (tamoxifen)
c. Includes one study of CT + IT + hormonal therapy (tamoxifen)
d. Preoperative radiotherapy
e. (1) RT alone vs Preoperative RT (2) Preoperative RT vs Postoperative RT vs RT alone
f. Head and neck tumors, soft tissue sarcomas, pediatric solid tumors, brain tumors

TABLE II
PRINCIPAL PARAMETERS OF STRATIFICATION USED IN ADJUVANT TRIALS

Tumor Type	Total No. of Trials	Stratification: Parameter	No. of Trials	% of Total
Breast	15	Node Status	11	73
		Age or Menopausal Status	13	87
Gastrointestinal	11	Depth of Tumor Invasion	6	55
		Location	3	27
		Extent of Surgery	2	18
		Time from surgery to adjuvant therapy	2	18
Lung	7	Clinical Stage	6	86
Bone Sarcomas	7	None	3	43
		Location of Primary	3	43
		Classical vs Atypical sarcoma	2	29
Melanoma	7	Sex	4	57
		± Node Dissection	2	29
		Time elapsed since surgery	2	29

TABLE III
REGIMENS MOST COMMONLY INVOLVED IN ADJUVANT TRIALS

Tumor Type (Total Trials)	Regimen	No. of Studies	% of Total Trials
Breast (15)	L-PAM	5	33
	L-PAM + 5-FU	4	27
	CMF	6	40
Gastrointestinal (11)	5-FU ± MeCCNU	10	91
Lung (7)	CCNU	4	57
Bone sarcomas (7)	Adriamycin	7	100
	Cyclophosphamide	6	86
	Vincristine	5	71
	High dose Methotrexate	4	57
Melanoma (7)	DTIC	4	57
	BCG	2	29
	C. Parvum	2	29
Genitourinary (6)	Radiotherapy	4	67
Ovarian (5)	L-PAM	4	80
	Radiotherapy	3	60

DISCUSSION

Patient entry criteria are relatively well defined in all the studies, with heavy reliance on cell type (lung tumors) and anatomic stage of disease. Most studies require histologic diagnoses and exclude patients with prior therapy. Thus, the trend is toward better defined patient groups and eventually this should lead to more consistent and accurate results in most studies.

A major finding in this analysis is that adjuvant therapy in many tumor types is dominated by only 1 or 2 treatment regimens, and many trials have only slight variations on a common theme. (Table III). This is certainly true in breast cancer where L-PAM ± 5-FU and CMF based regimens are used in the overwhelming majority of studies and is also true in GI cancer where 5-FU plus MeCCNU appears in all of the CT protocols. Similar trends can be seen in lung cancer, bone sarcomas, melanoma, and ovarian cancer.

Standarization of treatment regimens is desirable if adjuvant therapy is successful. However, in colon and lung cancer and for other tumor types, adjuvant studies have not yet shown consistently promising results and, perhaps, little would be lost by initiating studies with other active agents or agent combinations.

For the future we hope that increasing knowledge of tumor biology will allow study designs with more uniform criteria for patient entry and, in particular, for stratification. We expect increasing use of immunotherapy. Finally, we hope that in diseases where current adjuvant therapy is suboptimal, new agents successful in advanced disease will be introduced into adjuvant trials.

REFERENCES

1. Staquet, M. (1975) Cancer Therapy: Prognostic Factors, and criteria of Response, Raven Press, New York.
2. Sears, M., et al. Melphalan in Advanced Breast Cancer, Cancer Chemotherapy Reports 50:271, 1966 (No. 5)
3. Ansfield, F., et al. Five Drug Therapy for Advanced Breast Cancer: A Phase I Study. Cancer Chemotherapy Reports 55:183, 1971 (Part 1, No.2)
4. Cooper, R. Combination Chemotherapy in Hormone Resistant Breast Cancer. Proceedings American Association Cancer Research 10:15, 1969
5. Carter, S.K., et al. Integration of Chemotherapy into Combined Modality Treatment of Solid Tumors, Part II: Large Bowel Carcinoma, Cancer Treatment Reviews 1:111, 1974
6. Moertel, C.G. Therapy of Advanced Gastrointestinal Cancer with Nitrosoureas. Cancer Chemotherapy Reports 4:27, 1973
7. Baker, L.H., et al. 5-FU vs 5-FU and MeCCNU in Gastrointestinal cancers. A Phase III study of the Southwest Oncology Group. Proceedings American Society Clinical Oncology 16:229, 1975
8. Gutterman, J.U., et al. Active Immunotherapy with BCG for Recurrent Malignant Melanoma. Lancet 1:1208, 1973

Adjuvant Therapy of Cancer, S.E. Salmon and S.E. Jones eds.
© 1977 Elsevier/North-Holland Biomedical Press, Amsterdam

IMMUNOTHERAPY OF HUMAN CANCER: AN OVERVIEW

By Evan M. Hersh, M.D., Jordan U. Gutterman, M.D., Giora M. Mavligit, M.D., and Samuel G. Murphy, Ph.D., M.D., Department of Developmental Therapeutics, The University of Texas System Cancer Center, M. D. Anderson Hospital and Tumor Institute, Houston, Texas, 77030. Supported by Contract N01-CB-33888 and Grant CA-05831, from the National Cancer Institute, National Institutes of Health, Bethesda, Maryland 20014.

During the last seven years, clinical trials of various immunotherapeutic modalities have been intensively investigated as an additional modality of cancer treatment. Immunotherapy appears to have immunological and clinical activity in several human malignancies, including breast cancer, colon cancer, lung cancer, malignant melanoma, malignant lymphoma, and several of the leukemias. Immunotherapy originally appeared to be most active when the tumor burden was small. However, newer data from animal models and the recent clinical studies, suggests that immunotherapy may show activity even in patients with advanced or metastatic disease and a large tumor burden. Newer approaches to systemic adjuvant immunotherapy administered by the intravenous route are encouraging in this regard. The ultimate role of immunotherapy in the management of human malignancy cannot be determined at this time. Immunotherapy is in its earliest developmental phases. The available agents are crude and poorly defined. In addition, rapid developments in other adjuvant approaches, particularly adjuvant chemotherapy and new approaches to adjuvant radiotherapy make the future role of immunotherapy uncertain. In this paper we will outline some of the approaches to and principles of immunotherapy. An overview of the current status of the positive trends in immunotherapy of several human malignancies will be detailed. We will briefly review some of the highlights of our adjuvant studies in the immunotherapy of malignant melanoma. Finally, newer approaches to immunotherapy which have the potential for clinical application to human cancer will be reviewed.

Table 1 shows a classification of the various approaches to immunotherapy. Active-non-specific immunotherapy refers to the use of microbial or synthetic materials with adjuvant activity which can boost general immunocompetence, increase cell-mediated or humoral immunity, and most important, activate macrophages[1]. The chemical agent levamisole was originally classified as a member of the non-specific immunotherapeutic reagents. However, it should be considered in the category of immunorestorative agents which can, acting through the cyclic nucleotide system, increase the numbers of circulating maturity lymphocytes and restore deficient T-lymphocyte functions such as delayed hypersensitivity in immunologically incompetent individuals[2]. Active-specific immunotherapy refers to immunization with tumor cells or tumor antigen. Adoptive and cellular product immunotherapy refers to the transfer of general immunocompetence or specific tumor immunity or both from a competent or immune donor to an incompetent or non-immune patient using lymphocytes or lymphocyte products such as transfer factor, immune RNA, thymic hormones, interferon, or lymphokines. Passive immunotherapy refers to the use of antibody directed against the tumor cell surface antigens which can function in a variety of ways including direct cytotoxicity, facilitation of anti-tumor attack of lymphocytes or macrophages, or by deblocking through the removal of blocking substances from the blood. Local immunotherapy refers to the direct intralesional injection of active-non-specific or adoptive immunotherapeutic reagents directly into primary or metastatic tumors[3]. Tumors are killed by a bystander effect of the delayed hypersensitivity reaction by the macrophages activated by the adjuvant and in the process, more extensive antitumor immunity may be induced.

TABLE 1

APPROACHES TO THE IMMUNOTHERAPY OF MALIGNANT DISEASE

APPROACH	MECHANISM OF ACTION	COMMONLY USED REAGENT	DISEASES WHERE ACTIVITY DEMONSTRATED
Active Non-specific (Immunostimulation)	Increase general immune competence, activate macrophages, possible cross immunogenecity with tumor antigens	BCG C. parvum MER	Melanoma Leukemia Colon Ca. Lung Ca. Breast Ca.
Immuno-restoration	Restore immunocompetence	Levamisole Thymosin	Lung Ca. Breast Ca.
Active specific	Increase specific cell-mediated and humoral anti-tumor immunity	Tumor Cells Tumor Antigens	Leukemia Lung Ca.
Adoptive	Transfer tumor immunity from immune to hypo-immune subjects	Immune Cells Transfer Factor Immune RNA Lymphokines	None with certainty ? Sarcoma ? Melanoma
Passive	Transfer of cytotoxic, deblocking, opsonizing, ADCC or drug or isotope transporting antibody	Allogeneic or xenogeneic natural or induced antibody	None with certainty
Local-regional	Locally activate macrophages, kill tumor by bystander effect of DTH, induce specific tumor immunity	BCG C. parvum PPD DNCB	Lung Ca. Melanoma Breast Ca.

At the present time, only active-non-specific and local immunotherapy have been investigated in any detail. Even these modalities of immunotherapy have been very inadequately explored in man. Immunotherapeutic effects demonstrated thus far have been relatively weak. There have been a few studies suggesting some activity for chemical immunostimulants and active-specific immunotherapy.

There is essentially no evaluable data regarding adoptive or passive immunotherapy.

Table 2 lists some of the objectives of immunotherapy. These objectives are based on the evidence that there are tumor associated antigens and tumor associated immune responses in at least some cancer patients, that there is a correctable immunological deficiency associated with malignancy or induced by its treatment, and that there are clinical circumstances in which these therapeutic modalities can be both rationally and ethically applied. Immunotherapy can be designed to restore the immunocompetence of deficient patients or patients whose immunity is depressed by treatment. Active-non-specific immunotherapeutic reagents, such as BCG or C. parvum[1], or better, immunorestorative agents such as levamisole[2], or thymic hormones[4] are active in these circumstances. Active-specific immunization against tumor associated antigens can be used to induce or heighten specific tumor immunity, particularly when the tumor burden is low. Immunotherapy may also be designed to modulate immune responses for specific objectives. Since it has recently been demonstrated that activated macrophages can kill tumor cells, and that activation of macrophages and of the reticuloendothelial system is important in host defense against cancer and is part of the mechanism of action of microbial adjuvants[1]. The use of agents which can specifically modulate host defense mechanisms to activate macrophages and the reticuloendothelial system seem particularly appropriate. This can be best accomplished at present by the intravenous administration of microbial adjuvants.

TABLE 2

OBJECTIVES OF IMMUNOTHERAPY

1. Restore Immunocompetence of Immunodeficient Patient
2. Prevent or Reverse Immunosuppression Induced by Surgery, Radiotherapy, Chemotherapy
3. Induce Specific Tumor Immunity if Absent
4. Heighten Specific Tumor Immunity if Weak
5. Modulate Immune Response for Selected Objectives
    - Augment Cell-Mediated Immunity
    - Increase Cytotoxic Antibody
    - Activate Macrophages
    - Increase RES Clearance of Particles
        - Reduce Blocking Factors
        - Reduce Antigen-Antibody Complexes

In an overview of the clinical trials of immunotherapy in human cancer, there is evidence in several classes of cancer that immunotherapy has activity. However, for each of the disease categories and approaches to immunotherapy, negative trials have also been reported, and the utility of immunotherapy in these diseases is not generally accepted.

In malignant melanoma (Table 3), responses to immunotherapy have been reported for patients with primary disease as well as for patients with metastatic disease.

TABLE 3

IMMUNOTHERAPY OF MALIGNANT MELANOMA IN MAN

STAGE (ANDERSON) AND EVIDENT DISEASE (YES OR NO = y or n)		TYPE OF IMMUNOTHERAPY	CONCURRENT CHEMOTHERAPY	RESULT OR RESPONSE
I	y	Vaccinia IL then Surgery	No	↑DFI & S
I	y	BCG IL then Surgery	No	Too Early
I	n	BCG (Cutaneous)	No	Too Early
III	n	BCG (Cutaneous)	No	↑DFI & S
III	n	BCG plus Allo. Irr. cultured TC	No	↑DFI & S
IVA	n	BCG (Cutaneous)	No	↑DFI & S
IVB	y	BCG (Cutaneous)	Yes	↑Remission Duration & S.
IVB	y	BCG plus Autolo. Irr. TC	No	Regression in 40%
IVB	y	BCG plus Allo. Irr. TC	Yes	Remission in 60%
IVB	y	C. parvum IV for 14 days	Yes	Increased Remission Rate Duration & S
IVB	y	BCG (Oral)	No	Tumor Regression & ↑S
IVB	y	Cross Grafting and Cross Leukocyte Transfusion	No	Tumor Regression in 26/123
IVB	y	Transfer Factor	No	Tumor Regression in 40%
IVB	y	Transfusion of Remission Serum	No	Tumor Regression
IVB	y	Transfusion of Antibody Bound Drug	Yes	Increased Remission Rate
IVB	y	Levamisole	Yes	Increased Survival

Abbreviations and Definitions: Stage I, primary III: regional lymph node metastases; IVA: distant metastases no evident disease: IVB: distant metastases evident disease; IL: intralesional; DFI: disease free interval; S: survival; Allo.: allogeneic; Irr.: irradiated; TC: tumor cells; IV: intravenous.

The administration of intralesional vaccinia[5] prior to surgery produces a modest prolongation of disease-free interval and survival. BCG administered cutaneously with or without tumor cells and with or without chemotherapy to patients who have had stage III or stage IV disease removed surgically may also increase the post-surgical disease-free interval and survival[6]. In patients with metastatic melanoma, the administration of BCG cutaneously appears to increase remission duration and survival when added to chemotherapy[7], while the administration of C. parvum appears to also increase the remission rate. Of great interest, certain approaches to immunotherapy when administered alone to patients with metastatic disease can induce remissions in melanoma. Thus, in pilot studies vaccines of tumor cells mixed with BCG[8], the intravenous administration of C. parvum[9] or the administration of transfer factor[10], have been associated with transient remissions in 20% to 40% of the patients. However, a number of investigators have been unable to confirm some of these preliminary observations in more extensive studies.

In lung cancer (Table 4), there is evidence that immunotherapy has activity. However, this group of studies to be mentioned must be confirmed before the current results can be accepted. The most important study is that of McKneally, in which intrapleural BCG following surgery has prolonged both the disease-free interval and the survival in patients with stage I lung cancer[11]. The post-surgical disease-free interval and survival of stage I patients is apparently also prolonged by the administration of tumor antigen mixed with complete Freund's adjuvant[12] or by the pre- and post-operative administration of levamisole[13]. Each of these modalities of immunotherapy is ineffective in patients with stage II or III disease at least to the extent that they have been tested. There are, however, several reports of immunotherapy showing activity in patients with advanced disease which could not be completely removed surgically. A BCG water extract and a modified tumor cell vaccine in complete Freund's adjuvant both seemed to prolong survival. These studies, however, have not yet been confirmed. Finally, in patients with advanced regional or distant metastatic disease, survival of patients receiving chemotherapy appears to be prolonged if they also receive immunotherapy with subcutaneous C. parvum[14], with BCG cell wall skeleton[15], or with OK432[16]. All of these studies must be confirmed and extended.

TABLE 4

IMMUNOTHERAPY OF LUNG CANCER IN MAN

STAGE AND EVIDENT DISEASE (y or n)		TYPE OF IMMUNOTHERAPY	CONCURRENT CHEMOTHERAPY	RESULT OR RESPONSE
I	n	BCG, Intrapleural	No	↑DFI
II,III	n	BCG, Intrapleural	No	No Effect
I-II	n	BCG, Cutaneous	No	↑DFI & S
I-IV	n, y	BCG CWS-oil Multiple Routes	Yes	↑Survival
III	y	BCG Water Extract	No	Partial Remission
III,IV	y	C. parvum (SC)	Yes	↑Survival
III,IV	y	OK432	Yes	↑Survival
II,III	y	Modified Auto. TC plus CFA	No	↑Survival
I	n	PAGE Purified Tumor Antigen + CFA	Yes	↑DFI
I	n	Levamisole	No	↑DFI & S
II,III	n	Levamisole	No	No Effect

Abbreviations: BCG; Bacillus Calmette Guerin; DFI: disease-free interval; S: survival; CWS: cell wall skeleton; PAGE: polyacrylamide gel electrophoresis; CFA: complete Freund's adjuvant; TC: tumor cells.

A variety of studies have also shown that immunotherapy may have activity in leukemia (Table 5). The classical study of Mathè and co-workers in which children with ALL received either BCG, allogeneic irradiated tumor cells or both after the end of chemotherapy resulted in an increased disease-free interval and survival[17]. This study has never been confirmed but none of the several attempts to reproduce it followed the original experimental design. This study is important, however, because it was the report which prompted much of the modern development of the field of immunotherapy.

TABLE 5

IMMUNOTHERAPY OF LEUKEMIA IN MAN

HISTOLOGIC TYPE	TYPE OF IMMUNOTHERAPY NON-SPECIFIC	SPECIFIC	RESULT OR RESPONSE
ALL	BCG	Allo. Irr. TC	Increased DFI & S
ALL	B. pertussis	None	Increased DFI
AML	BCG	Allo. Irr. Tc	Increased DFI & S
AML	BCG	None	Increased S
AML	MER	None	Increased DFI S & Remission Rate
AML	Pseudomonas Vaccine	None	Increased DFI & S
AML	None	Allo. Neura-minidase treated TC	Increased DFI & S
CML	BCG	Allo. Irr. Cultured Lymphoid Cell Line	Increased S
CLL	None	Anti-allotype Serum	Hematological Improvement

Abbreviations: ALL: acute lymphatic leukemia; AML: acute myelogenous leukemia; CML: chronic myelogenous leukemia; CLL: chronic lymphatic leukemia; BCG: Bacillus Calmette Guerin; Allo.: allogeneic; Irr.: Irradiated; TC: tumor cells; MER: methanol extraction residue; DFI: disease-free interval; S.: Survival. NOTE: In ALL, most attempts at immunotherapy have not been effective. See text.

In AML there are now a number of studies suggesting that BCG alone[18], BCG plus allogeneic irradiated tumor cells[19], MER[20], Pseudomonas vaccine[21], or allogeneic neuraminidase-treated tumor cell vaccine[23] can improve the survival of leukemia patients. Of interest, only a few of these studies show an effect on remission duration. The reason for this is unclear, but it presumably relates to an easier ability to induce second remissions. Immunotherapy is apparently also active in CML although the original study in this area awaits confirmation[23]. Immunotherapy of various types has also shown activity in a variety of other human tumors. These are outlined in Table 6.

TABLE 6

IMMUNOTHERAPY OF OTHER MALIGNANT DISEASES IN MAN

HISTOLOGIC TYPE	STAGE AND EVIDENT DISEASE (y or n)		IMMUNOTHERAPY	CONCURRENT CHEMOTHERAPY	RESULT OR RESPONSE
Hodgkin's	I-IV	n	BCG	No	↑DFI
Non-Hodgkin's lymphoma	III-IV	n	BCG	No	↑DFI
Osteogenic sarcoma	I	n	TC Homogenate	No	↑DFI & S
Osteogenic sarcoma	I	n	BCG + Allo. Irr. Cultured TC	No	No Effect
Osteogenic sarcoma	Advanced	y	Transfer Factor	Yes, No	Stabilization
Soft Tissue sarcoma	I	n	BCG + Allo. Irr. Cultured TC	Yes, No	↑DFI & S
Breast Ca.	II	n	BCG	Yes	↑DFI & S
Breast Ca.	III	n	Auto. Irr. TC	No	↑S
Breast Ca.	III	n	Levamisole	No	↑DFI & S
Breast Ca.	IV	y	Transfer Factor	No	Partial Remission
Breast Ca.	IV	y	BCG or MER	Yes	↑Remission Duration & S
Colon Ca.	Dukes' C	n	BCG or FU-BCG	Yes	↑DFI & S
Colon Ca.	Dukes' D	y	BCG or MER	Yes	No Effect
Head & Neck Ca.	Advanced	y	BCG	Yes	↑Remission Rate or Survival
Renal Ca.	Advanced	y	BCG	No	Partial Remission in 40%

Abbreviations: BCG: Bacillus Calmette Guerin; DFI: disease-free interval; S: survival; Allo.: allogeneic; Irr.: irradiated; TC: tumor cells; Auto.: autologous; MER: methanol extraction residue; FU: 5-fluorouracil.

The experience with immunotherapy of malignant melanoma at the M. D. Anderson Hospital and Tumor Institute is of interest because it illustrates some of the principles of immunotherapy. Table 7 summarizes this work. Patients with clinical stage III disease that is, regional node metastases, who were brought to a state of no evident disease by surgery were treated with BCG immunotherapy after surgery and compared to historical controls. In a study comparing the administration of BCG by scarification weekly for three months, and then every other week by rotation to the four extremities to the historical control, two doses of BCG were investigated. Overall, the high dose of BCG, 6×10^8 organisms per scarification, was effective in prolonging remission and survival while a low dose of BCG, 6×10^7 organisms was not effective. However, for patients who had trunk primary melanoma, metastatic to regional lymph nodes, and who were rendered free of disease by surgery, both the high dose and the low dose were effective. A significant improvement in disease-free interval was observed and it was estimated that 40% of the patients on immunotherapy were still in remission at 50 months, compared to 20% among the historical control. In contrast, patients with head and neck primary tumors did not benefit from BCG. Their remission duration and survival was identical to that of the historical controls. Since BCG was administered into the proximal portions of the upper and lower extremities, it was not introduced into the regional lymphatic drainage of the primary tumor in these patients. In contrast to our data in this regard, in the studies reported by Morton[24], BCG was administered over the primary lesion and efficacy for BCG in patients who originally had head and neck primaries was seen. The conclusions from these studies are that BCG has activity, that the activity is not great, that the dose of immunotherapy is critical, and that the administration must be in the regional area of the disease.

TABLE 7

EFFECTS OF IMMUNOTHERAPY OF MELANOMA ILLUSTRATING PRINCIPLES OF IMMUNOTHERAPY

STAGE AND SITE	EVIDENT DISEASE	IMMUNOTHERAPY			RESULT
		AGENT	DOSE	ROUTE	
IIIB All Sites	No	BCG	High	Skin (arms & legs)	↑DFI & S
IIIB All Sites	No	BCG	Low	Same	No Effect
IIIB Trunk	No	BCG	High or low	Same	↑DFI & S
IIIB Head & Neck	No	BCG	High or low	Same	No Effect
IVB	Yes	BCG	High	Same	↑RD & S
IVB	Yes	C.parvum	High	IV	↑RR,RD & S

High dose BCG = 6×10^8 viable units, low dose = 6×10^7, high dose C. parvum = 2 mg/m^2/day. DFI = disease-free interval; S=survival, RR=remission rate; RD= remission duration, IV=intravenous.

Immunotherapy has also shown activity as an adjunct to chemotherapy for advanced metastatic melanoma. Leads obtained from the treatment of metastatic disease are rationally applied to the adjunctive treatment of earlier disease. When BCG immunotherapy was added between courses of DTIC chemotherapy for metastatic malignant melanoma, several important observations were made[6]. First, the addition of BCG to DTIC did not significantly influence the response of disease in visceral sites like lung or liver. However, the addition of BCG improved responses to chemotherapy in lymph nodes and subcutaneous sites from 18% to 55%. This again showed the regional effects of BCG. Also, BCG did have an overall effect on survival. A significant improvement in survival was noted compared to historical controls receiving chemotherapy alone, although there were few long term survivors. It is reasonable to assume that more potnet immunotherapeutic reagents given by improved routes, doses, or schedules, might have a greater immunotherapeutic effect.

From these observations, and the work of other investigators, the limitations of BCG immunotherapy are becoming clear. There is variability among different lots and suppliers in the number of viable BCG organisms per milliliter. Different strains vary in virulence and genetic change in virulence and other strain characteristics have been noted. While systemic BCG disease is rare, we have observed it in several patients receiving BCG by scarification. It is difficult to administer an accurate dose of BCG by the cutaneous route. The remission rate on BCG is not greatly increased compared to conventional therapy. Finally, at least part of the effects of BCG are regional and disease in visceral sites, which is most important clinically, is least affected by the cutaneous application of BCG. For these reasons, we have begun to investigate intensive intravenous C. parvum therapy before and between courses of chemotherapy for metastatic malignant melanoma. In experimental models, intravenous immunotherapy with agents which can activate macrophages does effect visceral disease[25]. In a pilot study at M. D. Anderson Hospital (unpublished observations), we observed an increase in response of liver metastases among patients receiving C. parvum in addition to chemotherapy. Finally, pilot studies by Pierre Band[26] and Lucien Israel[27] have suggested that C. parvum can itself cause the regression of visceral metastases and that it may increase the sensitivity to chemotherapy.

With this in mind, we designed a protocol in which patients received intravenous C. parvum daily for 10 to 14 days, followed by cycles of DTIC or DTIC + actinomycin chemotherapy. Between courses of chemotherapy, the patients received subcutaneous C. parvum, and every three months, daily intravenous C. parvum was repeated (unpublished observations). This therapy was well tolerated. The response rate to chemotherapy in patients receiving a dose of C. parvum approximating 2 $mg/m^2/day$ approaches 40%. This is a significant improvement over our previously observed overall response rate of 26% on DTIC-BCG, and 15% on DTIC alone[6]. The survival of these patients was also markedly improved with approximately 90% being alive at 6 months, compared to 75% on DTIC-BCG and 55% on DTIC alone. Our conclusion is that systemic administration of microbial adjuvants intravenously, where host defense mechanisms can be activated in visceral tumor sites such as liver and lungs, may improve the prognosis of patients receiving chemotherapy. Furthermore, application of intravenous systemic adjuvant immunotherapy to patients with earlier stages of disease should be even more beneficial. As purification of the active subcomponents of microbial adjuvants procedes, active non-toxic preparations for intravenous use should become available.

Several newer approaches to immunotherapy are showing great promise for the future (Table 8). One of these is active-non-specific immunotherapy with natural or synthetic purified microbial subfractions which can be given regionally or systemically. These include various combinations of the active granuloma-forming components of BCG, namely trehalose dimycolate, other esters of trehalose and relatively non-toxic mutant derivatives of endotoxin, such as Re glycolipid from the various strains of Salmonella[28]. Other approaches include active-specific immunotherapy with purified tumor antigen preparations and the application to patients with immunodeficiency of immunorestorative agents, such as thymosin or levamisole. Ribi and co-workers have been investigating the immunotherapy activity of microbacterial fractions[28]. One of the active components of BCG appears to be various esters of trehalose. The critical feature is that the trehalose be esterified to relatively long chained branched fatty acids such as mycolic acid which is found in mycobacteria or corynomycolic acid, which is found in corynebacterium such as C. parvum. Ribi has studied a number of these in the guinea pig hepatoma model. The activity of BCG or BCG cell wall in causing regression of the primary tumor and clearing of disease in regional lymph nodes can be completely mimicked by a combination of trehalose esters and Re mutant endotoxin. Virtually 100% cures are obtained with this combination. The individual components show almost no activity. These materials are important because they are non-viable, can be formulated precisely, and the dosage can be accurate. Their entry into clinical trials is awaited with great anticipation.

TABLE 8

NEWER APPROACHES TO IMMUNOTHERAPY

APPROACH	AGENT	MECHANISM
Active-non-specific	Trehalose dimycolate Trehalose dicorynomycolate Re mutant endotoxin	Adjuvant and macrophage activation
Immunorestoration	Levamisole Thymosin Thymic Humoral Factor	Restore T-lymphocyte function to normal
Active specific	Tumor antigen purified by column chromatography and PAGE*	Boosts specific humoral and cell-mediated immunity

*PAGE=Polyacrylamide gel electrophoresis

In active specific immunotherapy, purified tumor antigens are receiving attention. Stewart and Hollinshead and co-workers[12] reported that immunization with tumor antigen in complete Freund's adjuvant with or without chemotherapy prolonged the disease-free interval and survival in patients with stage I lung cancer. Small numbers, short follow-up, and lack of a confirmatory study prevent complete interpretation of that data. However, active-specific immunization with purified tumor antigen can boost reactivity to autologous tumor. Thus, we have observed the blastogenic responses of the lymphocytes of patients in remission from AML to their own leukemic cells increases significantly and specifically after repeated immunization with purified allogeneic leukemia antigen (unpublished observations). A variety of doses of pooled allogeneic antigen are effective. The conclusion that the response is specific, is based on the fact that blastogenic responses to mitogens and other antigens did not increase.

Immunorestoration with thymosin or thymic humoral factor is of increasing interest[4]. Since many cancer patients have deficiencies in the number and function of T-lymphocytes, and since these are important to host control of cancer, their restoration to normal by agents like thymosin and levamisole could be important. In our clinic we have noted significant boosting of in vitro lymphocyte blastogenic responses and the numbers of circulating T-lymphocytes among immunodeficient cancer patients who have received thymosin[29]. Thus, there seems to be a rationale for the use of this agent and clinical trials with it have started. The in vivo administration of levamisole is apparently also associated with improved immunological function in cancer patients. We have observed an increase in in vivo delayed hypersensitivity among immunoincompetent patients after even a single dose of levamisole[30]. Levamisole may already have been proven to have activity in human cancer. In the data published by Amery and coworkers[13], in a study of levamisole versus placebo immunotherapy in stage I lung cancer, the relapse rate among patients on immunotherapy after removal of relatively large tumors was significantly diminished, compared to the appropriate control. A similar observation has been made in stage III breast cancer after radiotherapy.

In summary, immunotherapy has been actively investigated recently. A number of biological and clinical observations indicating activity have been made. We must realize that immunotherapy is in its early developmental stages. Immunotherapy today is where chemotherapy was in 1950. While in our clinic we feel that immunotherapy is unequivocally indicated in a number of specific disease categories, this is a controversial point-of-view at this time. The immunotherapeutic agents available to us today are weak. We do not understand their mechanisms of action. We do not know their optimum timing, dose, route, or schedule of administration. In addition, immunotherapy may have detrimental as well as beneficial effects, and may under certain circumstances be associated with tumor enhancement. Finally, the role of immunotherapy particularly relative to the role of other adjuvant approaches such as chemotherapy cannot be determined at this time, and should be the subject of a variety of comparative studies. It is our opinion that the multimodality approach will eventually prevail. In spite of these reservations, certain principles of immunotherapy are becoming apparent. Immunotherapy must be considered adjunctive to conventional therapy at present, although it is conceivable that it may become the primary therapy of the future. There are three broad approaches to immunotherapy which should be tailored to these specific objectives. These include local immunotherapy, regional immunotherapy, or what is most exciting, systemic intravenous immunotherapy. Maximum tumor burden reduction should be carried out preceding or at least concurrent with the immunotherapy. In immunocompetent patients, immunopotentiation and macrophage activation seem to be the optimal approaches. In immunoincompetent patients, immunorestoration should be carried out prior to or concurrent with other approaches to therapy. I feel that immunological monitoring is extremely important, has been done haphazardly at best in most immunotherapy trials, and probably not with the optimal tests. It is extremely important that animal work go on concurrent with clinical studies and that extensive biomathematical support be provided to the immunotherapist.

REFERENCES

1. Weiss, D.W., et al. (1976) Mode of action of micobacterial fractions in antitumor immunity. Ann. N.Y. Acad. Sci. 276:536.
2. Tripodi, D., et al. (1973) Drug-induced restoration of cutaneous delayed hypersensitivity in anergic patients with cancer. N. Engl. J. Med. 289:354.
3. Rosenberg, S.A., et al. (1976) Intralesional immunotherapy of melanoma with BCG. Med. Clin. N. Amer. 60:419.
4. Goldstein, A.L., et al. (1970) Influence of thymosin on cell-mediated and humoral immune responses in normal and immunologically deficient mice. J. Immunol. 104:359.
5. Everall, J.D., et al. (1975) Treatment of primary melanoma by intralesional vaccinia before excision. Lancet 2:583.
6. Gutterman, J.U., et al. (1973) Active immunotherapy with BCG for recurrent malignant melanoma. Lancet 1:1208.
7. Gutterman, J.U., et al. (1974) Chemoimmunotherapy of disseminated malignant melanoma with Dimethyl Imadazole Carboxamide and Bacillus Calmette Guerin. N. Engl. J. Med. 291:592.
8. Currie, G.A., et al. (1975) Active immunotherapy as an adjunct to chemotherapy in the treatment of disseminated malignant melanoma. A pilot study. Brit. J. Cancer 31:143.
9. Israel, L., et al. (1975) Brief communication. Daily intravenous infusion of Corynebacterium parvum in twenty patients with disseminated cancer. A preliminary report of clinical and biological findings. J. Natl. Cancer Inst. 55:29.
10. Vetto, R.M., et al. (1976) Transfer factor therapy in patients with cancer. Cancer 37:90.
11. McKneally, M.F., et al.(1976) Regional immunotherapy of lung cancer with intrapleural BCG.
12. Stewart, T.H.M., et al. (1976) Immunochemotherapy of lung cancer. Ann. N.Y. Acad. Sci. 277:436.
13. Amery, W.K. (1976) Double-blind levamisole trial in resectable lung cancer. Ann. N.Y. Acad. Sci. 277:216.

14. Israel, L. (1974) Clinical results with Corynebacteria. In: Recent Results in Cancer Research: Investigations and Stimulation of Immunity in Cancer Patients, Springer-Verlag, New York.

15. Yamamura, Y. et al. (1976) Immunotherapy of cancer with cell wall skeleton of Mycobacterium bovis Bacillus Calmette Guerin. Ann. N.Y. Acad. Sci. 277:209.

16. Kimura, I. et al. (1976) Immunotherapy in human lung cancer using a streptococcol agent OK432. Cancer 37:2201.

17. Mathé, G. et al. (1969) Active immunotherapy for acute lymphoblastic leukemia. Lancet 1:697.

18. Vogler, W.R. et al. (1974) Prolongation of remission in myeloblastic leukemia by Tice strain Bacillus Calmette Guerin. Lancet 2:128.

19. Powles, R. et al. (1973) Immunotherapy for acute myelogenous leukemia. Brit. J. Cancer 28:365.

20. Weiss, D.W., et al. (1975) Treatment of acute myelocytic leukemia (AML) patients with the MER tubercle bacillus fraction. A preliminary report. Transplantation Proc. 7:545.

21. Gee, T.S. et al. (In Press) Pseudomonas aeuruginosa vaccine in a treatment protocol for adult patients with acute non-lymphoblastic leukemia. A preliminary report. In: Immunotherapy of Cancer: Present Status of Trials in Man.

22. Bekesi, J.G. et al. (1976) Therapeutic effectiveness of neuraminidase treated tumor cells as an immunogen in man and experimental animals with leukemia. Ann. N.Y. Acad. Sci. 277:313.

23. Sokal, J.E. et al. (1976) Immunotherapy in well-controlled chronic myelocytic leukemia. N.Y. State J. Med. 73:1180.

24. Morton, D.L. et al. (1974) BCG immunotherapy of malignant melanoma. Summary of seven years experience. Ann. Surg. 180:635.

25. Scott, M.T.: (1974) Corynebacterium parvum as an immunotherapeutic anticancer agent. Sem. Oncol. 1:367.

26. Band, P.R. et al. (1975) Phase I study of Corynebacterium parvum in patients with solid tumors. Cancer Chemo. Rep. 59:1139.

27. Israel, L. et al. (1975) Brief Communication. Daily intravenous infusion of Corynebacterium parvum in twenty patients with disseminated cancer. A preliminary report of clinical and biological findings. J. Natl. Cancer Inst. 55:29.

28. Ribi, E. et al. (In Press) Structural requirements of microbial agents for immunotherapy of the guinea pig line-10 tumor. In: Present Status of BCG in Cancer Immunotherapy.

29. Schafer, L.A. et al. (1976) In vitro and in vivo studies with thymosin in cancer patients. Ann. N.Y. Acad. Sci. 277:609.

30. Lewinski, U.H. et al.(1977) Interaction between repeated skin testing with recall antigens and temporal fluctuations of in vitro lymphocyte blastogenesis in cancer patients. Clin. Immunol. Immunopathol. 7:77.

Adjuvant Therapy of Cancer, S.E. Salmon and S.E. Jones eds.

CORRELATION OF CHEMOTHERAPY ACTIVITY IN ADVANCED DISEASE WITH ADJUVANT RESULTS

Stephen K. Carter, M.D., Director
Northern California Cancer Program
770 Welch Road, Suite 190
Palo Alto, California 94304
U. S. A.

INTRODUCTION

Chemotherapy combined with surgery and/or radiotherapy to eradicate postulated micrometastasis after local and regional tumor control is currently under widespread investigation. The experimental logic underlying this approach has been reviewed previously.[1] One of the cornerstones of the assumptions on which this strategy is predicated is that activity with a drug or regimen in advanced disease will be predictive for activity in the adjuvant setting. If a drug regimen can cause objective regression (>50% shrinkage) of an advanced disease lesion then it should be even more effective against the smaller tumor cell burden which is postulated to remain after curative resection in so many cases of Stage II breast cancer, Dukes C large bowel cancer, osteosarcoma and ovarian cancer just to name a few examples which are under vigorous clinical investigation.

Combined modality trials involving surgery plus drugs have now been on-going for several years and we can now begin to make some correlations between activity in the advanced disease situation and in the adjuvant setting. It is the purpose of this paper to briefly review some of the current combined modality study results and match these to the known data for the regimens when utilized in the clinically evident disease situation for that same tumor.

BREAST CANCER

Breast cancer has been the one major solid tumor which has been widely reported to prove the effectiveness of the combined modality use of adjuvant chemotherapy. The studies of Fisher[2] with L-PAM and Bonadonna[3] with CMF in preliminary literature reports were reported to be causing statistically significant diminished recurrence rates. The authors cautioned about the preliminary nature of the results since neither survival data, nor long term chronic toxicity data were available but the results were picked up with enthusiasm by both the press, the public and a good deal of the professional community. Untreated control groups are no longer seen in any on-going clinical trial for Stage 2 breast cancer post-mastectomy.

Unfortunately, further analysis of both studies has shown that any benefit, in terms of diminished relapse rates, has disappeared for women who are post-menopausal.[4,5] Post-menopausal women make up more than half the women in both of the trials. The results for premenopausal women are still positive and when combined with the rest of menopausal women the total trial can still be viewed as positive at this time. It is now likely however that the result in the premenopausal situation is due to the drugs causing a chemical ablation of ovarian function and may not be due to actual tumor cell kill by the drugs. It is possible that the tumor cell burden and/or the kinetics of the tumor cells in premenopausal women are more favorable than in the post-menopausal women, but this can only be speculation given our current state of knowledge.

L-PAM has a 20% response rate in advanced breast cancer[6] while CMF has a 50-60% response rate in several studies.[6] In a controlled comparison of the two regimens the East Cooperative Oncology Group showed a superiority for CMF in terms of both response rate and duration of response. When the L-PAM and CMF studies were felt to be clearly positive this was highly encouraging for the success of the concept in general. This was particularly true because L-PAM with its 20% advanced disease response rate was well within the range of activity for chemotherapy regimens in other tumor types. If we now reevaluate the situation and consider that even CMF as given is not clearly active in Stage 2 breast carcinoma, then one has to become somewhat more pessimistic. Advanced breast cancer is one of the more responsive of the solid tumor types to chemotherapy. If a regimen with a greater than 50% objective response rate cannot make a meaningful impact on an adjuvant trial, then the possibilities for gastrointestinal cancer, lung cancer and other tumors becomes more questionable with existing drugs and regimens.

A wide range of trials are currently on-going in breast cancer. None are utilizing a regimen which is clearly more active in advanced disease than CMF. Some are adding immunotherapy and other hormonal therapy to the picture. Adriamycin containing combinations cause worry about long-term cardiac toxicity effects. The lack of surgery only groups will complicate matters greatly for interpretation as controls of L-PAM and CMF will now have to be compared to the NSABP or Milan studies in order to get some feeling about the validity of utilizing their untreated arms as "historical controls."

LARGE BOWEL CANCER

For many years the standard chemotherapy for advanced disease has been 5-Fluorouracil (5-FU). This drug has given an overall 21% response rate when over 2,000 cases from the literature are totalled up.[7] There have been five controlled clinical trials utilizing 5-FU as adjuvant to surgery in patients with Dukes C lesion after curative resection.[8] None have shown any benefit in terms of relapses or survival. It is of interest to note that a recent trial utilizing a "historical control" was reported as positive.[9] It is clear that an ≈20% response rate in advanced disease has not translated to anything meaningful in the adjuvant situation. Recently the combination of methyl CCNU plus 5-FU either alone or with Vincristine has been shown to be more active than concomitant controls of 5-FU. In the Mayo Clinic study the 3 drug combination gave a 43% response rate[10] as compared to 19% for 5-FU but survival was not improved. In the study of the Southwest Oncology Group the two drug combination gave a 30% response rate as against 9% for a low dose weekly 5-FU regimen which gave minimal toxicity.[11] There are at least five major trials underway looking at methyl CCNU + 5-FU adjuvant treatment after curative resection for Dukes B_2 and C lesions.[12] These studies are all too early to meaningfully report on, but will add another strong piece of data to the correlation analysis.

LUNG CANCER

There have been many trials of the alkylating agents, especially cyclophosphamide, in combination with curative resection surgery in the hopes of improving the relapse and survival rates.[13] If one looks at the overall objective response rate for cyclophosphamide in lung cancer, it approximates 30%.[14] Much of the cumulative data comes from earlier studies in which response criteria were not as stringent as they are today. Lung cancer data are complicated by the various histological types, the critical variables of performance status, extent of disease and prior therapy as well as the fact that shrinkage on the x-ray can be due to diminished pneumonitis secondary to reduced atelectasis rather than meaningful cell kill. Some recent studies have reported response rates of under 20% or even 10%. Given this low order of objective response (and minimal survival improvement if any) it is not surprising that single alkylating agent trials have been negative. With the exception of oat cell cancer no combinations have been proven superior to single agents so that the immediate future for adjuvant studies is clouded. While oat cell lesions do respond, this is now considered disseminated disease at diagnosis and so surgical adjuvant studies are difficult to contemplate. Combinations with radiation are under study but none to date have been shown to give an improved result in a controlled setting.

OSTEOGENIC SARCOMA

Osteogenic sarcoma is another tumor in which chemotherapy in the combined modality setting is considered successful. Studies at Sydney Farber Cancer Center with high doses of Methotrexate and Citrovorum Factor Rescue (HDMTX-CF)[15] and by Cancer and Leukemia Group B with Adriamycin[16] have been reported as having a dramatic impact on disease free survival at two years. In the advanced disease setting both HDMTX-CF and Adriamycin have been reported to have response rates in the 20-30% range. The interpretation of adjuvant studies is clouded by the fact that historical controls were used and the possibility exists that more stringent diagnostic criteria for exclusion of metastases and more careful case selection may have been used in the newer studies in comparison with the large retrospective analysis used for historical control purposes. There is data from the Mayo Clinic[17] indicating that the two year disease free interval in the kind of cases currently selected for adjuvant trials may be twice that reported in the series of Marcove[18] and others[19] utilized as historical controls. Preliminary reports of adjuvant activity for materials such as Interferon, transfer factor and anticoagulation make one uneasy that with more careful case selection combined with early data analysis almost anything can be seen to be positive when compared to the earlier data base. We need a more careful delineation of the critical factors known to affect survival, e.g., histology, size of lesion, surgical procedure, location of lesion, etc., in the current series as compared to older series before we can feel absolutely confident about the correlations we would like to make in this disease.

OTHER TUMORS

A broad range of trials are on-going in other disease areas[20] which hopefully when analyzed will add to our ability to make the critical correlations which hopefully will add to our ability to design better trials in the future. In ovarian cancer and head and neck cancer, single agents which have a roughly 50% response rate (L-PAM and Methotrexate)[14] are now being evaluated after surgery and/or radiotherapy. In gastric cancer the combination of Methyl CCNU plus 5-FU which has a 40-50% response rate[21] is being tried after curative resection by several groups. In lung cancer the nitrosourea CCNU is being tried either alone (response rate 10-20%)[14] or in combination with hydroxyurea where advanced disease data for response rate are not available.

DISCUSSION

How should the clinician approach the choice of drugs for adjuvant usage? Screening for surgical adjuvant drugs can be approached in two ways. One approach is to use experimental systems to test for a potentially positive therapeutic interaction among a selected universe of drugs. The number of drugs that should be in this universe and their sources relate to where the clinicians are choosing drugs for human studies.

One approach to the question is to select drugs based purely on their postulated mechanism of action as supported by either experimental data or nonspecific clinical activity. Examples of such approaches being used today are in the field of immunotherapy where a range of materials such as bacillus Calmette-Guérin (BCG) and Corynebacterium parvum are being given in postsurgical situations based on their experimental activity and their ability to apparently enhance immunologic responsiveness in some patients. The clinical "activity" is non-specific in that it is not disease oriented and, in many cases, these materials are being employed in adjuvant situations in the face of almost no previous clinical data for the specific tumor. Other examples that might occur in the future in a similar manner involve possible antimetastasis compounds and reverse transcriptase inhibiting drugs.

Another approach is to choose clinically active drugs that have shown the ability to kill tumor cells in advanced disease. Again, the question could be raised as to whether this activity should or should not be disease specific. Should investigators evaluate a drug postsurgically in breast cancer based on activity in lymphomas or malignant melanoma, or should activity against advanced breast cancer be required?

In actuality, the combining of cytotoxic drugs with surgical treatment has almost always been along disease-oriented lines using a drug that has some degree of activity against the tumor in the advanced state. One of the critical questions that needs to be answered is what degree of activity in advanced disease is required of a drug or regimen before a significant gain in survival can be expected in the adjuvant situation where the drug is given in the hope of eradicating microscopic disease after local and regional tumor ablation by surgery and/or radiotherapy. Based on our evaluation of the data to date it appears that a response rate in excess of 50% (CR + PR) will be required for a regimen to be active. The data to date would indicate that single agents in the 20-30% activity range will not be enough. The latest analysis of the CMF data has to make us consider that a 50% response rate may not be enough. Obviously the available data are still minimal and the essential questions of duration of therapy, intensity of therapy, schedule of therapy, etc., have not been addressed. The choice of our adjuvant therapy regimens and their schedules, durations and intensities have been much more empirical than any of us might care to admit. We need to begin to think more carefully about experimental models and to setting up foci of critical analysis of on-going and planned studies so that we can learn from what we have done in the past and hopefully not repeat our mistakes.

BIBLIOGRAPHY

1. Carter, S. K. and Soper, W. T. Integration of chemotherapy into combined modality treatment of solid tumors. 1. The overall strategy. Cancer Treat Rev, 1:1-13, 1974.
2. Fisher, B., et al. L-Phenylalanine mustard (L-PAM) in the management of primary breast cancer. A report of early findings. N Engl J Med, 292:117-122, 1975.
3. Bonadonna, G., et al. Combination Chemotherapy as an adjuvant treatment in operable breast cancer. N Engl J Med, 294: 405-410, 1976.
4. Fisher, B. Personal Communication.
5. Bonadonna, G. Cancer. In press.
6. Carter, S. K. The integration of chemotherapy into combined modality treatment of solid tumors: Adenocarcinoma of the breast. Cancer Treatment Reviews.
7. Carter, S. K. Large Bowel Cancer--the current status of treatment. J Natl Cancer Institute, 56:3-10, 1976.
8. Moertel, C. G. Flourouracil as an Adjuvant to Colorectal

Surgery: The Breakthrough that Never Was. JAMA, 236: 1935-1936, 1976.

9. Li, M. C. and Ross, S. T. Chemoprophylaxis for Patients with Colorectal Cancer. JAMA, 235:2825-2828, 1976.

10. Moertel, C. G., et al. Therapy of advanced colorectal cancer with a combination of 5-Fluorouracil, Methyl CCNU and Vincristine. J Natl Cancer Inst, 54:69-71, 1975.

11. Baker, L. H., et al. Phase III comparison of the treatment of advanced gastrointestinal cancer with bolus weekly 5-FU vs. Methyl CCNU plus Bolus weekly 5-FU. Cancer, 38:1-7, 1976.

12. Carter, S. K. Current protocol approaches in large bowel cancer. Seminars in Oncology, 3:433-443, 1976.

13. Legha, S., et al. Adjuvant Chemotherapy of Lung Cancer: Reviewed Prospects. Cancer. In press.

14. Wasserman, T. H., et al. Tabular analysis of the clinical chemotherapy of solid tumors. Cancer Chemother, Part 3, 6: 399-419, 1975.

15. Jaffe, N., et al. Adjuvant methotrexate and citrovorum factor treatment of osteogenic sarcoma. N Engl J Med, 294:994-997, 1974.

16. Cortes, E. P., et al. Amputation and adriamycin in primary osteosarcoma. N Engl J Med, 291:998-1000, 1974.

17. Ivins, J. C., et al. Transfer factor versus combination chemotherapy: A preliminary report of a randomized postsurgical adjuvant study in osteogenic sarcoma. Annals of N. Y. Acad of Sci, 277:558-574, 1976.

18. Marcove, R. C., et al. Osteogenic sarcoma under the age of 21: A review of 145 operative cases. J Bone Joint Surgery, 52: 411-423, 1970.

19. Friedman, M. and Carter, S. K. The Therapy of Osteogenic Sarcoma: Current Status and Thoughts for the Future. J Surg Oncology, 4:482-510, 1972.

20. Carter, S. K. and Wasserman, T. H. Interaction of experimental and clinical studies in combined modality treatment. Cancer Chemother Rep, Part 2, 5:235-241, 1975.

21. Carter, S. K. Gastric Cancer: The current status of treatment. J Natl Cancer Institute. In press.

Adjuvant Therapy of Cancer, S.E. Salmon and S.E. Jones eds.

SECOND MALIGNANCIES FOLLOWING FIRST BREAST CANCER IN PROLONGED THIOTEPA ADJUVANT CHEMOTHERAPY

Paul Y. M. Chan, Leonard Sadoff, and John H. Winkley

Kaiser Permanente Medical Center, 1510 North Edgemont Street, Los Angeles, California 90027.

Supported by Kaiser Foundation Research Grant.

INTRODUCTION

Since we presented our preliminary data on this subject in 1974,[1] we have now completed this retrospective study of 1,265 patients with operable carcinoma of the breast at five Kaiser Foundation Hospitals in Southern California between 1953 and 1967. The purpose of this paper is to report the incidence of second primary malignancies developed after first carcinoma of the breast treated with surgery and prolonged thiotepa adjuvant chemotherapy. During this period, the treatment policy of operable mammary cancer was radical mastectomy with and without postoperative external radiotherapy or simple mastectomy with radiotherapy. In October 1960, triethylenethiophosphoramide or thiotepa adjuvant chemotherapy was added to the surgical procedure. Thiotepa was given during surgery as surgical adjuvant chemotherapy and was maintained for two years as prophylactic chemotherapy. This approach was inspired by the pioneer work in adjuvant chemotherapy by Dr. Warren H. Cole and his associates.[2,3] In reviewing our data, it may be possible to determine whether or not prolonged use of thiotepa adjuvant chemotherapy enhances the development of new cancers.

MATERIALS AND METHODS

All patients with histopathological diagnosis of carcinoma of the breast treated with simple or radical mastectomy with and without postoperative radiotherapy between 1953 and 1967 at five Kaiser Foundation Hospitals in Southern California were reviewed for this study. According to the modes of treatment, patients were divided into four groups. Group I consisted of patients receiving thiotepa with surgery; Group II, thiotepa, surgery, and radiotherapy; Group III, surgery and radiotherapy and Group IV, surgery only.

Radical mastectomy of the Halsted type was the standard surgical procedure in this study. However, simple mastectomy and radiotherapy were employed occasionally. Operability was generally considered as mobile tumor mass confined to the breast with or without clinical axillary involvement, provided no evidence of lymphedema of the arm, inflammatory changes of the breast, distant or visceral metastases demonstrated in preoperative survey. The anatomic staging of the disease was based on the final pathological identification of axillary contents. Stage I was designated for disease confined to the breast without axillary metastases, wheras Stage II, showed evidence of axillary involvement. Radiation therapy was given with either 250 KV Machine or CO^{60} teletherapy.

Prior to 1960, postoperative radiotherapy was a routine treatment procedure for Stage II disease or for medial quadrant lesions. Since 1960, the majority of patients of Stage II disease were treated with adjuvant and prophylactic thiotepa for two years instead of radiotherapy. The treatment fields were to encompass the entire chest wall and immediate lymphatic drainage sites, including internal mammary chains, supraclavicular fossa and axilla. The irradiation schedule was 200 to 250 rads per day and five fractions per week. Total tumor dose was 4,500 - 5,000 rads given in 4½ to five weeks.

Thiotepa was given to patients with either Stage I or Stage II diseases. At surgery, thiotepa of 0.4 mg/kilo was given at the completion of the surgical procedure. During the first and second postoperative days thiotepa of 0.1 mg/kilo was given in each day. The total dosage of perisurgical adjuvant chemotherapy was 0.6 mg/kilo. Postsurgical prophylactic thiotepa chemotherapy was then continued three months after surgery and was repeated every three months for two years. The dosage of thiotepa was 1 mg/kilo which was administered in 2 divided doses in consecutive days. The total dose of thiotepa in every three-month period was not to exceed 60 mgms. Thiotepa was not given when white blood corpuscular count was below 3,500 per mm^3, hemoglobin below 10 gm%, and platelets below 100,000 per mm^3. Thiotepa was discontinued when there was evidence of recurrence or metastasis, severe side effects, or patient's refusal of further therapy.

Data was obtained from patients' records and was analyzed by BMP 115 Computer Program at the Health Science Computing Facility, University of California in Los Angeles.

TABLE 1

INCIDENCE OF CARCINOMA OF THE BREAST AT 5 KAISER FOUNDATION HOSPITALS IN SOUTHERN CALIFORNIA (1953 - 1967)

YEAR	NON-THIO-TEPA GROUP	THIOTEPA GROUP
1953	19	
1954	32	
1955	33	
1956	42	
1957	40	
1958	48	
1959	53	
1960	52	18
1961	16	66
1962	28	99
1963	38	93
1964	47	94
1965	59	109
1966	51	88
1967 (Sept.)	74	66
TOTALS	632	633

TABLE 2

SECOND MALIGNANCIES DEVELOPED AFTER INITIAL CARCINOMA OF THE BREAST

Groups	No. of Pts. 1st Breast Carcinoma	Second Breast Ca.	Second Ca., Non-Breast
I THIOTEPA + SURGERY	588	34 (5.8%)	37 (6.3%)
II THIOTEPA + SURGERY + RADIOTHERAPY	45	2 (4.9%)	3 (6.6%)
III RADIOTHERAPY + SURGERY	225	10 (4.4%)	5 (2.2%)
IV SURGERY ONLY	407	27 (6.6%)	29 (7.1%)
TOTAL	1,265	73 (5.8%)	74 (5.8%)

RESULTS

Table 1 shows the total number of reviewed patients in this study at five Kaiser Foundation Hospitals in Southern California between 1953 and 1967. All patients were followed between 5 to 10 years. There were nine patients lost to followup between the third and fifth years. Six hundred thirty-two patients who did not receive thiotepa served as historic control. Since 1960, a total of 633 patients received thiotepa. The average age of patients in the historic control was 50.8 years, range 19 to 78. The average age in the thiotepa treated patients was 51.5 years, range 25 to 77. The majority of patients (over 85%) had infiltrating ductal carcinoma of the breast.

Second primary malignancies developing after first carcinoma of the breast are listed according to the modes of treatment in Table 2. There were 588 patients treated with thiotepa and surgery. Thirty-four patients or 5.8% developed carcinoma of the opposite breast and 37 patients or 6.3% developed second malignancy in other primary sites.

In Group II, 45 patients received thiotepa, surgery, and radiotherapy. Only two patients or 4.9% developed second breast cancer, and 3 patients or 6.6% developed second other primary malignancies. Among 225 patients in Group III, the radiotherapy and surgery group, 10 patients or 4.4% developed second breast cancer and 3 patients or 2.2% developed other primary malignancies. In Group IV, 407 patients were treated by surgery only. Twenty-seven patients or 6.6% developed second breast cancer whereas 29 patients or 7.1% developed other primary malignancies. The overall incidence of second primary malignancies was 11.6%, and half of these new cancers developed in the remaining breast (5.8%).

TABLE 3

INCIDENCE OF SECOND MALIGNANCY AND CUMULATIVE DOSE OF THIOTEPA IN 633 PATIENTS *

No. of Patients	No. of Courses	Median Cumulative Dose	Second Breast Ca.	Second Non-Breast Ca.
65	Adjuvant only	38 mg	1 (0.2%)	3 (0.5%)
71	1-2	136 mg	4 (0.6%)	5 (0.7%)
65	3-4	258 mg	5 (0.7%)	4 (0.6%)
66	5-6	390 mg	6 (1.0%)	7 (1.1%)
366	7,8,9	522 mg	20 (3.2%)	21 (3.4%)
		TOTAL	36 (5.7%)	40 (6.3%)

* 45 PATIENTS RECEIVED RADIOTHERAPY

TABLE 4

DURATION BETWEEN FIRST AND SECOND BREAST CARCINOMA

DURATION IN YEARS	THIO-TEPA GROUP		HISTORIC CONTROL	
	No.	%	No.	%
Less than 2 years	15	2.4	12	1.9
2-4	8	1.2	6	0.9
4-6	9	1.4	6	0.9
6 or more	4	0.7	13	2.0
Total Second Primary	36	5.7	37	5.7
No Second Primary	597	94.3	595	94.3
TOTALS	633	100.0	632	100.0

The incidence of second malignancy and cumulative dose of thiotepa is shown in Table 3. Sixty-five patients received perioperative adjuvant chemotherapy only. The median cumulative dose of thiotepa of this group was 38 mgms. One patient (0.2%) developed cancer in the opposite breast and 3 patients (0.5%) developed second cancer in another primary site. Three hundred sixty-six patients received high doses of thiotepa and the median cumulative dose was 522 mgms. Twenty patients, 3.2% developed second primary breast cancer and 21 patients (3.4%) developed second primary cancers of other sites. The duration between first and second breast cancers among the thiotepa treated patients and the historic control is shown on Table 4. In the first two years of postmastectomy period, 15 patients (2.4%) developed second breast cancers in the thiotepa treated patients as compared with 12 patients (1.9%) in historic control. The total incidence of second primary malignancies were identical in both groups, i.e. 5.7%.

TABLE 5

DURATION BETWEEN FIRST BREAST CA AND SECOND NON-BREAST MALIGNANCY

DURATION IN YEARS	THIO-TEPA GROUP		HISTORIC CONTROL	
	No.	%	No.	%
Less than 2 years	9	1.4	5	0.7
2-4	13	2.1	8	1.3
4-6	7	1.1	7	1.2
6 or more	11	1.7	14	2.2
TOTAL SECOND MALIG.	40	6.3	34	5.4
NO SECOND MALIG.	593	93.7	598	94.6
TOTALS	633	100.0	632	100.0

The duration for the development of second malignancies in other primary sites is shown on Table 5. There was no definite pattern observed. In Table 6, second malignancies are listed according to various anatomic sites and tissue origins. Forty of 633 patients or 6.3% in the thiotepa group developed second new cancers as compared with 34 of 632 patients or 5.4% in the historic control.

TABLE 6

SECOND PRIMARY MALIGNANCIES ACCORDING TO ANATOMIC SITE

	THIO-TEPA GROUP (633 Patients) No.	CONTROL (632 Patients) No.
1. SKIN-BASAL CELL CA	12	7
MELANOMA	1	2
2. HEMATOPOIETIC SYSTEM		
LYMPHOMA	1	2
AML	1	0
CGL	1	0
CLL	0	2
3. GI SYSTEM		
STOMACH	3	3
COLON	6	2
4. LUNG CA	3	2
5. GU AND GYN SYSTEMS		
BLADDER	1	1
RENAL	0	1
CERVIX	1	2
OVARY	2	2
ENDOMETRIUM	4	4
6. BONE	0	0
7. CNS	0	1
8. MISCELLANEOUS		
THYROID	2	2
TONGUE	1	0
LARYNX	0	1
LIPOSARCOMA	1	0
9. TOTALS	40 (6.3%)	34 (5.4%)

DISCUSSION

Based on the concept that adjuvant chemotherapy is able to control microscopic metastasis, prolong relapse-free interval, and possibly improve survival rate, its use has become increasingly more popular. The major concern of this approach has been the carcinogenicity of anticancer agents. Numerous case reports have shown new cancers arising in patients treated with intensive chemotherapy for cancer or for immunosuppression in renal transplantation.[4,5] In general, anticancer agents which act by alkylation, such as nitrogen mustard and/or by binding tightly to DNA such as actinomycin D have been demonstrated to cause cancer in experimental animals and maybe carcinogenic in man.

Thiotepa which is closely related chemically and pharmacologically to nitrogen mustard, has been reported to induce second primary cancer in the treatment of chronic granulocytic leukemia, carcinoma of the lung and the breast. In the treatment of carcinoma of the breast, however, Donegan[6] reported his experience on extended surgical adjuvant thiotepa and stated that his data did not suggest protracted treatment with thiotepa predisposed to the development of new cancers. He observed 5.6% of second primary cancers, including breast and other primary sites in the thiotepa group as compared with 9.2% in the control group. In our series (Table 7), 76 patients (12%) developed second primary cancers as compared with 71 patients (11.1%) in the historic control. Our data is in agreement with Donegan's[6] observation. In spite of the suggested low carcinogenicity of thiotepa, our data further suggests that patients receiving higher cumulative doses had more tendency to develop second cancers than patients receiving lower doses of thiotepa (Table 3). This increase of incidence in second cancers could be due to the possibility of cause and effect relationship between dosage of carcinogen and carcinogenesis. However, in our data, patients receiving higher cumulative doses of thiotepa had the survival advantage and thus subjected themselves to a higher risk of second new cancers.

Table 7

INCIDENCE OF SECOND CA

	THIO-TEPA GROUP (633 patients)		CONTROL (632 patients)	
	No.	%	No.	%
SECOND BREAST CA	36	5.7	37	5.7
SECOND CA (Non-breast)	40	6.3	34	5.4
TOTAL SECOND PRIMARY	76	12%	71	11.1

Radiation is a powerful anticancer agent and is well known for its carcinogenic effects in man and in experimental animals. Recent clinical reports from the National Cancer Institute suggested an increased risk of second cancer arising in patients with Hodgkin's disease after intensive radiotherapy and MOPP chemotherapy.[7,8] Among 45 patients receiving thiotepa chemotherapy and postoperative radiotherapy in our study (Table 2), five patients, or 11.5% developed second primary cancers, i.e. one basal cell carcinoma of the skin, one lymphoma, one chronic granulocytic leukemia and two carcinomas of the opposite breast. Of 225 patients treated with surgery followed by postoperative radiotherapy, 15 patients or 6.6% developed second primary cancers, i.e. two basal cell carcinomas of the skin, one malignant melanoma, two gynecological cancers, and ten carcinomas of the opposite breast. It would seem that the addition of radiotherapy to thiotepa may increase the risk of second cancer. On the other hand, radiotherapy would appear to lower the risk of second cancer among patients treated with surgery and radiotherapy (Table 2). The decrease was mainly due to the fact that the majority of patients in this group had Stage II disease and, most of them, did not live long enough to develop second new cancers. It is apparent from our study that prolonged thiotepa adjuvant chemotherapy did not increase the risk of second carcinoma of the breast or of other anatomic sites and organs. It is our general belief that patients with first malignancy are prone to develop second new cancers. The risk of second cancers among cancer patients is unlikely increased by the prolonged use of thiotepa adjuvant chemotherapy but it is rather due to the inherent susceptibility of the host.

SUMMARY

A retrospective study of 1,265 patients with operable carcinoma of the breast was conducted to determine whether or not prolonged use of thiotepa for two years increases the risk of second primary cancer. According to the modes of treatment, patients were divided into four groups. Group I consisted of patients receiving thiotepa with surgery; Group II, thiotepa, surgery, and radiotherapy; Group III, surgery and radiotherapy and Group IV, surgery only. All but nine patients were followed between five to ten years. Thirty-four of 588 patients (5.8%) in Group

I developed second carcinoma in the opposite breast, 2 of 45 patients (4.4%) in Group II, 10 of 225 patients (4.4%) in Group III and 27 of 407 patients (6.6%) in Group IV. The overall incidence of second carcinoma of the opposite breast was 73 of 1,265 patients or 5.8%. There were 37 of 588 patients (6.3%) who developed second cancers of other primary sites in Group I, 3 of 45 patients (6.6%) in Group II, 5 of 225 patients (2.2%) in Group III and 29 of 407 (7.1%) in Group IV. No specific histopathologic cell type, organ or anatomic site were predominant in the development of second primary cancer. Our data suggests prolonged thiotepa adjuvant chemotherapy does not seem to increase the risk of second primary cancer. We feel that the inherent susceptibility of the host plays an important role in the oncogenesis of second primary cancer.

ACKNOWLEDGMENTS

The authors wish to acknowledge computing assistance obtained from the Health Sciences Computing Facility, UCLA, supported by NIH Special Research Resources Grant RR-3 under the supervision of Mrs. B. Carnahan. The secretarial assistance of Mrs. P. Singer, S. Tyson, and A. Moore is appreciated.

REFERENCES

1. Sadoff, L., Chan, P., Tyson, S. (1974) Incidence of second primary cancers in breast patients after prolonged thiotepa therapy. Proc. Am. Assoc. Cancer Res./Am. Soc. Clin. Oncol. 15:145.
2. Cruz, E. et al (1956) Prophylactic Treatment of Cancer: The use of Chemotherapeutic Agents to Prevent Tumor Metastasis. Surg. 40:291-296.
3. Mrazek, R. et al (1959) Prophylactic and Adjuvant Use of Nitrogen Mustard in the Surgical Treatment of Cancer. Ann. of Surg. (Oct.) 745-755.
4. Harris, C. (1976) The Carcinogenicity of Anticancer Drugs: A Hazard in Man. Cancer 37:1014-1023.
5. Penn, I. (1976) Second Malignant Neoplasms Associated with Immunosuppressive Medications. Cancer 37:1024-1032.
6. Donegan, W. (1974) Extended Surgical Adjuvant Thiotepa for Mammary Carcinoma. Arch. Surg. 109:187-192.

7. Arseneau, J. et al (1972) Nonlymphomatous Malignant Tumors Complicating Hodgkin's Disease. N. Engl. J. Med. 287:1119-1122.

8. Cancellos, G. et al (1975) Second Malignant Neoplasms Complicating Hodgkin's Disease in Remission. Conference on Delayed Consequences of Cancer Therapy: Proven and Potential. (Jan.) 9-11.

Adjuvant Therapy of Cancer, S.E. Salmon and S.E. Jones eds.

PERSONAL COMMENTS ON PROBLEMS OF INTERPRETATION OF CLINICAL TRIALS PRESENTED AT THE CONFERENCE ON THE ADJUVANT THERAPY OF CANCER*

Saul A. Rosenberg, M.D.
Division of Medical Oncology
Stanford University Medical Center
Stanford, California 94305

I feel I must respond to the question of the appropriate clinical trial design, the need for controls and the appropriateness of historical controls, especially for adjuvant trials. My perspective after 15 years of involvement with clinical trials gives me some credibility, if not responsibility, to speak out vigorously against what I perceive to be scientifically wrong. We have heard of some adjuvant trials at this meeting which are well controlled, carefully analyzed and conclusions and projections appropriate to the data presented. However, other reports are testing new methods of treatment, chemotherapy or immunotherapy or both, in the adjuvant setting in an uncontrolled trial and are very difficult to evaluate. The use of a historical group carries with it a number of very serious risks, not adequately expressed or appreciated by those who use them.

First, it is assumed that all important prognostic factors are understood and quantifiable by investigators and statisticians for malignant disease. This is naive and voiced most emphatically by statisticians and non-clinicians than by those who are experienced physicians. The usual staging systems rarely acknowledge even known variables, such as histopathologic variability, sites of metastases, patient symptoms or performance status, time from first symptoms to diagnosis, or time to recurrence, immunologic status, or indeed patient motivation.

Second, it is assumed that referral patterns to institutions in different regions are the same, or to the same institution over a period of years are constant. I believe this to be patently untrue. Patients are referred to study groups by primary physicians because of their bias of what they want done for the patient. In some cases the most favorable and cooperative patients are referred to experimental groups because cure is the goal of the referring physician. In other instances, unfavorable and advanced patients are referred to study centers because the primary physician sheds the responsibility of a difficult clinical problem by center referral. The patterns of referral behavior must be different in different localities and must change with time.

---

*Editors' Note: On the final day of the meeting, Saul A. Rosenberg, M.D., Professor of Medicine and Radiology at Stanford, made the following remarks imploring investigators to continue to use well-controlled and carefully conducted clinical trials to evaluate adjuvant treatment. His comments, prompted by the reports of others during the meeting who presented either pilot data or studies employing historical controls, were well received by the conference participants. In fact, they were loudly and resoundingly applauded. With Dr. Rosenberg's permission we are including his remarks here.

Third, diagnostic methods and accuracy are different in different institutions and change with time, sometimes dramatically. Even within the same institution new pathologic criteria or even new pathologists, new radiologic, imaging and surgical techniques make sequential group analyses invalid especially for prognostic subgroups.

Fourth, the bias of investigators must be acknowledged. Bias is a necessary and desirable characteristic of an investigator. I would predict that our most innovative and productive investigators are the very individuals with the greatest bias. It is necessary to have a bias to be committed and involved in these kinds of studies, but bias can significantly influence patient selection, staging designations, accuracy of followup and criteria of response. Anyone who denies this has not been a clinical investigaotr. Bias cannot be completely eliminated as a factor in the kinds of trials we are involved in, but concurrent randomized trials are the major safeguard against this important danger.

Adjuvant trials by their very nature must be carried out with the greatest scientific accuracy. Freedom from relapse data is not sufficient. Survival must be demonstrably improved both in duration and quality. A period of delay to recurrence occupied by difficult chemotherapy exposing some already cured patients, to acute and uncertain late complications is not good enough. The ever-improving salvage methods even resulting in cure of our patients thought to be previously incurable must be considered in interpretation of freedom from relapse figures. It is highly probable the very groups of investigators involved in adjuvant trials are the most successful in salvaging these patients after relapse. The use of historical controls or sequential series do not adequately consider the advances in salvage treatment programs.

It is most regrettable to me that some of the most able, vocal and prominent medical oncologists are the most guilty of ignoring or even condeminng the need for good controlled clinical trials. They set up straw men of ethics or morality on one hand, or hide behind statisticians on the other to justify their behavior. They say it is unethical to have an untreated control group. I have been told by a prominent investigator quoting an even more prominent one, that the use of MOPP chemotherapy was unethical because we must improve the results even further. This is an irresponsible statement.

There must always be two treatment methods which can be compared. In some trials, no treatment is the necessary control for an adjuvant approach. In others, two different methods might be more appropriate. But, if two new adjuvant programs are equally effective, the investigators must consider the possibility that neither has been.

The new specialty of medical oncology is in the spotlight, in the center of this stage of the drama of the fight against cancer. We have promised for years that chemotherapy will make great strides in controlling and curing cancer. The potential of adjuvant therapy has been accepted and is being exploited. The eyes of our surgical and radiotherapy colleagues, and of more importance, the public, are on us and they expect results. The results must be improved survival of good quality. Improved response rates, delays to recurrence, projections of results from months or even a few years of observation are not good enough. There is no justifiable reason to panic, to design poor trials, or to draw premature conclusions in the name of the serious problem of cancer. In the long run, more patients' lives will be prolonged if studies are designed that can be interpreted scientifically and thus accepted by the majority of the physicians who will have to utilize the methods for the greatest population of patients.

Adjuvant Therapy of Cancer, S.E. Salmon and S.E. Jones eds.
© 1977 Elsevier/North-Holland Biomedical Press, Amsterdam

ADJUVANT THERAPY - AN OVERVIEW

Vincent T. DeVita, Jr., M.D.
Director, Division of Cancer Treatment
National Cancer Institute
Bethesda, Maryland 20014

Presented at International Conference on the Adjuvant Therapy of Cancer,
March 2-5, 1977, Tucson, Arizona

One might conclude two things from listening to the papers presented at the symposium. (1) Adjuvant therapy is here to stay, and (2), that Clinical Investigators can be their own worst enemies. I will try to justify the first conclusion in my comments to follow. In regard to the second point, I would only emphasize that clinical investigation is extremely difficult, and the difficulties are often compounded by Clinicians for non-scientific reasons. Why is this so? Experiments designed by Clinical Investigators are not confined by the walls of the laboratory but rather are conducted in the universe occupied by patients with the multiple complex illnesses we call cancer. The numerous experimental variables are difficult to control at best and often go unappreciated. This added complexity of clinical research is, alas, unappreciated by many who have not had to deal with it and, unfortunately, sometimes even ignored by Clinical Investigators, as illustrated in many studies reported here. The precision of clinical trials was improved markedly by the use of the randomized clinical trial. However, randomization does not make up for ignorance about a disease or a new therapy. Failure to do randomized clinical trials, when the variables are appreciated, and failure to appreciate that randomized clinical trials performed too early are often erroneous, can both lead to useless repetition of clinical studies. Clearly, we still need more precision in the control of the variables of the clinical experiment.

As a prelude to comments on specific sections of the symposium, I would like first to try to attempt to put therapeutic research in focus because I think it helps us understand how we got here. I believe we are at the beginning of the end of an eighty year long therapeutic experiment. Three events happened at the turn of the century that were important to therapeutic research in the cancer field. First, the discovery of X-rays by Conrad Roentgen; second, the design of the radical mastectomy by Halsted, which was the first operative procedure developed on the basis of a hypothesis on the spread of human tumors; and third, the development of animal tumor model systems; the latter advance was important because it ultimately led to our ability to develop drug treatments for cancer in experimental systems. For most of the fifty years that followed we examined the use of surgery and radiotherapy in the treatment of human cancers, for mostly localized tumors. These types of treatments worked, and survival improved up until the 1950's, but they did not work as well as expected.

The global hypothesis that evolved as a result of the observations made in these early, crude clinical experiments was that treatment failure after local treatment is often related to the presence of micrometastases outside the treatment field. Most therapeutic trials, however, actually went in the direction of attempting to develop more aggressive local treatment to obviate the clinical failures, while observational evidence clearly continued to show that, for most visceral tumors, recurrences were indeed most often remote from the primary site. Examples of these data have been presented at this symposium in reference to breast cancer, malignant melanoma, colon and lung cancer. However, it should be noted that it took almost a century of clinical studies to validate this point.

By 1940 we were beginning to understand the biology of tumor growth. Tumor growth was clearly a dynamic interplay of dividing cells, static cells, and cells being shed during expansion of tumor volume. The working hypothesis that evolved from these observations was that the likelihood of having micrometastases increases with the size of the primary tumor and the degree of local extension. Again, the experimental setting was humans with cancer, particularly those with breast, malignant melanoma and colon cancer. It was on the basis of observations made in these diseases that the modern staging classifications you have heard discussed here have evolved. In addition, rather elegant experimental data have been developed by Drs. Skipper and Schabel and their co-workers at Southern Research Institute, and by numerous other investigators, indicating the same is true of both spontaneous and transplantable rodent tumors. As more elegant laboratory techniques have become available, cell kinetic studies have also shown that the rate of shedding of tumor cells (both viable and non-viable) increases with tumor size.[1] Thus, we can conclude rather firmly from observational evidence in humans and animals that this hypothesis is correct. The time span of these experiments was the past thirty to forty years. It has taken far too long to convince clinicians, particularly surgeons, of the validity of the hypothesis. Still, it was evident even at this symposium, that we still spend a great deal of time trying to reconvince ourselves of the adverse influence of local extension such as in patients with nodal involvement and Stage II breast cancer and Duke C colon cancer vis-a-vis survival. Dr. Livingston told us even more about lung cancer. In spite of the commonness of carcinoma of the lung, we are just now beginning to learn the prognostic variables that will undoubtably influence the design of future clinical trials in this disease.

In my view, these two hypothesis have now been amply proven. It should be clear that the greatest impact on survival of patients with cancer will come from the development of effective systemic treatment. For those investigators that appreciated this point, some years ago, there were really three options to pursue. First, chemotherapy; the Drug Development Program at the National Cancer Institute and other Institutions began on this basis more than twenty years ago; second, immunotherapy -- the evolution of immunotherapy really began approximately fifteen years ago with the recognition of tumor immunity and the evolving, precise, information about the dual nature of the immune system which could be exploitable for immunotherapy. Third, total body irradiation. Although not discussed at the symposium, this latter form of therapy has recently re-emerged as a potential form of systemic treatment with radiotherapy. Most studies, illustrated at this symposium concentrated on options 1 and 2.

Added momentum for the use of adjuvant therapy was the result of the most important experiment of all. Before toxic drugs could be accepted as treatment for patients in the postoperative period, it remained to be shown that cancer was, indeed, curable at all by drugs in humans. Most of the studies to test this hypothesis were pilot-type, uncontrolled trials using patients with widely disseminated universally fatal diseases, usually cared for in the specialty of internal medicine. The hypothesis that cancer in humans is curable by drugs has stood the test of time and experimentation. There are now numerous and convincing examples of success in curing patients with several types of advanced cancers using drugs alone.[2] The time span of this experiment was the past twenty years. The fact that during most of the past twenty years, therapeutic researchers were preoccupied with testing this hypothesis, and this hypothesis alone, is often unappreciated. The pace of this type of experimentation accelerated with the identification of each new active anticancer drug. The importance of the observation that drugs can cure advanced cancer cannot be over-emphasized since it was the substantiation of this hypothesis that allowed adjuvant therapy to proceed at its current pace.

Additional work of Drs. Skipper and Schabel, and their many co-workers at the Southern Research Institute, which was discussed in part by Drs. Schabel and Salmon in the opening session of this symposium, exerted a major influence in these studies in the early 1960's. These investigators hypothesized that the ability to eradicate cancer cells with drugs was dependent not only on the dose of the drug but on number of tumor cells present, and that a given dose of drugs will kill a constant fraction of tumor cells regardless of the size of the population. Thus, drugs killed tumor cells by first order kinetics. The implications of this hypothesis were enormous. It implied that in order to treat cancer more effectively, one would have to increase the dose of the agent, or agents used or treat earlier to take advantage of smaller tumor volumes. These ideas would have a major impact on the design of the clinical trials that led to the cure of many types of advanced cancer. The relationship of dose of drug to volume of tumor, and the fractional kill hypothesis, has certainly been clearly validated in animal tumors and appears true in some human situations.[3] Humans with advanced cancers, however, have high tumor volume, and volume, as a variable, cannot usually be controlled by the clinician. Because single drugs often reach limiting toxicity to one or another organ, as doses are increased, it became necessary to explore the simultaneous use of several effective drugs, and the observations made by Schabel and Skipper helped usher in the era of combination chemotherapy, for human advanced cancer, which as I have already alluded to, has been so successful.

Finally, these workers also hypothesized that sensitivity to drug treatment increases with decreasing volume of tumor cells. In general, this appears to be true in rapidly growing animal tumors. The attractiveness of this hypothesis is also readily apparent. If one had a treatment that was effective against advanced disease, it could well be expected it would at least be effective as an adjuvant treatment against micrometastases. It would also be likely one could use even less aggressive therapy than the type used in patients with the same but advanced cancer, which would be less toxic; with the mood of the time this was an important consideration. In fact, many of the studies presented at this symposium have employed the principle of using reduced levels of treatment in the adjuvant situation based on this hypothesis. Can we conclude this is true? The fractional kill hypothesis is clearly true for exponentially growing tumors. However, it appears most human tumors follow a gompertz growth curve. What is not generally appreciated is the fact that the fractional kill hypothesis, applied to tumors growing on a gompertz growth curve, would actually predict for a greater degree of response at the upper end of the growth curve then we actually see clinically, at least for cell cycle non-specific drugs.

Drs. Norton and Simon at the NCI have recently reexamined and questioned some aspects of these concepts. They have formulated a hypothesis which, I believe, if it stands the test of experimentation, could have an important impact on the design of future adjuvant studies.(4) First, the assumption is that most human tumors (and even most spontaneous animal tumors) grow in a gompertzian fashion. In gompertzian growth, tumor volume increases until it reaches a plateau. The instantaneous growth fraction, which in this case is a mixed function including the net effect of cell birth and cell loss, expressed as the increase in tumor volume per unit of time, decreases as tumor volume increases. Cell production rate, under these circumstances, is slowest at either end of the growth curve. This is illustrated in Figure 1. Note, that

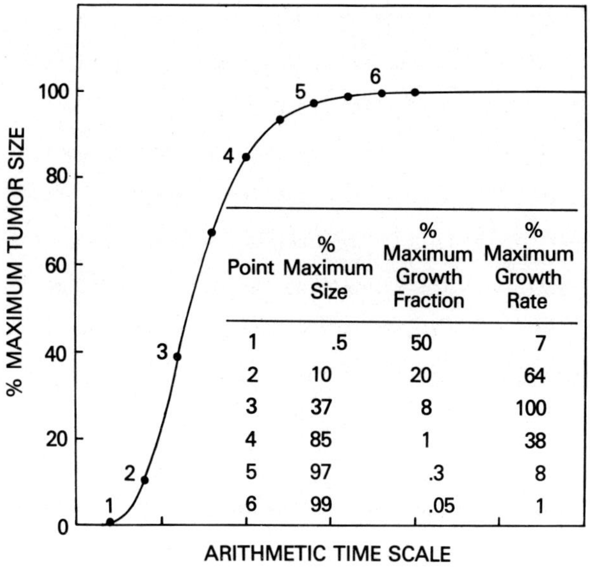

Point	% Maximum Size	% Maximum Growth Fraction	% Maximum Growth Rate
1	.5	50	7
2	10	20	64
3	37	8	100
4	85	1	38
5	97	.3	8
6	99	.05	1

Figure 1

although the growth fraction is larger at smaller volumes of tumor, the maximum growth rate, shown in the column on the right, occurs at point 3 on the curve, at the inflection point, when the tumor mass is approximately 37% of its maximum size. Relating this to the clinical situation, it would appear that most patients with metastatic tumor are probably somewhere on the high side of the curve between points 3 and 4. Thus Norton and Simon imply that a given level of effective treatment may take longer to achieve an equivalent effect on a smaller tumor mass than a moderately large one (at the inflection point of a growth curve) since "sensitivity to treatment", in their view, is a complex function of the interactions of the instantaneous growth fraction and tumor volume. Most clinical studies using combination chemotherapy of advanced cancer employ a relatively fixed number of cycles of treatment which, either by design, or because of toxic side affects, usually diminish in intensity with each subsequent cycle. Their model simply stresses that a therapy, effective in causing regression of advanced tumor, may not be as effective in dealing with microscopic disease if doses are reduced, and in fact, may only be effective in eradicating the residual cells if doses are actually escalated toward the end of therapy--a therapeutic "boost" if you will. Clearly this has not been the trend in most adjuvant studies. You will hear more about this hypothesis since experimental data in animal tumor systems suggests something like this is going on. As we proceed through this overview, I shall try to point out where I think these principles may be operative in some of the adjuvant studies reported at this symposium.

In reference to the value of cancer treatment, in general, I was troubled by a comment made by our colleague from Edmonton when he quoted Dr. Hayflick's statement that even if we could cure all patients with cancer, the life expectancy of humans in this country would only increase by some 2.1 years. It seems to me this suggests the impact of universally successful treatment would be slight. Quite the contrary. The potential population of patients that might benefit from the development of successful adjuvant treatment programs number some 400,000 in this country. Using very conservative estimates, the successful control of cancer in this cohort of patients would add, each year, 8 million person years of life, and 8 billion dollars to the economy. In addition, it would save some 20 billion dollars in medical expenses attributable to the care of dying cancer patients. These facts, of course, do not even take into consideration the impact of a cure on the individual patient. All this, in spite of the fact that the average life span would only be increased by some 2.1 years. In the same vein, Dr. Saul Rosenberg has made some calculations in reference to the impact of specific cancer treatment programs. He estimates there has been a 25% increase in relapse free survival in of patients with Hodgkin's disease at Stanford, coincident with the introduction of the MOPP chemotherapy program. In the USA, this would amount to curing some 2,000 additional patients per year. Since these patients have an average age of 30 at diagnosis, and can be expected to work and be productive for an additional 30 years, and might conservatively make (not considering inflation) an average annual income of $10,000.00, this, cohort of Hodgkin's patients, cured annually, should each add, in their lifetime, some six hundred million dollars to the economy of the United States. The annual taxes alone on this income could make the amount of money spent on the development of these treatment programs a very handsome investment for the United States government indeed. If one wishes, one could make very similar and even more striking calculations based on data on successfully treated young patients with acute leukemia, and osteogenic sarcoma, etc. In short, the economic impact of the development of successful treatment has often been overlooked but could be quite enormous.

Now to the studies presented here. The following trends seem to be apparent in the design of the adjuvant studies presented at this symposium. (1) Adjuvant treatment programs have become more aggressive; usually using one or more drugs with or without immunotherapy. The drugs used generally are already known to be effective in advanced stages of the same cancer. (2) The reluctance to carry out adjuvant therapy trials seems to be disappearing (well, almost). Notably absent from this symposium, and from our own list of ongoing adjuvant studies at NCI, are trials in prostate cancer, bladder cancer, ovarian cancer and head and neck cancer. I will return to some of these cancers in a moment. (3) Immunotherapy is often used alone, based on its hypothetical value, even in the absence of a known effect, in patients with advanced disease, something usually required of chemotherapy. This is done apparently because of its relative safety and the fact that it is somewhat physiological--after all, we all have an immune system (hopefully). (4) The use of adjuvant heat therapy was mentioned by Dr. Boone in the opening session. At the National Cancer Institute, we have felt that in order to fully explore heat as an adjuvant to chemotherapy, it would be necessary to heat the entire body. Accordingly, we have developed a heating garment which allows us to safely heat patients to a temperature of 41.8^{0} centigrade. We have just completed our Phase I trial and will be shortly embarking on a randomized controlled trial using a known effective therapy, probably in patients with metastatic sarcoma, with and without heat. The potential usefulness of heat as an adjuvantive therapy to drugs will await the outcome of trials such as these.

The first disease discussed in detail was breast cancer. Adjuvant studies are more advanced here. The following points can be extracted from the data presented primarily from the randomized controlled trials presented by Drs. Fisher and Bonadonna. (1) Adjuvant chemotherapy works in breast cancer. (2) L-PAM and CMF combination chemotherapy are clearly effective in premenopausal women with positive lymph nodes. The greatest effect is seen in those women who have 1-3 nodes positive, an effect we would have predicted, based on the lower volume of tumor. However, as I recall in the initial report by Fisher et al, of the L-PAM study, he indicated the effect was maximum in patients who had 4 or more positive lymph nodes, the population with the worst prognosis (and higher tumor volume). It is likely that the reversal is due to the fact that the control population with 1-3 involved lymph nodes, having a smaller tumor volume, takes a longer time to relapse, making the later data in this group more significant than the early data. (3) A hormonal effect of chemotherapy, or a combined hormonal-chemotherapeutic effect, cannot be totally ruled out in premenopausal women. This controversy still has to be sorted out. (4) Contrary to what most have been led to believe, a positive effect of adjuvant chemotherapy is readily apparent in postmenopausal women with 4 or more lymph nodes involved. (5) These effects, regardless of how long they last, are likely to have an impact on survival. We should remember the old thiotepa data from the first NSABP study. Although the effect of thiotepa in preventing recurrences was only observed between the 18th and 36th months, a survival advantage persisted in this group up to 9 years. This fact was, and still is, often overlooked. And, ultimately, an effect was also noted in post-menopausal women as well. (6) We would have expected the CMF combination to produce results superior to L-PAM, based on the ECOG comparison of the two treatments, and, in general, indirect comparisons indicate this is true. The data presented by Dr. Fisher from the NSABP studies are also showing a trend toward better disease free survival with the addition of other drugs to L-PAM. (7) At the moment there appears to be no evidence that immunotherapy adds anything to the adjuvant treatment of breast cancer. We, however, should keep in mind that the best studies examing this point, such as the randomized trial in progress at UCLA are too early to fully evaluate the effect of immunotherapy. (9) My own bias is that the adriamycin-cytoxan combination, presented here by the Arizona group, is somewhat risky in patients with Stage II disease because of the long-term risk of cardiotoxicity, unless it is shown to be superior to existing combination therapies, which has not yet been done. (10) Adjuvant therapy in patients with Stage I breast cancer was only briefly discussed here, but it may be risky for another reason. These drugs, particularly alkylating agents, are potentially carcinogenic, and we are as yet, unable to assess the true risk of developing second cancers in treated patients. I will return to this point later. (11) The use of postoperative radiotherapy was only discussed briefly here but a statement was made, by at least one investigator, that his group did not feel it was ethical <u>to withhold</u> it from their patient population and, therefore, they designed its use into all phases of their clinical trial. In my view, this statement requires an expanded comment.

I do not believe there is any longer a place for routine postoperative radiotherapy in the treatment of breast cancer.[5] What all of us would like to see is an expansion of the study reported by Hellman at the Harvard Joint Center for Radiation Therapy examining the use of radiotherapy as the primary treatment of breast cancer; this approach was not discussed here.[6] We hope someday that perhaps the NSABP group would consider doing such a trial since with their current study designs they appear headed in this direction. What are the facts about postoperative radiotherapy. First, it clearly does not improve survival; no knowledgable investigator ever argues this point anymore. Second, it does, in fact, decrease local recurrences; there is also no argument on this point, as Dr. Fisher stressed in the panel discussion on breast cancer. But what are the facts about local recurrences in breast cancer? Only 1/3 of operated patients, left untreated by radiotherapy, will develop local recurrences. Fully 2/3 of those who do develop them can be successfully treated with radiotherapy when they occur. Thus, only 1/9 of all patients not treated with postoperative radiotherapy will have local tumor present at the time of their death and in the overwhelming majority of these patients it will not be the cause of their death. If one examines the available data in patients treated routinely with postoperative radiotherapy, it is interesting to note that approximately 1/9 of the treated population will also have developed local tumor in the treatment field by the time of their death, and it will also not usually be a contributing factor to their death. While it seems acceptable to test the use of postoperative radiotherapy as an adjuvant to chemotherapy, to determine if further reduction in tumor volume by radiotherapy will be of benefit to patients, there are not many studies like this in progress and none were presented here. We should also take into consideration the fact that we know very little about the correct sequence in which to administer radiotherapy and chemotherapy. It is conceivable that the use of both together will obviate the beneficial

effects of drugs. Dr. Schabel told us, in the opening session, that he has ample evidence in animal tumor systems that many transplantable tumors, when innoculated in small numbers, will not grow unless they are supplemented with "feeder cells", cells of the same tumor line which have been lethally irradiated. While he presented these data in a positive sense, that this enhanced growth of viable cells by lethally irradiated cells might be exploited chemotherapeutically we should also consider a potential reverse effect. In short, I think it is time we put to rest the practice of using postoperative radiotherapy routinely. (12) Not discussed here, and not in progress anywhere that I know of, are studies to explore the use of prophylactic castration, essentially repeating previous negative studies, in that population of patients who have evidence of estrogen binding proteins. (13) We have heard several papers discussing the use of various adjuvant programs in private practice and I will return to these at the end of my presentation.
Genito-Urinary Tumors: Not a great deal was presented on this subject at this symposium, but this was not a unique feature of this meeting. It has simply been difficult to get adjuvant studies started in patients with GU tumors because of lack of access to the proper patient population. It was sad to note that although we have had the rationale and tools for adjuvant treatment in testicular tumors since as early as 1960, we still have not sorted out how to use them. It seems reasonable that patients with this very drug responsive tumor should be treated with drugs in the postoperative period if they are in Stage II, particularly the Stage IIB of Peckum, and have embryonal, terato or choriocarcinoma. The bigger question in my mind is the true role of adjuvant radiotherapy in those patients with positive retroperitoneal lymph nodes. Do we need it? Have the proper studies been designed to answer this question?

An even greater opportunity to explore the value of adjuvant chemotherapy exists in patients with ovarian cancer. We have also had good drugs in this disease for years and many patients with ovarian cancer have resectable tumors, and resectable patients often develop recurrent tumors. Some work on this subject was presented here, but we all eagerly await the recently implemented, large, controlled clinical trials now being conducted under the auspices of the National Cancer Institute by the Ovarian Tumor Study Group at five instutions.

Colorectal cancer: I disagree with Dr. Carter's comments about the efficacy of 5-Fluorouracil as an adjuvant treatment in colon and rectal cancer. I think it is time we admit that 5-Fluorouracil works as an adjuvant therapy. There are two good studies on this point. One presented here, from the old Central Oncology Group, by Dr. Grage, and one not presented here from the VA Surgical Adjuvant Group. Dr. George Higgins, the Chairman of the VA Surgical Adjuvant Group, kindly supplied me with an updated version of the VA study. They examined the effectiveness of 5-Fluorouracil first given in a short course and then, in a subsequent study, as prolonged intermittent therapy. The data now clearly show there is a significant difference in both groups, when compared to untreated concurrent controls, which begins to manifest itself from the third to the fifth year. The effect is more striking in the patients who receive prolonged intermittent treatment as we would have expected. Again, it seems likely that the delayed expression of the beneficial effect of 5-Fluorouracil in the postoperative period relates to the fact that the drug may be exerting its effect primarily on patients with a relatively small volume of tumor; again, the control populations with small residual tumor volumes also takes a longer time to recur and thus the late splaying of the curves. You can argue the clinical significance of these findings (as some did in the panel on colorectal cancer) but the biologic significance is clear; these data should impact on the design of future adjuvant studies in colon cancer.

Therefore, it seems reasonable to control other adjuvant treatments in colon cancer against the use of 5-Fluorouracil. BCG may also have some effect in the postoperative period on the recurrence rate in colorectal cancer, as reported by the group from the M.D. Anderson Hospital. Because of the implications of these data, this study needs confirmation in randomized controlled clinical trials, some of which are now in progress. None of the studies using Methyl CCNU and 5-Fluorouracil, with or without vincristine, were presented here, but Dr. Louis told us a significant number are in progress. Since this treatment program is more effective than 5-Fluorouracil in producing responses in patients with advanced disease, we all eagerly await the results of the adjuvant studies which should be coming available in the next year or two.

Please note that the results of adjuvant treatment in colon and breast cancer, although positive, are not as effective as would have been predicted on the basis of the effect of these drugs against patients with advanced disease and theories purporting the enhanced sensitivity of micrometastases of the same tumor to the same drugs. Is the hypothesis proposed by Norton and Simon operating here? I will cite other examples shortly.

Melanoma: This capricious neoplasm seems to be responding to immunotherapy. The study presented by Dr. Morton, from UCLA, seems to be showing an effect of BCG, although it must be admitted there does not appear to be any significant advantage to adding a tumor cell vaccine to the mix. Not presented here, is the WHO study showing that BCG, and BCG plus DTIC, the imidazole carboxamide derivative, are better than no treatment at all in patients with Stage II disease. DTIC alone, however, was not effective. Please note, that although DTIC, or DTIC plus BCG are effective in patients with advanced melanoma, especially in those patients with soft tissue metastases (but relatively large volumes of tumor) DTIC has not yet been reported to be effective in any adjuvant study when used by itself. Again, this suggests a greater resistance of micrometastases to chemo therapy than has been previously appreciated. Finally, Dr. Monsour presented what has to be the easiest way to treat melanoma, by local treatment with DNCB. Although this study has only a small group of patients, the apparent affect on some patients with deeply invasive melanoma is of great interest. This is essentially a replica of the guinea pig hepatoma model experiment. A similar study is in progress at the National Cancer Institute using BCG rather than DNCB.

I believe real progress has been made in the treatment of osteosarcoma. Most of the data shows a consistent 60-70% disease free survival in patients treated with adjuvant therapy of one sort or another, and the increased response to high dose methotrexate in patients with advanced disease, when used weekly, rather than tri-weekly, reported from the Sydney Farber Center is indeed impressive. In contrast to most other adjuvant treatment schedules, the treatment used in the postoperative program is extremely vigorous and commensurate with the previously dire prognosis in surgically treated patients with osteosarcoma. An important trend toward the use of lesser amounts of surgery was reported here--a very important change and, as several investigators commented, a change that has taken place apparently without adversely effecting survival. There does appear to be a dose response affect of drugs used in the postoperative period, as has been previously noted by Dr. Holland using Adriamycin. Supporting this point of view were data from several sources; in one abstract it was mentioned that Adriamycin alone did not work well as an adjuvant at the M.D. Anderson Hospital, while at Mt. Sinai in New York and at the Cancer Institute in Milan, Italy, it appeared to be useful. Methotrexate appears to work well at the Sydney Farber Cancer Center, but our own study at the NCI does not show the same positive affects. In all cases, if one examines the data closely, it seems the different effects can be explained by the intensity in which the therapy was employed. Thus, there does appear to be a dose response effect and surprisingly it is occurring within the high dose range of each of the drugs used. Again, intensity of the treatment in the postoperative period appears important, suggesting this is another example where small volumes of tumor are not as sensitive to drugs as we would have predicted. The Mayo Clinic data, not presented here, stands alone, in the USA, in showing that the prognosis of patients with osteosarcoma is improving using surgery alone. The only other study showing a similar affect, was also not presented here, and comes from Sweden where the apparent positive effect of postoperative interferon treatment has to be balanced against an improvement in survival of controls treated at the same time with surgery alone at different hospitals. Two final points representing my own personal bias. I do not believe I could recommend an untreated control arm in operable patients with osteosarcoma. The second point is that there are only about 1,000 patients with osteosarcoma in this country each year, and it seems prudent to recommend that all of them should be referred to centers studying the use of these rather difficult and intensive treatment programs which require the amassment of impressive amounts of support services.

The same points can be made about soft tissue sarcomas. Several studies now show an increasing capacity to salvage limbs without compromising survival; one was reported here, a similar study is in progress at the NCI and both, in their early stages, are showing impressive results. Here again, the intensity of the adjuvant treatment seems appropriate to the prognosis of patients with these tumors in the past. Thus far, in all the sarcomas, no one has reported a positive effect from the application of immunotherapy, either alone, or in combination with chemotherapy.

I won't say a great deal about pediatric neoplasms except to emphasize the following point. Pediatric oncologists have had the advantage over the rest of us for a long time; they have had drugs that worked, tumors ideal for adjuvant therapy, a small population of patients, usually seen by physicians who work well together, and they have clearly demonstrated, as Dr. Sutow pointed out to us, that combined modality therapy is effective in most childhood tumors; the exception seems to be neuroblastoma.

Lung Cancer: One clear message came across to me in the presentations at this meeting--something is going on with the use of BCG in epidermoid carcinoma of the lung, particularly in those patients with resectable disease, as shown by the work presented by McNeally, and the French group headed by Professor Mathe. These results, and those previously reported using Levamisole, are important, and because they are so important they bear repetition; such studies are now in progress. One such study was also presented here employing not only BCG, but Levamisole, and the two agents used in combination. This study will be of interest when sufficient numbers of patients are accumulated to truly evaluate the results. However, we are only talking about some 15% of all patients with lung cancer and the patient with advanced epidermoid carcinoma of the lung still has no useful therapy. Dr. Livingston clearly pointed out to us how long it takes to learn the important clinical variables in lung cancer even though it is such a common disease. Many controlled clinical trials in the past bear repetition because in most of them not even histology was considered in the randomization. We are all slow to do this because, in general, we do not like to repeat older negative studies. In some cases the repeat trials may be important, particularly in evaluating the use of postoperative radiotherapy in those patients with epidermoid carcinoma and positive mediastinal lymph nodes.

Most of the exciting studies employing combination chemotherapy for the treatment of oat cell lung cancer were not discussed here; one was, and, in general, the results show we are now able to achieve a quite high complete response rate with drug combinations and we are even beginning to see some long term disease free survivals beyond two and even three years. Clearly the progress has been dramatic with the use of drugs; it may now be safely stated that most other therapies for oat cell carcinoma of the lung are adjunctive to the use of drugs.

There is not much to say about head and neck cancer because only a few papers were presented here. This again is not unique to this meeting, but rather a statement of the activity in the field of head and neck cancer in general. I will say this, however, no where is there a more noble venture than attempts to reduce the extent of surgical treatment of head and neck cancer. What we heard here were some preliminary attempts to do this exploring methotrexate in the perioperative period. All of us will await further results with interest.

Lymphomas: Dr. Rosenberg reported that overall survival of patients with Hodgkins disease at Stanford has increased 25% with the use of MOPP chemotherapy in addition to radiotherapy in patients classified as Stages I, II and III. It is still unclear whether MOPP and total nodal x-irradiation are best used together or in sequence because of the potential risk of carcinogenesis with both used together. There is however, a definite trend toward better overall survival with both used together. Frankly, at the moment, it seems prudent to use radiotherapy alone in patients with relatively localized, good histologic subtypes (lymphocyte predominant and nodular sclerosing) of Hodgkin's disease, and try and salvage those who fail with the MOPP program. The data from Stanford now clearly show that MOPP chemotherapy is substantially better than total nodal irradiation in patients with Stage IIIB disease, something others have felt was true for some time. Current data from the Stanford controlled trial show only a 7% disease free survival in patients with Stage IIIB disease compared to their past experience (uncontrolled) of 40% disease free survival. When radiotherapy and chemotherapy were used together, in patients with Stage IV disease, in a controlled comparison to MOPP chemotherapy alone, it appeared that adjunctive radiotherapy adds nothing to chemotherapy in Stage IV patients in contrast to some results reported elsewhere. There is still some controversy about the treatment of Stage IIIA disease. At Stanford, patients treated with both radiotherapy and MOPP have essentially a 100% response rate and 100% relapse free survival while in those IIIA patients treated with radiotherapy alone, a 73% disease free survival was noted. At the NCI, all patients with IIIA and IVA disease treated with MOPP alone have achieved a complete remission and none have relapsed with followup up to 12 years.(7) These data are further substantiated by those reported for our Baltimore Cancer Research Center and those previously reported by other workers with one exception. A study recently reported from England showed radiotherapy superior to MOPP in patients with IIIA disease.(8) The administration of the chemotherapy by numerous investigators is suspect in this latter exception, I am told, but it cannot be fully judged since details were not given in the report. Although one has to compare the morbidity of the two programs, it seems that the potential 25% advantage in relapse free survival offered by MOPP in patients with Stage IIIA disease ought to attract our attention, and favors chemotherapy as the treatment of choice. If necessary, further trials should be conducted to confirm or deny this observation. The data from Stanford clearly show the power of a controlled clinical trial when the therapies being evaluated are relatively well defined as was the case in total nodal irradiation and MOPP therapy, both of which were evaluated in uncontrolled trials, to a great degree, before institution of the current Stanford studies.

In the non-Hodgkin's lymphomas, the most interesting results, to me, were those reported by Bonadonna showing a significant advantage of the use of CVP chemotherapy in patients with Stage I and II disease, in a randomized controlled trial, comparing its use with radiotherapy to radiotherapy alone. This is the first concrete evidence of the successful addition of drugs to x-irradiation in the early stages of some types of non-Hodgkin's lymphomas. In a way, these results are surprising since CVP would now be considered one of the least effective combinations used in non-Hodgkin's lymphoma patients, particularly in those with diffuse histologies. One can only hope that when a similar study is done with one of the more effective combinations, the results will be even more remarkable. Although the Stanford data, presented by Dr. Glatstein, does not show a similar effect, there are significant differences in study design at Stanford, particularly in the extent and manner of delivery of radiotherapy, which could adversely affect the impact of the use of drugs. More studies on the use of drugs in patients with localized stages of the non-Hodgkin's lymphoma are clearly indicated, some of which are already in progress. Although studies were presented using BCG as immunotherapy for patients with non-Hodgkin's lymphoma, there are currently insufficient data to draw any firm conclusions. At this point in time it cannot be said that immunotherapy is of any benefit in patients with lymphoma and until further data are available, it should be used only in the study format.

In the acute leukemia, further arguments were presented supporting the use of chemo-immunotherapy. To date, there are still no data to indicate immunotherapy adds anything to chemotherapy in patients with lymphocytic leukemia, although, as Dr. Mathe pointed out, this may well be related to our failure to adequately define subpopulations of patients with this disease according to the cell of origin. Further studies will undoubtably be needed to clarify this point. There continues to be suspicion that immunotherapy may play a greater role in patients with acute myelocytic leukemia, although its interaction with chemotherapy is proving to be very complex as Dr. Holland pointed out. A brief mention was made of an ongoing trial by Dr. Holland's group which shows much more dramatic affect of immunotherapy, in this case MER, than has previously been reported.

Important considerations in the design of adjuvant studies and some of the problems inherent in their evolution was discussed by Dr. Carter, but I would like to re-emphasize some of these points from my own point of view. There is a great need to identify the types and stages of each tumor suitable for adjuvant therapy; it is surprising that in 1977 it is even necessary to say this. We need to identify all the subtle variables such as histology, stage, sex, the effect of increasing numbers of lymph nodes involved with tumor, etc. Many variables not known to influence the outcome of patients with metastatic disease appear to become important in the adjuvant situation and have not been previously appreciated.

The subject of the use of controls has been alluded to throughout the meeting and was discussed in great detail by Dr. Rosenberg. I can add very little to what he said except that I agree with him. When one is treating blind, as is the case in adjuvant treatment protocols, it is almost invariably necessary to have an untreated control population, at least in the early studies, with the proviso that one is using a therapy which in itself is not replete with variables; thus the need for reliance on "known to be effective" treatment programs in adjuvant protocols. The real problem appears to be the link between the pilot study, showing efficacy in patients with advanced disease, and the controlled clinical trial and the same treatment as an adjuvant. If too much time takes place between the two types of studies, results of pilot trials tend to be believed too soon, too eagerly; the opinion of investigators then

becomes fixed, according to their biases, and controlled clinical trials, in many cases, may become unethical in their minds. I have listened to speaker after speaker try to convince the audience of the validity of their adjuvant study based on historical controls. It simply didn't work. If part of our responsibility is to convince the universe of physicians and the public with cancer about the effectiveness, or lack of effectiveness, of a given treatment, then we must make greater use of controlled clinical trials at appropriate points in the development of a new treatment. However, I would not want these comments to be misinterpreted by those who believe it is proper to use concurrent controls for every study. There is a place for pilot studies. I do not believe a controlled trial is appropriate during the developmental stages of many new treatments. Most of these studies are conducted in patients with advanced disease where the mortality is striking enough that a significant impact of a new treatment is readily noted without a concurrent control, and until the variables of the new treatment are appreciated, it is usually inefficient to embark directly on a controlled trial. There are exceptions in adjuvant studies as well. For some types of very aggressive tumors, patients treated with surgery alone have uniformly done so poorly it may be unreasonable and unnecessary to insist on an untreated control, especially if one is looking for sizable differences. In colon and breast cancer, however, as we have seen, controls are necessary because those diseases evolve more slowly along several well recognized lines of evolution. To emphasize this point, it should be noted that prior to the institution of the L-PAM study, by the NSABP group, there were 7 clinical trials using adjuvant drug treatment reported as positive, most of which were either uncontrolled or poorly controlled; none of them had a significant impact on the use of adjuvant therapy until the study of Dr. Fisher, and the subsequent study of Bonadonna, were completed and reported.[5]
Dr. Carter tried to come to grips with the question of the level of

effectiveness of drugs in advanced disease necessary to suggest their usefulness as an adjuvant treatment. Dr. Schabel, early on in the program, even suggested that drugs with no affect against advanced disease, at least in animal models can, in fact, be useful in the adjuvant situation. In the clinic it seems likely that any drug, or combination of drugs, capable of producing complete remissions in patients with advanced disease should be considered strong candidates for adjuvant treatment in resectable tumors with a propensity to recur. Drugs capable of producing partial responses in as few as 25% of patients with advanced disease may not be effective, but some of them have been, for example L-PAM. In the absence of any better drug, they should be reasonable candidates for clinical trials. At the moment, it is difficult to understand how to select an "inactive" compound for use in adjuvant studies primarily because the choice of inactive compounds is very wide and there is potential harm from immunosuppression caused by a drug that ultimately proves to have no anti-tumor effect. Because of the long duration of adjuvant studies in humans, an adverse effect from an inactive drug may not be noted until far too late. If we are to use drugs not known to be active in advanced disease, we need to develop better biochemical rationale than we now have, for doing so.

We need to continue to try to identify the long term risks of adjuvant therapy since it must always be remembered that a fraction of each population of patients treated with postoperative drug therapy would not have developed recurrent cancer if left alone. At the National Cancer Institute, a central registry of the more significant adjuvant studies is being established. The intent is to establish baseline data, calculating expected incidences of specific tumors, against which the actual incidence can be compared as they occur. In my view, it is not a question of whether we will see an increase incidence of second tumors, it is a question of how much. Dr. Chan from the Kaiser Hospital reported that the alkylating agent, thiotepa, used for two years in operated breast cancer patients, caused no increased risk of second malignancy. There was no opportunity to review these data in detail, and they will warrant considerable examination. If true, they suggest there are differences in carcinogenic potential amongst the alkylating agents since L-PAM has often been implicated as a leukemogen in man. Dr. Einhorn from Radiumhemmet, reported data from 472 cases of advanced ovarian cancer treated with L-PAM. Four patients developed acute myelocytic leukemia, and they were extracted from the 40 who survived three to ten years, or, further, from the twelve who recieved greater than 800 mgs. of L-PAM as a total dose. Not presented here are unpublished data collected by Drs. Young and Reimer at The National Cancer Institute from some 5,000 patients of the Gynecologic Oncology Group treated with L-PAM. Thirteen cases of acute leukemia have been found. Ten of the thirteen had both drugs and X-ray treatment and the incidence appeared to be increasing over the duration of the study. The data are soft since they are not derived from patients treated in the adjuvant situation, in which otherwise healthy patients are treated with these compounds for a finite period of time. They do, however, suggest up to one hundred times the normal incidence of acute myelocytic leukemia might be seen. This could add up to an incidence of acute myelocytic leukemia of about 10% at ten years. While this incidence of leukemia should have no effect on the use of adjuvant therapy in Stage II patients with carcinoma of the breast, it might give us pause before developing adjuvant programs with alkylating agents in patients with Stage I disease. For the time being, in fact, it might be more appropriate to consider the use of antimetabolites, in Stage I patients, if they can be established to be effective in controlled clinical trials in patients with Stage II disease. Another fruitful area of research we are now expanding, is the attempt to develop methods of circumventing the carcinogenic potential of anticancer drugs.

There are other problems surrounding the development of adjuvant chemotherapy programs not all of which are scientific. They are:

1. Specialty competition--who will be the oncologist of the future? This is not a trivial question and is affecting the design of clinical trials. Investigators seem unwilling to design a clinical trial that might move the treatment of a disease outside their specialty. And yet, such trials are necessary.

2. Skepticism and optimism--the failure to appreciate the true risk-benefit ratio. I will return to the latter point in a moment. As Dr. Fisher pointed out there are those investigators who believe everything and those who believe nothing even if the results come from a controlled clinical trial. Hopefully, there are sufficient numbers of investigators in the middle to provide a modicum of sanity to the development of these investigations.

3. Unavailability of patient material: I have already alluded to this in urology and gynecology, but it exists in other areas as well. Some categories of cancer are compartmentalized within a surgical subspecialty, and are not readily available for adjuvant trials initiated and requiring the collaboration of other specialists. It has been reported in one study that only 10% of patients with ovarian cancer were managed by gynecologists located at centers. The rest were treated in the community. For these reasons and others, it has been difficult to set up adjuvant studies even when the opportunities offered by the availability of effective systematic treatment exist.

4. Group and investigator ego. One of the most serious problems in study design in clinical trials is the failure to capitalize on the results of others. Clinical investigators often lose the opportunity to leap frog over each others data because either a group of investigators or a single investigator wishes to promulgate programs

developed within his or her own sphere of influence. This leads to wasteful repetition just for the sake of doing something. No where is this more true in adjuvant programs where some institutions report such studies with such small numbers they can never have any significant impact on the evolution of adjuvant treatment. Another aspect of group and investigator ego, and a most serious one in my view, is the tendency to modify known effective treatments without considering the impact of doing so. This is a common practice in large colloborative programs, again, seemingly related to either the tendency to want to identify programs with a particular cooperative effort or a result of a compromise necessitated by a large group effort. This leads to wasteful repetition since most negative studies designed this way eventually have to be repeated if the question posed is important enough.

I would like now to turn to the role of the practicing physician in the development and use of adjuvant drug programs and make a few comments. While every practicing physician should reserve the right to pick and choose the best therapy for his patient, he cannot do so if the information is not available. When a field is in a state of transition, as it is for many of the diseases discussed here, these data are best obtained by taking part in a clinical trial. Practicing physicians can and should take part in the research effort. However, I quite frankly, was disappointed in the abstracts presented here using adjuvant therapy in the community. I think the designers of these studies lost sight of the important questions they should have been asking. All, without exception, reduced doses and modified the therapeutic program without considering the effect of doing so, in spite of the fact that sufficient clinical and animal data exists to indicate this will very likely be harmful to the program in question. Dr. Schabel reviewed some of these data in the opening session. One community adjuvant program used a combination of drugs given by the oral route when data have already been published showing these same drugs are ineffective, or less effective, against advanced disease when they are given orally rather than intravenously.

Dead patients don't complain of side effects. It seems to me too much emphasis was placed on what have to be trivial side effects compared to the toxicity of dying prematurely. If you don't believe the question or the therapy being posed are valid, ethical, or useable, then you shouldn't take part in such a study. If you do take part, you should do so in a whole hearted fashion. Physician motivation is at least as important as patient motivation. In one study, nausea and vomiting were said to be the limiting toxicity when the protocol drugs were used at 1/3 of the doses originally reported by others. Even when used at full doses, nauseau and vomiting with this particular program (CMF) were not limiting toxicities and yet the patients treated in the original study were human too.

Finally a word about cost. The cost of a new treatment is an unimportant question. If it works, its cost will diminish, as Dr. Frei emphasized in the opening panel. If it works, even if it remains expensive, the return to society of a productive citizen is the best investment we can make, and I have already cited the example of the financial benefit derived from the salvage of a young patient with Hodgkins disease or osteosarcoma.

I would like to conclude these comments by stating that the ultimate goal of cancer treatment research today is to develop methods of treatment that will result in not only live but intact patients. I believe we are well on our way to achieve this. Examples cited at this symposium such as the treatment of osteosarcoma, soft tissue sarcomas, and breast cancer clearly illustrate the trend. This symposium was timely, even though many of the studies presented are in their early stages. It will be of great interest to have a repeat symposium in a few years to measure the progress in the field, and I personally look forward to it.

References

1. DeVita, V.T.: Cell Kinetics and the Chemotherapy of Cancer. Cancer Chemother. Rep. 2:23-33, 1971.
2. DeVita, V.T., Young, R.C. and Canellos, G.P.: Combination Versus Single Agent Chemotherapy. Cancer 35:98-110, 1975.
3. DeVita, V.T. and Schein, P.S.: The use of drugs in combination for the treatment of cancer: Rationale and results. N. Eng. J. Med. 288:998-1006, 1973.
4. Norton, L. and Simon, R.: Tumor size, sensitivity to therapy, and the design of treatment schedules. Cancer Chemother. Rep. (in press).
5. DeVita, V.T.: Carcinoma of the breast: Status of adjuvant medical treatment. Frontiers of Radiation Therapy & Oncology 11:42-58, 1976.
6. Weber, E. and Hellman, S.: Radiation as primary treatment for local control of breast carcinoma. J.A.M.A. 234:608-611, 1975.
7. DeVita, V.T., Canellos, G.P., Hubbard, S., Chabner, B.A. and Young, R.C.: Chemotherapy of Hodgkin's Disease with Nitrogen Mustard, Oncovin, Procarbazine and Prednisone (MOPP): A ten year progress report. Proc. of 12th Annual Meeting of ASCO 17:269, 1976.
8. British National Lymphoma Investigation: Initial treatment of Stage IIIA Hodgkin's disease: Comparison of radiotherapy with combined chemotherapy. Lancet 2:991-995, 1976.

Author Index